health

the science of human adaptation

health

the science of human adaptation

second edition

charles carroll
ball state university

dean miller
university of toledo

wcb

Wm. C. Brown Company Publishers
Dubuque, Iowa

wcb

Wm. C. Brown   *Chairman of the Board*
Larry W. Brown   *President, WCB Group*

Book Team

John Stout   *Editor*
Marilyn A. Phelps   *Designer*
Mary Heller   *Visual Research Editor*
Edit, Inc., Chicago   *Production Services*

Wm. C. Brown Company Publishers, College Division

Lawrence E. Cremer   *President*
Richard C. Crews   *Publisher*
Robert Nash   *Executive Editor*
Raymond C. Deveaux   *Director of Sales and Marketing*
David Wm. Smith   *National Marketing Manager*
James Farrell   *Director of Marketing Research*
David A. Corona   *Director of Production Development and Design*
Ruth Richard   *Production Editorial Manager*
Marilyn A. Phelps   *Manager of Design*

Consulting Editors

Health
Robert Kaplan
The Ohio State University

Physical Education
Aileene Lockhart
Texas Woman's University

Parks and Recreation
David Gray
California State University, Long Beach

Contents

Preface and Acknowledgments

In any given field the leaders are rarely those who have entered the professional life with the largest amount of practical information, but rather those who have breadth of understanding, critical judgment, and especially discipline of learning. The intellectual equipment most needed is that which makes it possible to adapt readily to new situations, as they constantly arise in the ever-changing world.*

We do not work in isolation. As integrated beings, we combine hereditary, historical, biological, environmental, psychological, sociological, and other factors in developing both our conscious and subconscious selves. All of these factors act, react, and adapt more or less simultaneously throughout our lives. The renowned René Dubos probably summarized this view best in his statement "Man's physical and mental state, in health and disease, is always conditioned by all the multiple determinants of his nature."†

Beginning with conception, this book follows the human life cycle from "seed to sod" and beyond. From considerations of conception it moves to birth, growth and development, communicable disease, personality and mental health, lifestyle, environment, chronic disease, and death, finishing on a positive note with a chapter on the future of quality life. This approach has a number of advantages. Initially, it permits us to open with an exciting chapter, rather than the more customary one on definitions and general principles. We delve directly into content. Secondly, the life-cycle approach helps us view the human experience in a functional way: we treat the human individual as an adapting organism. We try to explain many of his health behaviors, not just examine them. We see man as a developing, experimenting dynamic complexity—one capable of drawing upon virtually unlimited resources in attempting to cope with the day-to-day demands of our biocultural environment. The stage for this approach is set early. Following our opening chapter on "Welcome to Earth: The Seed Is Sown," we immediately move into one on "Genetics: The Science of Involuntary Adaptation," in which we examine the complex interaction of heredity and environment. Equipped with essential concepts and vocabulary, we move next to a consideration of the communicable diseases that affect us throughout the life cycle, and

---

*John W. Gardner, *Excellence: Can We Be Equal and Excellent Too?* (New York: Harper & Row, 1961).
†René Dubos, *Man Adapting* (New Haven: Yale University Press, 1965), p. 2.

then on to youth. Here an understanding of one's personality and related mental health along with matters of psychosexual development and coping skills are extremely important. Smoking, drinking, drug-taking, dating, and mating follow as we recognize the complex interactions between youth and various groups demanding their allegiance. Reference groups are examined within the context of the eternal struggle to gain independence in an environment which literally breathes expectations from within and without.

We take up marriage, family, and population only after examining the alternatives. In maintaining our life-cycle approach, we have included human sexual response in the chapter on marriage, recognizing, of course, that not all teachers or readers may wish to follow our sequence exactly. Chapters on consumerism, nutrition, weight control, physical fitness, noncommunicable diseases, environment, and health care delivery systems follow as we continue the cycle with the beginning of yet another generation. Finally, we examine aging, a phenomenon forgotten in most texts, but one accorded major status here. Death, dying, and coping with death follow, before we examine the future of quality life, ending on a note of hope for those who are willing to accept the challenge. Let us hope enough of us are!

The text presents a great number of facts, theories, and hypotheses. The facts and theories are, of course, well-documented, but the hypotheses are often original attempts to provide plausible explanations for our health behavior. You are encouraged to challenge them. The explanations offer a rational, realistic base for discussion . . . but by no means are they unassailable.

Hardly a typical health education textbook, this work goes far beyond the simple exploration of health science. It tries to stimulate the reader to gain wisdom. Wisdom cannot be taught, it must be learned over time. Nor is wisdom communicable, for

> The wisdom which a wise man tries to communicate always sounds foolish. . . . Knowledge can be communicated but not wisdom. One can find it, live by it, be fortified by it, but one cannot communicate and teach it.*

As a reader, then, you alone are responsible for developing wisdom. Our text is an excellent source of information. A health educator may guide you through it, but you alone will determine its impact on your own health behavior. The degree to which you ultimately engage in positive health behavior is the true measure of the success or failure of this process. Health knowledge is of little benefit if one's health behavior is detrimental to one's self or to others.

In our view, health education is aimed at more than just the individual reader. Its purpose is to develop an informed and vigilant public, one that is aroused to protect the health interests of society. Health education moves beyond people, and strives to modify or reinforce all of those factors that affect the ecosystem. It promotes the "good life" for the many, but never at the expense of the few. It views man as a continually adapting creature, and all states of health or disease as expressions of the success or failure of the organism in its attempts to adapt.

*Hermann Hesse, SIDDHARTHA, translated by Hilda Rosner. Copyright 1965 by New Directions Publishing Corporation. Reprinted by permission of New Directions Publishing Corporation, New York.

In writing this book we gratefully acknowledge the contributions of many people. Initially, mention must be made of the contributions of Dr. Robert Kaplan of The Ohio State University. The germination for the concept of this book originated with Dr. Kaplan. It was through his efforts that the writing team was brought together. Then his often critical analysis of the manuscript made for a much better final result.

Of invaluable help was Professor Nicholas Iammarino of Rice University. Professor Iammarino developed the entire Instructor's Resource Manual, wrote the guiding questions, and prepared the glossary. Grateful acknowledgment is also made to Dr. Eileen Metress, The University of Toledo, for rewriting chapter 25 and part of chapter 17.

Valuable assistance in the preparation of the text and important contributions to the text were given the authors by Mr. Wallace F. Janssen, historian of the Food and Drug Administration (Mr. Janssen reviewed the material in his private capacity, and no official support or endorsement by the U.S. Food and Drug Administration is intended nor should it be inferred), the American Cancer Society, Inc., the American Heart Association, the Arthritis Foundation, the American Lung Association, and the Center for Disease Control, Public Health Service, and are gratefully acknowledged.

Special thanks to our colleagues in the health education field who reviewed the manuscript and provided valuable criticisms and suggestions: Professor Eileen Broomell, Highland Community College, Washington; Professor Tom Crum, Triton College, Illinois; Professor Karen J. Dowd, Central State University, Oklahoma; Professor Robert Neeves, University of Delaware; Professor Patrick Earey, University of North Carolina; Professor Calvin Garland, East Tennessee State University; Dr. Robert Baum, Western Kentucky University.

We are especially indebted to our families, who encouraged and sustained us; to our students and colleagues, who inspired and tolerated us; and to those who have already completed their life cycle and whose memory will always be cherished.

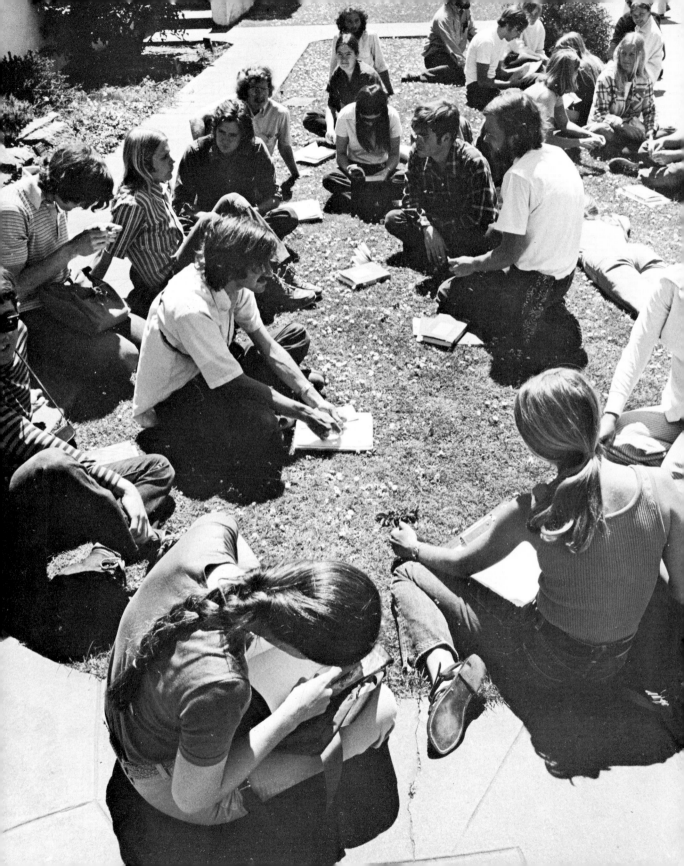

Interaction and Adaptation: An Introduction

Health is a process of continuous change or adaptation throughout the human life cycle. From conception to death, you are confronted with countless forces that influence your growth, development, general state of welfare, and your eventual decline. In addition to genetic factors, there are varying degrees of deprivation, adequacy, and in some instances excesses, of food, medical care, environmental hazards, love, mental stress, physical activity, germs, self-fulfillment, and so forth. Both favorable and unfavorable, these dynamic, interacting, hereditary, personal and environmental factors determine the level of well-being or of disease that any one person might experience at any given time—as a helpless infant, a growing child, an indestructible and invincible college student, a maturing, middle-aged person, or a terminally ill senior citizen.[1]

Such ecological interactions are continuous and evoke accommodations or adaptations within your physical-mental-spiritual being. Thus health and disease are viewed as ever-changing processes involving various interactions and adaptive responses throughout your life cycle—from cradle to grave.

Health, then, is not just the absence of disease or discomfort, but your ability ". . . to function effectively, happily, and as long as possible in a particular environment."[2] But since the internal and external environments keep changing, ". . . good health is a process of continuous adaptation to the many microbes, irritants, pressures, and problems which daily challenge man."[3] Common physiological adaptations include the constriction of peripheral blood vessels to prevent loss of body heat; shivering and secretion of the hormone, epinephrine, to combat cold; panting to pay the oxygen debt following exercise; and scarring to promote healing. These particular adaptations are coordinated by the nervous system and by body-regulating chemicals, the hormones. They are also examples of *homeostatic mechanisms* that serve to maintain the body's internal environment in its original state of constancy and evenness. Other adaptations involve the active physical process of deeper breathing to compensate for a rarefied atmosphere and psychological acceptance of or mental resignation to some irritating psychosocial situation or physical stress. In addition, genetic changes that in time affect body shape and skin pigmentation, and chemical alterations of the mind to achieve feelings of ecstasy or to forget one's troubles could be identified as adaptive processes. And think also of the many adaptations in equipment and behavior made by both design engineers and the astronauts themselves that made

Concepts of Health and Disease

Indestructible and invincible young adults—somewhere in their life cycle between cradle and grave

1

it possible for humans to survive in outer space and walk on the moon. *Such measures helped humans adapt to the environment or adapted the environment to human advantage.*

Evidently, human adaptations are essential factors in the prevention of diseases and in the preservation of one's health. In addition, certain changes or adaptive responses can foster higher levels of well-being in which the quality of health is elevated beyond the mediocre. From a developmental point of view health can enable a person to function more effectively and efficiently, to improve interrelationships, to achieve self-actualization or fulfillment, to live more fully, and to serve best in socially constructive endeavors. It is this enhanced dimension of health that we identify as *wellness.*

Dr. John W. Travis of the Wellness Resource Center offers the following explanation of wellness.

The ideas of measuring wellness and helping people attain high levels of wellness are relatively new. Most of us think in terms of illness and assume that the absence of illness indicates wellness. This is not true. There are many degrees of wellness as there are many degrees of illness. The diagram below is a model used by well medicine.

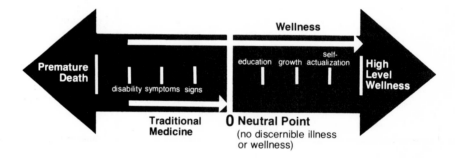

Moving from the center to the left shows a progressively worsening state of health. Moving to the right of center shows increasing levels of health and well-being. Traditional medicine is oriented towards curing evidence of disease, but usually stops at the midpoint. Well medicine begins at any point on the scale with the goal of helping a person to move as far to the right as possible.

Many people lack physical symptoms but are bored, depressed, tense, anxious or generally unhappy with their lives. These emotional states often lead to physical disease through the lowering of the body's resistance. The same feelings can also lead to abuse of the body through smoking, drinking and overeating. These behaviors are usually substitutes for other more basic human needs such as recognition from others, a stimulating environment, caring and affection from friends, and growth towards higher levels of self-awareness.

Wellness is not a static state. It results when a person begins to see himself as a growing, changing person. High level wellness means giving good care to your physical self, using your mind constructively, expressing your emotions effectively, being creatively involved with those around you, being concerned about your physical and psychological environment and becoming aware of other levels of consciousness.[4]

The questionnaire that follows will give you some idea about where you are presently on the wellness scale. It also will identify many human adaptations as they relate to your life-style and responsibilities in the prevention of illness and injury, as well as in the promotion of health and higher levels of wellness.

The Wellness Inventory
(Copyrighted 1977 by John W. Travis, M.D.,
and used with his special permission)

Instructions: Place a mark in the box before each statement which is true for you. Total each section, then copy the subtotals into the appropriate box at the conclusion of the inventory on page 8. Add up your total score. Average total scores range from 65 to 75 points, although no precise measurement should be interpreted as either ideal or failure.

1. Productivity, Relaxation, Sleep

00 ☐ I usually enjoy my work.
01 ☐ I seldom feel tired and rundown (except after strenuous work).*
02 ☐ I fall asleep easily at bedtime.
03 ☐ I usually get a full night's sleep.
04 ☐ If awakened, it is usually easy for me to go to sleep again.
05 ☐ I rarely bite or pick at my nails.
06 ☐ Rather than worrying, I can temporarily shelve my problems and enjoy myself at times when I can do nothing about solving them immediately.
07 ☐ I feel financially secure.
08 ☐ I am content with my sexual life.
09 ☐ I meditate or center myself for 15 to 20 minutes at least once a day.*

☐
Total
Checked

2. Personal Care and Home Safety

10 ☐ I take measures to protect my living space from fire and safety hazards (such as improper sized fuses and storage of volatile chemicals).
11 ☐ I have a dry chemical fire extinguisher in my kitchen and at least one other extinguisher elsewhere in my living quarters. (If very small apartment, kitchen extinguisher alone is adequate).*
12 ☐ I regularly use dental floss and a soft toothbrush.*
13 ☐ I smoke less than one pack of cigarettes or equivalent cigars or pipes *per week.*
14 ☐ I don't smoke at all (if this statement is true, mark item above true as well).
15 ☐ I keep an up-to-date record of my immunizations.
16 ☐ I have fewer than three colds per year.*
17 ☐ I minimize my exposure to sprays, chemical fumes or exhaust gases.*
18 ☐ I avoid extremely noisy areas (or wear protective ear plugs).*
19 ☐ I am aware of changes in my physical or mental state and seek professional advice about any which seem unusual.

*An asterisk at the end of a statement indicates that there is a footnote for that statement at the end of the inventory.

Women

100 ☐ I check my breasts for unusual lumps once a month.
101 ☐ I have a pap test annually.

Men

☐
Total
Checked

102 ☐ If uncircumcised, I am aware of the special need for regular cleansing under my foreskin.
103 ☐ If over 45, I have my prostate checked annually.

3. Nutritional Awareness

20 ☐ I eat at least one uncooked fruit or vegetable each day.*
21 ☐ I have fewer than three alcoholic drinks (including beer) per week.
22 ☐ I rarely take medications, including prescription drugs.
23 ☐ I drink fewer than five soft drinks per week.*
24 ☐ I avoid eating refined foods or foods with sugar added.
25 ☐ I add little salt to my food.*
26 ☐ I read the labels for the ingredients of the foods I buy.
27 ☐ I add unprocessed bran to my diet to provide roughage.*

☐
Total
Checked

28 ☐ I drink fewer than three cups of coffee or tea (with the exception of herbal teas) a day.*
29 ☐ I have a good appetite and maintain a weight within 15% of my ideal weight.

4. Environmental Awareness*

30 ☐ I use public transportation or car pools when possible.
31 ☐ I turn off unneeded lights or appliances.
32 ☐ I recycle papers, cans, glass, clothing, books and organic waste (mark true if you do at least three of these).
33 ☐ I set my thermostat at 68° or lower in winter.
34 ☐ I use air conditioning only when necessary and keep the thermostat at 76° or higher.
35 ☐ I am conscientious about wasted energy and materials both at home and at work.
36 ☐ I use nonpolluting cleaning agents.
37 ☐ My car gets at least 18 miles per gallon. (If you don't own a car, check this statement as true).

☐
Total
Checked

38 ☐ I have storm windows and adequate insulation in attic and walls. (If you don't own your home or live in a mild climate, check this statement as true).
39 ☐ I have a humidifier for use in winter. (If you don't have central heating check this statement as true).*

5. Physical Activity

40 ☐ I climb stairs rather than ride elevators.
41 ☐ My daily activities include moderate physical effort (such as rearing young children, gardening, scrubbing floors, or work which involves being on my feet, etc.).
42 ☐ My daily activities include vigorous physical effort (such as heavy construction work, farming, moving heavy objects by hand, etc.).
43 ☐ I run at least one mile twice a week (or equivalent aerobic exercise).*
44 ☐ I run at least one mile four times a week or equivalent (if this statement is true, mark the item above true as well).*

45 ☐ I regularly walk or ride a bike for exercise.
46 ☐ I participate in a strenuous sport at least once a week.
47 ☐ I participate in a strenuous sport more than once a week (if this statement is true, mark the item above true as well).
48 ☐ I do yoga or some form of stretching-limbering exercise for 15 to 20 minutes at least twice per week.*
49 ☐ I do yoga or some form of stretching exercise for 15 to 20 minutes at least four times per week (if this statement is true, mark the item above true as well).

☐
Total
Checked

6. Expression of Emotions and Feelings

50 ☐ I am frequently happy.
51 ☐ I think it is OK to feel angry, afraid, joyful or sad.*
52 ☐ I do not deny my anger, fear, joy or sadness, but instead find constructive ways to express these feelings most of the time.*
53 ☐ I am able to say ''no'' to people without feeling guilty.
54 ☐ It is easy for me to laugh.
55 ☐ I like getting compliments and recognition from other people.
56 ☐ I feel OK about crying, and allow myself to do so.*
57 ☐ I listen to and think about constructive criticism rather than react defensively.
58 ☐ I would seek help from friends or professional counselors if needed.
59 ☐ It is easy for me to give other people sincere compliments and recognition.

☐
Total
Checked

7. Community Involvement

60 ☐ I keep informed of local, national and world events.
61 ☐ I vote regularly.
62 ☐ I take interest in community, national and world events and work to support issues and people of my choice. (If this statement is true, mark both items above true as well.)
63 ☐ When I am able, I contribute time or money to worthy causes.
64 ☐ I make an attempt to know my neighbors and be on good terms with them.
65 ☐ If I saw a crime being committed, I would call the police.
66 ☐ If I saw a broken bottle lying in the road or on the sidewalk, I would remove it.
67 ☐ When driving, I am considerate of pedestrians and other drivers.
68 ☐ If I saw a car with faulty lights, leaking gasoline or another dangerous condition, I would attempt to inform the driver.
69 ☐ I am a member of one or more community organizations (social change group, singing group, club, church or political group).

☐
Total
Checked

8. Creativity, Self-Expression

70 ☐ I enjoy expressing myself through art, dance, music, drama, sports, etc.
71 ☐ I enjoy spending some time without planned or structured activities.*
72 ☐ I usually meet several people a month who I would like to get to know better.
73 ☐ I enjoy touching other people.*
74 ☐ I enjoy being touched by other people.*
75 ☐ I have at least five close friends.
76 ☐ At times I like to be alone.
77 ☐ I like myself and look forward to the future.
78 ☐ I look forward to living to be at least 75.*
79 ☐ I find it easy to express concern, love and warmth to those I care about.

☐
Total
Checked

9. Automobile Safety

If you don't own an automobile and ride less than 1,000 miles per year in one, enter 7 points in the box at left and skip the next 10 questions. (If you ride more than 1,000 miles per year but don't own a car, answer as many statements as you can and show this copy to the car's owner.)

80 ☐ I never drink when driving.
81 ☐ I wear a lap safety belt at least 90% of the time that I ride in a car.*
81a ☐ I wear a shoulder-lap belt at least 90% of the time that I ride in a car. (If this statement is true, mark the item above true as well.)*
82 ☐ I stay within 5 mph of the speed limit.
83 ☐ My car has head restraints on the front seats and I keep them adjusted high enough to protect myself and passengers from whiplash injuries.*
84 ☐ I frequently inspect my automobile tires, lights, etc. and have my car serviced regularly.
85 ☐ I have disc brakes on my car.*
86 ☐ I drive on belted radial tires.*
87 ☐ I carry emergency flares or reflectors and a fire extinguisher in my car.
88 ☐ I stop on yellow when a traffic light is changing.
89 ☐ For every 10 mph of speed, I maintain a car length's distance from the car ahead of me.

☐
Total
Checked

10. Parenting

If you don't have any responsibility for young children, enter 7 in the box at left and skip the next 10 questions. (If some of the questions are not applicable because your children are no longer young, answer them as you would if they were youngsters again.)

90 ☐ When riding in a car, I make certain that any child weighing under 50 pounds is secured in an approved child's safety seat or safety harness similar to those sold by the major auto manufacturers.*
91 ☐ When riding in a car, I make certain that any child weighing over 50 pounds is wearing an adult seat belt/shoulder harness.*
92 ☐ When leaving my child(ren), I make certain that the person in charge has the telephone numbers of my pediatrician or a hospital for emergency use.
93 ☐ I don't let my children ride escalators in bare feet or tennis shoes.*
94 ☐ I do not store cleaning products under the sink or in unlocked cabinets where a child could reach them.
95 ☐ I have a lock on the medicine cabinet or other places where medicines are stored.
96 ☐ I prepare my own baby food with a baby food grinder—thus avoiding commercial foods.*
97 ☐ I have sought information on parenting and raising children.
98 ☐ I frequently touch or hold my children.
99 ☐ I respect my child as an evolving, growing being.

☐
Total
Checked

Enter subtotals in the scoring section following the footnotes.

Footnotes

Numbers before each statement refer to a statement above.

01. Fatigue without apparent cause is not a normal condition and usually indicates illness, stress or denial of emotional expression.
09. Meditation or centering greatly enhances one's sense of well-being.

11. Many injuries and much damage can be prevented by putting out fires when they first start. Dry chemical or CO_2 fire extinguishers are necessary for oil, grease and electrical fires.

12. Regular flossing and using a good soft toothbrush with rounded tip bristles prevent the premature loss of teeth in one's 40s and 50s. Be sure to learn the proper techniques of use from a dental hygienist or dentist.

16. If you have more than three colds a year, you may not be getting enough rest, eating a good diet or meeting other energy needs properly.

17. All such toxins have a harmful effect on the liver and other tissues over long periods of time.

18. Very loud noises which leave your ears ringing can cause permanent hearing loss which accumulates and is usually not noticeable until one reaches 40 or 50. Small cushioned ear plugs (not the type designed for swimmers), wax ear plugs and acoustic ear muffs (which look like stereo headphones without wires) can often be purchased in sporting goods stores.

20. Fresh fruits and vegetables provide vitamins, minerals, trace nutrients and roughage which are often lacking in modern diets.

23. Soft drinks are high in refined sugar which provides only "empty" calories and usually replace foods which have more nutritional value. Artificially sweetened soft drinks consumed in excess may have long-range consequences as yet not known. (Both types of soft drinks contain caffeine or other stimulants.)

25. Salting foods during cooking draws many vitamins out of the food and into the water which is usually discarded. Heavy salting of foods at the table may cause a strain on the kidneys and result in high blood pressure.

27. Wheat bran, usually removed in the commercial milling of wheat, is the single best source of dietary fiber available. The use of approximately two tablespoons per day (individual needs vary) can substantially reduce colon cancer, diverticulosis, heart disease and other conditions related to refined food diets.

28. Coffee and tea (other than herbal teas) contain stimulants which, if abused, do not allow one's body to function normally.
    Environmental Awareness. Taking care of your environment affects your own wellness as well as everyone else's.

39. Humidified heated air allows one to set the thermostat several degrees lower and still feel as warm as without humidification. It also helps prevent many respiratory ailments. House plants will require less watering and will be happier too.

43, 44. Vigorous aerobic exercise (such as running) must keep the heart rate at 150 beats per minute for 12 to 20 minutes to produce the "training effect." Less vigorous aerobic exercise (lower heart rate) must be maintained for much longer periods to produce the same benefit. The "training effect" is necessary to prepare the heart for meeting extra strain.

48. Such exercise prevents stiffness of joints and musculo-skeletal degeneration. It also promotes a greater feeling of well-being.

51. Basic emotions, if repressed, often cause anxiety, depression, irrational behavior or physical disease. People can relearn to feel and express their emotions with a resulting improvement in their well-being. Some people, however, exaggerate emotions to control and manipulate others; this can be detrimental to their well-being.

52. Learning ways to constructively express these emotions (so that all parties concerned feel better) leads to more satisfying relationships and problem solving.

56. Crying over a loss or sad event is an important discharge of emotional energy. It is, however, sometimes used as a manipulative tool, or as a substitute expression of anger. Many males in particular have been erroneously taught that it is not OK to cry.

71. Spending time spontaneously without relying on an external structure can be self-renewing.

73, 74. Physical touch is important for the maintenance of life for young children and remains important throughout adult life.

78. With proper self care, most individuals can easily reach this age in good health.

81. Shoulder/lap belts are much safer than lap belts alone. (Shoulder belts should never be worn without a lap belt.)

83. Whiplash injuries can be prevented by properly adjusted head restraints. These are required, in the U.S., on the front seats of all autos made since 1968 but are often not raised high enough to protect passengers and driver.

85. Disc brakes provide considerably better braking power than conventional drum brakes.
86. For most cars, radial tires maintain firmer contact with the road and improve braking and handling better than bias ply tires. They also have less rolling friction and give better gas mileage.
90, 91. Over 1,000 young children a year are killed in motor vehicle accidents in the U.S. Many deaths can be prevented by keeping the child from flying about in a car crash. Most car seats do not provide enough protection—as government standards are very low. Check consumer magazines for up-to-date information. Never use an adult seat belt for a child weighing less than 50 pounds.
93. The bare feet of young children are often injured at the end of escalators. Wearing tennis shoes is equally dangerous because their sturdy long laces get pulled into the mechanism and their thin canvas walls offer little protection.
96. Commercial baby foods contain high amounts of sugar, salt, modified starches and preservatives which may adversely affect a baby's future eating habits and health. Federal legislation has been introduced to help correct this problem. Portable baby food grinders and blenders can be used to prepare for an infant the same food as eaten by the rest of the family. Individual servings can be packaged and frozen for future meals.

Scoring

Enter subtotals from each section and compute your total score.

1. ☐ Productivity
2. ☐ Care & Safety
3. ☐ Nutrition
4. ☐ Environment
5. ☐ Physical
6. ☐ Emotions
7. ☐ Community
8. ☐ Creativity
9. ☐ Auto
10. ☐ Parenting

Total _____

There are, nevertheless, limitations to your human adaptive responses in meeting environmental challenges. Sometimes the adjustment or accommodation fails to return your internal environment to its original state. On occasion, the adaptation may not be conducive to your welfare. *The consequences of such maladaptations are often manifest as disease.*[5] For instance, the process of scarring ordinarily functions to promote healing following injury. However, when scar tissue invades the liver and results in cirrhosis or immobilizes a joint as in rheumatoid arthritis, the adaptive response resulted in another health problem. Adaptation can overwhelm the person!

In some instances the adaptation is inadequate. Such was the case of the native Hawaiians who had never developed natural immunities or defenses to the disease-causing germs carried by the early explorers and missionaries who "contaminated" the Pacific islands. Hundreds of thousands of the natives were decimated by measles. Thus, *disease* may also be viewed as ". . . a *failure to respond appropriately to challenge.*"[6]

The challenge of disease comes in a variety of forms:

Hereditary defects are manifest in such diseases as phenylketonuria (or PKU, failure of body chemistry resulting in mental retardation), sickle-cell anemia (a

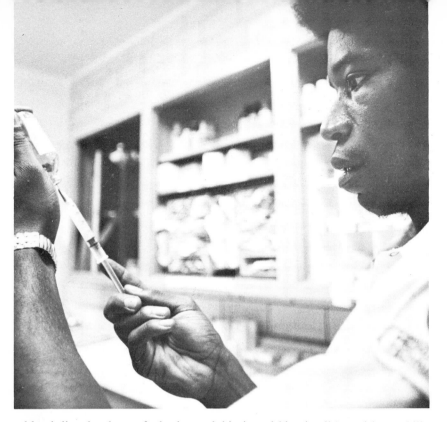

Fig. I.1. Development of immunization procedures and the discovery and use of effective chemotherapeutic and antibiotic drugs are two factors that extended average life expectancy and modified the ranking of the major causes of death.

blood disorder due to faulty hemoglobin in red blood cells), and hemophilia (bleeders' disease marked by a lack of blood-clotting factors).

Environmental insults of air and water pollutants, insecticides, harmful radiations, dangerous drugs, cancer-causing substances, and safety hazards take their toll in ailments ranging from respiratory difficulties to accidents. Recent additions to campus health problems related to the environment and changing life-styles are '' . . . more bicycle injuries, leg burns from motorcycle exhausts, and complaints by bra-less coeds of breast bruises.''[7]

Stress generators of frustrating jobs, unrewarding interpersonal relationships, overcrowding, emotional threats, competition, and anxiety are often translated into tension headaches, peptic ulcers, high blood pressure, arthritic conditions, and asthma (severe airway obstruction). While worry and tension by themselves cannot make everyone sick, '' . . . they and other emotions play a vital part in how our bodies feel, how illness develops, and how the individual copes with and recovers from sickness.''[8]

The wear and tear of daily life does contribute to the gradual deterioration and loss of function of certain body organs. Diseases and disorders of aging involve the heart, kidneys, gastrointestinal tract, muscles, endocrine glands, and respiratory system. However, effects of aging are often accelerated by a life-style of physical inactivity and personal irresponsibility. Even superstition and psychosocial taboos are cited as reasons behind the decline of sexual interest and functioning decades before physical incapacity occurs.[9]

Malnutrition abounds in underdeveloped nations but persists even in the midst of affluence in the form of anemia (iron deficiency), blindness (vitamin A deficiency), rickets (vitamin D deficiency), goiter (iodine deficiency), kwashiorkor (protein deficiency), and growth retardation.[10]

Overnutrition has become even more of a deadly affliction in America. Obesity is increasingly associated with the incidence of heart and blood vessel diseases, and diets rich in animal fats are frequently implicated as factors in coronary artery disease.

Infection or invasion of the human body by harmful organisms results in signs and symptoms of specific diseases, such as the common cold, infectious mononucleosis, polio, cholera, tetanus, tuberculosis, gonorrhea, and syphilis.

Mortality and Morbidity

Vital statistics are an indication of the success or failure of humans to meet environmental and hereditary challenges. Since 1900, some significant changes have occurred in the major causes of death (mortality). These variations are shown in table I.1.

Table I.1 Leading Causes of Mortality in the United States in Order of Decreasing Death Rates for the Years 1900, 1940, 1975

1900	1940	1975*
1. Pneumonia, influenza	1. Diseases of the heart	1. Diseases of the heart
2. Tuberculosis	2. Cancer, other malignant neoplasms	2. Cancer, other malignant neoplasms
3. Diarrhea, enteritis, intestinal ulceration	3. Intracranial lesions of vascular origin	3. Cerebrovascular diseases
4. Diseases of the heart	4. Nephritis	4. Accidents (all)
5. Intracranial lesions of vascular origin	5. Pneumonia, influenza	5. Influenza, pneumonia
6. Nephritis	6. Accidents (excl. motor vehicle)	6. Diabetes mellitus
7. Accidents (all)	7. Tuberculosis	7. Cirrhosis of the liver
8. Cancer, other malignant neoplasms	8. Diabetes mellitus	8. Arteriosclerosis
9. Senility	9. Motor vehicle accidents	9. Suicide
10. Diphtheria	10. Premature birth	10. Diseases, disorders of early infancy

Source: John H. Dingle, "The Ills of Man," *Scientific American* 229 (September 1973): 82–83. National Center for Health Statistics, *Monthly Vital Statistics Report,* Final Mortality Statistics, 1975 (Washington: U.S. Government Printing Office, February 11, 1977).

Table I.2 Leading Causes of Death by Selected Age Groups in the United States in Order of Decreasing Death Rates

1–14 yrs.	15–24 yrs.	35–44 yrs.	55–64 yrs.	75–84 yrs.
Accidents	Accidents	Heart Diseases	Heart Diseases	Heart Diseases
Cancer	Homicide	Cancer	Cancer	Cancer
Congenital Defects	Suicide	Accidents	Cerebro-vascular Diseases	Cerebro-vascular Diseases
Influenza, Pneumonia	Cancer	Suicide	Cirrhosis of the Liver	Influenza, Pneumonia
Homicide	Heart Diseases	Cirrhosis of the Liver	Accidents	Diabetes Mellitus

Source: National Center for Health Statistics, *Monthly Vital Statistics Report,* Final Mortality Statistics, 1975 (Washington: U.S. Government Printing Office, February 11, 1977).

At the turn of the century, the top three causes of death were diseases of infection that could be transmitted to other persons—the communicable diseases. By 1940, three noninfectious diseases assumed the top positions. Incidence of heart disease and cancer rose sharply, while pneumonia and tuberculosis deaths declined dramatically. From 1940 to the present, the noninfectious diseases have become more prominent, and as of 1975 influenza and pneumonia were the only category of infectious-communicable diseases among the top ten causes of mortality.

An analysis of the leading causes of death by selected age groups as seen in table I.2 reveals a quite different picture of the successes or failures of college-aged persons in meeting the challenges of life. For persons between the ages of fifteen and twenty-four years, diseases actually claim relatively few lives when compared with the much greater probability of death by accident, homicide, or suicide. Malignant neoplasm, or cancer, ranks fourth as a leading cause of death in this age group because of the rather high incidence of leukemia (cancer of the blood) in young adults.

The prevalence of accidents as the fourth leading cause of death in the United States is a perplexing situation, despite various adaptations of the environment and engineering technology to assure safer living. Injuries actually present a greater threat to persons ages one to forty years, during which time accidents are the number one killer and are responsible for more than 50 percent of deaths in the fifteen to twenty-four-year-old age group.

Accidents:
A Leading Cause
of Death

In addition to 46,000 motor vehicle deaths each year, falls, drownings, fires, burns, poisonings, respiratory obstructions, firearms, electrical current, falling objects, air and rail crashes, and medical complications claim 57,000 more lives.[11]

Accidents are also responsible for an estimated 10.7 million disabling injuries per year. Of this number, 380,000 prove to be permanent impairments. Although a price cannot be applied to human life, the cost of accidents in terms of lost wages, medical expenses, insurance costs, property damage, fire losses, and indirect losses from work accidents amounted to more than $47 billion in one recent year. On a national level, accidents are expensive!

By definition, an accident is "... that occurrence in a sequence of events which usually produces unintended injury, death, or property damage."[12] Traditionally, connotations of fate, chance, and unexpectedness are associated with accidents. In rejecting such commonly held ideas, one source contends that:

> ... the notion of "fate" is inappropriate, because injuries can be prevented or
> reduced in their severity; they are not "chance" or random events but the
> predictable results of specific combinations of human and environmental
> factors; and they are no more "unexpected" than most diseases.[13]

Research has revealed numerous causative factors of accidents: inadequate knowledge of potential hazards and safety rules, insufficient skills of persons participating in any activity, environmental hazards, faulty habits and attitudes, and unsafe behavior.[14] When any one or more of these factors contributes to an unsafe act or condition, injury, death, or property damage is more likely to occur.

While the physical environment presents many situations with a high potential for accidents, investigations suggest that mental and emotional factors play significant roles in accidents. Resentment, worry, carelessness, frustration, anger, and immaturity typically characterize the person who lacks emotional control. Such individuals are prime candidates for accidents, especially if they have a low regard for safety and frequently take unnecessary risks. Errors in judgment also claim many victims, for example, when persons overestimate their ability to swim long distances or underestimate how long it will take them to drive past slow-moving vehicles by going left-of-center as oncoming traffic approaches.

An analysis of social determinants of accidental injuries reveals that accidents tend to occur more frequently among the following groups:[15]

1. Infants and young children who are not able to care for themselves and are not supervised adequately.
2. Young adults who drive automobiles or who engage in hazardous and body contact sports or hazardous occupations.
3. Elderly persons who are infirm and have various impairments of hearing, vision, or walking, or who suffer from debilitating conditions such as diabetes, cardiovascular disease, and mental illness.
4. Persons with relatively low incomes and education, such as laborers, craftsmen, and other operatives, who are engaged in hazardous jobs.
5. Those who drink alcoholic beverages and then drive automobiles.

In identifying young males between twenty and twenty-four as an extremely high risk group for motor vehicle accidents, injuries, and death, a major task force report concludes that:

> This risk is associated with their propensity for driving automobiles rapidly and hazardously, and for drinking before driving. In many cases, this behavior is part of a pattern of young male behavior in our society which is supported, encouraged, and perpetuated by the behavior of peer groups. To many young men, the automobile is a symbol of power and an outlet for hostility and aggression, discourtesy, emotional conflict, and revolt.[16]

Initial efforts in preventing accidents focused on the "three Es" of safety: (1) *education* to help people live and act in a safe way; (2) *environment* improvement to eliminate accident hazards and protect human life; and (3) *enforcement* of legislation, rules, and regulations conducive to safe behavior. However, recognizing the limitations of both education and enforcement in changing human behavior, strategists recently have promoted products and practices aimed at preventing various forms of energy (mechanical, thermal, electrical, and ionizing radiation) from reaching people at rates or in amounts that are harmful.[17]

These adaptations to reduce human losses due to injuries are identified as *phases* and are described as follows:

Preevent Phase (before the accident occurs)—activities or processes that eliminate or reduce the source of energy or potential energy that could damage a person. Emphasis is placed on reducing the number of drinking drivers, separating pedestrians from motorized traffic and cars from heavy trucks on highways, placing handrails on stairs, childproofing matches and medicine containers, erecting fences around swimming pools, draining ponds, covering electrical outlets, and venting explosive gases.

The Event Phase (the person interacts with an energy source)—countermeasures that prevent a harmful energy exchange, even when an accident occurs. Activities include placing guardrails and breakaway signposts beside highways, packaging automobile occupants, installing door locks and windshields on automobiles to prevent ejection of passengers, utilizing of circuit breakers and proper fuses, making clothing that is flame retardant, drownproofing individuals by training them to swim, float, and tread water, and making available fire nets and life jackets.

Postevent Phase (after the accident occurs)—efforts used to increase human survival once the actual damage or injury has taken place. This phase includes making available and utilizing trained ambulance crews who can use lifesaving techniques and the effective use of burn centers, poison information centers, and detoxification centers. These activities represent society's response to emergencies and the provision of subsequent medical care and treatment.

Although these preventive strategies have been employed in the past to reducing human losses due to diseases, their application to the reduction of injuries resulting from accidents have only recently been adopted.

What the statistics on mortality fail to show, but what medical science has now confirmed, is that many disease processes responsible for death in older individuals originate in their strong, robust, invincible youth. Quite often the life-style you adopt now and in the immediate future will contribute significantly to morbidity and mortality. Consider the gradual decline in cardiovascular (heart/blood vessel) fitness that occurs as you become more sedentary. And just think that ten years from now, when many of you can at last afford to eat ''high off the hog'' and enjoy all those mouth-watering goodies in abundance, your caloric requirements will probably be less and your metabolic rate of food utilization will have declined. How many skin cancers will develop because of the periodic or frequent overexposure of human hide to the sun for the sake of a tan? No one will ever know for sure.

The average life expectancy at birth also has increased from forty-seven years in 1900 to over seventy-one years in the 1970s. Reasons for this marked increase, as well as for the changes in the major causes of death, are complex and overlapping.[18] They include the following developments:

1. Improvements in environmental sanitation
2. Better housing, clothing, and nutrition
3. Control of infectious diseases of infancy and childhood
4. Development of immunization procedures against certain communicable diseases.
5. Eradication of tuberculous cattle
6. Activities of health officials in case-finding techniques and in health education
7. Discovery and use of effective chemotherapeutic and antibiotic drugs in treating communicable diseases

Both human and environmental adaptation have made possible an extended life span. This is the situation in the United States, where the general population has experienced a long-term decline in mortality rates and significant changes in the leading causes of death. However, in comparison with other nations, including Canada and the Scandinavian countries, the age-adjusted death rates for the United States are considerably higher.

This less favorable position of the United States is related to excessive deaths due to heart, blood vessel, and kidney diseases, homicide, cirrhosis, suicide, lung cancer, diabetes mellitus, and motor vehicle accidents. In thirteen major disease categories, Canadian death rates, for example, exceed those of the United States in only three—tuberculosis, pneumonia, and nonrespiratory cancer. Of course, in the final analysis, the death rate for all humans is still 100 percent. But these statistics do suggest that populations vary in their capacity to adapt either their environment or themselves to life-threatening challenges.

When indicators other than leading causes of mortality are considered, a different view of human ills emerges.[19] For instance, musculoskeletal disease (particularly arthritis) *limits* the *activity* of more persons than any other disease category. *Hospital admissions* are led by persons suffering digestive system disorders, excluding cancer. More *days of bed disability* are due to upper respiratory infections (colds and influenza) than any other major condition—nearly twice as many as for heart disease, the next highest. In *days of hospitalization*, heart disease is followed closely by fractures, dislocations, and mental disorders.[20]

The most prevalent health problems of the living (morbidity) are not the well-known causes of death.[21] College students suffer broken arms and mono. They contract colds and flu and the so-called creeping crud. They may have sustained rheumatic fever as children and only recently have been found to have heart valve damage. Mental pressures sometimes generate mental anguish and cause students to drop out of school. Apathy, ignorance, or lack of money may be responsible for undernutrition and malnutrition. Sharing "pads" can result in more than endearing relationships; some persons get "crabs" or even gonorrhea.

Fortunately, many of these diseases and disabling conditions can be remedied, cured, or controlled. Some of them could have been prevented. On your journey through life, you will have the opportunity to influence and, in some measure, determine your health status. We hope you will be able to make health-promoting adaptations so that you can function with personal and social effectiveness and with a reasonable degree of happiness as you meet the challenges of living.

Notes

1. Howard S. Hoyman, "An Ecological View of Health and Health Education," *Journal of School Health* 35 (March 1965): 112-15.
2. René Dubos, *Man Adapting* (New Haven: Yale University Press, 1965), p. 263.
3. René Dubos, Maya Pines, and the Editors of *Life* magazine, *Health and Disease* (New York: Time Incorporated, 1965), p. 10.
4. John W. Travis, *Wellness Inventory* (Mill Valley, Calif.: Wellness Resource Center, 1977), facing p. 1.
5. Dubos, *Man Adapting*, p. 257.
6. Dubos, Pines, and the Editors of *Life* magazine, *Health and Disease*, p. 13.
7. "What Ails the Young," *Time*, 7 February 1972, p. 13.
8. Michael Halberstam, "Can You Make Yourself Sick?" *Today's Health* 50 (December 1972): 27.
9. James Leslie McCary, *Human Sexuality*, 2d ed. (New York: D. Van Nostrand Company, 1973), pp. 256-68.
10. F. Glen Loyd, "Finally, Facts on Malnutrition in the U.S.," *Today's Health* 47 (September 1969): 33.
11. National Safety Council, Statistics Division, *Accident Facts* (Chicago: The Council, 1976), pp. 3, 6–7.
12. Ibid., p. 97.
13. Susan P. Baker and William Haddon, "Injuries," *Preventive Medicine USA: Theory, Practice and Application of Prevention in Environmental Health Services—A Task Force Report* (New York: Prodist, 1976), p. 54.
14. W. Wayne Worick, *Safety Education: Man, His Machines, and His Environment* (Englewood Cliffs, N.J.: Prentice-Hall, Inc., 1975), pp. 23–25.
15. "Social Determinants of Accidental Injuries," *Preventive Medicine USA: Social Determinants of Human Health—A Task Force Report* (New York: Prodist, 1976), pp. 104–6.
16. "Social Determinants of Accidental Injuries," *Preventive Medicine USA*, p. 104.
17. Baker and Haddon, "Injuries," *Preventive Medicine USA*, pp. 54–59.
18. John H. Dingle, "The Ills of Man," *Scientific American* 229 (September 1973): 83–84.
19. Measures of ill health are based on principal disease categories defined by the World Health Organization and derived from data available from the U.S. Center for Health Statistics.
20. Kerr L. White, "Life and Death and Medicine," *Scientific American* 229 (September 1973): 24–26.
21. For an eye-opening statistical account of illnesses, accidental injuries, disability, use of hospital, medical, dental, and other services, and other health-related topics, based on data collected in a continuing national household interview survey, the reader should consult National Center for Health Statistics, *Current Estimates From the Health Interview Survey*. Washington: U.S. Government Printing Office, 1977 (Series 10, No. 115).

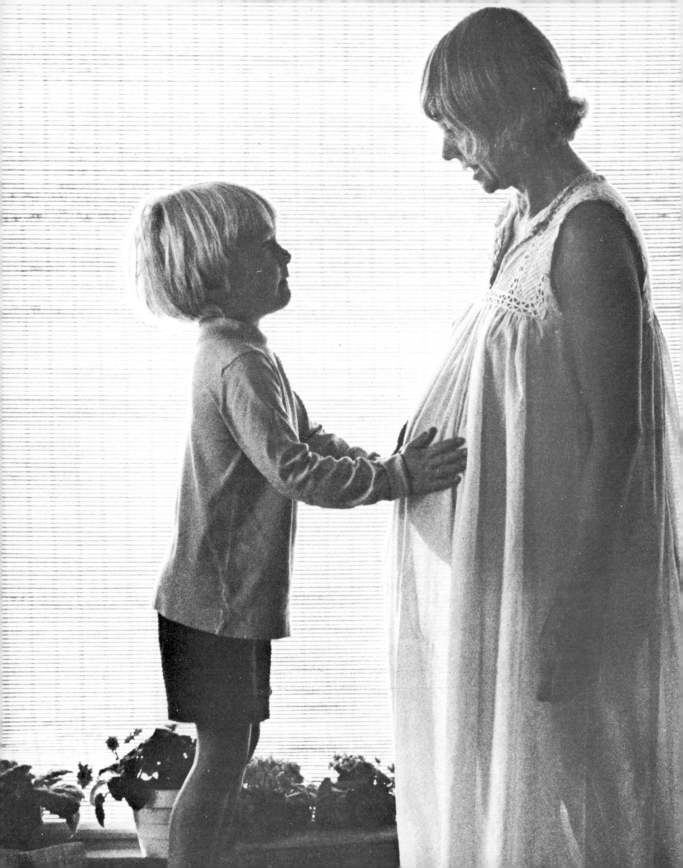

Welcome to Earth: The Seed Is Sown

A few years ago one could safely explain that a child was always conceived through the act of sexual intercourse, when a healthy sperm from the father united with a viable ovum (egg) from the mother. The newly fertilized ovum (biologically known as a *zygote*) quickly began to reproduce itself as it traveled down the fallopian tube and prepared to implant itself in the wall of the uterus.

Today the explanation is not always so simple. Artificial insemination, mechanical wombs, "test-tube babies," ovarian transplants, and even *cloning* (reproduction of another human being from a single body cell of the individual, such as a skin cell) are all within our grasp. The renowned embryologist Robert Francoeur has predicted that self-reproduction may be possible, even within this century, and that virtually all of the seemingly incredible literary creations in Aldous Huxley's *Brave New World* may in fact be realized.* Certainly one fact is abundantly clear—sexual intercourse is not the only way to induce conception.

The assumption that continuation of the human race is insured through our instinctive sexual urges and the pleasure they bring when fulfilled through sexual intercourse is no longer plausible. Sexual intercourse and reproduction are not essential partners—each can and does exist alone. Although it is unlikely that the human sexual encounter will diminish in incidence, the number of times that it leads to reproduction is most likely to decline. Contraceptives, abortion, artificial insemination, and test-tube reproduction may someday bring about a permanent separation between the seemingly indivisible partners of coitus (sexual intercourse) and reproduction. Nevertheless, the process of bisexual reproduction (one male, one female) remains relatively stable, and until cloning becomes a reality, we can assume that a viable egg, a healthy sperm, and a suitable environment are still essential for reproduction to take place.

The Conception Process

Conception occurs when one of the body's largest cells, the ovum, and one of its smallest cells, the sperm, fuse to produce a zygote. From conception to birth requires about 266 days, or nine and one-half lunar (twenty-eight-day) months. The normal range is great, however, running from 240 days to over 300 days.

*Francoeur is an associate professor of experimental embryology and interdisciplinary studies at Fairleigh Dickinson University. His theories are expressed in several thought-provoking books, including *Principles in Evolution, Eve's New Rib, Utopian Motherhood,* and *Hot and Cool Sex.*

A simple method for predicting the baby's due date is to subtract three months from the first day of the female's last menstrual period, that is, the first day of bleeding and add seven days.

Due Date

> To determine due date:
>
> | | |
> |---|---|
> | Take first day of last menstrual flow | November 18, 1979 |
> | Subtract three months | August 18, 1979 |
> | Add seven days, and that is the due date | August 25, 1980 |

Such calculations are estimates only, since they are based on averages. For the first birth in particular, allow an error of plus or minus two weeks in the calculated due date. Fluctuation in the timing of ovulation for first births tends to make accurate prediction difficult. The first perceptible movement by the fetus around the end of the fifth lunar month gives a better indication of its actual stage of prenatal development.

In the case of twins, the confinement is frequently about a month shorter; for triplets it is shorter still. The earlier the infant is born, the lower its birth weight, and the greater the risk. Twins occur only once in every eighty human births; triplets once in every 6,400 (80 × 80); quadruplets once in every 512,000 (80 × 80 × 80), and so forth. According to Guinness[1] the largest human multiple birth involved a "litter" of fifteen fetuses, five male and ten female, that were removed from the womb of a thirty-five-year-old Italian housewife. None survived. The woman had used a fertility drug, which probably was responsible for such a unique instance of quindecaplets.

Conception takes place when the egg and sperm fuse. Since nature is indifferent to how each arrives at the site of fusion, the race, marital status, previous experience, opinions, religion, vocation, and other characteristics of the parents are quite incidental. The most common way for pregnancy to occur is by sexual intercourse, although other methods of human reproduction are becoming available. The other methods include artificial insemination, cloning, womb transplants, and even the use of artificial wombs.

"Virginity" is not a total barrier to conception. A young woman with an intact hymen can get pregnant through artificial insemination, or in very rare instances through heavy petting, when sperm left at the vaginal opening make their way through the perforation, into the uterus, and ultimately up the fallopian tubes.

What Determines Fertility?

Age, health, sperm count, internal chemistry, timing, and many other factors affect the ability of men and women to produce viable sperm and ova. In general, women are capable of producing children during their mid-teens to mid-forties; men are relatively unaffected by age after puberty. Before puberty, *spermatogenesis*, or the production of sperm, is usually incomplete, and although ejaculation may be possible, the sperm are immature. Reports of new fathers over eighty years of age are not common but do exist; on the other hand, no new

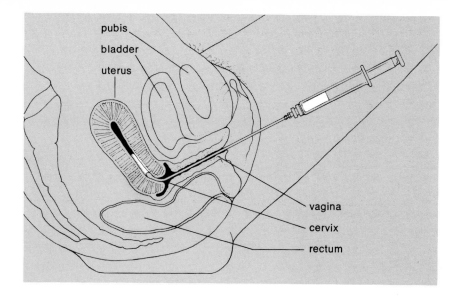

Fig. 1.1. In conception through artificial insemination, semen is collected from the husband or donor and stored (usually frozen). Eventually, the semen is sucked into a syringe and released into the uterus of the mother at or near the time of ovulation.

mothers over the age of fifty-six have been reported. More detailed discussions on fertility are included in chapter 12. For now we shall deal solely with the matter of pregnancy.

How Is Pregnancy Diagnosed?

For the female who menstruates regularly, the most common presumptive sign of pregnancy is a missed menstrual period. Unfortunately, few young women are really regular, and the menstrual cycle varies somewhat with state of health, tension, and so forth. As a consequence, it may be necessary to seek other signs. Some nausea may occur quite early in pregnancy, frequently after eating. This has been referred to by many as "morning sickness."

Vomiting is not particularly common, but does occur. Fortunately, self-diagnosis is now possible within a few days of a missed menstrual period and can be over 95 percent accurate. Test kits can be bought in the drug store, and a urine sample taken early in the morning can be tested for the presence of HCG (Human Chorionic Gonadotropic Hormone). If the hormone is present, the evidence is that a viable *blastocyst* (a hollow, fluid-filled sphere formed by the cells of a fertilized ovum in early pregnancy) is developing in the uterus.

Regardless of the outcome of this test, however, when pregnancy is even suspected, a doctor should be consulted. The early weeks of pregnancy are critical in the overall development of the fetus, and the total health of the mother is vitally important. Further, the doctor can assess more accurately the uterine condition and make a positive diagnosis of pregnancy through additional tests.

A new test to determine pregnancy is the Saxena blood test. Developed by Dr. Brij B. Saxena of Cornell University Medical College, this test, like the self-diagnostic test, measures levels of HCG. The Saxena test makes it possible to

Welcome to Earth: The Seed Is Sown   19

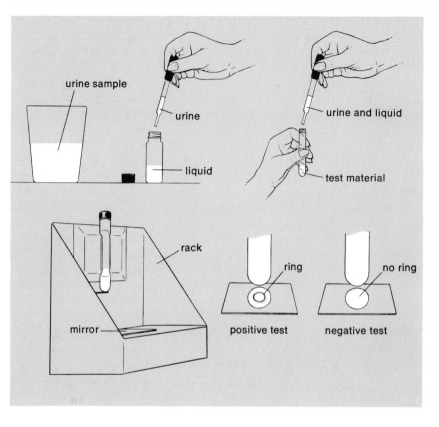

Fig. 1.2. Self-Diagnostic Pregnancy Test
1. Collect a small amount of your first urine in the morning. Within two hours, empty a measured amount of urine from dropper into vial containing liquid and shake well.
2. Add required amount of mixture from vial to tube containing test material. Recap the tube and shake vigorously.
3. Place tube in slot above mirror at back of rack and let stand undisturbed for two hours.
4. Read test two to four hours after placing tube in rack. If a ring forms in botton of tube, and is seen in the mirror, the test is positive. The HCG hormone is present.

ascertain pregnancy as early as six to eight days after conception. Most previously developed and presently used blood tests for pregnancy do not give reliable results until the second week after a missed menstrual period.

In addition to identifying whether the woman is pregnant, the Saxena test gives warning of imminent spontaneous abortion, ectopic pregnancy, and other abnormalities. Low levels of HCG produced during the first trimester of pregnancy often result in spontaneous abortion. Early diagnosis may offer opportunity for needed therapy.

Presently the Saxena test is performed only in laboratories or hospital clinics. This is because the procedure requires the use of a gamma counter. Dr. Saxena hopes that eventually the test may be conducted in a physician's office.

Imaginary Pregnancy

Imaginary pregnancy, medically known as *pseudocyesis,* is not uncommon, particularly among very hopeful or "child-starved" women. Cases of pseudocyesis can be traced back for centuries. One well-known case involved Queen Mary of England in the sixteenth century. When she was thirty-nine, she developed many signs of pregnancy, including lactation (milklike secretions from the breast). She sewed baby clothes and prepared the Royal Suite for the expected arrival. The physicians, midwives, and wet nurses came, stayed, and finally left when Queen Mary still failed to deliver two months after her due date. Eventually her physical condition returned to normal, and she was bitterly disappointed at her psychosomatic experience.

Instances of false pregnancy are not uncommon, nor are cases of male ''pregnancy,'' or couvade. Some primitive males, as well as some North American males today, go through many of the symptoms of pregnancy just as their wives do, and reach their peak of pain during the wife's actual delivery.[2]

In fact, couvade, usually in a very minor form, is reported more frequently today than in the past. One might expect this in a situation where the male may feel relatively helpless and useless throughout the nine-month period. Couvade may in some ways be indicative of the empathy a husband shares with his wife, and in that respect might be considered both normal, and even desirable, particularly when the couple is together throughout the confinement. Cases of father-absent couvade are not unknown, however. A considerable number of such instances were reported during the Korean conflict, when American soldiers complained of abdominal pain and nausea at the precise time their wives were delivering back home. In some instances the husband didn't even know his wife was pregnant.

Gestation

Fertilization generally occurs in the upper one third of the fallopian tube. The zygote (fertilized egg) multiplies rapidly as it travels for two to four days down the four- to five-inch tube and waits in the womb while the uterine wall completes its preparations. Finally, between the eighteenth and twenty-third days of the

Fig. 1.3. Fertilization and implantation

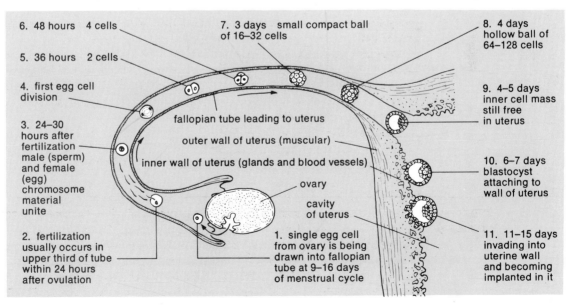

6. 48 hours   4 cells

7. 3 days   small compact ball of 16–32 cells

8. 4 days hollow ball of 64–128 cells

5. 36 hours   2 cells

9. 4–5 days inner cell mass still free in uterus

4. first egg cell division

fallopian tube leading to uterus

3. 24–30 hours after fertilization male (sperm) and female (egg) chromosome material unite

outer wall of uterus (muscular)

inner wall of uterus (glands and blood vessels)

ovary

10. 6–7 days blastocyst attaching to wall of uterus

cavity of uterus

2. fertilization usually occurs in upper third of tube within 24 hours after ovulation

1. single egg cell from ovary is being drawn into fallopian tube at 9–16 days of menstrual cycle

11. 11–15 days invading into uterine wall and becoming implanted in it

menstrual cycle, the zygote, now a fluid-filled, cellular mass called a blastocyst, begins to implant itself. (For a more detailed account of the menstrual cycle see chapter 4.)

Cell multiplication in the blastocyst continues after implantation until an internal layer, the *endoderm*, begins to separate. The endoderm helps form the respiratory and gastrointestinal tracts of the body. Cells of the outer layer gradually form the *exoderm*, destined to develop the external structures, such as the hair, nails, skin, and nervous system. The middle layer, the *mesoderm*, eventually becomes the muscles, bones, blood, kidneys, and sex organs. These three layers further differentiate and grow to become the human animal.

The zygote multiplies for days before forming the blastocyst; within a week this cell mass becomes the embryo. Only near the beginning of the third month is it called a fetus.

Although most women consider themselves to be one-month pregnant when they miss their first period, they probably conceived only about fourteen days earlier because ovulation probably occurred fourteen days prior to the date menstruation would ordinarily have begun. This fact should be remembered in reading the month-by-month development of the fetus as outlined in table 1.1.

Table 1.1   The First Nine Months

	Period	Development
Embryo	0–4 weeks	Zygote undergoes multiple cell devision, developing into a blastocyst that attaches itself to the uterine wall. Placenta and umbilicus develop. Head, spine, and limbs form.
	5–8 weeks	Embryo is unmistakably human. Primitive heartbeat. About 1 inch long, the embryo has a large head, webbed hands and feet, and noticeable limbs.
Fetus	9–12 weeks	Fetus now over 3 inches long. Sex is distinguishable, and almost all systems are developed.
	13–16 weeks	Length doubles again. Movement may be detected by the mother (quickening). Bones solidify.
	17–20 weeks	Length 9½ inches, weight about 11 ounces. Fetus wakes and sleeps. Fetal heartbeats become obvious.
	21–24 weeks	Skin wrinkled and red. Eyes open and move. Grasp reflex present. All systems except respiratory system are quite well developed. External survival chances poor.
	25–28 weeks	Length about 2 feet, weight 3 pounds or more. External survival chances are reasonably good.
	29–32 weeks 33–36 weeks 37–40 weeks	The respiratory system develops still more. Fat forms over the body, and the finishing touches are put on the organs and systems. Hair grows. Survival chances increase rapidly from now to full term.

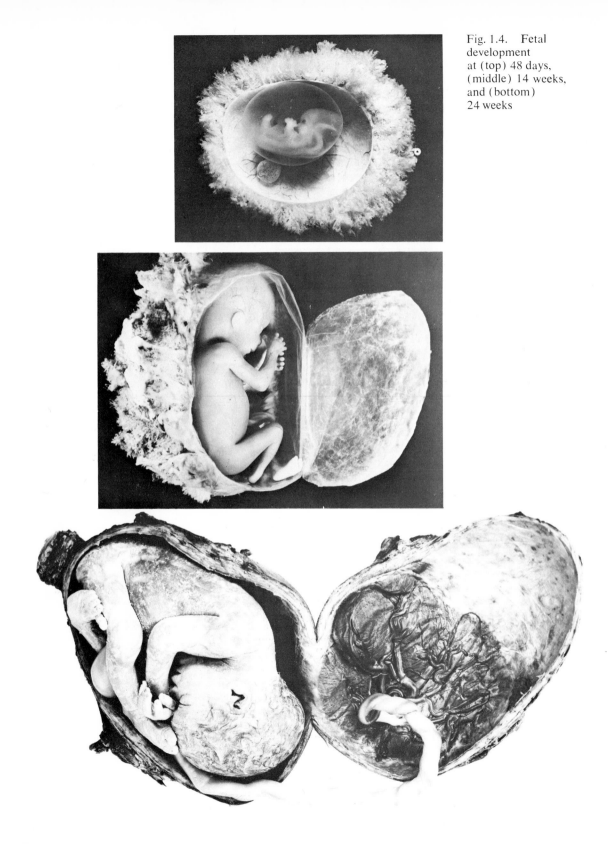

Fig. 1.4. Fetal development at (top) 48 days, (middle) 14 weeks, and (bottom) 24 weeks

| Influences on the Fertilized Ovum | Normal development of the fertilized ovum depends upon a normal environment both inside and outside each cell in the growing embryo. Maternal nutrition, for example, has a direct effect on the developmental process, as do infection, radiation, internal chemistry, and external drugs. All of these factors and many others influence the gestation process; some of them cause birth defects. A closer examination of the most prominent influences on the fertilized ovum follows. |

Maternal Age Although it is true that the ideal ages for maternity appear to be between twenty and thirty, and that both stillbirths and children born with birth defects are more common in mothers over thirty, there is increasing hope for "late" mothers. Evidence indicates that women over thirty-five have as good a chance as younger women of giving birth to a live infant. They may have more cesarean deliveries, more mongoloid babies, and more multiple births, but the chances of live birth are still very good—and a real encouragement to late starters.

Nutrition The old saying that a pregnant woman should eat more because she is eating for two has done much more harm than good. The critical question is one of quality of food, not quantity. It is true that children born underweight tend to be weaker than normal, but their status in terms of vitamins and minerals is far more important than weight. Physicians frequently prescribe vitamin and mineral supplements as insurance against shortages of them in the fetus, particularly when the conscientious mother-to-be is restricting her calorie intake. She should gain weight, but not an unnecessarily large amount, since the fetus requires sound nutrition.

The National Research Council Committee on Maternal Nutrition (1970)[3] recommends an average weight gain during pregnancy of twenty to twenty-five pounds. The recommended daily calorie intake should be only 200 more than the woman consumes when she is not pregnant. Pregnancy is no time for an already overweight woman to go on a diet in the hope that her fetus will consume her excess weight. Daily intake is essential for both the mother and the growing baby.

Rh Factor Formerly a serious problem for parents with an Rh incompatability (more than 10,000 fetal or newborn deaths were attributed to it in 1969), the condition of *erythroblastosis fetalis*, or hemolytic disease, in the newborn child is now almost completely controllable. Since blood tests have become automatic for pregnant women, early detection is probable and treatment can be prescribed.

A blood-clotting factor originally discovered in blood of the *Rh*esus monkey, Rh is a protein found in the red blood cells of 85 percent of all adults; that is, they are Rh positive. The remaining 15 percent are Rh negative. Rh incompatibility occurs in approximately one out of every eight marriages. When the factor *does not exist* in the mother and *does exist* in the father, it is possible that the baby is Rh positive. If some of the fetus's Rh-positive blood finds its way into the mother's bloodstream, it acts as an antigen, and the mother's blood produces antibodies to combat the foreign Rh factor. (See the discussion on immunization in chapter 3.) Should these antibodies reach the fetus, hemolytic disease may

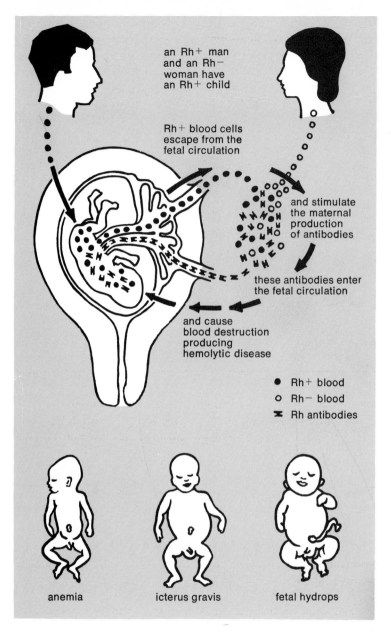

an Rh+ man
and an Rh−
woman have
an Rh+ child

Rh+ blood cells
escape from the
fetal circulation

and stimulate
the maternal
production
of antibodies

these antibodies enter
the fetal circulation

and cause
blood destruction
producing
hemolytic disease

● Rh+ blood
○ Rh− blood
✖ Rh antibodies

anemia   icterus gravis   fetal hydrops

Fig. 1.5.   Hemolytic disease
of the newborn only occurs when
an Rh− mother carries an Rh+ fetus.
The fetus may suffer from anemia,
icterus gravis (severe jaundice),
or fetal hydrops (abnormal
accumulation of fluids in the
tissues).
(From *Rh* by Potter, E. L. Copyright
© 1947 by Year Book Medical
Publishers, Inc., Chicago.
Used by permission.)

develop, causing the destruction of the child's red blood cells. Without treatment, the child could die from jaundice or anemia.

The child's Rh factor may reach the mother through the placenta, or, more frequently, during delivery. In the former case, the amounts are usually very small and may not cause the mother to react. In the latter instance, however, enough of the factor may reach her to stimulate the development of antibodies. If she has been stimulated once, even minute amounts of Rh-positive antigen in the future will cause her to produce new antibodies. This is why the disease usually affects children of second and later pregnancies more than the first.

Although transfusions for the child are possible, either during gestation (the fetus is temporarily removed from the uterus, its blood replaced, and the fetus returned to complete its development) or immediately after delivery, such a procedure is uncommon today. It is far more common to immunize Rh-negative mothers immediately after delivery, miscarriage, or abortion with Rhogam, which is gamma globulin that already possesses antibodies. These antibodies quickly combine with any fetal Rh-positive antigen and neutralize it before the mother begins to develop her own antibodies. Within a few weeks this foreign mixture is washed out through the mother's kidneys, and she is left free of antibodies that might threaten her next pregnancy.

Infection   Women who develop German measles (rubella) during the first three months of pregnancy have a 15 percent chance of giving birth to a defective child. The heart, ears, and lungs are the most commonly affected organs. Vaccines are now available to prevent German measles.

Many other infections are of concern to the pregnant woman, but they generally can be treated. Regular measles (rubeola), infectious hepatitis, smallpox (even fresh smallpox vaccine), and syphilis can be transmitted to the unborn child, and they all require immediate attention when detected in the mother.

Noise   Noise has been receiving widespread publicity as a pollutant with potential pathological repercussions in man. Undoubtedly, much of this publicity has been a reaction to hard rock music of the past two decades. On the other hand, a number of recent reports attest to infants' postnatal reactions to prenatal experiences with noise. The Japanese scientists Ando and Hattori[4] noticed that the way babies reacted to aircraft noise depended on the length of the mother's stay in Itami City, near the Osaka International Airport. Infants exposed to the noise while developing in the uterus responded more passively to it after birth. This effect was even more pronounced when the mothers were exposed to the noise very early in their pregnancy.

Radiation   Exposure to radiation may have serious, detrimental effects on the unborn. The reproductive organs—the ovaries and the testes—are very sensitive to radiation. Sperm cells in the male's testes may be damaged on exposure to even low levels of radiation. The same is true for the developing embryo. Whenever possible, dental and medical X rays should be avoided during pregnancy. Radiation has a predilection for tissues that are dividing and is particularly harmful to the structure of DNA (genes) during embryonic and fetal development, which are both periods of prolific cell replication.

Recent Japanese reports of blind and paralyzed newly born children have given us a new fear of chemical pollution. The stricken children were all born to mothers who ate fish taken from water with high mercury pollution. New research is underway to check reports on other chemicals, such as diethylstilbestrol (DES) found in meat and polychlorinated biphenyls (PCBs) found in industrial products and wastes.

Since the tragic crippling of thousands of unborn children in the late 1950s by the tranquilizer thalidomide, the use of drugs during pregnancy has become a highly controversial issue. Pharmacogenetics, a new science combining pharmacy and medicine, has become an increasingly important specialty.

Thalidomide was prescribed as a mild sedative for pregnant women until its disastrous side effects became obvious. The history of this drug has shown why it is impossible to rely solely on animal tests in studying the effects of drugs in pregnant women. Humans were found to be over 700 times more sensitive to thalidomide than hamsters, for example. Even enormous doses of the drug given to several species of animals failed to produce the severe crippling, disfigurement, and limb deletion that the drug causes in humans.

The effects of drugs on the fetus depend upon the particular drug (or combination of drugs), the dosage, and, most importantly, the stage of fetal development. Embryonic cells multiply and grow rapidly while food exchange and waste elimination occur through simple diffusion. Therefore, drugs capable of rapid cellular diffusion introduced during this period may cause significant embryonic alterations.

Between the fifth and eighth weeks, drug action can cause abnormal tissue and/or organ differentiation. Timing is vital, with the most severe effects occurring in the nervous system between days fifteen to twenty-five; in the heart days twenty to forty; in the legs between days twenty-four to thirty-six; and in the eyes between days twenty-four to forty.[5] The major parts of the body have usually been differentiated by the eighth week of pregnancy and the danger of drugs diminishes. Some effects, like smoking, are cumulative, however.

The evidence linking low birth weight with smoking mothers is unquestioned these days, but some argument persists. Although it is true that infants weighing 2½ pounds or less have a neonatal mortality rate more than twenty times as high as that for infants of normal weights, and that babies of smoking mothers have average birth weights of 200 grams (or approximately 7 ounces) less than normal, infant mortality in the children of smokers may be no higher than average. Yerushalmy,[6] for example, reported a lower incidence of neonatal death within the smoking group; Butler,[7] on the other hand, found a highly significant increase of late fetal and neonatal deaths amounting to 28 percent in offspring of smoking women.

Nicotine and carbon monoxide, two main constituents of tobacco smoke, are the most likely causes of retarded growth in the fetus. Nicotine appears to be most responsible for the cardiovascular effects of smoking, and in smoking pregnant women, it may affect the fetus in one or more ways: (1) by decreasing the appetite and caloric intake of the mother; (2) by altering the maternal and/or fetal metabolism; (3) by constricting the uterine blood vessels, thereby diminishing fetal blood supply; (4) by increasing uterine contractility.

Marijuana (*cannabis*) also affects the fetus, although in nonspecific ways. Two factors must be considered here, the techniques used in taking the marijuana, and the effects of the drug itself. If cannabis is smoked, the smoking action may have effects similar to those of cigarettes. On the other hand, the active ingredient of cannabis is tetrahydrocannabinol (THC). Studies indicate that it does cross the placenta, but its effects on the fetus are undetermined.

Although much has been written about *lysergic acid diethylamide* (*LSD*), a thorough, four-year California study concluded that LSD ingested in moderate doses does not damage the chromosomes nor cause detectable genetic damage,[8] nor does it cause limb displacement nor cancer in man. Coupled with its exhaustive review of literature, the California study concluded that since spontaneous abortions are clearly linked with use of illicit (and possibly impure) LSD, the drug should be avoided during the gestation period, but otherwise "there is no present contraindication to the continued controlled experimental use of pure LSD."[9] However, other scientists hold opposite views, thus perpetuating the controversy over the potential harmful effects of LSD on the human organism.

As far as opiates (heroin) are concerned, New York City hospitals reported more than 700 cases of children born with heroin dependence during 1971, and the incidence is increasing annually. What more need be said?

Most authorities now recommend that ingestion of all drugs and medications, including over-the-counter and prescription drugs, be kept to a minimum or totally eliminated during all stages of pregnancy, unless such medications are considered necessary by the physician.

Miscarriage

Spontaneous abortion or miscarriage occurs in at least 30 percent of all conceptions. Miscarriage is believed to be nature's way of eliminating an imperfect embryo—one in which the egg or sperm is defective and/or the implantation on the uterine wall is incorrect. Since miscarriages are so common and natural, they might be looked upon with gratitude rather than annoyance in that they prevent the birth of a defective child. Spontaneous miscarriage is technically an abortion, although we tend to avoid this term because of its controversial connotation.

Miscarriages normally are not caused by automobile trips, strenuous physical activity, falls, or emotional shocks. On the other hand, they may well be related to general body disorders. Complete medical examinations early in pregnancy may help prevent miscarriages in both the current and future confinements.

Some women are chronic miscarriers. This unfortunate condition requires both specialized medical investigation and considerate counseling. The "fault" may be nature's and not the parents', as in cases of imperfect implantation of the blastocyst in the uterus, unusual development of the embryo, early dilatation of the cervix, or hormonal abnormalities.

One term should be cleared up immediately—"congenital" does not have the same meaning as "genetic." "Congenital" means "present at birth" and does not signify the cause of a disorder. Many congenital conditions are not genetic. For example, urogenital syphilis, spina bifida (open spine), and many genetic diseases, like Huntington's chorea and cystic fibrosis, are not congenital. The appearance of a particular disease in more than one member of a family is not necessarily an indication that it is hereditary—it may be due more to a shared environment and/or a genetic predisposition, such as obesity.

Fortunately, most babies with defective development die before they are born. Of the million or so miscarriages that take place yearly in the United States, most occur in the first month before the woman herself is even aware of being pregnant. Other miscarriages occur after a few months and are the body's way of cleaning a defective fetus out of the uterus. About 250,000 defective babies are

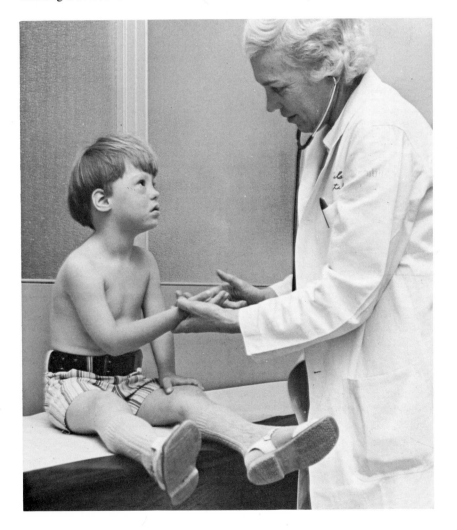

Fig. 1.6. This four-year-old boy has the typical facial characteristics and the prominent crease across the palm of the hand that are associated with Down's syndrome. One out of every 600 children is a mongoloid.

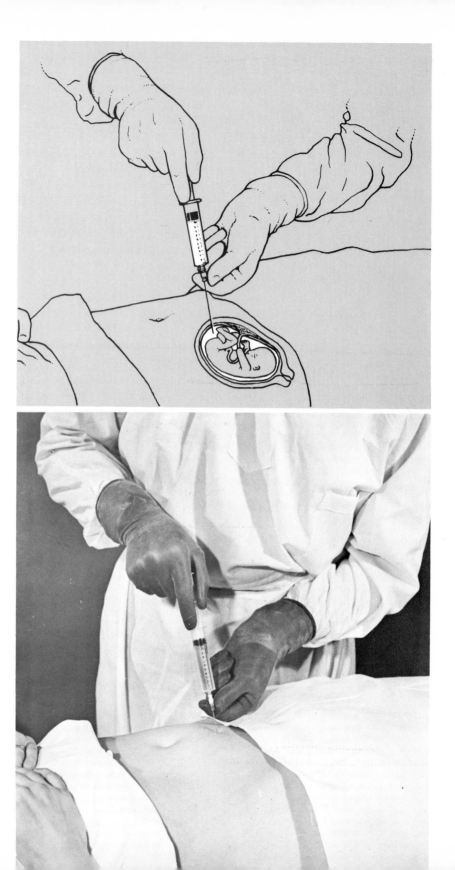

Fig. 1.7.
Amniocentesis is
usually performed
during the fourteenth
to sixteenth weeks
of pregnancy. A
hypodermic needle is
inserted through the
abdomen into the
uterus of the pregnant
woman, and a small
amount of amniotic
fluid is withdrawn.
This amniotic fluid
contains cells
from the fetus. These
cells are then grown
in tissue cultures
and examined
for biochemical and
chromosomal
abnormalities.

born every year, and many of these die within a year of birth. Unfortunately, many defective fetuses survive full term and are born as children with limited human potential.

Most birth defects are unavoidable and are clearly the fault of nature, with parents and child being the innocent victims. Science is at work even now trying to overcome such circumstances. As our knowledge of genetic disorder grows, so does the potential for treatment.

Diagnostic tests, some of which can be done directly on the amnion surrounding the developing fetus as early as the first few weeks of pregnancy, are now possible through amniocentesis. This technique involves the removal of a few ounces of amniotic fluid, which usually contains some cells from the fetus (figure 1.7). The cells are then grown in a tissue culture. The chromosomes are examined for evidence of Down's syndrome (mongolism), Turner's syndrome, and many other disorders. In cases where treatment for such disorders is possible, it may be started early; in other cases, pregnancy could be terminated.

For all diseases, of course, prevention remains the primary weapon. In the instance of genetic aberration, prevention involves identifying the problems in potential parents and preventing conception. The identification of current genetic anomaly and the prevention of future occurrences lie in the field of genetic counseling. The research into and the biological treatment for such disorders is known as genetic engineering.

Although many birth defects are clearly unavoidable, some steps can be taken to optimize potential for a healthy delivery. A physician should be consulted as soon as pregnancy is suspected, and any medication, even vitamins, should be taken only under medical supervision. An adequate, balanced diet should be followed, with supplements taken only upon the advice of the presiding physician. Radiation should be avoided wherever possible, and heavy smoking and the use of drugs should be discontinued. In addition, genetic counseling should be sought in cases where the birth of a healthy, normal child is in doubt. Such instances might be: (1) where blood relationships between husband and wife are suspected, and (2) when potential parents have a history of genetic disorder, such as diabetes, hemophilia, or sickle-cell anemia.

We shall return to this subject, in both this chapter and the next, but first let us deliver the baby.

Sometime near the end of pregnancy, the mucus "plugs" from the base of the uterus will be expelled. The mucus will likely be flecked with bright red blood and may be accompanied by amniotic fluid. Labor is likely to start shortly after the amniotic sac (or bag of waters) ruptures. Normal and painless, the breaking of this sac often precedes a shorter and easier labor. Some contractions may also occur around this time, either as the result of nervous tension or natural pushing and reaction by the uterine wall. Real labor pains occur at regular intervals, usually 15 to 20 minutes apart. Normally mild and rhythmic, pains increase steadily in frequency, intensity, and duration. Total muscular relaxation occurs between pains in a relaxed mother-to-be.

Parturition—
The Process of
Childbirth

Single Birth,
Full Term

A dilation of the cervix (from ⅛ inch to about 4 inches) should occur at this stage to permit the emergence of the baby into the vagina. As the cervix reaches complete dilation, the second stage of labor begins. The first stage may last about 16 hours for the first baby, but it is usually less and grows much shorter with future births. (See figure 1.10.)

Each contraction moves the fetus downward, gradually forcing the cervix open. Complete dilation of the cervix starts the second stage of labor, the actual expulsion of the fetus.

If the amniotic sac has not yet ruptured, the obstetrician will break it surgically. The head of the fetus by now is pressing on the mother's lower vagina and bowel, producing reflexive muscle actions that help to expel the fetus. As the baby's head passes through the cervix, the mother's natural inclination is to "bear down" and "push" the baby out of the vagina. Such a reaction is noted even under light anesthetic.

As the head emerges from the vagina, it turns naturally to the right or left, depending upon its own shoulder position. Using a ball-type syringe, the obstetrician immediately removes any blood, amniotic fluid, or watery mucus that may have accumulated in the infant's nose and mouth. Crying may begin any time now.

Holding the head in both hands (or by use of forceps if necessary), the attendant guides the expulsion while the shoulders emerge, one at a time, and the baby rotates. The rest is easy, since the largest parts are now outside. The umbilical cord is tied, and the newly breathing, loudly crying baby is welcomed to the world of harsh reality.

Shortly after the baby's birth, the placenta or afterbirth is delivered. Muscular contractions shrink the uterus and the area of placental attachment. The placenta is detached and expelled through the uterus. The umbilical cord should not be cut until after the pulsation of blood flow has ceased and/or the placenta is expelled. This is particularly important in emergency, nonprofessional deliveries, such as those that take place in taxicabs, in kitchens, or the out-of-doors. The delivery of the placenta is the third and final stage of labor.

Fig. 1.8. Before the invention of forceps, the use of any "instruments" to aid childbirth was synonymous with the child's death, and often the mother's as well. Here low forceps are used to assist both mother and child in the birth process.

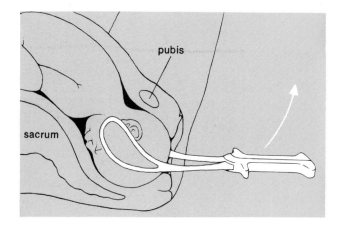

Common Delivery Practices   The mother is frequently half asleep during the delivery, thanks to the use of a light (gaseous) anesthetic. For the mothers who request complete consciousness, a low spinal anesthesia, known as a "spinal" or "saddleblock," is available. Combinations of anesthetics frequently are used. For those requesting "no aids," intensive pretraining sessions are recommended. These sessions include education and practice in labor breathing, process, and procedures. Natural childbirth may include light anesthesia to reduce discomfort but not inhibit natural processes.

Low forceps are frequently used to assist the expulsion and should not be confused with the popular conception of an "instrumental delivery." Further, an *episiotomy,* or surgical incision, is frequently made to prevent undue stretching and tearing of the tissues around the vaginal opening. The incision is repaired with sutures, and the vagina size soon returns to normal.

Cesarean Section   Instead of the normal delivery through the birth canal, the fetus is sometimes removed directly through the abdomen. A relatively safe operation, even during the course of labor, this procedure may be required for any number of reasons: a small pelvic opening in relation to the baby's head size, malpresentation of fetus for delivery, placenta previa wherein the placenta blocks the cervix and causes a heavy blood loss with labor, previous use of cesarean section making rupture of earlier incisions possible, weak heart, diabetes, and others.

Lamaze Method of Childbirth   Natural childbirth has gained in popularity in recent years. This method helps the mother have a more positive attitude toward the process of childbirth. It has been suggested that fear of the unknown is responsible for much of the pain related to the birth process.[10]

A technique developed by a French physician, Fernand Lamaze, is now widely used among young couples in the United States. The woman is taught what to expect during the birth of her child and learns a series of exercises that will help her relax and relieve the pain normally associated with childbirth.

The father is prepared through instruction to be with his wife during childbirth and to assist her. He can encourage her to relax, massage her, and inform her of

Fig. 1.9. About 6 to 7 percent of North American births are by cesarean section. A steady decline in perinatal mortality has accompanied the increase in cesarean births.

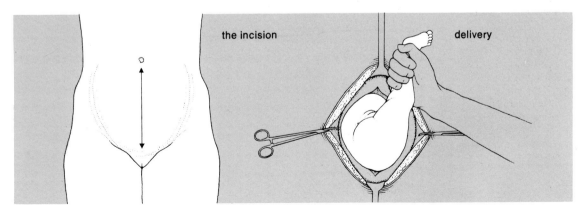
the incision   delivery

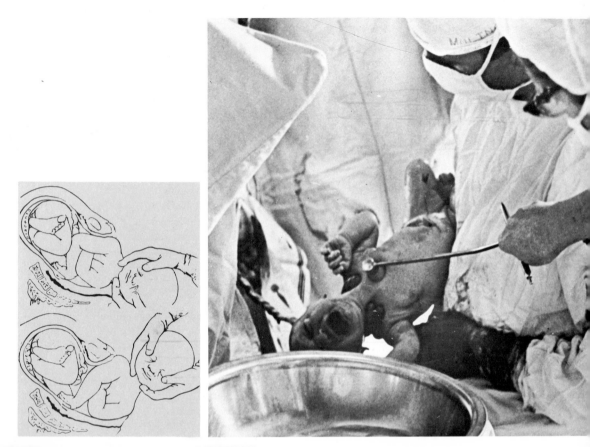

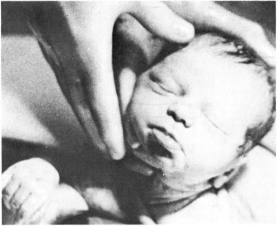

Fig. 1.10. The first stage of labor begins with the first true labor pain and ends with the cervix completely dilated. As shown in the drawings at left above, the baby's head, which has been lying close to the opening of the cervix, is forced into the vagina. The second stage of labor is shown in the picture at left, with the head being expelled. The picture above shows the end of the second stage of labor, with the birth of the baby and the placenta still attached. One minute after birth, the infant's hearbeat is checked.

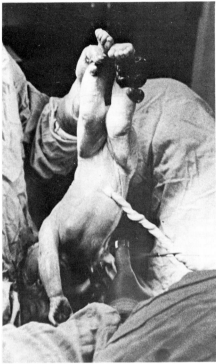

At the same time the umbilical cord is being cut, another team of doctors is taking care of the expulsion of the remaining placenta from the mother. This is all called the third stage of labor. In the picture at the right, the doctor has just cut the umbilical cord.

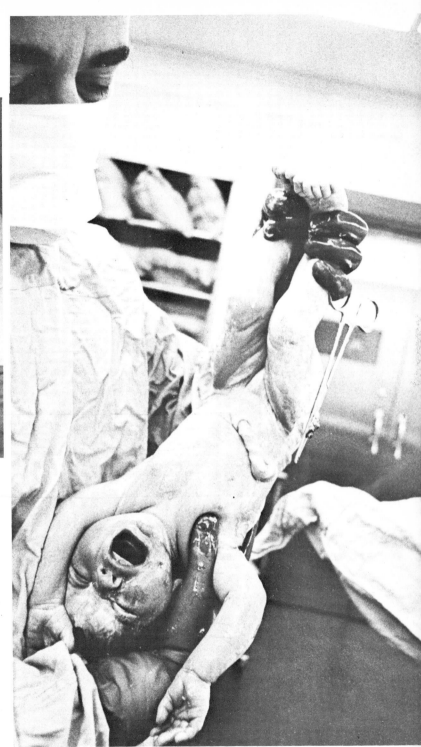

the progress. The father is as much a participant in the birth process as the mother. Using the Lamaze method, a woman does not require medication and is fully aware of the process as it occurs.

Leboyer Technique   Another procedure followed in childbirth is the Leboyer method.[11] The French obstetrician Dr. Frederick Leboyer focuses on the nonviolent birth of the baby. He recommends that an infant have a gentle entry into the world. He feels that there should be lowered light and sound levels in the delivery room. Reducing light and noise levels will make the environment less threatening for the baby.

The umbilical cord should not be severed immediately on birth, according to Leboyer. The baby should begin breathing gradually. This means the cord should not be cut at the moment of birth nor should the baby be held by the heels and spanked to force air into its lungs. Leboyer recommends that the newborn be bathed in warm water shortly after birth.

Leboyer's concepts are questioned by some American doctors. However, these techniques constitute another adaptation in the modern age to the process of childbirth.

Multiple Conceptions and Deliveries

Multiple births occur about once in every 80 to 89 births. They may result from the fertilization of two or more eggs, from the splitting of a single egg, or from a combination of both.[12] Interestingly, the larger the number of fetuses, the smaller are the sizes of the fetuses, and the greater is the number of females. Fraternal (nonidentical) twins are more common than identical twins. This ratio persists through triplets, quadruplets, and up.

What causes multiple births? Heredity, age of mother, and racial factors appear to be significant. Multiple births occur more frequently in some families, to women over thirty-five, and among blacks.

Identical twins develop from a single fertilized ovum that undergoes *mitosis* and splits completely. Each half then divides and multiplies independently until birth. Siamese twins, therefore, are the result of an incomplete separation. They are always identical and like all identical twins are provided for by a single placenta.

Fraternal twins develop from two separate ova, both of which are fertilized at approximately the same time. An ovary may expel two or more mature ova, or ova from two or more follicles may develop to maturity simultaneously. Fraternal twins can be of the same or of the opposite sex, will have separate placentas, and will bear no more resemblance to each other than they would as separately born siblings.

Generally, twins follow the normal pattern of parturition and are born at or about the same time. Unusual cases have been recorded, however. Case histories tell of twins who have arrived forty-eight days apart; mothers who have given birth to babies of two different races, fathered, of course, by two different men (the conceptions having taken place within a short time); and at least one set of twins has been born with different blood types.[13]

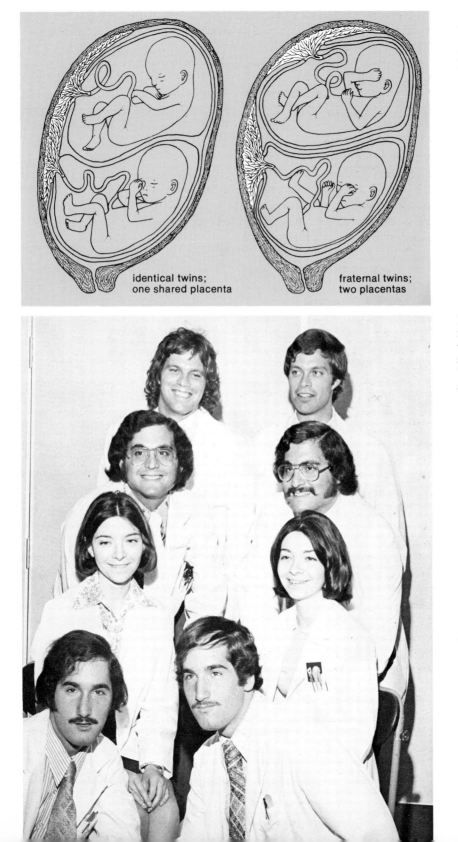

identical twins;
one shared placenta

fraternal twins;
two placentas

Fig. 1.11. Identical twins *in utero* (in the uterus) share one placenta, while fraternal twins have separate placentas.

Fig. 1.12. These four sets of twins were medical students at Thomas Jefferson University at the same time.

Although one commonly hears that sexual intercourse should be avoided for six weeks before and six weeks after childbirth, the figures are misleading. Some caution is certainly essential during the late stages of pregnancy, but the critical considerations are usually purely physical. Deep penetration may be hazardous to a dilating cervix, and female orgasm may adversely affect normal uterine processes at this stage. Similarly, the major limiting factors after delivery are slight vaginal bleeding and some pain about the vagina as the incisions or small tears begin to heal. When conditions are ''back to normal,'' full sexual relationships may resume, but with certain cautions.

Children spaced two or more years apart are associated with the lowest incidence of late fetal and newborn mortality. Contrary to popular belief, women can get pregnant very soon after delivery, in spite of breast-feeding! Although breast-feeding usually delays the onset of menstruation, the extent of effectiveness cannot be accurately estimated. Whenever ovulation occurs, conception is possible. A woman may ovulate prior to her first menstruation after pregnancy.

Should all mothers breast-feed? Certainly there can be many advantages, both physical and emotional. Breast milk is usually free from contamination and has superior protein balance, greater amounts of iron and vitamin C, and immunity-imparting qualities, compared with cow's milk. Obviously, it is considerably less expensive! Breast-fed babies endure fewer respiratory infections and fewer allergies. Conversely, cow's milk contains more protein, thiamin, riboflavin, and calcium. In North America, however, any of these nutritional deficiencies, as well as others, can easily be made up through food supplements.

Many psychiatrists claim that breast-feeding is psychologically advantageous for both mother and child, particularly in terms of intimacy and a warm, affective relationship. It is also undoubtedly true that the woman who is unhappy breast-feeding her baby will have a more harmful relationship with the child than if she had bottle-fed it. Furthermore, working women, high-anxiety women, and heavy-smoking, drinking, or drug-taking women should clearly weigh the consequences of breast-feeding carefully. In such cases, bottle-feeding might be of greater benefit to both mother and child. Further, a woman should not nurse who has had breast cancer or has had a breast-cancer history in her family. Viruslike particles have been detected in human milk and may be passed on to the baby.[14]

What Lies Ahead?

Three significant advances have occurred in the field of genetics in the past few years: (1) *amniocentesis,* (2) *culture growth,* and (3) *chromosome staining.* In amniocentesis (see figure 1.7), a needle is inserted through the abdomen into the uterus to extract a small amount of amniotic fluid. The fluid may contain enzymes, amino acids, and cells from the fetal skin, trachea, bronchi, and gastrointestinal tract. Cells from the fluid grow rapidly in cell cultures (culture growth) and can be examined for the presence or absence of chromosome abnormalities, respiratory pathology, or particular diseases, such as mongolism, Tay-Sachs disease, or Rh incompatibility. The later in pregnancy amniocentesis is performed, the better the diagnostic potential. On the other hand, the earlier it is performed

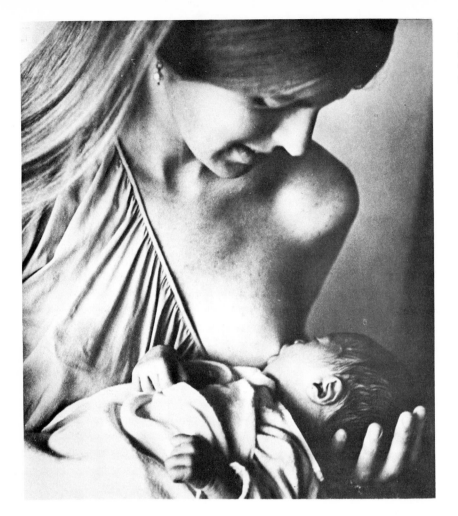

(rarely before the fifteenth week), the more useful it can be in decisions of pregnancy termination.

Although amniocentesis is quite safe, it is never performed without just cause. Simply to satisfy the parents' curiosity concerning the sex of a fetus is not considered a justifiable reason for the procedure to be undertaken. To assist a female carrier of an X-linked disorder in deciding whether to keep or to abort a male fetus may be sufficient cause for amniocentesis in some cases.

New staining techniques make it possible to identify accurately every chromosome in the human *karyotype* (chromosomal chart). Chromosomes treated with a fluorescing compound can be viewed under fluorescent microscopes to see the stripes, or banding. The pattern of banding is specific for each chromosome and is the same in the cells of all people. Such banding permits the identification of chromosomal anomalies and is proving invaluable in the tedious process of identifying gene patterns in chromosomes.

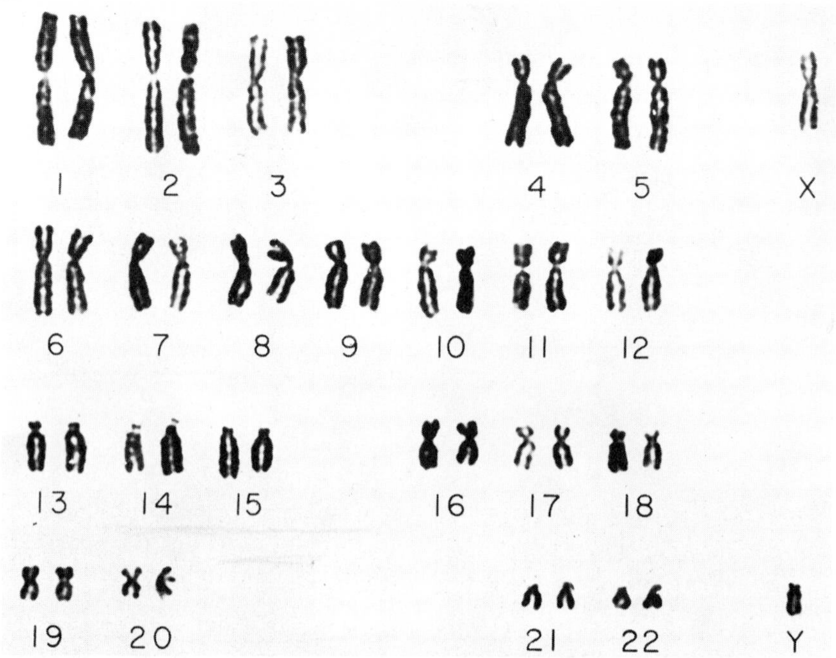

Fig. 1.14. This karyotype of a normal human male has the X and Y chromosomes, while the karyotype of a female has two X chromosomes.

The next step will be the development of techniques to correct flaws detected in utero—this is a major task in the field of genetic engineering.

As mentioned before, amniocentesis is one way of detecting the sex of a child before it is born. A close examination of the cells can determine the number of X chromosomes a fetus has. A dark area called the Barr body is in the female cells; no such area exists in the male. Sex determination of an unborn child, therefore, can be made with relative ease—although, again, such is never done without just medical cause.

However, the truly critical question is—can the sex of a child be controlled before it is conceived? Many believe this is possible, and such a theory is not new. In a *Scientific American* article, Manuel Gordon[15] pointed out that an Egyptian papyrus over 1,000 years old predicted that women manifesting a greenish cast were certain to produce boys, and that the Talmud forecast of placing a marriage bed along the north-south axis virtually guaranteed the production of boys.

Although techniques of sex determination have not yet been perfected, no major biological or chemical breakthroughs appear to be necessary. Scientists have found a clear difference in the X and Y sperm: the female-producing X chromosome is clearly larger than its counterpart, and X-carrying sperm are clearly larger than Y-carrying sperm. Any number of techniques may be used to separate the X-carrying, female-producing *gynosperm* from the Y-carrying, male-producing *androsperm*, including centrifugation, electrophoresis (separation in an electrical field), electrolysis, staining, and others. Not all sex prediction models involve artificial insemination either.

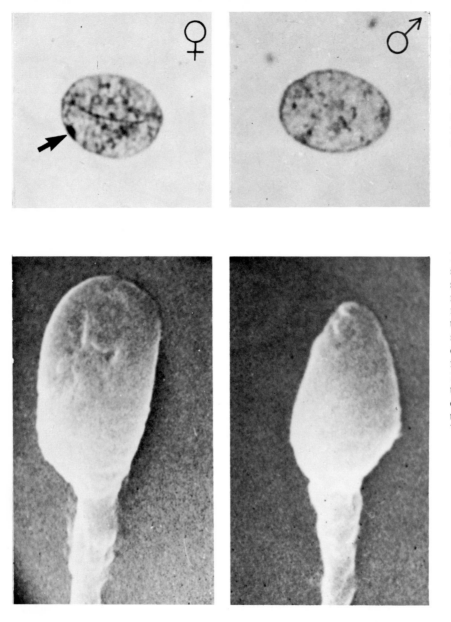

Fig. 1.15. The arrow in the photo at the left points to the Barr body, or sex chromatin, found in the female cell. As you can see, no such dark spot is found in the male cell shown at the right.

Fig. 1.16. Human sperm seen through a scanning electron microscope are magnified 56,000 times. The larger sperm on the left carries the female-producing X chromosome and the smaller sperm on the right carries the male-producing Y chromosome.

In the widely read article, "You Can Choose Your Baby's Sex" (*Look,* 1970), Dr. Landrum B. Shettles outlined an operational model for predetermining the sex of a child while still using intercourse as the method of sperm transport into the uterus. Recognizing, from the vast stores of literature on artificial insemination and sperm research, that low sperm counts appeared to be associated with a predominance of female offspring and high sperm counts with male offspring, he suggested a number of procedures that could be used without prior analysis.

For Female Offspring   The procedure for producing females is as follows.

1. *Have frequent intercourse up to two or three days prior to ovulation.* A low sperm count increases the potential for female births. Frequent intercourse up to two or three days before ovulation may help keep the sperm count low.
2. *Intercourse should be immediately preceded by a mildly acidic douche* (two tablespoons of white vinegar added to a quart of water). The acidic environment tends to immobilize the androsperm.
3. *The woman should try to avoid orgasm.* Orgasm increases the flow of alkaline secretions and neutralizes the environment.
4. *Sperm should be deposited low in the vaginal tract, that is, away from the cervix.* This insures maximum exposure to the acidic vaginal environment.

For Male Offspring   The procedure for producing males is almost the reverse of that for females.

1. *Intercourse should take place as close to ovulation as possible.* Prior abstinence is necessary, even to the point of avoiding intercourse from the onset of menstruation until the day of ovulation.
2. *Intercourse should be immediately preceded by an alkaline douche* (two tablespoons of baking soda thoroughly dissolved in a quart of water). Androsperm favor an alkaline environment.
3. *The wife should try to achieve orgasm, preferably prior to the moment her husband ejaculates.* This will maximize the flow of alkaline secretions.
4. *Sperm should be deposited as close to the cervix as possible.* Vaginal penetration from the rear is the recommended position.

Sound mechanical? It may, but Shettles claims a very high success rate.[16] Couples should consult the doctor first, however, to avoid the fate of one couple who, desiring a sister for their three-year-old son, read the Shettles article, purchased a basal thermometer, litmus paper, white vinegar, and a douching device. Finally, everything was ready and the grand strategy planned. Before starting, however, the husband insisted that his wife have a medical checkup. She did, and the doctor pronounced her healthy and fit—and six weeks pregnant. They had a second boy! The Shettles plan may work for people planning pregnancy but not for those already pregnant.

Summary

Conception occurs when, with the help of an enzyme, one tiny, male sperm penetrates a female ovum, and the nuclei fuse. Virtually all genetic potential is contained within the zygote and will eventually develop into a new human being. In the preceding pages we have looked at factors that control and influence conception, gestation, and childbirth.

After birth, numerous entities come into play in determining the physical characteristics of each child. The process of adaptation clearly begins even before birth. We now turn to the interactions of genetics and environment and the role of each in the nature-nurture question.

1. How is fertilization without sexual intercourse possible?
2. What are the signs of pregnancy?
3. Name the various types of pregnancy tests. Which are the most popular?
4. Distinguish between legal, therapeutic, and illegal abortions.
5. What are the major influences on the developing embryo and fetus?
6. In the past, what were the major causes of most birth defects?
7. How does the Rh factor affect the unborn child?
8. How do marijuana, LSD, heroin, and alcohol affect the unborn child?
9. What are the effects of nicotine and carbon monoxide on the fetus?
10. Discuss the idea of genetic counseling.
11. Explain the stages of labor. What is natural childbirth? How and why are forceps used in most births?
12. What is an episiotomy? — *surgical incision*
13. Discuss the reasons for performing a cesarean section.
14. Explain the principles underlying the Lamaze method of childbirth.
15. What is the genetic difference between fraternal and identical twins?
16. What advances have been made in the area of genetics in recent years? What can we expect within the next decade? The next century?

Notes

1. Norris McWhirter and Ross McWhirter, *Guinness Book of World Records*, Revised and Enlarged Edition (New York: Bantam Books, 1975), p. 31.
2. H. Diner, *Mothers and Amazons* (New York, 1965), p. 113.
3. National Research Council Committee on Maternal Nutrition (1970), "On Recommended Average Weight Gain During Pregnancy," as cited in "Pregnant Weight Watchers Risk Harm to Babies," *Public Health Reports* 85, no. 11 (November 1970): 94.
4. Y. Ando and H. Hattori, "Effects of Intense Noise During Fetal Life upon Postnatal Adaptability," *Journal of the Acoustical Society of America* 47 (April 1970): 1128–30.
5. B. L. Mirkin, "Effects of Drugs on the Fetus and Neonate," *Postgraduate Medicine* 47, no. 1 (January 1970): 91–95.
6. J. Yerushalmy, "Mother's Cigarette Smoking and Survival of Infant," *American Journal of Obstetrics and Gynecology* 88, no. 4 (February 15, 1964): 505. "Infants with Low Birth Weight Born before Their Mothers Started to Smoke Cigarettes," *American Journal of Obstetrics and Gynecology* 112, no. 2 (January 15, 1972): 277.
7. N. R. Butler, H. Goldstein, and E. M. Ross, "Cigarette Smoking in Pregnancy: Its Influence on Birth Weight and Perinatal Mortality," *British Medical Journal* 2, no. 5806 (April 15, 1972): 127–30.
8. N. J. Dishotsky et al., "LSD and Genetic Damage," *Science* 172, no. 3982 (April 1971): 439.
9. Dishotsky's conclusion is based on the study by W. H. McGlothin et al., "Effects of LSD on Human Pregnancy," *Journal of the American Medical Association* 212, no. 9 (June 1970): 1483–91.
10. Grantly Dick-Read, *Childbirth without Fear*, 4th ed. (New York: Harper & Row, 1972).
11. Frederick Leboyer, *Birth without Violence* (New York: Alfred A. Knopf, Inc., 1975).
12. L. J. Carbary, "The Fascinating Facts about Twins," *Sexology* (February 1966): 478–81.
13. Ibid.
14. H. Vorherr, "Suppression of Postpartum Lactation," *Postgraduate Medicine* 52, no. 1 (July 1972): 145.
15. Manuel J. Gordon, "The Control of Sex," *Scientific American* 197 (November 1958): 87.
16. L. B. Shettles, "Predetermining Children's Sex," *Medical Aspects of Human Sexuality* 5, no. 6 (June 1972): 178.

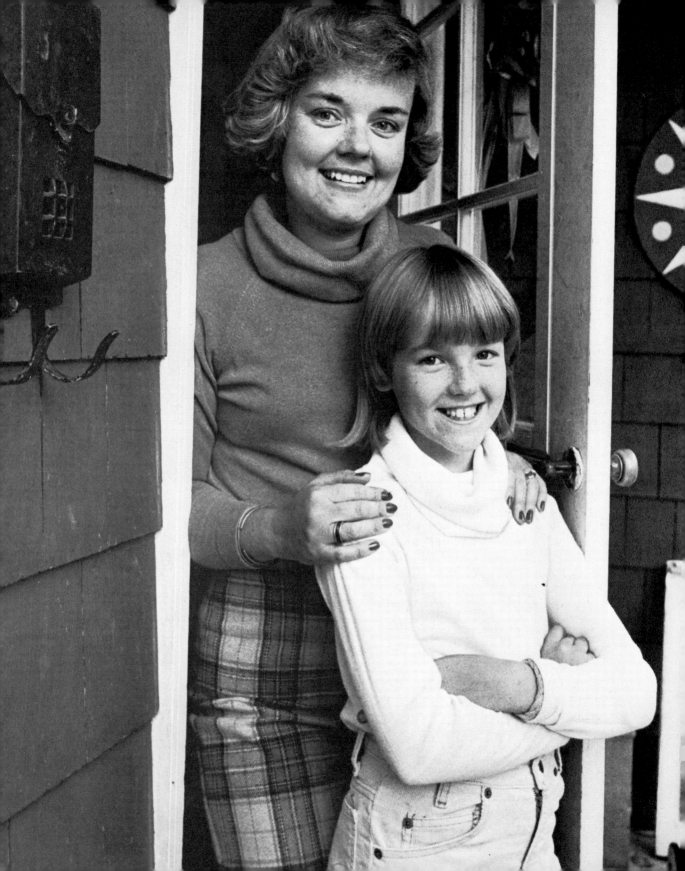

Genetics: The Science of Involuntary Adaptation

2

- *John Fitzsimmones lifted weights for three years prior to permitting himself to father a child–he wanted to insure the birth of a strong son.*
- *Marion Plutarch, a young factory worker with slighly below average intelligence, read Plato's* Republic *aloud throughout her pregnancy in an attempt to give her unborn child an intellectual head start.*
- *When Jeremiah Pederson's son was born with a cleft palate, he blamed himself, claiming the defective child was God's punishment for his promiscuous premarital conduct.*

Myths like these will be discussed throughout this chapter on the age-old question of which is more important, *heredity* or *environment*. Genetics is the science that analyzes the transmission of hereditary factors from one generation to the next. The science is extremely complex, yet its laws remain consistent throughout all levels of the biological phylum, from microbe, to fish, to plant, to animal, to man. Genetics does not work alone.

Long before birth and throughout one's lifetime, environment plays a major role. Occasionally maternal illness during pregnancy, such as rubella (German measles), or influences before pregnancy, such as exposure to radiation and resultant genetic mutation, adversely affect the still-to-be-conceived child. Certainly much of what a person will be during his or her life is determined after birth and depends upon the environmental conditions under which postnatal development takes place and on how the individual utilizes genetic and environmental potential. The question, then, is not whether the individual is influenced by both heredity and environment, but how much an individual is influenced by each.

Historical figures like Hitler and Rousseau believed that heredity was the all-important determinant of potential greatness in any given person. Others like Stalin, Skinner, and Watson have given the balance of credit to environment. Today the argument seems ludicrous—obviously both are intricately involved. From the same parental pair have come giants and dwarfs, idiots and geniuses, single births and triple births, blonds and brunettes, live births and stillbirths. Brothers and sisters sometimes resemble the parents; sometimes they do not clearly resemble anyone in the family. How is this possible?

Traits are passed on from generation to generation by tiny protein structures called *genes*. Nevertheless, identical twins born with the same genes do not always remain identical. One would hardly expect identical twins, separated at birth and raised in entirely different environments, to still look alike after a number of years—for example, one twin raised in the foothills of Kentucky, pursuing a rugged, physically demanding life-style, and the other twin raised in an upper-class city environment, following a pampered, intellectually stimulating but physically nondemanding life-style. Even the measured IQs of such twins are likely to be considerably different. Still part of them, namely their genetic composition, would remain identical even though their physical appearance would be markedly different. Interestingly enough, if each twin could undergo spontaneous self-reproduction, as in *cloning*, the offspring from each twin would be identical twins. If these offspring were raised in a common environment, the identical cousins would grow, develop, and change in essentially the same fashion—and probably still would resemble each other very much even late in life.

Often, visible features (phenotype) vary from the genetic bases or fundamental heredity constitution (genotype) in man. While physical appearance reflects the development of genetic potential, its expression is the result of interaction between heredity *and* environment.

How Do the Genes Function?

The basic unit of all life is the *cell*. Cellular protoplasm provides the chemical life for the cell and houses a number of ministructures, or *organelles*, the largest of which is the *nucleus*. Within the nucleus are *chromosomes*, composed of long strands of genes, the agents of heredity. The chromosomes are actually highly concentrated packages of DNA (deoxyribonucleic acid). In the form of double-strand coils of chemicals, DNA biologically determines all of man's hereditary characteristics. The coils contain the blueprints for the body's production of proteins, which can reproduce DNA when necessary, engineer the body's chemistry, and provide an individual with his characteristic shape, size, internal functions, and external appearance.

All living cells within a single person contain this same DNA; each cell has a complete set of blueprints. Yet, not all cells behave in the same way nor are all committed to the same structure or function. The process of differentiation, which is essentially the assignment of different roles to different cells, permits skin, blood, liver, kidney, lung, and other tissues to acquire their own particular appearance and function even though every cell composing them has in fact the same potential abilities. Given a different direction, a skin cell could just as easily become part of the kidney or part of the spleen. The genotype of all body cells is the same.

Genetically speaking, there are only two kinds of cells in the human body: (1) germ cells, which are the sex-determining cells (the ova or sperm), and (2) somatic, or body cells, which form all the other body tissues. In each germ cell are twenty-three single chromosomes; in each somatic cell are twenty-three pairs of chromosomes.

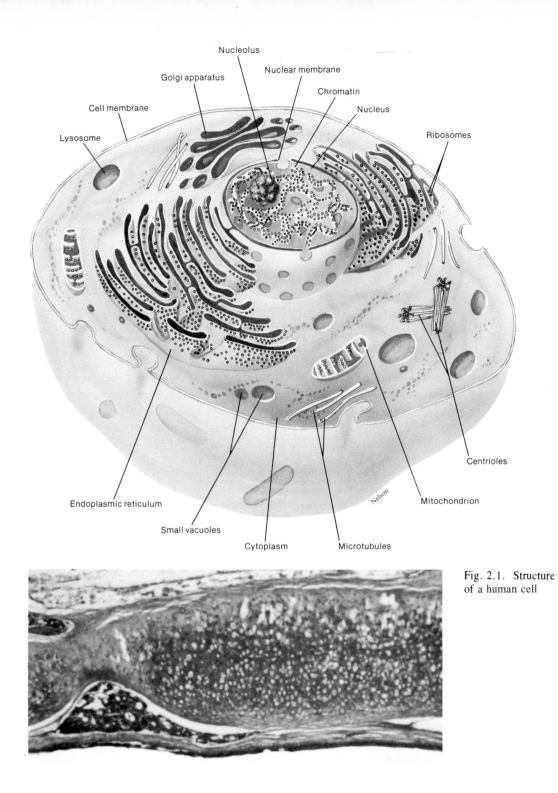

Nucleolus

Golgi apparatus

Nuclear membrane

Chromatin

Cell membrane

Nucleus

Lysosome

Ribosomes

Centrioles

Endoplasmic reticulum

Mitochondrion

Small vacuoles

Cytoplasm

Microtubules

Nelson

Fig. 2.1. Structure of a human cell

Genetics: The Science of Involuntary Adaptation

47

All cells are reproduced by the process of *mitosis*. The chromosomes duplicate and line up along a central axis. Each pair then splits in opposite directions, the wall between the two parts pinching in at the center and forming two "mirror image" cells—each containing twenty-three pairs of chromosomes. Although one day it may be possible to reproduce an entire human being by "nurturing" any one of these complete somatic cells (cloning), we shall not concern ourselves with that just yet. All human beings to date have been formed by "sexual" reproduction.

If each parent contributed a somatic cell instead of a germ cell to each offspring, their children would be born with forty-six pairs of chromosomes per cell (twenty-three pairs from each parent). In turn, their children's offspring might be born with ninety-six pairs per cell, and so on. Clearly, such biological anomalies do not exist. Why not?

Like body cells, germ cells do undergo mitosis. Unlike body cells, however, they undergo a second process, a reduction-division called *meiosis*. The once-divided cells divide a second time, but this time without the chromosomes duplicating. Four daughter cells result—each with half of the chromosomes of the parent. Since germ cells undergo reduction-division, each contributes only twenty-three single chromosomes in the human reproduction component. The resulting zygote, then, is composed of twenty-three pairs of chromosomes and is clearly distinct from its parent cells, having received half of its genes from the mother and half from the father. Of these chromosomes, twenty-two pairs are known as *autosomes,* while the remaining pair constitutes the sex chromosomes, XX for the female and XY for the male. In each pair of corresponding chromosomes except the XY pair, the various genes of one chromosome have their individual counterparts in the other chromosome. Such paired genes are called *alleles.*

Identical alleles are said to be *homozygous* for the gene in question. Differing alleles are called *heterozygous.* All humans are composed of both types of alleles—hence our individuality. Homozygous alleles perpetuate a common quality, such as blue eyes; heterozygous alleles are more complex. In some instances one allele clearly overrules another, making the stronger one the dominant trait and its partner allele the recessive trait. An example of this occurs in eye color. If the fetus has received a "brown" gene from one parent and a "blue" gene from the other, the baby will be brown-eyed. Brown is a dominant trait. In other instances codominance may exist, as in blood types where A and B are both dominant traits. When one parent contributes an A blood-type gene and the other parent contributes a B gene, the child will in fact have an AB blood type (see table 2.1).

Although many human traits, such as skin color and blood type, are each controlled by a small number of genes, other traits, such as body type and intelligence, are quite complex and are said to be polygenic, that is, under the influence of many genes. Polygenic traits have a range of potential and are subject to past, present, and future influence. This raises the question, "Which is more important, heredity or environment?" The question cannot be answered in simple terms.

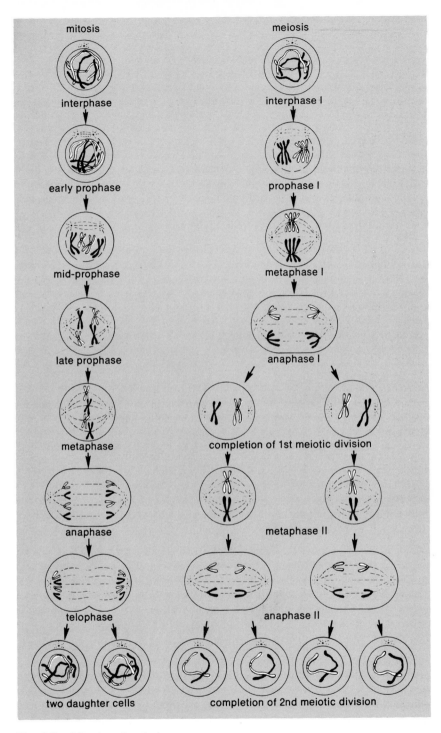

Fig. 2.2   Mitosis and meiosis

Table 2.1 Inheritance of Blood Type

Parents' Phenotypes*		Possible Children Phenotypes	Impossible Children Phenotypes
Father	*Mother*		
A	A	A, O	AB, B
A	B	A, B, AB, O	
A	AB	A, B, AB	O
A	O	A, O	AB, B
B	B	B, O	A, AB
B	AB	A, B, AB	O
B	O	B, O	A, AB
AB	AB	A, B, AB	O
AB	O	A, B	O, AB
O	O	O	A, B, AB

*O=O/O; A=A/A or A/O; B=B/B or O/B; AB=A/B

Note: Among North American Blacks, 47% are O; 28% are A; 20% are B; and 5% are AB. Among North American whites, 45% are O; 41% are A; 10% are B; and 4% are AB.

The Constant Interplay— Heredity and Environment

As late as a decade ago, people still argued that some human traits are clearly hereditary in origin, while others are entirely environmental. Belief in this dichotomy is symptomatic of a misunderstanding of the roles of social conditions, medicine, and education. "Hereditary diseases are incurable," the notion goes, "but those contracted through exposure to some noxious environment can be cured," or "If the IQ of a child depends upon his schooling, then IQ cannot be hereditary." Such statements, based on a dichotomy of hereditary and environmental traits, are untenable. In principle, any trait can be modified by changes in the genes and/or manipulation of the environment.

Within the cell core the DNA stamping process is complex and is affected by its own environment. Each cell with its nucleus, each strand of DNA in the nucleus, and each chemical substructure within the DNA, all function within a microenvironment and are influenced by it. As a consequence, no individual is the result of the genotype alone. Cell division, with its resultant increase in the number of cells and growth of the organism, forces the constituents of the genotype to continuously duplicate themselves—and the materials for such continuous duplication can only come from the environment. A single zygote weighing well under a millionth of an ounce grows into an adult of 180 pounds, at first within the environment of the uterus, and later without. Development of all life occurs within, and draws upon, an environment.

A look at genetic disorder should still the argument entirely.

Abnormal mitosis and meiosis, radiation, and chemicals, as well as unexplainable spontaneous mutations, may lead to errors in the physical or chemical structure of a chromosome. Frequently, such deviations from the normal create problems for the individual. Severe metabolic disturbance may occur when alteration of the micro-acid chain in a defective gene results in the inability of the body to produce a specific protein, be it an enzyme, hormone, or vitamin. This is known as an inborn error of metabolism, and over 1,500 such errors have been cataloged. The vast majority of them involve recessive alleles, spread by heterozygous carriers and manifest in homozygous pairings.

Abnormalities in Chromosomal Structure

In sickle-cell anemia, for example, a hereditary chemical disorder affecting the blood of almost 10 percent of American blacks, the hemoglobin (protein) of red blood cells is adversely affected. In afflicted individuals these cells assume a sickle shape and tend to clog up the small capillaries in the circulatory system, cutting off the supply of oxygen to surrounding tissues and thereby causing both

Sickle-Cell Anemia

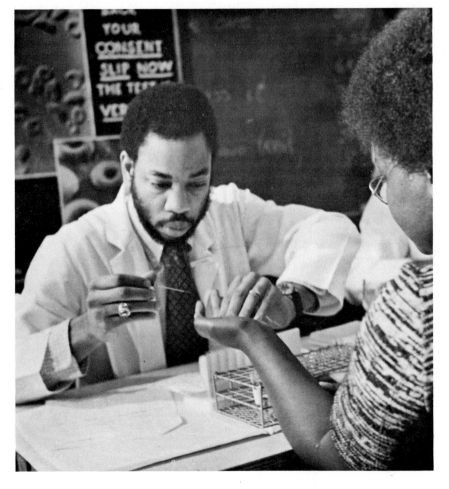

Fig. 2.3. Blood tests can show some genetic disorders. This woman is being tested to see if she carries the sickle-cell trait.

tissue damage and pain. To make matters worse, the spleen tends to destroy these cells more quickly than the body can manufacture them, thus creating an anemic condition.

Although sickle-cell anemia develops only under homozygotic conditions, even carriers may be affected at high altitudes or after extreme hemorrhaging.

Besides reduced oxygen-carrying capacity of blood cells (chronic anemia), victims of the sickle-cell disease suffer recurring bouts of pain called "crises," weakness and exhaustion, occasional growth retardation, increased susceptibility to certain infections, and a shortened life expectancy. Blood circulation to the liver, spleen, bones, kidneys, and brain is impaired by sickle cells that obstruct the small blood vessels, thus severely complicating treatment. In general, symptoms are not present at birth, but appear between the second and fourth years of life.

There is a distinctive racial distribution and prevalence associated with sickle-cell anemia.[1] The disorder affects blacks primarily, although it also occurs in "blacks passing as whites" and in persons of Mediterranean, Middle Eastern, and Near Eastern origin. These are people whose genotype is Negroid, but whose phenotype is tan or even white.

For anemia to develop, both parents must relay to the child a gene for producing abnormal hemoglobin. Usually both parents of such a child have what is known as the *sickle-cell trait,* an essentially benign carrier state without signs or symptoms. The patterns of *hereditary transmission* are as follows:

- If both parents have the sickle-cell trait, each child born to these parents has one chance in four of having sickle-cell anemia; one chance in two of only carrying the trait; and one chance in four of having neither the anemia nor the trait.
- If just one parent has the trait, none of the children will have sickle-cell anemia, but each child has one chance in two of carrying the trait.
- If one parent has sickle-cell anemia and the other has neither the disease nor the trait, all their children will carry the trait but not have anemia.
- If one parent has sickle-cell anemia and the other carries the trait, all of their children will have either the anemia or the trait.

The trait occurs in approximately one out of every ten blacks in the United States, or about two million individuals.[2] Individuals with the trait do not develop sickle-cell anemia and do not require special medical treatment themselves, except in unusual situations. Detection of the trait usually occurs when carriers parent a child with sickle-cell anemia. However, laboratory blood tests have been developed that now detect hemoglobin abnormalities in trait carriers. Genetic counseling or personalized education of carriers has proven controversial because of the implied need for birth control to eliminate hereditary sickle-cell anemia.[3]

Although there is no cure for sickle-cell anemia, it is effectively treated with pain-killing drugs, blood transfusions, proper nutrition and health care, bed rest, and protection against infection and other stresses that may precipitate the "crises" of this disease.

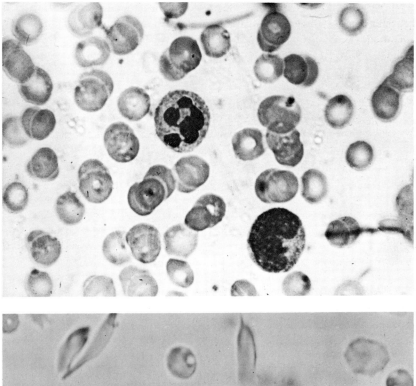

Fig. 2.4. Normal red blood cells are round, as seen in the top picture, but in sickle-cell anemia the affected red blood cells have a sickle shape that is typical of the disease, as shown in the bottom picture.

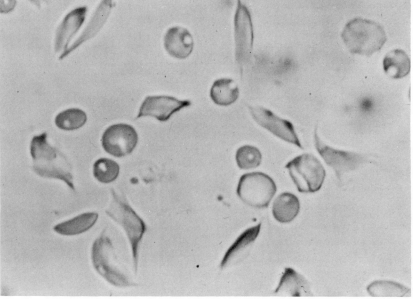

Another example of a disease caused by an inborn metabolic disorder is phenylketonuria (PKU), an inherited disability linked to mutant genes that prevent the production of a vital liver enzyme, or cause it to be produced in an inappropriate form. This progressive disease that causes severe mental retardation is a recessive disorder, occurring only when both parents transmit the abnormal gene.

Phenylketonuria

PKU victims lack phenylalanine hydroxylase, an enzyme normally produced in the liver. This enzyme is needed to convert phenylalanine (an essential amino acid) into tyrosine (another amino acid). When unconverted phenylalanine builds up in the blood and urine, so do levels of abnormal and characteristic degradation products, including phenylketone bodies. It is these bodies that cause all the damage.

If not detected and treated early, PKU can cause mental retardation. Children with PKU who are not put on special diets early in life accumulate dangerous quantities of phenylalanine and its chemical by-products in the blood. These harmful substances can cause permanent and irreversible brain damage.

PKU occurs in about 1 out of every 16,000 persons in the United States, with relatively high incidence among individuals of European origin. People of Negroid and Ashkenazi Jewish ancestry, however, have low PKU incidence rates.

Originally urine testing was used to screen infants six to eight weeks old for PKU. Presently, blood tests for PKU have been perfected for administration within a few days after birth. Most Canadian provinces and states in the U.S. have laws requiring such screening. If the condition is detected, special formulas and recipes are used to reduce phenylalanine intake as much as possible, while still providing enough protein and amino acids for normal growth and tissue repair. Such dietary management is usually maintained for an extended period of time, and it has proved to be quite successful in countering PKU.

Tay-Sachs Disease

Another enzyme deficiency disease that is caused by a recessive gene is Tay-Sachs disease. This condition is found almost exclusively among young Jewish children of Eastern European ancestry. Tay-Sachs disease impairs a child's physical development, usually after the sixth month of life. Mobility is affected, sight and speech do not develop normally, and the central nervous system is destroyed. Rarely will a child with this affliction live beyond the fifth year.

Since the gene responsible for Tay-Sachs is recessive, both parents must be carriers for an infant to be affected. One of every thirty Jews of Eastern European ancestry is a carrier; hence, the condition is rare, but of great enough concern to necessitate a blood test. If both parents are carriers, then genetic counseling becomes necessary.

Abnormalities in Chromosomal Number

Normally there are forty-six chromosomes in the human soma cell, or twenty-three pairs of chromosomes. Occasionally there are more, sometimes there are fewer. Generally unusual numbers of chromosomes reveal themselves in genetically linked diseases that are readily definable.

There are two phases in biological development when chromosomal disorders can occur naturally—during meiosis and mitosis. Such development is normally beneficial in terms of human welfare. In some instances it is restorative. There are times when chromosomal disorders may be negative and result in varying abnormalities.

Changes in chromosomal structure usually occur spontaneously, and are either externally induced (for example, by exposure to radiation) or internally developed (by *chromosomal breakage,* wherein DNA structure is upset and may be altered while mending, or by chromosomal exchange). *Translocation* occurs when a piece of one chromosome slides into another, noncorresponding chromosome. Also, on occasion, fragments simply break off, and become ''lost.''

Usually zygotes containing abnormal chromosomes die or are spontaneously aborted. Occasionally they survive, however, and the individual profits from, or more likely suffers, the consequences—consequences that may be passed on to future generations.

Occasionally during meiosis the chromosomes of a particular pair fail to separate, and one new cell receives both chromosomes, leaving the other deficient. This happenstance is called *meiotic nondisjunction;* it may occur in either the first or second division. Should the deficient germ cell (*gamete*) mate with a normal partner during fertilization, the zygote and all cells developed through its replication will have forty-five chromosomes instead of the customary forty-six. Conversely, should an overabundant gamete mate with a normal one, the resultant zygote would possess forty-seven chromosomes.

Fig. 2.5. Chromosomal translocation

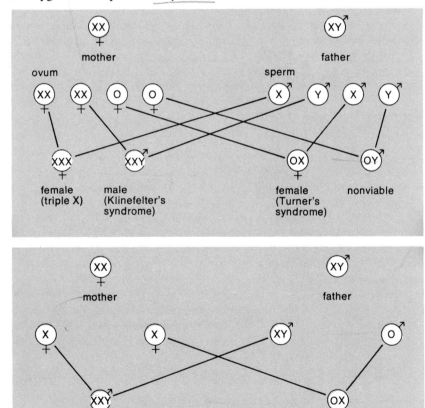

Fig. 2.6. When nondisjunction occurs in the mother, ova have either two X chromosomes or none at all.

Fig. 2.7. When nondisjunction occurs in the father, sperm have either both X and Y sex chromosomes or none at all.

A triple zygotic chromosome produced by an overabundant gamete is appropriately labeled *trisomic*, and a single zygotic chromosome out of a deficient gamete is called *monosomic*. Both factors can occur in autosomal and/or sex chromosomes; the results are interesting.

The most common trisomic autosomal abnormality is found in the twenty-first chromosome; it is one cause of Down's syndrome (commonly referred to as mongolism). Such individuals are characterized by physical and mental retardation, poor muscle development, an enlarged tongue, slanted eyes, and a flattened forehead. Mongoloid children are far more common from pregnancies in older women. The chances of producing a mongoloid child appear to increase with maternal age, after thirty. The risk is about 1 in 800 for new mothers ages 35 to 39, about 1 in 100 for new mothers 40 to 44, and about 1 in 40 for those over 44. Over one half of all mongoloid children are born to women over thirty-five.[4]

Nondisjunction of the sex chromosomes results in four major types of chromosomal abnormality, regardless of which parent contributes the aberrant cell. The types are XXY, OY, XXX, and OX.

In males, Klinefelter's syndrome (abnormally small testes, no mature sperm) is associated with an XXY sex-chromosome set. The Klinefelter male is usually sterile, and though often normal looking, is frequently mentally retarded.

Complete absence of an X chromosome in the male (OY) always results in death of the zygote.

Cases of XXX as occuring in the "super" female are rare and usually cause this female to be incapable of normal functioning.

OX chromosomal types are quite viable, an interesting fact for those prone to debate which is the stronger sex! An OX zygote can develop into an individual who has *Turner's syndrome*. This is a disorder in which the child develops as a female but never menstruates and never develops any secondary sexual characteristics, such as breasts and hips. The Turner's girl does not grow to normal height, often exhibits deformities of the arms, and has a webbed neck.

As noted, in all of the above cases the victim is usually sterile, and as a consequence the hereditary transmission of disorders is unlikely.

The XYY Controversy

When Richard Speck, the 1966 murderer of eight Chicago nurses, was found to have an abnormal number of sex chromosomes (XYY), interest in the behavior of such individuals increased. The incidence of XYY is relatively low, and roughly the same as XXY (Klinefelter's syndrome), but the presumed association with violence has led to some rather hasty and emotion-laden conclusions. Whereas prisoners do exhibit a slightly higher incidence of both XXY and XYY abnormalities than the normal population (.20 percent to .13 percent), still members of the "normal" population also exhibit both traits. XYY is not automatically associated with violence; the majority of violent crimes are committed by chromosomally normal persons. However, the increased frequency of XYY individuals among perpetrators of crimes does suggest that an extra Y chromosome may predispose the individual toward aggressive behavior. Such predisposition has proven insufficient before the law as grounds for exoneration from any particular crime committed in North America (it did provide a successful defense in

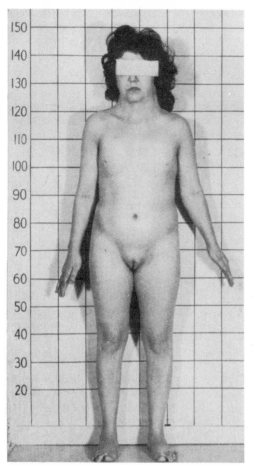

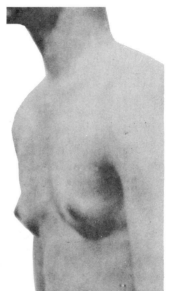

Fig. 2.8. Sexual infantalism, webbed neck, and short stature are typical features of Turner's syndrome in this 22-year-old woman.
(From M. Bartalos and T. A. Baramki, *Medical cytogenetics*, 1967. The Williams & Wilkins Co.)

Fig. 2.9. Enlarged breasts in males are one symptom of Klinefelter's syndrome. The man at left is one of the original cases described in 1942 by Dr. Henry Klinefelter. (From M. Bartalos and T. A. Baramki, *Medical cytogenetics*, 1967. The Williams & Wilkins Co.)

an Australian court), but the finding has led to interesting speculation. How closely is the Y chromosome linked to aggressiveness? Is it the Y chromosome that gives males a more aggressive nature than females? Innovations in detection techniques, such as fluorescent staining, have made mass testing for sex chromosomes more feasible and should provide more accurate data soon. In short, the XYY sex-chromosome set appears to contribute little more than a slightly heightened tendency toward aggression. Certainly, it is not a legitimate excuse for violence.

Sex-Linked Genes

Some genes are carried only on the X chromosome. A female receives one X chromosome from her mother and one from her father. Since it is unlikely that both Xs would ever contain the same recessive gene, the female is relatively safe from X-linked diseases. A male receives one X chromosome from his mother and a Y from his father. If the X chromosome contains a recessive allele, it will act as a dominant trait, and the son will be affected.

Table 2.2 Selected Birth Defects, U.S.A.

Birth Defect	Type	Annual Incidence*	Prevalence†	Cause	Detection‡	Treatment‡	Prevention‡
Down's syndrome (mongolism)	functional/structural: retardation often associated with physical defects	5,100	44,000	chromosomal abnormality	chromosome analysis, amniocentesis	corrective surgery, special physical training and schooling	genetics services
Low birthweight/prematurity	structural/functional	248,000	NA	hereditary and/or environmental: poor prenatal care, maternal disorder	prenatal monitoring, visual inspection at birth	intensive care of newborn, high nutrient diet	proper prenatal care, genetics services
Muscular dystrophy	functional: impaired voluntary muscular function	unknown (late-appearing)	200,000	hereditary: often recessive inheritance	apparent at onset	physical therapy	carrier identification, genetics services
Congenital heart malformations	structural	24,800	248,000	hereditary and/or environmental	examination at birth and later	corrective surgery, medication	proper prenatal care, genetics services
Clubfoot	structural: misshapen foot	9,300	149,000	hereditary and/or environmental	examination at birth	corrective surgery, corrective splints, physical training	genetics services
Polydactyly	structural: multiple fingers or toes	9,300	184,000	hereditary: dominant inheritance	visual inspection at birth	corrective surgery, physical training	genetics services
Spina bifida and/or hydrocephalus	structural/functional: incompletely formed spinal canal; "water on the brain"	6,200	53,000	hereditary and environmental	prenatal X ray, ultrasound, maternal blood test, examination at birth	corrective surgery, prostheses, physical training, special schooling for any mental impairment	genetics services
Cleft lip and/or cleft palate	structural	4,300	71,000	hereditary and/or environmental	visual inspection at birth	corrective surgery	genetics services
Diabetes mellitus	metabolic: inability to metabolize carbohydrates	unknown (late-appearing)	90,000	hereditary and/or environmental	appears in childhood or later; blood and urine tests	oral medication, special diet, insulin injections	genetics services
Cystic fibrosis	functional: respiratory and digestive system malfunction	2,000	10,000	hereditary: recessive inheritance	sweat and blood tests	treat respiratory and digestive complications	carrier identification, genetics services

*Incidence: the number of new cases diagnosed within a specific time period. Above statistics based on 1971 data.

†Prevalence: total number living who have been diagnosed as having defect. Above statistics based on number less than 20 years of age.

‡Last three columns list possible means now known for detection, treatment, and prevention. The techniques may not necessarily be applicable or successful in every case.

Birth Defect	Type	Annual Incidence*	Prev- alence†	Cause	Detection‡	Treatment‡	Prevention‡
Sickle-cell anemia	blood disease: malformed red blood cells	1,200	16,000	hereditary: incomplete dominance—most frequent among Blacks	blood test	medication, transfusions	genetics services
Hemophilia (classic)	blood disease: poor clotting ability	1,200	12,400	hereditary: sex-linked recessive inheritance	blood test	medication, transfusions	genetics services
Congenital syphilis	structural: multiple abnormalities	(newborn only) 313	NA	environmental: acquired from infected mother	blood test, examination at birth	medication	proper prenatal care
Phenyl-ketonuria (PKU)	metabolic: inability to metabolize a specific protein	310	3,100	herditary: recessive inheritance	blood test at birth	special diet	carrier identification, genetics services
Tay-Sachs disease	metabolic: inability to metabolize fats in nervous system	30	100	hereditary: recessive inheritance—most frequent among Ashkenazi Jews	blood and tear tests, amniocentesis	none	carrier identification, genetics services
Thalas-semia	blood disease: anemia	70	1,000	hereditary: incomplete dominant inheritance	blood test	transfusions	carrier identification, genetics services
Galacto-semia	metabolic: inability to metabolize milk sugar galactose	70	500	hereditary: recessive inheritance	blood and urine tests, amniocentesis	special diet	carrier identification, genetics services
Erythro-blastosis (Rh disease)	blood disease: destruction of red blood cells	2,600	NA	hereditary and environmental: Rh— mother has Rh+ child	blood tests	transfusion: intrauterine or postnatal	Rh vaccine, blood tests to identify parents at risk, genetics services
Turner syndrome	structural/ functional	575	3,100	chromosomal abnormality	chromosome analysis, amniocentesis	corrective surgery, medication	genetics services
Congenital rubella syndrome	structural/ functional: multiple defects	varies with occur- rence of disease; less than 50	NA	environmental: maternal infection	antibody tests and viral culture	corrective surgery, prostheses, physical therapy and training	rubella vaccine, good prenatal care

* Incidence: the number of new cases diagnosed within a specific time period. Above statistics based on 1971 data.

† Prevalence: total number living who have been diagnosed as having defect. Above statistics based on number less than 20 years of age.

‡ Last three columns list possible means now known for detection, treatment, and prevention. The techniques may not necessarily be applicable or successful in every case.

The Foundation's experts estimate that among Americans of all ages, birth defects afflict 2.9 million mentally retarded; 4 million with diabetes; 1 million with congenital bone, muscle, or joint disease; 500,000 born completely or partially blind; 750,000 with congenital hearing impairment; 350,000 with heart or circulatory defects; 100,000 with severe speech problems; millions of others with defects of the nervous, digestive, endocrine, urinary, and other body systems. Courtesy The National Foundation/March of Dimes, 1975

Genetics: The Science of Involuntary Adaptation

59

Sex-linked diseases are relatively common, and much more frequent in males. Hemophilia, the "bleeding" disorder caused by the lack of essential blood-clotting components in the blood, can be traced back for centuries. The family of Queen Victoria is perhaps the most famous example. Since a mother with hemophilia must be homozygous, she passes the trait on to all of her children. Her sons will all have the disease. Her daughters may be saved by the father's normal X, but all will be carriers.

Other sex-linked genes are responsible for red-green color blindness, myopia, juvenile dystrophy, and at least twenty-five other known diseases. All are carried only on the X chromosome, and all are far more prevalent in males than females.

"Dominance" in genetic traits is a value-free term. Some dominant traits are considered beneficial—the normal allotment of hair in the female, normal vision, freedom from hemophilia; some are harmful—webbed fingers, dwarfism, migraine headaches; and still others are neutral—brown eyes, dark hair, the Rh factor. By that same logic, some recessive traits are beneficial (five fingers on each hand, normal blood pressure, attached ear lobes), some are of questionable benefit (baldness in females, straight hair), and others are definitely harmful (congenital deafness, diabetes mellitus, hemophilia). The critical step for us is to identify the traits, genetically map them, and develop techniques to correct the undesirable ones. Does this seem impossible? To many, it may seem to be beyond comprehension; yet many outstanding feats have been accomplished by mankind in genetics, as well as in the whole field of science, and genetic alterations may become commonplace one day.

Genetic Counseling

Science is continually learning more about human genetics. Much of this knowledge may be useful to couples who are planning families. As a means of interpreting medical information about genetics and thereby preventing birth defects, *genetic counseling* has become increasingly common.

Genetic counseling can be of help to any couple. However, it should be particularly useful to couples who already have a child with a birth defect. Often these parents are confused and bitter. Genetic counseling can help them understand the factors related to birth defects, and, in cases of families with histories of abnormalities, can help them make important decisions in their family planning.

In addition to helping individuals understand the probabilities of genetic defects, genetic counseling identifies carriers of potentially harmful traits. For example, rather simple blood tests can be used to identify carriers of the traits for Tay-Sachs disease and sickle-cell anemia. If one or both parents are carriers of a trait, genetic counseling helps the couple decide whether to have a baby or not.

When a woman becomes pregnant and certain genetic defects are suspected, amniocentesis is performed. Much can be learned about the developing fetus from the amniotic fluid. Not all birth defects can be identified through amniocentesis; however, it is extremely useful in detecting defects resulting from chromosome error.

Genetic counseling helps couples decide whether to have a child or to continue a pregnancy and teaches them what to expect if a baby is born with a defect.

We have examined the basic concepts of inheritance and the interplay of heredity and environment in shaping the ultimate product of conception. We have examined some disorders of chromosome structure, and considered both sickle-cell anemia and phenylketonuria in some detail. Disorders of chromosome number have been examined, and particular attention was accorded the XYY phenomenon. What does all this mean? How far can we go in manipulating our genes? Do we want a *Brave New World* society of identical beings? Is total genetic equality within the population a desirable end? Do we have a right to tamper with such fundamental genetic differences? At what point do we stop tampering? The questions are clear; the answers easy! Yet research continues. How long will it be before we create a "monster" that we cannot control? How long will genetic concerns play on the emotions of prospective parents?

Review Questions

1. Name and describe the two types of cells found in the body.
2. In what ways can the environment affect a child before birth? after birth?
3. Differentiate between meiosis and mitosis. What genetic problems result when these processes are incomplete? *chromosomal abnormalities*
4. Which do you believe has the greater effect upon an individual, heredity or environment? Explain your answer.
5. What is sickle-cell anemia? How does it affect the body?
6. Describe the metabolic disorders of PKU and sickle-cell anemia.
7. Describe the effects of meiotic nondisjunction on individuals. How are these effects outwardly manifested?
8. What role can genetic counseling play in a couple's family planning?

Readings

Bartalos, M., and Baramki, T. A. *Medical Cytogenetics*. Baltimore: The Williams & Wilkins Co., 1967.
Hook, E. B. "Behavioral Implications of the Human XYY Genotype," *Science* 179 (1973): 139–50.

Notes

1. U.S. Department of Health, Education, and Welfare, *Sickle Cell Anemia* (Washington, D.C.: U.S. Government Printing Office, 1972), p. 2.
2. National Heart and Lung Institute, *Sickle Cell Disease* (Washington, D.C.: The Institute, 1973), p. 1.
3. C. Pochedly et al., "Sickle-Cell Trait: A New Medical and Social Dilemma," *Journal of the American College Health Association* 21 (April 1973): 276–77.
4. Benjamin, A. Kogan, *Human Sexual Expression* (New York: Harcourt Brace Jovanovich, Inc., 1973), p. 188.

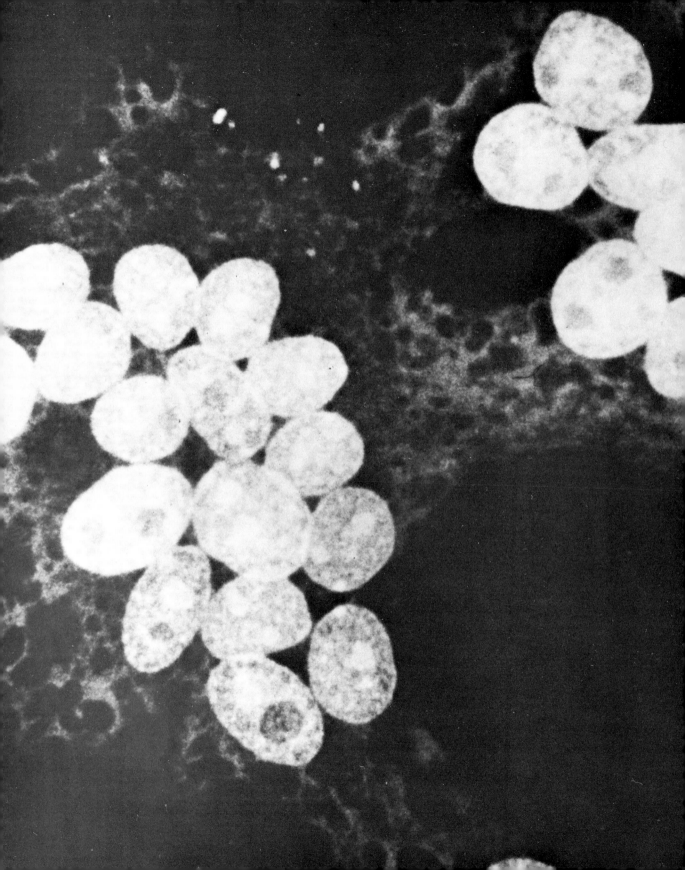

Communicable Diseases: From Host to Host

3

Throughout the life cycle, a human must cope with many diseases that can spread from one person to another. The agents of disease pose a continual threat to the well-being of each individual before birth and until the termination of life. Disease-causing organisms that invade a human host can cause an unfavorable adaptation or maladaptation in that person—a response known as disease.

Since many such maladaptations occur first in infancy and childhood, it seems reasonable to present our discussion of communicable diseases at this point as we consider health status in the life cycle. It should be remembered, however, that increasing age is no guarantee of freedom from the diseases to be discussed here. Adults can and do contract the so-called children's diseases, and children are quite susceptible to what many people formerly called adult diseases.

Communicable diseases might be called the "ho-hum" illnesses of modern society. They rarely excite the general population, which largely accepts the common cold and flu as inevitable. Seldom are such diseases dramatized as much more than bothersome ailments of childhood or the expected consequences of impoverishment confined to some distant underdeveloped or war-torn nation.

Unfortunately, we have a long way to go in health science before the eradication of communicable diseases becomes a reality. The threat of diseases that can be spread from person to person still persists even in America and in Western Europe where disease control measures have been developed and used for many years. During the early 1970s epidemics of diphtheria occurred in Florida, Arizona, and Texas. A measles outbreak erupted on the Texas-Arkansas border. German measles afflicted college students in North Dakota, while polio crippled schoolboys in Connecticut.[1] A disaster of major proportions also struck in southern Italy when cholera caused great suffering, took a heavy toll of human life, and snuffed out a thriving tourist business. In parts of India smallpox continued in epidemic proportions until the mid-1970s. Although smallpox transmission has been interrupted since 1977 and many nations have been certified smallpox-free, an isolated case of laboratory-acquired smallpox was reported in England during 1978.

Recently, the United States has witnessed an outbreak of so-called Legionnaires' disease, a sometimes fatal ailment that attracted worldwide notice during a 1976 American Legion convention in Philadelphia. Resembling pneumonia, the disease appears to be caused by an organism that infects groups in close quarters, such as persons attending conventions or confined to hospitals.[2] Fortunately, the disease is hard to catch, as the causative microbe is not

A group of living cells being invaded by measles, causing the nuclei to cluster together and the cytoplasm to fuse.

easily transmitted in the general population. Nevertheless, sporadic cases of Legionnaires' disease have occurred in at least twenty-seven states since 1976,[3] including Bloomington, Indiana, and New York City, with a fatality rate sometimes approaching 25 percent.

The cost of communicable diseases to human health generally is expressed in temporary pain and discomfort, feeling below par, personal inefficiency, doctor and drug bills, time off from job or school, missed social or employment opportunities, and sometimes even dropping out of college. While not usually fatal to the young adult, these illnesses can and do interfere with reaching the immediate and often the future goals of life. If you have any doubts, just ask a friend who has had mono, the flu, or viral hepatitis.

Microorganisms in the Environment

Tiny living agents or materials that are not visible to the naked eye abound in our environment. These agents are referred to as *microorganisms* or *microbes*. Some of these microorganisms live on the surface of the human body. Others normally reside in various parts of the body, such as the digestive tract, and are necessary for the maintenance of health. As long as a state of "biological coexistence" is maintained, the microbes thrive in and on the *human host* that provides subsistence or lodging. In turn, the microbes cause no harm.

Pathogens: Agents of Disease

Microorganisms that can harm or injure the human host in some way are called *pathogens*, disease-causing agents. Popularly known as germs, pathogens can invade the deeper tissues of the human host where they produce a body reaction manifest as disease. This invasive capability of microbes is known as infection. When the human host is infected by a pathogenic agent, the resulting disease is described as an infectious one.

Some pathogens normally live in the soil and infect the human host through a wound or break in the skin. Others can be transmitted from one person to another or from an infected animal to a human host. These latter microbes produce a host reaction known as a *communicable disease*, ". . . one whose causative agent is directly or indirectly transmitted from host to host."[4] The term *contagious* is often used to describe a disease that can spread easily from person to person. Although we say that we have "caught a cold," in reality we have caught the pathogens that produce in our bodies the host reaction known as a cold.

Not all microorganisms cause diseases in humans. Widely distributed in nature, some of them actively promote life activities of plants and animals. Others have the capability of causing a characteristic referred to as pathogenicity.

Among the major groups of pathogens are the following: bacteria, viruses, fungi, protozoa, rickettsiae, and metazoa.

Bacteria

Extremely small, single-cell microorganisms, *bacteria*, are one of the lowest forms of plant life. They can be seen only with a microscope. Although there are more than 1,500 known species, only about 100 are pathogenic in humans. Bacteria are able to utilize food materials in soluble form only because they have a

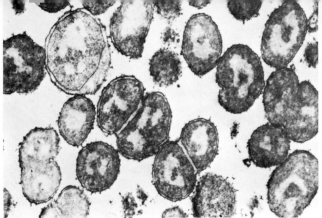
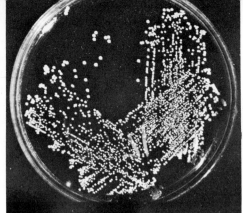

Fig. 3.1. (Left) *Neisseria gonorrhoeae*, the cause of gonorrhea, and (right) *Staphylococcus*, the cause of such pus-producing infections as boils and acne, are spherical bacteria.

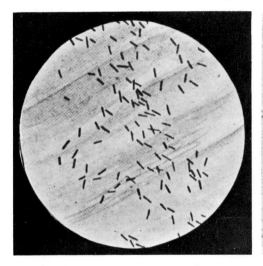
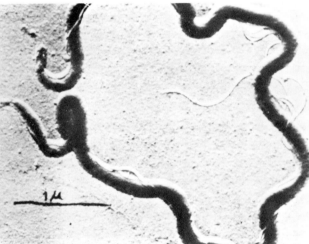

Fig. 3.2. Rod-shaped *Escherichia coli* bacteria are one cause of epidemic diarrheal disease.

Fig. 3.3. The spiral bacteria *Treponema pallidum* causes syphilis.

rigid cell wall. They occur in three basic shapes: spherical (coccus), rod-shaped (bacillus), and spiral-shaped. Among bacteria-caused diseases are tuberculosis, syphilis, gonorrhea, diphtheria, and strep throat.

The smallest of all pathogens, *viruses*, can be seen only with an electron microscope. Each virus particle contains a central core of nucleic acid surrounded by a protein coat. Because they neither respond to stimuli nor carry on typical chemical functions of cells, they are not considered living entities.[5] Yet, within living

Viruses

cells, viruses reproduce themselves. Since they must rely on other living organisms to complete their life cycles, they are termed *obligate intracellular parasites*. Virus-caused diseases include the common cold, influenza, polio, smallpox, measles, chicken pox, and rabies.

Fungi

Fungi include the plantlike organisms known as molds and yeasts. They vary in size from microscopic single-cell entities to large, multicellular, easily visible mushrooms and toadstools. Fungi contain no chlorophyll as do other plants and must function as *parasites*—living on, in, or at the expense of another viable organism—or sustain themselves on the dead remains of organic material. Fungal infections (mycoses) result in two basic types of disease: (1) superficial skin diseases, such as ringworm and so-called athlete's foot, and (2) systemic infections of the respiratory and intestinal tracts. A fungus infection of the lungs, *histoplasmosis*, is a systemic disease especially prevalent in the central Mississippi Valley and in the Ohio Valley in the United States.

Protozoa

The simplest of animal forms, *protozoa*, are mostly microscopic in size and usually occur as single cells. Classified as to their means of locomotion, the protozoans include amebas, ciliates, flagellates, and sporozoans. Some of these are parasitic and pathogenic in humans and cause such disorders as amebic dysentery, malaria, African sleeping sickness, and trichomoniasis (a common nonfatal chronic disease of the urogenital tract manifest in women by vaginitis and a foul-smelling yellowish discharge). In men this fungus disease rarely produces symptoms.

Rickettsiae

Very small microorganisms that resemble both bacteria and viruses are called *rickettsiae*. They are obligate intracellular parasites and are with few exceptions transmitted to humans through the bite of fleas, lice, mites, and ticks. Among diseases caused by rickettsiae are Rocky Mountain spotted fever, typhus fever, scrub typhus, Q fever, and rickettsialpox.

Metazoa

Other pathogenic agents include the *metazoa*, or multicellular animal organisms, that can infect human beings. Among these are the beef tapeworm, the pork tapeworm, and the larva of intestinal roundworms. Because of their relatively large size and visibility, they are not considered microorganisms. Usually these pathogens gain entry to the host when food or fluids containing them are consumed.

Chain of Infection

A communicable disease is spread by the escape of a pathogen from its *host reservoir* (any human, animal, plant, or inanimate matter in which an infectious agent normally lives and multiplies) and its entrance into another susceptible person, the *new host*.[6] Pathogens leave the body through definite routes of discharge called *portals of exit*. These include discharges from the mouth, nose, and throat, sneezing and coughing, fecal wastes, possibly urine, saliva, blood, mucous membranes, open wounds, sores, and insect bites.

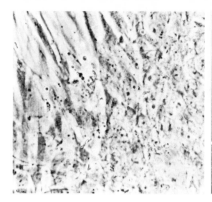

Fig. 3.4. The virus *Briarcus varicellae* causes chicken pox. These connective cells are infected with varicella.

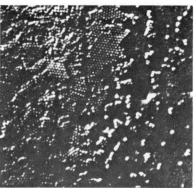

Fig. 3.5. The Coxsackie virus causes acute aseptic meningitis.

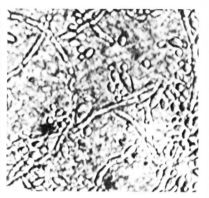

Fig. 3.6. This is a *Candida albicans* fungal infection in a skin scraping. *Candida* also affects mucous membranes, nails, mouth, vaginal tract, bronchi, and lungs.

Fig. 3.8. The protozoan *Plasmodium vivax* causes benign tertian malaria (attacks occur every other day). Malaria is transmitted from man to man by infected mosquitos, and this particular type is found in temperate areas of the world.

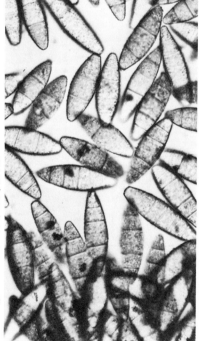

Fig. 3.7. *Trichophyton gallinae*, one of five groups of *Trichophyton* fungi, is responsible for infections commonly called ringworm.

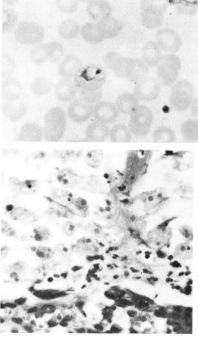

Fig. 3.9. The intestinal *Entamoeba histolytica* protozoan causes amebic dysentery.

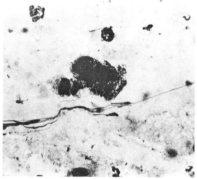

Fig. 3.10. *Rickettsia mooseri* causes endemic typhus. It is transmitted to man from rats via fleas and is common along seacoasts.

Once removed from its host reservoir, the pathogen must be able to survive in an unfavorable environment until the agent infects a new host. The survival rate is influenced largely by the method of pathogen transmission from host to host. There are several methods of transmission.

Transmission Methods

Direct Contact   This may be through contact with skin or mucous membrane by kissing or sexual intercourse; through droplet infection in the fine spray of a cough or sneeze; or through blood transfusions.

Indirect Contact   These contacts can be made by drinking milk or water, or eating food, or using toys, towels, bedding, or hypodermic needles that have been contaminated with pathogenic microorganisms from the host reservoir.

Airborne Transfer   Pathogens are carried in the evaporated residue of human discharges and in dust arising from contaminated bedding or from the soil.

Vector Transfer   Crawling and flying insects, particularly the house fly, carry the pathogens on their feet or other body parts, or impart an infection by biting first the sick reservoir and then a new host.

In addition to a favored portal of exit, each species of pathogenic microorganism has a preferred invasion route termed a *portal of entry*. Among portals of entry are the skin (usually broken by injury or bite), mucous membrane lining body openings, the nose, mouth, urogenital system, and the placenta.[7]

Thus, the *chain of infection* consists of the following "links":

the *pathogen*
  in a *human reservoir*,
    escape of pathogen via *portal of exit*
      into an *environment*,
        transmission to a new host,
          invasion of host via *portal of entry*,
            establishment of disease in *new host*.

Control of any communicable disease is based upon breaking any one or more of the links in this chain of infection.

Fig. 3.11. The chain of infection

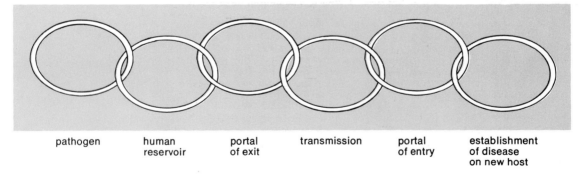

pathogen   human reservoir   portal of exit   transmission   portal of entry   establishment of disease on new host

Upon the entry of pathogens into a new host, two opposing forces come into play:

1. The microorganisms attempt to set up residence in the deeper body tissues and become parasites, living at the expense of the host; and
2. The host strives to defend itself through a series of biochemical adaptations to stop the invasion and destroy the pathogens.

"If the body wins the contest, the microbes are destroyed and the body suffers no ill effects. If the microbes win, infection occurs."[8] This process of interaction between host and parasite is typical of infectious diseases.

As the infection progresses, the pathogens begin to multiply and eventually cause harm or injury by adversely affecting normal structure or function in the host. Pathogens display their capacity to cause disease by damaging or destroying host cells, by producing a mechanical blockage of blood vessels, by releasing poisonous chemicals (toxins) that travel to all parts of the body through the bloodstream, or by interfering with normal reproduction of host cells.

How pathogens succeed

Most host-parasite interactions follow a pattern or course of progression marked by the specific stages described below:

Incubation Stage   The period between initial infection and the appearance of particular signs and symptoms characteristic of disease is called the *incubation stage*.

Prodromal Stage   This is the short interval that often follows the incubation period. This stage is marked by nonspecific complaints (symptoms) of fever, headache, malaise, general aches and pains, and that "feeling of impending illness" that most people experience just before signs and symptoms of a specific disease occur. During this stage the disease is already contagious.

Acme Stage   The period during which specific outcomes of any particular disease (the observable signs and symptoms of complaint) reach their highest peak or intensity is the *acme stage*. Communicability of the disease-causing organisms is most probable during this period of typical illness. Depending upon the defensive powers of the host, this stage is followed by recovery or death.

Convalescence Stage   The period during which the evidence of disease subsides, and the host regains normal functioning unless permanent damage has been sustained is called the *convalescence stage*. The disease may still be contagious during this stage. The defensive powers of the host, often with the assistance of drug therapy, eventually win out over the infecting pathogens. Sometimes after recovery, the host may still be a reservoir of pathogens although signs and symptoms of discharge are not apparent. Such a host is described as a *carrier* of the disease.

Communicable diseases also display various patterns of incidence within the larger community. When an occasional case of a particular disease occurs, the disease is referred to as a *sporadic disease*. The constant presence of a particular communicable disease to a lesser or greater degree in any given population is termed *endemic*. A sudden increase in the prevalence of a disease constitutes an *epidemic*, and when a disease becomes epidemic in many countries at the same time, the situation is referred to as a *pandemic*.[9]

In Self-Defense

If the human host were not so well equipped to survive the onslaught of pathogens, the death rate due to communicable diseases would eliminate the need to keep statistics on most other illnesses. Fortunately, constitutional and environmental factors can assist humans in defending themselves against infectious microorganisms. The defensive adaptations collectively known as *general resistance* to disease are defined as:

> the sum total of body mechanisms which interpose barriers to the progress of invasion or multiplication of infectious agents, or to damage by their toxic products.[10]

Constitutional and Environmental Factors

Constitutional factors of age, sex, hormones, and genetic predisposition apparently influence the host's response to infection.[11] The young typically survive the common childhood diseases, such as mumps, measles, and chicken pox, with much less disturbance than do adults. Gonorrhea, though still extremely damaging in females, seems to cause a more severe initial reaction in males. Estrogen (a female sex hormone) renders the vaginal lining more resistant to bacterial invasion, while testosterone sensitizes the male testes to the mumps virus. Human resistance to diseases, such as malaria and tuberculosis, may be genetically determined through natural selection.

The environment frequently determines the spread of infection by affectioning both host and parasite. Have you noticed that influenza epidemics tend to occur more often in autumn, winter, and early spring? Changes in humidity and temperature have some impact on the daily life activities of the host, the state of the respiratory system, and the survival of the pathogen prior to infection. The standard of personal health activities, including nutrition, rest, and relaxation, is related to the general resistance of the host. Both the external environment and the host's internal environment are important factors in determining whether a disease develops. While infectious, pathogenic agents are necessary causes of communicable disease, their presence within a host is not a sufficient cause of disease. Consequently,

> in order for infection to progress into disease, the parasite must be capable of damaging the host; the environment must be suitable; and finally the host must be susceptible to the damage inflicted.[12]

The evolution of an infection into a host-parasite interaction is now viewed as a progressive failure of various body defense mechanisms. As long as structural, cellular, and chemical defenses are functioning and are not overwhelmed, health status is maintained.

Structural Defenses Included in structural defenses are unbroken skin, the "first line of body defense," that presents an effective barrier to the invasion of many pathogens; nasal hairs that filter incoming bacteria from inspired air; and tiny, hairlike cilia that line the respiratory passageways and sweep up from the deeper portions of the respiratory system airborne debris that has been entrapped by mucus.

Cellular Defenses Cells provide additional protective mechanisms. They show true adaptive responses to the presence of pathogenic agents within the host. Shortly after infecting pathogens injure host cells, the local inflammatory reaction begins. Characterized by swelling, redness, fever, and pain, this adaptation to cell damage is beneficial as it concentrates a number of dissolved chemical substances in the blood at the damage site. These substances kill some pathogens, prevent the growth of others, and make certain ones more susceptible to attack by white blood cells. Inflammation also works to wall off the infected area with specialized host cells and other chemicals that will function later in scar formation and healing. Fever itself speeds up the destruction of some pathogens by increasing the action of white blood cells. Known as *phagocytes*, these white blood cells engulf and destroy individual pathogens. Such cellular activity is termed *phagocytosis*, an important protection against bacterial invaders. Increased blood and lymph flow of the inflammatory reaction also dilutes and flushes away toxic substances.

Chemical Defenses Several substances that tend to combat infectious microorganisms are involved in the chemical defenses of the host. Among these are body fluids, such as saliva, tears, gastric juice, bile, perspiration, and the sebaceous secretions on the skin, all of which have a general, nonspecific antimicrobial action. One chemical, *lysozyme*, found in tears and mucus, is particularly effective in dissolving the cell walls of certain bacteria. *Interferon*, a protein, also functions as an antiviral defense. It interferes with virus reproduction, thus blocking viral infection of additional host cells.

However, the only chemical defense that can be influenced significantly by human intervention—and thus contribute to human adaptation in an environment of pathogens—is the formation of a protein called *antibody*. Unlike all the other structural, cellular, and chemical nonspecific defense mechanisms, these blood serum protein molecules, known as *antibodies*, confer specific resistance to specific infection agents and provide the basis for the concept of immunity to disease.

In general, the term *immunity* is described as host resistance to specific diseases. As an adaptive response, immunity helps the human host to maintain ". . . structural and functional integrity and to ward off certain kinds of injury."[13] Furthermore, the infecting pathogenic microorganisms evoke this adaptive response that, if successful, will function to inactivate or kill the foreign invaders.

Immunity

Pathogenic microorganisms function as antigens in the human host, i.e., the infecting agents when introduced into the body stimulate certain host tissues to produce antibodies. *Antigens*, therefore, *are antibody generators*. After antibodies are formed from a type of blood protein, they act as chemical defenders of the host and react with the foreign antigens (pathogens) in some demonstrable way. The formation of antibodies in response to antigens is termed the *antigen-antibody reaction*. Moreover, this reaction is highly specific. Invading polio viruses acting as antigens evoke antibodies that will combat the polio antigens only. Polio antibody will not have any effect on the diphtheria antigen.

Chemically, antibodies react with antigens in a variety of ways: Antibodies (1) neutralize antigens, thus rendering them noninfective; (2) immobilize motile microorganisms and aggregate (clump) them for phagocytic action; (3) dissolve antigen cell walls; (4) combine with microbes so as to enhance the likelihood of phagocytosis; and (5) kill certain pathogenic agents.[14]

If the production of antibodies—as detected by laboratory procedures— is the only host response to infection and no recognizable clinical signs or symptoms of disease appear, the condition is often referred to as *inapparent disease*. Inapparent disease is a subclinical response to infection.

The basic antigen-antibody reaction is operable in at least two other instances: (1) the development of *Rh disease* in a fetus or newborn infant possessing the Rh blood factor, the mother being Rh−, or without the Rh factor; and (2) the success or failure of *organ transplantation*. Too often, the host rejects a donor's organ because it is biochemically perceived as a foreign invader threatening the host's self-identity and integrity.

Immunization

The development of immunity (immunization) can be achieved in several ways.

Natural Acquired Immunity   This immunity may be conferred: (1) *Actively*, by sustaining an actual disease and developing antibodies against the infecting agent during recovery or as the result of inapparent disease, or (2) *Passively*, by the transfer of preformed antibodies across the placenta from immune mother to fetus or via the mother's colostrum to her breast-fed infant.

Artificial Acquired Immunity   This immunity may be developed: (1) *Actively*, by the administration of a suitable *vaccine* or *toxoid* that stimulates host production of its own antibodies. "Active immunity develops over a period of days or weeks but tends to persist, usually for years."[15] Once formed, antibody production can be renewed and increased upon subsequent reinfection or ". . . may be maintained through the repeated use of doses of antigens given at properly spaced intervals."[16] Both vaccines and toxoids are used to develop artificial, acquired active immunity. *Vaccines* are preparations of weakened or killed pathogens that can stimulate antibody formation without causing observable signs and symptoms of disease. *Toxoids* are preparations of altered, yet antigenically active, bacterial poisons or toxins that do not cause signs or symptoms of disease. Or (2) *Passively*, by the reception of preformed antibodies in a preparation derived from the blood serum of immune human beings or animals. Passive immunity confers temporary resistance for a duration of a few weeks or months at most. Because antibodies are being broken down constantly and no antigen-antibody reaction has ever occurred as in active immunity, passive immunization is "... used to provide immediate protection in cases of known exposure to infection or during epidemics."[17]

Immunization for many specific diseases is available: smallpox, mumps, typhoid fever, tuberculosis, typhus, yellow fever, rabies, cholera, and the plague. Recently, pharmaceutical research has developed a vaccine that offers protection against pneumococcal pneumonia and a more effective rabies vaccine that has fewer side effects than the type presently used. However, in America, only the following immunizations are routinely recommended for infants and preschool children: diphtheria, tetanus (lockjaw), pertussis (whooping cough), poliomyelitis (polio), measles, mumps, and German measles (rubella). Once established, immunization to these and other diseases throughout the life cycle should be maintained according to the schedule recommended by the American Medical Association (see table 3.1).

Obviously, immunizations are effective only if they are used, and only if anti-body levels are maintained. Unfortunately, immunity to the common diseases listed in table 3.1 has dropped recently to dangerously low levels. Current esti-mates indicate that only 65 percent of young children have received recom-mended inoculations, leaving one in three preschoolers without protection. Con-sequently, "... these preventable diseases continue to afflict more than 100,000 children each year, killing some and leaving many more permanently disabled."[18] Thus, epidemics are likely to occur in unprotected populations and lead to loss of life, suffering, mental crippling, and decreased years of productivity, as well as unnecessary physician visits, hospitalizations, and absences from school.

Fig. 3.12. Infants and preschool children may be immunized against many specific diseases, such as mumps, measles, polio, and diphtheria.

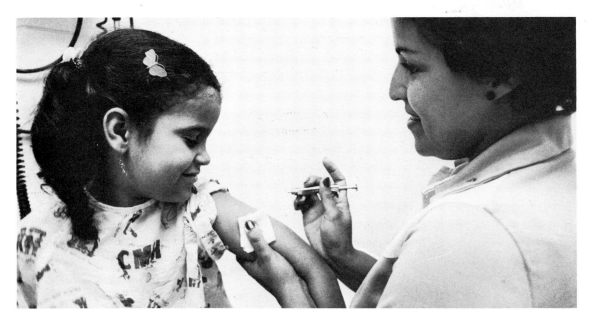

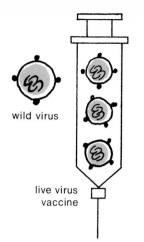

wild virus

live virus
vaccine

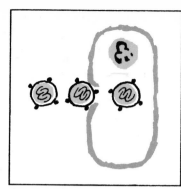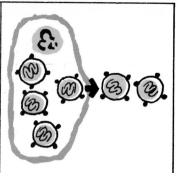

Attenuated virus
from live virus vaccine
is absorbed by host cell.

Attenuated virus is
replicated by host cell,
but without injury to
cell, unlike wild virus.

Fig. 3.13. Immunization against
wild virus by administration
of tamed live virus vaccine
(Reprinted with the permission
of Pfizer Laboratories Division)

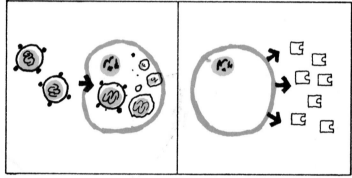

New viruses encounter
plasma cell, are engulfed,
and then broken down
to component chemicals.

Stimulated plasma
cell yields an army of
antibodies designed to
combat specific invader.

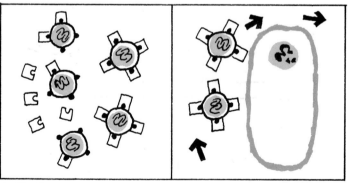

Antibodies are now
ready to attack and
neutralize invading
wild virus.

Wild virus neutralized
by antibodies is unable
to replicate and is
eliminated by the body.

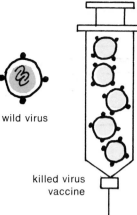

wild virus

killed virus
vaccine

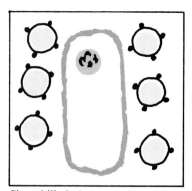

Fig. 3.14. Immunization against
wild virus by administration
of killed virus vaccine
(Reprinted with the permission
of Pfizer Laboratories Division)

Since killed virus
contains inactivated nucleic
acids, it does not invade
the natural host cell.

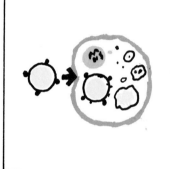

When killed virus
encounters plasma cells,
however, it is engulfed
and destroyed.

The plasma cell is
stimulated and produces
an army of antibodies.

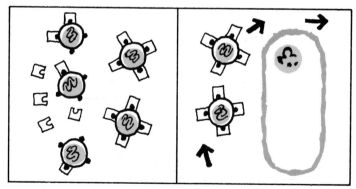

Upon later invasion
with wild virus, the body
produces more antibodies
to meet the new threat.

Antibodies neutralize
the virus to prevent
development of disease.

Table 3.1 Immunization Schedules for Various Infectious Diseases

Disease	Age at First Dose	Material (Antigen) and Dosage	Booster Doses	Adult Immunization
Diphtheria Tetanus Whooping Cough (Pertussis)	2 mo. through 6 yr.	Children—2 mo. to 6 yr.: 3 doses at 4- to 6-wk. intervals, fourth dose approximately 1 yr. after third injection (DTP) School children & adults: 3 doses of tetanus-diphtheria (adult) with second dose 4–6 wk. after first and third dose 6 mo. to 1 yr. after second	Children 3–6 yr.: 1 injection DTP intramuscularly All other persons: Tetanus-diphtheria (adult) every 10 yr. If dose administered sooner as part of wound management, next booster shot not needed for another 10 yr.	Tetanus-diphtheria (adult) every 10 yr. If dose administered sooner as part of wound management, next booster shot not needed for another 10 yr. Pertussis not indicated after sixth year
Poliomyelitis	2 mo.	Sabin Oral Polio Vaccine Types I, III, and II in that order; or trivalent oral vaccine, 3 doses, at 6- to 8-wk. intervals	1 dose of trivalent oral vaccine at 12–15 mo. and 1 dose on entering school	Adults subject to unusual risk, military service, or foreign travel should receive 2 doses of trivalent oral vaccine 6–8 wk. apart

German Measles (Rubella)	All children between 1 yr. and puberty Desirable for unimmunized adolescent girls and adult women	Live rubella virus vaccine—1 dose	Probably not needed	Contraindications:
				  Pregnancy
				  Altered immune states
				  Severe fever
				  Hypersensitivity

Mumps	12 mo. of age or older	Live mumps virus vaccine—1 dose	Probably not needed	Adolescent and adult males who have not had mumps
Smallpox		Routine vaccination in unexposed populations no longer recommended since September 1971		Routine immunization of health personnel, travellers to and from areas where smallpox still exists

Disease	Age at First Dose	Material (Antigen) and Dosage	Booster Doses	Adult Immunization
Measles (Rubeola)	12 mo. of age or older (6 mo. in epidemic exposure)	Live attenuated measles vaccine, 1 dose, or live attenuated measles vaccine plus measles immune globulin (MIG), 1 dose each	Children vaccinated before age 9–10 mo. (especially if vaccine was administered with MIG): revaccinate with live measles vaccine. Routine vaccination not routinely needed for children vaccinated at 10–12 mo. of age or older	Vaccination of adult rarely necessary. Precautions: Severe febrile illness. Active tuberculosis. Marked hypersensitivity to vaccine components. Contraindications: Altered immune states. Pregnancy
Typhoid Fever	Only when needed; routine immunization not indicated in USA	Typhoid vaccine 2 injections 4 or more wk. apart, or according to manufacturer's recommendations	At 4-yr. intervals a single injection up to 2 boosters	Only when needed. Typhoid vaccine, 2 injections with single boosters at 4-yr. intervals. Only for persons subject to risk or foreign travel
Influenza	Annual vaccination for persons with chronic debilitating conditions	Primary Series: 2 doses administered subcutaneously, preferably 6–8 wk. apart, to be completed by mid-Nov.	Single subcutaneous dose of bivalent vaccine before mid-Nov.	Precaution: Not administered to persons clearly hypersensitive to ingested or injected egg protein

Schedules may change with development of new vaccines and new medical discoveries.
A physician will make any appropriate changes that revised recommendations make necessary.
Reprinted with permission of American Medical Association.

There are many additional procedures presently available that either help human beings adapt to their disease-threatening environment or modify the environment itself to promote well-being rather than the spread of communicable diseases. Some of these adaptations require professional medical assistance or community-based support and action. Others depend upon individuals to exercise personal responsibility in preventive health practices affecting the person and the family.

Other Adaptive Countermeasures

Chemotherapy   The use of drugs in the treatment of disease is referred to as *chemotherapy*. Whether taken orally, by injection, or through some other means, the function of the drug used is to destroy or inactivate the pathogenic microorganism without damaging the host's cells. Examples of chemotherapeutic agents:

Quinine—for malaria-causing parasites.

Emetine—for treatment of amebic dysentery.

Sulfonamides—the sulfa drugs. Now largely replaced by antibiotics because of the toxic potential of sulfa drugs, they were formerly used against bacteria. They are still important in treating meningitis (inflammation of the membranes surrounding the brain) and certain urinary-tract infections.

Isoniazid—for tuberculosis.

Para-aminosalicylic acid—effective in treating tuberculosis, often in combination with isoniazid.

Nitrofurans—synthetic drugs used to inactivate bacteria, fungi, and protozoa.

Antibiotics—chemical substances derived from either fungi or bacteria that have the capacity to inhibit or destroy bacteria and certain fungi and rickettsiae. Among antibiotic drugs are penicillin, streptomycin, chloramphenicol, and tetracycline. Complications of antibiotic therapy include the development of *hypersensitivity* or *allergy* in the host and the induction of *bacterial resistance,* i.e., "... the drug is no longer effective in suppressing the growth and multiplication of the microorganisms."[19]

Antivirals—drugs used experimentally to induce the production of interferon within the host cells.

Sanitary Engineering   The modification of the environment to remove microorganisms and thereby establish conditions more favorable to health takes various forms. Significant sanitary measures to improve public health involve adequate garbage and waste disposal techniques, treatment of sewage, periodic street cleaning, installation of underground sewers, chlorination of public water supplies, insect and rodent (vector) control programs, and pasteurization of milk and dairy products (a special method of heating liquids whereby undesirable microorganisms are destroyed without altering the composition or food value of the material itself). Other measures include official inspection of public eating places and certain food products—to eliminate environmental reservoirs and the transmission of microbes—and the maintenance of health-promoting conditions.

Preventive Health Practices   While sanitary engineering focuses on the general public, the activities of preventive medicine are often concentrated on the individual. Emphasis is placed both on attacking microorganisms in contaminated areas and on excluding microbes, thus preventing the spread of infectious agents.[20] Techniques used particularly in hospitals include antiseptic presurgical measures that prevent the growth of bacteria; sterilization of surgical instruments, gowns, masks, and gloves to free such articles from living microorganisms and their products; and the use of disinfectants, such as phenol and alcohol, to destroy disease-producing organisms.

Recommended individual practices include the promotion of general, non-specific resistance to disease through proper nutrition, sleep, rest, and exercise; maintenance of immunity to specific diseases through periodic "booster shots"; washing hands after use of toilet facilities and before meals; self-isolation from others when infected or ill; and the avoidance of possible reservoirs, such as sick persons, crowds during an epidemic, and promiscuous sexual partners who may harbor venereal diseases. Available for general use and mandated for certain populations are *screening tests* to detect evidences of infection by microorganisms that cause tuberculosis and syphilis. Of course, when common danger signals of infection occur or persist, such as a sore throat, high fever, festering sore, skin rash, frequent coughing or sneezing, enlarged lymph nodes (swollen glands), and repeated diarrhea and vomiting, the wise person should seek out and accept medical advice.

Among the most frequent causes of disability is the *common cold*, ". . . an acute, highly communicable infection of the upper respiratory tract due to viruses. . ."[21] Colds usually localize in the head, throat, or chest. Fortunately, colds are usually self-limiting. However, such viral infections sometimes predispose a susceptible host to bacterial invasion of the lower respiratory tract, resulting in pneumonia. Ear infections, sinusitis, and laryngitis are frequent complications of a cold.

The Common Cold

Any one of more than one hundred different viruses can infect and produce a swelling of the lining membranes of the nose and throat. Mucus is produced in great quantity and eventually becomes thick and filled with pus. Well-known observable signs and symptoms (complaints) are: sneezing, watery eyes; chills; sore throat; stopped-up, runny nose; sore chest; coughing; and the "ache-all-over" feeling. Although none of these symptoms in itself is indicative of a cold, together this group of signs and symptoms forms the cold *syndrome*.

The incubation period of a cold is from one to three days. In addition, communicability seems to be greatest at the onset of the disease and for the first three days of symptoms. Contrary to popular belief, people do not catch more colds in winter; only 35 percent of the annual upper respiratory infections occur in winter.[22] Seasonal highs have been identified as autumn (shortly after school resumes), mid-winter, and during spring, around Easter time.

Because antibiotics, such a penicillin, have no effect against viruses, the treatment of a cold is aimed at the relief of symptoms. Popular "cold tablets" and other cold preparations usually contain:

First, an antihistamine, which is thought to reduce the reaction of the local tissues to the infecting virus; and second, a chemical related to epinephrine (adrenalin) which shrinks the blood vessels, and so relieves congestion in the nose and upper respiratory passages.[23]

Some cold medicines also contain aspirin to relieve aching and discomfort and to reduce fever. Caution is advised in the use of nasal decongestants during and after the onset of the cold because such use may actually help spread the infection down the respiratory tract.

Prevention of the common cold cannot be assured since no vaccine is available to reduce susceptibility. However, three suggestions to minimize the chances of infection are offered:

1. Keep general body resistance high to maintain nonspecific body defense mechanisms through good nutrition and adequate rest.
2. Keep the humidity at a comfortable level during the winter season when Americans tend to overheat their homes. Such superheating dries the mucous membranes of the nose and throat. Although:

   There is no experimental evidence indicating that dryness necessarily leads to more colds, . . . many doctors believe that an effective mucous membrane shield may trap viruses before they have a chance to infect the body.[24]

3. Avoid exposure to viruses as much as possible.

Although Nobel prize-winner Linus Pauling contends that relatively high doses of vitamin C are helpful in preventing colds, most medical authorities disagree with him.

Influenza

One of the most severe diseases caused by a respiratory virus is influenza. Spread by droplet infection, direct contact, or by contaminated objects, the flu is characterized by a high fever (between 101° F. and 104° F.), chills, headache, muscular aches in back and limbs, a dry cough without much sputum (lung secretion) production, flushed face, nasal discharge, and a sore throat. The illness usually "knocks out" the victim for two or three days. An overly tired feeling and a loose cough may persist for a week or more.

Families or types of flu virus have been responsible for numerous epidemics throughout the world, including the 1918 *pandemic* with more than twenty-one million fatalities.[25] Many readers of this chapter have been victims of the flu virus, the type A_2 (Asian) strain and/or the Hong Kong strain in particular. One of the difficulties in combating the influenza virus is its ability to change its own nature from time to time. As a consequence, few people will have built up immunity to a particular strain, and whole populations remain susceptible. One possible exception is the swine flu virus.

During 1976 and 1977, the federal government initiated a massive program to vaccinate millions of Americans against swine flu, after an outbreak of several hundred cases at a large army base. There was great fear that the swine flu virus—so named because the virus apparently flourishes among hogs—would cause another worldwide epidemic similar to the 1918 epidemic.

Anticipating an outbreak of major proportions, the U.S. Public Health Service prepared to immunize nearly everyone in the country with a newly developed vaccine. After millions of persons had received their swine flu shots, the federally funded effort was curtailed because of unfortunate side effects among elderly persons who had received the vaccine. Perhaps another reason for the program's early demise was that an epidemic failed to occur in the unprotected population. Nevertheless, many Americans have some residual protection against this strain.

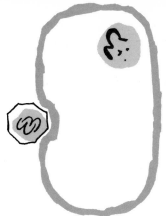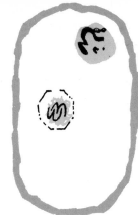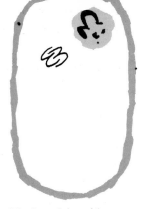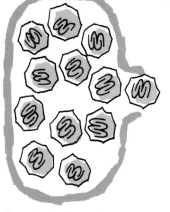

| Invading virus comes in contact with cell which absorbs it in the feeding process, or pinocytosis. | Inside the cell, the protein shell of the virus is metabolized by cell enzymes. The nucleic acid of the virus is not affected by this enzymatic action. | Viral nucleic acids are superimposed on the DNA of the cell. In what might be termed "the ultimate parasitism," the cell then begins producing amino acids for new virus particles which eventually may lead to its own destruction. | Completely formed new virus particles erupt from invaded cell ready to infect a widening area of host cells. |

Complications of influenza are pneumonia (a sometimes fatal lung inflammation), bronchitis, sinus trouble, and infections of the ear. Therefore, preventive flu shots (vaccines) are recommended for persons with chronic heart disease, arteriosclerosis, high blood pressure, or serious lung disorders. Influenza vaccines are now from 50 to 75 percent effective in offering protection.[26] *Polyvalent vaccines* containing several different antigens which are effective against the principal types of flu virus are now available and are frequently administered to military and law enforcement personnel and to pregnant women.

As in the case of the common cold, there is no specific treatment for influenza, although experimental antiviral drugs hold great promise for future use. Contrary to popular belief, penicillin and other

antimicrobial drugs are not effective against the virus, do not prevent bacterial infection, and may be needed later if bacterial infection does occur.[27]

Among recommended home treatment procedures are bed rest, keeping warm, drinking plenty of liquids, and taking regular doses of aspirin. If fever persists or if breathing or pulse rate is affected, medical advice should be sought.

Fig. 3.15. How a virus attacks a cell, characteristic of the common cold and influenza (Reprinted with the permission of Pfizer Laboratories Division)

An acute infectious disease, *mononucleosis* is characterized by a sore throat, fatigue, headache, fever, and swollen lymph glands at the side of the neck. Signs and symptoms generally persist for several days, and sore throat and weakness often last for a period of weeks.

Infectious Mononucleosis

Mononucleosis remains something of a mystery disease because its exact cause has not been identified. It is likely that the Epstein-Barr virus (EBV), a family member of the herpes virus group that causes fever blisters, is the causative agent.[28] The method of transmission is probably from one infected person to a susceptible host via the mouth and the transfer of saliva. As a consequence, mono has often been called the ''kissing disease.'' Its occurrence is most often noticed in youth and young adults in the more advanced and affluent countries of the world. It might also be termed the ''college disease'' because it is ''. . . at least three times more likely to hit college students than other young adults.''[29]

In some individuals the disease is so mild that illness is never suspected. An estimated one third of the college patients never have to be confined to bed rest, and, of the remainder, less than 2 percent require bed rest for more than two weeks.[30] However, the resulting fatigue is a variable factor from person to person, with some patients recovering their full strength only after a period of months.

Permanent disability or death following an attack of mono is rare. However, in addition to the disease's impact on loss of academic time, complications can be serious. Bacterial infection of the throat may require antibiotic treatment. Precaution against rupture of the spleen must be taken in a third of the cases in which the spleen becomes enlarged. As a consequence, some individuals will need to limit physical exertion so as to avoid blows to the chest or abdomen.

Because the signs and symptoms of infectious mononucleosis resemble those of strep throat, polio, and diphtheria, positive identification of the illness is based on two blood tests that detect atypical white blood cells and the ability of the host's blood serum to react with the red blood cells of some other species.

There are no specific treatments in terms of medication, and no vaccine is available. The only blessing of mononucleosis is that one infection apparently confers a high degree of acquired active immunity to the causative organism.

Viral Hepatitis   Hepatitis is a broad term that describes an inflammatory condition of the liver. Yellowing of the skin (jaundice) and abnormal liver functioning are the major characteristics of this virus-caused illness.

Two types of viruses are considered responsible for such inflammations: (1) The virus of *infectious hepatitis,* and (2) the virus of *serum hepatitis.* The end result of both infections is the same: liver damage. However, there are considerable differences in the manner in which these viruses are spread from one host reservoir to a new susceptible host. Both infections may be either acute (and clinically recognized) or subacute (i.e., the disease occurs without jaundice). Because so many cases go unrecognized, the true incidence of viral hepatitis is unknown.[31]

Infectious Hepatitis   Present in the blood and feces of the human host, the virus of infectious hepatitis is likely spread from person to person by the fecal-oral route. Contaminated milk, water, and food are possible vehicles of infection. Poor sanitation and inadequate treatment of human waste are also factors in the transmission of the disease. Unfortunately, neither chlorination nor pasteurization is completely effective in the destruction of these viral microorganisms.

In addition to suffering liver damage, malfunctioning of the liver, and jaundice, the victim usually sustains fever, malaise, loss of appetite, nausea, and abdominal discomfort. Infection results in the antigen-antibody response, although the duration of active immunity is unknown. There is no vaccine for active immunization, but immune serum globulin does provide passive immunity to exposed individuals during epidemics that can occur in such localities as low-cost housing projects and rural areas and among military forces during wartime conditions.

Serum Hepatitis

This illness of serum hepatitis closely resembles the signs and symptoms of infectious hepatitis. However, these viruses are transmitted by the transfusion of blood and other blood products from an infected donor to a susceptible recipient. Significantly, serious outbreaks have originated in clinics and physicians' offices among patients who received injections from contaminated and inadequately sterilized syringes and needles.[32] Serum hepatitis also has been traced to tattoo parlors. The disease has become increasingly prevalent among individuals who have developed a physical drug dependency, especially to narcotics. Addicts frequently use and share their unsterilized and contaminated hypodermic needles. While "passing the needle," they often "pass the virus."

Since there is no vaccine and passive immunization is of no demonstrated value, prevention must focus on strict discipline in blood banks to reject donors who have a history of viral hepatitis and who show evidence of drug addiction.[33] Sterilization of syringes, needles, and other equipment used in inoculation or venipuncture is a must. From the consumer's point-of-view, the best advice is " . . . to patronize only reputable physicians and seek all medical laboratory work in approved facilities."[34]

Tuberculosis

Still a significant public health threat in North America, *tuberculosis* (TB) is concentrated in large urban ghettos, in Appalachia, on certain Indian reservations, and along the Mexican border.[35] Primarily a bacterial infection of the lungs, tuberculosis is a communicable disease that can spread also to the bones, joints, kidneys, or skin. Infection is due to inhalation of bacteria present in tiny droplets expelled from a human reservoir by sneezing, coughing, or speaking.

Although caused by a specific bacterial agent, the *tubercle bacillus,* TB infection and reinfection are often related to overcrowding, poor ventilation, substandard living conditions, faulty nutrition, inadequate sleep, and emotional stress. These factors adversely affect general body resistance and play a role in the development of *active disease* following infection.

Tuberculosis is a form of "rot" or tissue decay in which bacteria destroy parts of various body organs.[36] After initial infection, the host attempts to wall off the foreign invaders by surrounding the bacteria with white blood cells and then layers of other cells to form the characteristic *tubercle.* The tubercle or healed *lesion* (tissue injury) becomes calcified with lime deposits, thus forming a firm

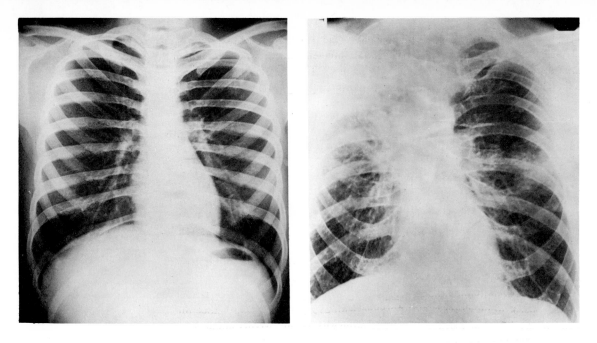

Fig. 3.16. The tubercules of TB appear as white spots on X rays. The left chest X ray of the lungs reveals a patient with minimal tuberculosis tissue decay. The right chest X ray shows advanced tuberculosis.

lump in the spongy lung tissue that resembles the knots on tuberous plants. These tubercles appear as the white spots on X rays. As long as general body resistance remains high, the infection is contained. However, "active" TB may develop years later when the tubercle bacilli in old scars "wake up" and begin to multiply and spread to other tissues.[37] An estimated 92 percent of all new cases of TB develop precisely in this way—in persons infected in the past.[38]

While tuberculosis is no longer the scourge of Western civilization, there are presently a quarter million cases under medical supervision in the United States. In addition, approximately sixteen million Americans are probably infected with the TB-causing microorganism. In many of these infected persons the disease will likely become active during their lifetimes.[39]

Unfortunately, there are no signs or symptoms of either the initial infection or the earliest stage of active pulmonary (lung) tuberculosis. By the time symptoms do occur—fatigue, weakness, irritability, fever, night sweats, coughing, spitting blood, and loss of weight—the active disease has already made considerable progress. However, two methods of detection are very effective in uncovering TB: (1) a *tuberculin skin test,* which is specific for determining TB *infection* only; and (2) the *X ray of the chest,* which can determine the *activity* of the infection, the extent of the tissue damage, and the tissue changes occurring during treatment.

In some countries, the BCG (Bacillus Calmette-Guérin) vaccine is given to uninfected persons who stand a high risk of infection. The vaccine, which confers active immunity, also renders the individual "tuberculin positive," thereby destroying the usefulness of the skin test. Thus it is not used widely in the United States. Where modern detection methods, isolation procedures, and treatment are available, as in North America, the use of drugs in controlling TB has been most successful. Chemotherapeutic agents include isoniazid (INH), para-aminosali-cylic acid (PAS), and streptomycin. Treating infected persons who have a high risk of developing active disease is more precise in blocking transmission of TB infection in the United States today than in vaccinating large numbers of nonreactors to the skin test.[40]

Venereal Diseases

Communicable diseases transmitted primarily through sexual intercourse or other sexual practices are known as *venereal diseases*, or sexually transmitted diseases. The term *venereal* is derived from Venus, goddess of love. Gonorrhea, syphilis, and genital herpes are the most common venereal diseases in the United States. Less common venereal infections include chancroid and granuloma inguinale (both bacteria-caused diseases) and virus-caused lymphogranuloma venereum.

Each of the venereal diseases is caused by a separate, distinct type of infecting microorganism. Therefore, an individual may be infected with two or more of these microbes at the same time and display signs and symptoms of both diseases simultaneously. Reinfection is also possible with every new exposure since immunity to the venereal diseases does not ordinarily occur. Myths about toilet seats, door handles, and soap dishes being responsible for transmission of venereal disease (VD) have been discounted by scientists. The pathogenic agents of gonorrhea and syphilis—both delicate bacteria—cannot exist outside the dark, warm, moist environment found within the human body, especially the reproductive tract. Venereal disease is transmitted almost exclusively from one person to another through intimate sexual contact.

Tragic Controversy

Few diseases raise as much controversy as does VD. In the mind of the general public, venereal disease has become confused with the method of its transmission. Indeed, "we have so consistently identified this disease with illegitimate sex that anybody who gets it feels as though he were a criminal, no matter how he got it."[41] Some people claim there is never an "innocent party" to venereal disease. But how else would you classify the husbands and wives who do contract VD from a "cheating spouse"? Some infected persons develop so much guilt that they do not seek medical care. Others fear the public or private censure sometimes dispensed by health professionals so they avoid treatment. The tragedy of VD is two-fold: while gonorrhea and syphilis are both curable and preventable, they are not being cured in millions of cases, and they are not being adequately prevented!

Many people are convinced that the epidemic of VD in America is evidence of widespread immorality and the decline of civilization. Some are more concerned that hundreds of thousands of untreated individuals are harboring dangerous and damaging pathogens that possibly will be transmitted to unsuspecting victims. Others view the increasing numbers of VD cases reported to public officials as evidence of increased personal and social responsibility. Hopefully, infected people seek help because they want to be cured and do not wish to give the disease to someone else. Still others look upon the alarming statistics of incidence and attribute the current epidemic to better case-finding and reporting techniques. Perhaps all viewpoints have some merit. One thing is certain: most people are not going to stop having sexual relations. If they do get VD and are not treated early, they are likely to suffer severe physical damage, perhaps even death.

Incidence and Trends

The occurrence of reported gonorrhea cases has nearly doubled in the United States within a recent ten-year period. Currently there are about one million cases per year. But with so many cases of infection never detected and so many cases treated but never reported to public health officials, estimates of gonorrhea incidence range as high as 2,600,000 cases each year.[42] In some large urban areas, it is likely that 10 percent of the sexually active population has had or is presently infected with VD. Although the number of cases of primary and secondary syphilis reported each year is approximately 24,000, estimates of actual occurrence range as high as 82,000 cases per year.

Because of the differences in male and female body structure, signs and symptoms of both gonorrhea and syphilis are more easily noticed in males. Women are strictly at a disadvantage! "As a matter of fact, women with gonorrhea usually don't have any complaints or clinical signs early in the course of the disease."[43] Lesions or tissue damage may occur within the female's vagi-

Fig. 3.17. Gonorrhea and syphilis case rates per 100,000 population, 1919–1976

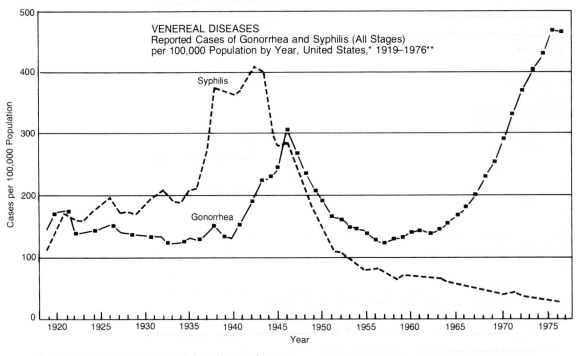

*Beginning in 1939, all states are included in the reporting area.
(Military cases included 1919–1940, excluded thereafter.)
**1919–1940 fiscal years: twelve-month periods ending June 30 of year specified
1941–1976 calendar years

Chapter Three

na or on the cervix, thus contributing to the large reservoir of undetected gonorrhea and "hidden" symptoms of syphilis.

Based on reported cases, gonorrhea and syphilis rates are highest in the 20–24 year age group. Significantly high rates of both diseases also occur in the 15–19 and 25–29 year age groups. Statistics also reveal a higher incidence of both gonorrhea and syphilis in nonwhites than in whites. However, it is common knowledge that VD is grossly underreported by private physicians and nearly completely reported by public clinics.

> The socioeconomically deprived (of whom nonwhites comprise a disproportionate segment) tend to seek medical care from public clinics and are far more likely to be reported than those treated by private physicians.[44]

VD is no respecter of race, color, creed, sex, economic status, or social standing. It has become a national disease for the United States with a case of gonorrhea occurring about every fifteen seconds around the clock.[45] While the occurrence of gonorrhea remains extremely high, the number of reported cases of syphilis has actually declined in recent years.[46] Public health officials believe that a turning point has been reached at last in the battle against the national epidemic of venereal diseases.

Often referred to as "clap," "strain," "morning dew," or "the drip," gonorrhea is caused by the *gonococcus* bacterium. The pathogenic agents are transferred between human hosts via the moist, mucous membrane lining of the genitals, the mouth, and the rectum.[47] Gonorrhea is spread from person to person by sexual contact, specifically intercourse and heterosexual and homosexual oral sex and anal sex. However, the underside of the eyelids may be infected nonsexually, ". . . from mother to offspring either during delivery or later through poor sanitation procedures."[48] Such an infection can damage the cornea of the eye and result in blindness.

Gonorrhea

In the *male* the first indication of the infection is usually a thick, yellowish puslike discharge from the urethra and a burning sensation upon urination. These are often sufficient to motivate most males to seek medical relief. However, the asymptomatic male—one who is infected with gonorrhea but who shows no common signs of the disease and experiences none of the symptoms—is occurring with increasing frequency. If the infection is not controlled, the organisms may spread to the prostate gland, the vas deferens, and the epididymis, and cause sterility. Untreated gonorrhea can result eventually in heart disease and arthritic conditions, although death is rare.

In the *female* initial signs and symptoms may include an itching or burning feeling in the genital area and a slight pus discharge from the vagina or urethra. It is more common, though, for the female to be without symptoms or with symptoms so mild that they are readily dismissed as insignificant. Untreated infections often invade the upper parts of the reproductive system, specifically the fallopian tubes and ovaries, and result in acute inflammation of the abdominal cavity. This condition is referred to as pelvic inflammatory disease, which constitutes a major threat to the life of the female. Complications of chronic (long-term) infections are similar to those experienced by the male.

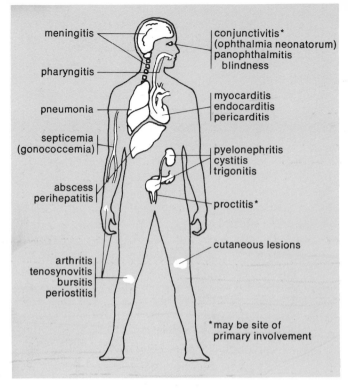

Fig. 3.18. Distant
complications
of gonorrhea in the
male and in the female

meningitis

pharyngitis

pneumonia

septicemia
(gonococcemia)

abscess
perihepatitis

arthritis
tenosynovitis
bursitis
periostitis

conjunctivitis*
(ophthalmia neonatorum)
panophthalmitis
blindness

myocarditis
endocarditis
pericarditis

pyelonephritis
cystitis
trigonitis

proctitis*

cutaneous lesions

*may be site of
primary involvement

Fig. 3.19. Female gonorrhea
is characterized by a slight
pus discharge from the vagina.
It is often undetected or does
not occur at all.

Fig. 3.20. Pus
discharge from the
penis is a common
sign of male gonorrhea.
It is often referred
to as the "clap" or
the "drip."

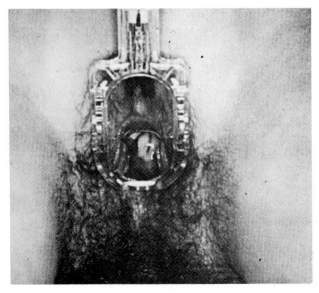

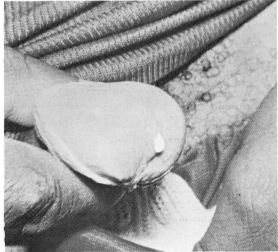

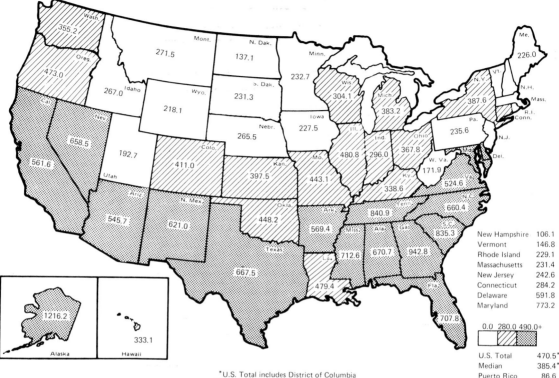

VENEREAL DISEASE
Reported Cases of Gonorrhea
per 100,000 Population by State,
Calendar Year 1976

New Hampshire	106.1
Vermont	146.8
Rhode Island	229.1
Massachusetts	231.4
New Jersey	242.6
Connecticut	284.2
Delaware	591.8
Maryland	773.2

0.0 280.0 490.0+

U.S. Total	470.5*
Median	385.4**
Puerto Rico	86.6
Virgin Islands	435.0

*U.S. Total includes District of Columbia
**Excludes Puerto Rico and Virgin Islands

Fig. 3.21. Gonorrhea case rates per 100,000 population. The 1976 United States total of 470.5 per 100,000 represents a very slight decrease (less than 0.1 percent) from the all-time high of 472.9 per 100,000 in 1975.

Until the advent of a rapid, reliable, and accurate blood test for gonorrhea, the disease must be detected by microscopic examination of the puslike discharge from either the urethra, vagina, cervix, throat, or rectum. Treatment with penicillin or other antibiotic (tetracycline or spectinomycin) is generally successful, although massive doses of more expensive medications are sometimes required to counter the problem of drug-resistant gonorrhea organisms. Routinely, a silver nitrate or antibiotic solution is placed in the eyes of all newborn infants to protect them from possible gonorrhea-induced blindness.

Because the advanced tissue destruction of syphilis simulates that of many other illnesses, this disease is known as the "great mimic." It is far more serious than gonorrhea because left untreated it can and does kill. Slang terms identifying syphilis include "siff," "lues," "bad blood," "pox," and "hair cut."

Syphilis

The causative organism is a fragile and sensitive bacterium, the *spirochete*, which can invade not only the mucous membranes of the host but also a break in the skin. However, the latter is only a remote possibility. Like the gonorrhea microorganisms, the spirochetes are transmitted most generally through heterosexual or homosexual practices, including intercourse, oral sex, and anal sex.

Spirochetes can cross over the placenta so that a fetus can receive an unwanted gift of damaging microorganisms from an infected mother. The condition is described as *congenital syphilis*. Left untreated, the disease usually results in a stillborn infant or in a seriously disfigured and diseased child. "Without treatment the pregnant syphilitic female has only one chance in six of delivering a normal healthy child."[49]

Stages of Untreated Syphilis

Without medical treatment, the initial infection typically progresses through distinct stages, each with characteristic signs and symptoms.

Primary Syphilis Between 10–90 days after infection, a *chancre* (a painless ulcer or sore that looks as if it should hurt) usually forms at the site of entry. Teeming with spirochetes, the chancre is evidence of the host-parasite interaction. The body's defense mechanisms generally win this first round of battle. Without treatment, the chancre disappears within four to six weeks. Observed easily on the male genitals, if it appears there, the chancre may remain hidden as in the female where the sore may be located on the cervix. Moreover, infection without any chancre is fairly frequent.[50] The disease is communicable during this stage.

Secondary Syphilis Spirochetes now spread throughout the body via the bloodstream and cause disturbances in the skin and mucous membranes of the host. These secondary manifestations may last only a few weeks or may persist for up to two years. Common signs and symptoms may include rashes on the hands,

Fig. 3.22. Chancre of the finger

Fig. 3.23. Benign cutaneous syphilis. The "saddlenose" is a complication of late syphilis.

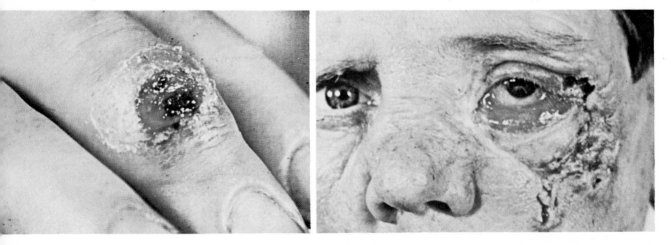

feet, or back; mucous patches (white blotches) in the mouth; loss of hair; low-grade fever; and a sore throat. In time, the spirochetes call a truce with the host, and even these secondary abnormalities disappear without treatment.

Latent Syphilis   The disease now enters a dormant or hidden stage, the latent period, during which there are no outward signs or symptoms. After about two years of latency, the host is not considered contagious. The spirochetes, however, are quietly at work destroying tissues of internal body organs, such as the heart, liver, and brain. Latency may continue for ten to twenty years or throughout life. Some untreated individuals eventually display the gross degeneration and disorders of the late stage of syphilis.

Late Syphilis   After years of latency, evidence of internal tissue destruction may be presented in the form of partial or complete paralysis, severe mental disturbances, blindness, bone destruction, liver damage, heart disease, and weakening of the walls of major arteries.

A reliable blood test to detect syphilis infection is available and is required in most states before a couple can be married. After all, no one would appreciate receiving syphilis as a wedding present. The test also aims to prevent congenital syphilis among newborn infants. Standard treatment with penicillin or other antibiotics has proved successful, although no medication can repair tissue that has been damaged or destroyed. Experimental vaccines indicate that an immunization against syphilis is a possibility of the future.

Genital Herpes

Many individuals develop cold sores or fever blisters around the mouth or lips. These conditions are caused by a virus identified as herpes simplex, type 1.* A closely related form, herpes type 2, can infect the genital areas of both men and women, causing painful blisters and lesions. Genital herpes is usually contracted through sexual contact. However, nonsexual transmission is also possible—for instance, when a person touches the genitals of an actively infected person, passing the virus to his or her own genitals by hand contact.

Since genital herpes is not yet a reportable communicable disease, there are no statistics on the number of persons infected annually. However,

> some doctors have come to think of sexually transmitted herpes as one of the top-ranking "venereal" diseases in terms of numbers of people infected, and there is increasing suspicion among scientists that herpes in the sex organs of women may be related to cancer of the cervix.[51]

Symptoms   According to the Center for Disease Control, symptoms of genital herpes will generally occur within one week after exposure to a person with an active infection. In women, small and painful blisters form around the vagina and soon break into open lesions (sores). Blistering can also occur in the anal area or on the cervix.

*Unless indicated otherwise, the information in this section was provided by the Center for Disease Control.

Other Sexually Transmitted Diseases

Chancroid (soft chancre)—An acute bacterial infection transmitted sexually and characterized by painful genital ulcers and swelling of the lymph nodes.

Granuloma inguinale—A chronic and progressive ulcerative disease involving the skin and the lymphatics of the genital and anal regions. Relatively uncommon in the United States, the disease is thought to be caused by bacterialike intracellular microorganisms known as Donovan bodies.

Lymphogranuloma venereum—A systemic infection of the lymph nodes and lymph channels caused by sexually transmitted bacteria and characterized by small ulcers on the penis, vagina, or rectum.

Nonspecific urethritis—Any inflammation of the male or female urethra (the passageway for urine) not caused by gonorrhea organisms. The condition is characterized by pain, discomfort, and a discharge of pus, although women are usually without symptoms.

Pediculosis ("crabs")—An infestation of the pubic area, especially the pubic hair, by crawling, bloodsucking lice that look like crabs when magnified.

The condition is marked by considerable itching and the appearance of pale blue spots on the skin. Crab lice are usually transmitted by intimate contact, but may also be spread by means of bedding and clothing.

Scabies—An infectious skin disease caused by a small mite and characterized by intense itching and by the appearance of pimples and blisters.

Vaginitis—Inflammation of the vagina due to various causes, some of which are organisms that can be transmitted by sexual intercourse. These organisms include a one-celled animal parasite that causes trichomoniasis and a yeastlike fungus responsible for moniliasis, often called candidiasis. These organisms also infect the male reproductive tract and give rise to the ping-pong effect in sexual relations—the back-and-forth infection between male and female.

Venereal warts—Virus-caused warts that appear on the external genitalia of males and females. Genital warts usually appear one to three months after intercourse with an infected partner.

In men, the sores develop on the shaft of the penis or around the anus. Additional symptoms in both men and women can include painful urination, generalized aching, and fever. These symptoms can last from two to six weeks before the sores heal spontaneously.

In many cases symptoms will not recur once the lesions have healed. However, some patients do have periodic flare-ups, which are often associated with nervous tension, emotional upset, fatigue, exposure to sunlight, and, in women, menstruation. Persons who experience frequent recurrences are often able to predict fairly accurately the events that are likely to bring on an attack and may be able to reduce the frequency by avoiding such situations. Recurrent infections are less severe than a primary infection and last one to two weeks.

If an active infection of genital herpes exists at the time of childbirth, the baby may acquire the virus as it passes through the infected birth canal. If the mother has an active case, a cesarean section may be advisable, since an infection in a newborn infant is often fatal. Active infections during pregnancy also increase the likelihood of spontaneous abortion and premature labor.

Treatment and Prevention   There is no proven, effective therapy for genital herpes at the present time. In general, anything that causes the blisters to dry up more quickly tends to alleviate symptoms. Wearing loose-fitting underwear may help keep the genital area dry.

During the active phase of the disease, when the blisters are present, and for at least two more weeks, the infected person should avoid sexual contact, or the male partner should use a condom during intercourse. This can decrease the likelihood of transmitting the disease.

Control of VD

If a case of either gonorrhea or syphilis comes to the attention of public health officials, they will make efforts to trace and contact all recent sexual partners of the infected host. When voluntary treatment is not obtained by the "contacts," medical examination and treatment are mandated by law and enforced by police action. Most states now have laws that authorize without parental consent the treatment of minors for VD or suspected VD.

Ultimately, the control of venereal disease is a personal responsibility. Refraining from promiscuous premarital and extramarital sexual activity is one sure way of avoiding infection. The male sex partner's use of a condom or "rubber" as a prophylactic (disease-prevention) measure will certainly reduce the chances of transmitting both syphilis and gonorrhea, provided the device is not broken and is properly applied. The condom tends to be more effective in protecting against gonorrhea than against syphilis.[52]

Although not guaranteed as absolutely effective, two additional actions can reduce a person's chances of getting a venereal disease: (1) washing one's hands and external sex organs with soap and water before and after sexual contact, and (2) urinating as soon as possible after sexual contact to flush out any infectious agents from the urethra.

If signs and symptoms of syphilis or gonorrhea appear, the responsible person will seek medical treatment and will warn other sexual partners of their possible infection, especially females who often have no warning signals of disease. Preventable, treatable VD is, after all, a people problem. Only the individual can break the chain of infection.

Summary

This chapter has included an explanation of pathogens and the chain of infection characteristic of communicable diseases, such as the common cold, influenza, infectious mononucleosis, viral hepatitis, tuberculosis, and the venereal diseases. The host-parasite interaction and various defense mechanisms of resistance, especially immunity, were examined along with other adaptive countermeasures. Personal and community health practices were also emphasized to indicate that prevention of communicable diseases is more desirable than attempting to cure those who have become infected with agents of disease.

As we draw this discussion to a close, one is forced to raise some questions about these person-to-person diseases. Will the time ever come when all such diseases can be conquered? Recent years have seen significant reduction in many communicable diseases. As we contemplate the years of your future, what can be expected regarding communicable diseases, their prevention, and their control?

1. How do communicable diseases affect a person other than physically?
2. Explain the term "biological coexistence."
3. Are all infectious diseases necessarily communicable or contagious?
4. List and differentiate between the major groups of pathogens.
5. Describe the ways in which pathogens are transmitted.
6. What is meant by the "chain of infection"? Describe it.
7. Discuss the four stages of disease.
8. Differentiate between sporadic, endemic, epidemic, and pandemic diseases. Name specific diseases that can be placed in each category.
9. How do external environmental factors promote or hinder the spread of disease? Internal environmental factors?
10. List and describe the defense mechanisms of resistance.
11. How do antibodies react with antigens to fight infection?
12. What types of immunization are still given children in the U.S.? Which are no longer administered? Why?
13. How have chemotherapy, sanitary engineering, and preventive health practices helped reduce the incidence of many infectious diseases?
14. Why is mononucleosis sometimes referred to as the "kissing disease" or the "college disease"?
15. Differentiate between syphilis, herpes type 2, and gonorrhea, the main types of venereal disease. Which is most dangerous? Most prevalent?

Notes

1. John J. Witte, "We're Not Immunizing Enough of Our Children," *Today's Health* (September 1973): 4–5.
2. "Legionnaires' Disease—In Perspective," *The Harvard Medical School Health Letter* (December 1977): 5.
3. Center for Disease Control, "Sporadic Cases of Legionnaires' Disease—United States," *Morbidity and Mortality Weekly Report* (November 11, 1977): 1.
4. Alice Lorraine Smith, *Microbiology and Pathology*, 10th ed. (St. Louis: C. V. Mosby Co., 1972), p. 75.
5. National Institute of Allergy and Infectious Disease, *Viruses: On the Border of Life* (Washington: U.S. Government Printing Office, 1970).
6. Michael J. Pelczar and Roger D. Reid, *Microbiology* (New York: McGraw-Hill Book Co., 1972), p. 511.
7. Smith, *Microbiology and Pathology*, pp. 75–77.
8. Ibid., p. 78.
9. Ibid., p. 81.
10. Abram S. Benenson, ed., *Control of Communicable Diseases in Man*, 12th ed. (Washington: American Public Health Association, 1975), p. 385.
11. A. Melvin Ramsay and Roland T. D. Edmond, *Infectious Diseases* (London: William Heinemann Medical Books, 1967), p. 2.
12. Harold J. Simon, *Microbes and Man* (New York: Scholastic Book Services, 1963), p. 44.
13. Smith, *Microbiology and Pathology*, p. 93.
14. Clois W. Bennett, *Clinical Serology* (Springfield, Ill.: Charles C Thomas Publisher, 1968), p. 11.
15. Ibid., p. 7.

16. Deward K. Grissom, *Communicable Diseases* (Dubuque, Iowa: Wm. C. Brown Co., 1971), p. 21.

17. Pelczar and Reid, *Microbiology*, p. 524.

18. "Preventable Diseases Still Strike Children," *HE-XTRA* (September 1977): 1.

19. Smith, *Microbiology and Pathology*, p. 149.

20. For a detailed explanation of asepsis and antisepsis, the reader should consult Betty McInness, *Controlling the Spread of Infection* (St. Louis: C. V. Mosby Co., 1973).

21. American Lung Association, *Introduction to Lung Diseases*, 5th ed. (New York: The Association, 1973), p. 7.

22. *The Cold: Its Causes and Symptoms* (Bloomfield, N.J.: Schering Corporation, 1971), p. 16.

23. American College Health Association, *Your Cold and What To Do about It* (Evanston, Ill.: The Association, 1971).

24. Nellie Gifford, "Don't Take Your Winter Ailments Lying Down," *Today's Health* (January 1972): 26.

25. American Lung Association, p. 12.

26. Gifford, "Don't Take Your Winter Ailments Lying Down," p. 24.

27. American Lung Association, p. 13.

28. K. Diem and C. Lentner, eds., *Pathogenic Organisms and Infectious Diseases* (Basle, Switzerland: Ciba-Geigy, 1971), p. 77.

29. "Mononucleosis and the College Student," *Consumer Reports* (October 1973): 650.

30. American College Health Association, *So You've Got Mono* (Evanston, Ill.: The Association, 1971).

31. Smith, *Microbiology and Pathology*, p. 293.

32. Benenson, *Control of Communicable Diseases*, p. 145.

33. Ibid., p. 146.

34. Grissom, *Communicable Diseases*, p. 30.

35. *Tuberculin Testing: A Critical Evaluation* (Pearl River, N.Y.: Lederle Laboratories, 1973), p. 2.

36. William W. Stead, *Understanding Tuberculosis Today*, 2d ed. rev. (Milwaukee: Marquette University Press, 1969), p. 3.

37. Ibid., p. 13.

38. Lung Association of East Central Indiana, *Board Bits* (September 1973), p. 4.

39. American Lung Association, p. 41.

40. Lung Association, *Board Bits*, p. 4.

41. William F. Schwartz, "Enlightening the Public," *The VD Crisis*. Proceedings of the International Venereal Disease Symposium (New York: Pfizer Laboratories Division, 1971), p. 68.

42. American Social Health Association, "Special Issue: VD Incidence Data," *VD News* (June 1976): 12.

43. Harry Pariser, "Asymptomatic Gonorrhea," *The VD Crisis*. Proceedings of the International Venereal Disease Symposium (New York: Pfizer Laboratories Division, 1971), p. 26.

44. American Social Health Association, *Today's VD Control Problem* (New York: The Association, 1973), p. 15.

45. William J. Brown, "The National VD Problem," *Medical Aspects of Human Sexuality* (February 1972), 161.

46. Center for Disease Control, "Reported Morbidity and Mortality in the United States, 1976," *Morbidity and Mortality Weekly Report: Annual Summary, 1976* (August 1977): 2.

47. John Grover, *VD: The ABC's* (Englewood Cliffs, N.J.: Prentice-Hall, 1971), p. 49.

48. Stephen J. Bender, *Venereal Disease* (Dubuque, Iowa: Wm. C. Brown Co., 1971), p. 27.

49. Ibid., p. 21.

50. Benenson, *Control of Communicable Diseases*, p. 314.

51. Joseph A. Chiappa and Joseph J. Forish, *The VD Book*, Educational ed. (New York: Holt, Rinehart and Winston, 1976), pp. 56–57.

52. American Medical Association, *Venereal Disease* (Chicago: The Association, 1972), p. 24.

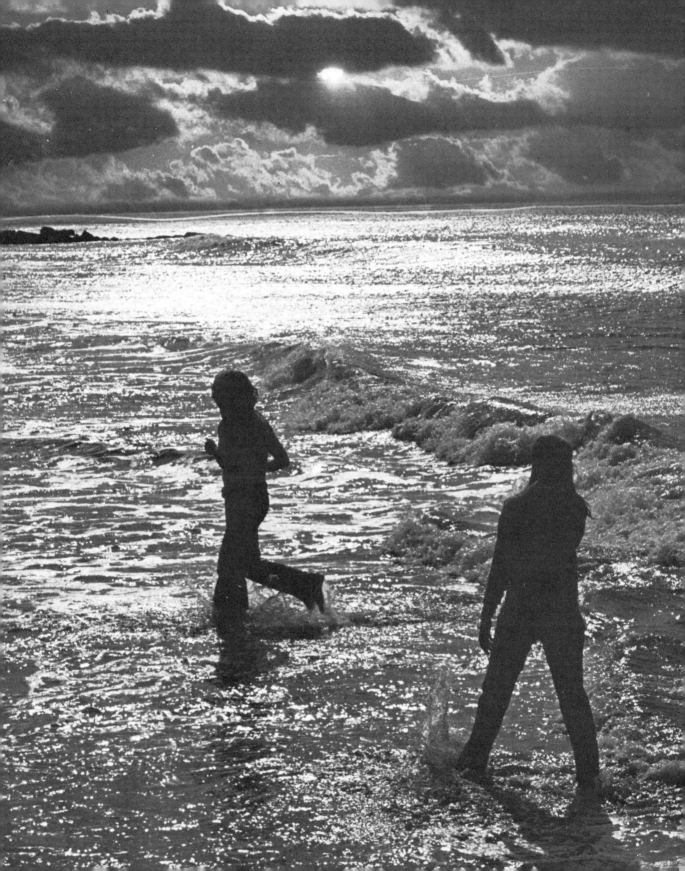

Puberty: Psychophysiological Consideration

4

Adolescence begins in biology and ends in culture.[1]

To no small degree the anxieties of youth are tied to the chemical, anatomical, and physiological changes of puberty. The spurt in growth, the changes in body size and shape, the development of organs and tissues, and sexual maturation combine to make the period from prepuberty through late teens traumatic and perplexing. And it all begins with a few small secretions from the pituitary gland.

Located immediately below the brain, the pituitary gland releases activating hormones of critical importance to body growth, development, and regulation. Among these several hormones are a thyroid-stimulating hormone (TSH), a follicle-stimulating hormone (FSH), an adrenocorticotrophic hormone (ACTH), and a growth-stimulating hormone (GSH). Frequently referred to as "the master gland," the pituitary secretes hormones that act both directly and indirectly on body organs and systems (see fig. 4.1).

Although the sequence of bodily development is consistent for all adolescents, the age of onset and rate of growth vary widely. The abrupt spurt in growth, for example, begins and ends at different times for the two sexes and for individuals within each sex. Beginning in early adolescence (somewhere between 7½ to 11½ years of age in girls and 10½ to 16 in boys), growth hits a peak of 2 to 5 inches per year and may continue for several years before returning sharply to pre-spurt rates.

The Sequence of Normal Development in Adolescence

The age of onset of the growth spurt and its duration are related to other physiological changes. Girls who experience an early growth spurt tend to reach *menarche* (first menstruation) early; boys who experience an early growth spurt tend to develop secondary sex characteristics early. Although there is a high correlation in an individual's height before and after the growth spurt, differences do exist. Tanner[2] attributes this variability primarily to differences in the hormones controlling growth before and during the adolescent growth spurt.

Figure 4.2 shows adolescent changes in males and females.

The rapid height and weight changes of adolescence are accompanied by changes in body proportions in both males and females. Although virtually all skeletal and muscular structures participate in the growth spurt, they do so at differing rates. Adult trunk length is achieved last, for example, and frequently

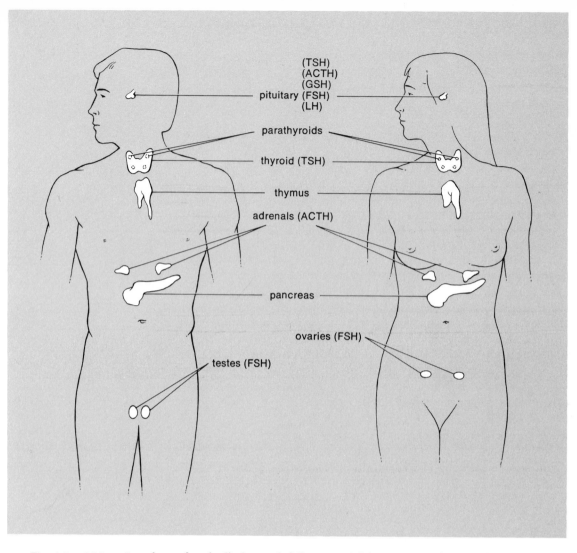

Fig. 4.1. Male and female endocrine systems

(TSH)
(ACTH)
(GSH)
pituitary (FSH)
(LH)

parathyroids

thyroid (TSH)

thymus

adrenals (ACTH)

pancreas

ovaries (FSH)

testes (FSH)

long after the limbs reach full range. A boy stops growing out of his trousers, at least in length, long before he stops growing out of his jackets! Such differences in rates of growth lead to some fascinating, and frequently embarrassing, problems for adolescents.

Muscles, Organs, and Fat

While the size of muscles increases, the percentage of body fat declines in adolescents, particularly in boys. Whereas prepubescent boys and girls have similar strength, adolescent boys tend to be much stronger than adolescent girls. Also, relative to their size, boys tend to develop larger hearts and lungs, greater oxygen-carrying capacity in the blood, lower resting heart rates, and a greater faculty for neutralizing the chemical products of muscular exercise, such as lactic acid.

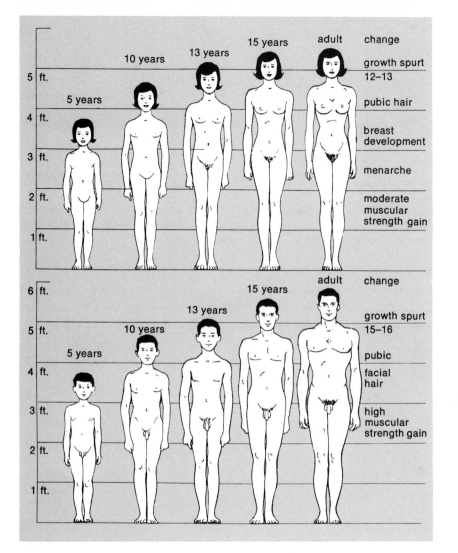

Fig. 4.2. Adolescent body development and sexual maturation in girls and boys (Adapted from Family Living. Sex Education transparency series, copyright 1968 by Hubbard Scientific Company, Northbrook, Illinois.)

By late adolescence boys' hearts and lungs tend to be significantly larger than girls', perhaps as a result of different activities and physiological stresses of the sexes. Similarly, boys tend to have higher basal metabolic rates than girls, undoubtedly due in part to greater muscular development requiring higher oxygen consumption.

Little growth takes place in the brain during adolescence. The child has acquired about 95 percent of his adult brain weight before his eleventh birthday.

Breast changes generally offer the first sign of sexual maturation in females, though some pubic hair may appear first in a few cases. Growth of the uterus and vagina and enlargement of the labia and clitoris occur simultaneously with breast development. Menstruation (menarche) occurs later, usually after the growth

Sexual Maturation: Female

spurt. Menstruation is not necessarily indicative of ovulation. Frequently it is a year or more after the menarche before the adolescent girl is physiologically capable of becoming pregnant.

Age of menarche varies from nine to sixteen and one-half years in the normal population; similarly, breast development can begin as early as age eight or as late as age thirteen. Breast size varies and does not appear to be related to the female's ability to produce milk.

The menstrual cycle affects almost every aspect of daily living for the female. Mood changes, activity levels, social relationships, and even family planning itself depend to some degree on her menstrual rhythm.

Menstruation is the regular discharge of blood and other body fluids from the uterus, and is the only instance in nature where loss of blood is a sign of good health. Menarche has occurred at an increasingly earlier age during the past century, probably because of better nutrition. In unusual cases, menstruation has begun as early as age two and as late as age twenty.

Fig. 4.3. Female reproductive system (Adapted from Family Living. Sex Education transparency series, copyright 1968 by Hubbard Scientific Company, Northbrook, Illinois.)

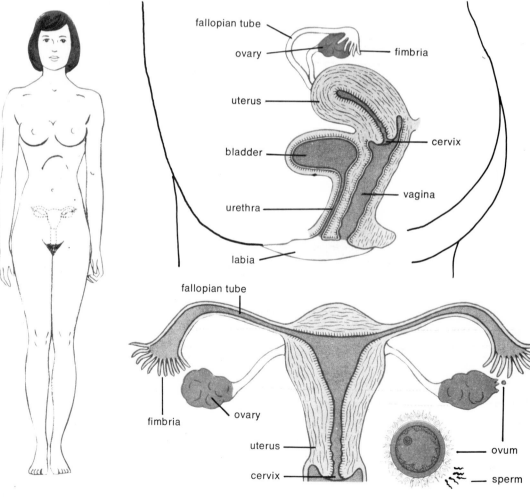

Chapter Four

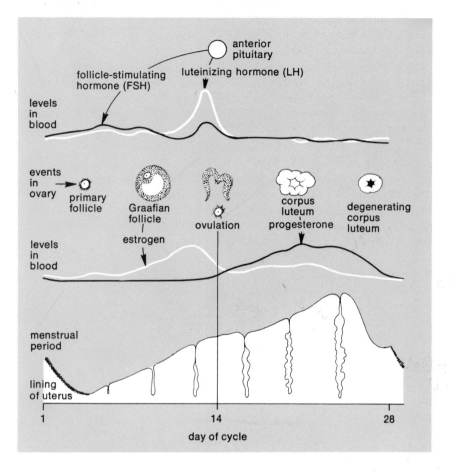

The average menstrual cycle lasts from twenty-seven to thirty-one days in most women, although complete cycles have been reported to have taken place in as few as seven days and as many as three hundred days. Menstrual flow generally continues for three to seven days. In the following analysis, we shall begin with day one of menstrual flow, and we shall assume a twenty-eight-day cycle.

Since conception did not take place during the previous cycle, the unfertilized egg gradually disintegrates, the progesterone level recedes, and menstruation begins the new cycle. Chemicals produced by the hypothalamus stimulate the anterior lobe of the pituitary gland, causing it to release a follicle-stimulating hormone (FSH) into the venous bloodstream. FSH activates the ovaries, and several ovarian follicles begin to mature.

The maturing ovarian follicles produce and release estrogen into the system. This, in turn, alerts the uterus to prepare itself for the next egg. (Indifferent to circumstances, the uterus automatically prepares itself for implantation, regardless of the female's marital status, sex life, or social position.) The inner layer of the uterus begins to thicken and continues to grow through ovulation in preparation for the expected zygote.

Puberty: Psychophysiological Consideration 101

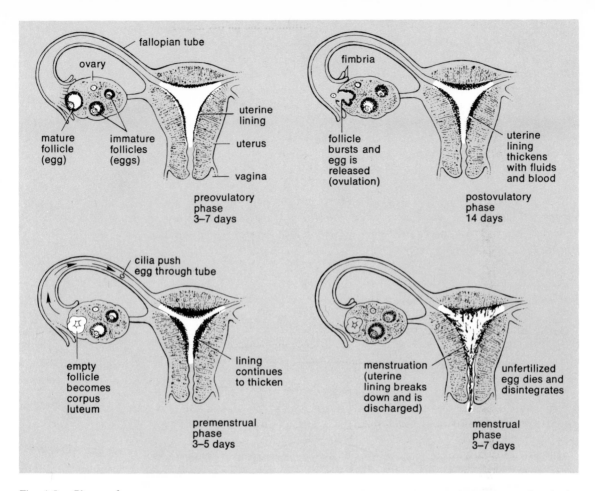

Labels in figure:

Top left (preovulatory phase 3–7 days):
- fallopian tube
- ovary
- uterine lining
- uterus
- vagina
- mature follicle (egg)
- immature follicles (eggs)

preovulatory
phase
3–7 days

Top right (postovulatory phase 14 days):
- fimbria
- follicle bursts and egg is released (ovulation)
- uterine lining thickens with fluids and blood

postovulatory
phase
14 days

Bottom left (premenstrual phase 3–5 days):
- cilia push egg through tube
- empty follicle becomes corpus luteum
- lining continues to thicken

premenstrual
phase
3–5 days

Bottom right (menstrual phase 3–7 days):
- menstruation (uterine lining breaks down and is discharged)
- unfertilized egg dies and disintegrates

menstrual
phase
3–7 days

Fig. 4.5. Phases of a twenty-eight day menstrual cycle. Note the overlap of the premenstrual phase with the postovulatory phase.

Around the tenth day after menstruation begins, rarely later, one developing follicle undergoes a growth spurt and completely matures within the next few days. The follicle moves to the surface of the ovary and prepares for release of the egg. Simultaneously, the anterior lobe of the pituitary gland releases the luteinizing hormone (LH) into the venous bloodstream; LH causes the mature Graafian follicle to rupture and release the egg.

Ovulation, then, occurs at about the middle of the menstrual cycle; there are usually fourteen days between ovulation and the next menstruation. Unfortunately for purposes of birth control, the time between menstruation and subsequent ovulation is far less predictable.

The released ovum is caught by the fingerlike fimbria at the end of the fallopian tube. Hairlike cilia lining the tube gently push the ovum toward the uterus (fig. 4.5).

Meanwhile, the LH causes the empty follicle to close, to increase in size, and to turn slightly yellow in color. Called the *corpus luteum,* this newly formed body produces the hormone progesterone (meaning "to promote pregnancy"), as does the egg itself. Progesterone causes the endometrium in the uterus to swell with rich nutrients in preparation for the fertilized ovum. If fertilization does not occur, the egg begins to disintegrate after about forty-eight hours and stops producing progesterone. About the twenty-fifth day in the cycle the corpus luteum also stops producing progesterone. Pieces of endometrium and mucus from glands in the uterus are carried off in the flow of menstrual blood.

If the egg is fertilized in the fallopian tube, the developing zygote progresses down the tube to the uterus, giving off progesterone as it awaits final preparation of the endometrium. Implantation usually takes place within a week after ovulation. The developing embryo then produces a gonadotropic hormone that stimulates the corpus luteum to continue producing progesterone.

Thus, the mature female is subject to hormonal changes throughout her menstrual cycle. She spends nearly a week menstruating, a week preparing for ovulation, and two weeks preparing for the possible implantation of the fertilized egg in the endometrium.

Personality fluctuations have been closely linked to the menstrual cycle. Such fluctuations vary tremendously both within and among individuals, and raise questions about the predictability of their effects. Highly motivated career women must obviously shield themselves from the adverse effects of the menstrual cycle, while taking advantage of the beneficial ones.

Beginning about day 22, the female may experience premenstrual tension, a condition characterized by anxiety, depression, irritability, and feelings of lowered self-esteem.[3] In contrast, as estrogen levels increase prior to ovulation, positive feelings tend to be high and self-esteem good. There is an increase in the frequency of accidents, absenteeism, and psychiatric counseling requests during the tense premenstrual period.[4] Interestingly, the contraceptive pill affects this phenomenon: the sequential pill complements it, and the combination pill tends to minimize it. "When the hormone levels are fairly constant during the cycle, as in women on combination pills, anxiety and hostility levels are correspondingly constant. When the hormone levels fluctuate during the cycle, emotions correspondingly fluctuate."[5]

Sexual Maturation: Male

The sudden appearance of nocturnal emissions (wet dreams), accompanied by penile erection and orgasm, may surprise and worry the uninformed pubescent boy. Most males experience such seminal flows during sleep at some time during their lives. Frequently this occurs in association with erotic dreams. What causes wet dreams? One must understand the male cycle to appreciate the significance of nocturnal emissions.

The male reproductive system consists of a pair of gonads (the testes) and accompanying excretory ducts: the epididymis, vas deferens, and ejaculatory ducts. These are assisted in function by the seminal vesicles, prostate gland, Cowper's glands, and penis (fig. 4.6).

In normal males the testes descend from the abdomen through the inguinal canal to the scrotum about two months prior to birth. Since sperm can only be produced at slightly less than body temperature, the scrotum is biologically essential for reproduction, and any undescended testes must be surgically assisted

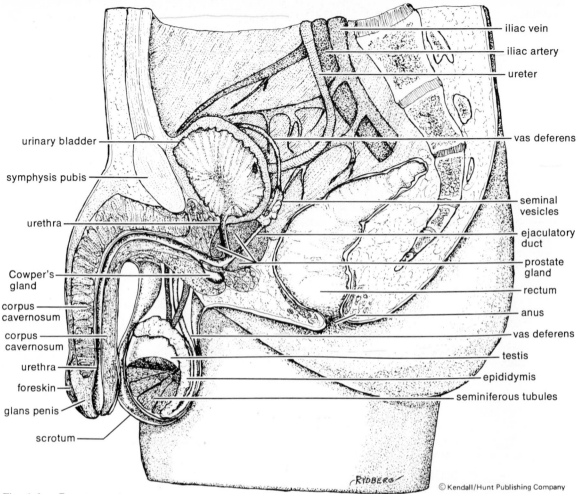

iliac vein
iliac artery
ureter
vas deferens
urinary bladder
symphysis pubis
seminal vesicles
ejaculatory duct
urethra
prostate gland
rectum
Cowper's gland
anus
corpus cavernosum
vas deferens
corpus cavernosum
testis
urethra
epididymis
foreskin
seminiferous tubules
glans penis
scrotum

RYDBERG

© Kendall/Hunt Publishing Company

Fig. 4.6. Cross section of the male reproductive system.

before adolescence to prevent possible sterility. The scrotum is relatively elastic, hanging loose when warm, but pulling up tight when exposed to coldness, such as cold water in swimming or in a shower, or to sexual stimulation.

The testes produce *spermatozoa* by the process of *spermatogenesis* in the germinal cells of the *seminiferous* (sperm-producing) *tubules*. These tubules would measure one to two feet in length if uncoiled, and each testicle contains several hundred of them. The walls of these tubules are lined with germinal tissue. It is here that sperm are continually produced. The space between the tubules is filled with interstitial tissue that, when stimulated by the luteinizing hormone (LH) of the pituitary gland, produces the male sex hormone testosterone.*

*The functions of testosterone are many. Testosterone is essential in the fetus for differentiation of male internal and external genitalia (in the absence of embryonic testosterone, male genitalia would not develop). It also causes the pubescent growth spurt in the genitals, as well as the voice change, anatomical alterations, and psychic responses.

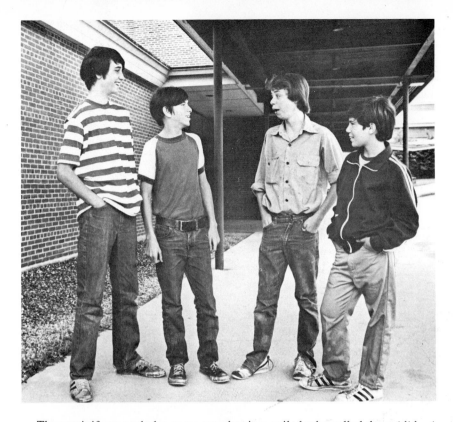

Fig. 4.7. Puberty comes to boys at different times with different results, as can be seen in these four thirteen-year-olds. Everything begins to happen at once—from dramatic increases in height, weight, and growth of sex organs, to less dramatic changes in voice, amount of body hair, skin texture, and emotional balance.

The seminiferous tubules come together in a coiled tube called the *epididymis* behind each testicle. Sperm pass into the epididymis, where they are stored temporarily before being transported by ciliary action to minute connecting ducts, the *vas deferens,* that pass into the abdominal cavity. The vas deferens serves both as a thoroughfare and as a storage vault, particularly near the upper end where it broadens into a pocketlike bag, called the *ampulla,* as it joins the seminal vesicle on either side of the body near the prostate gland. The two seminal vesicles, lying between the bladder and the rectum, secrete fluid as a vehicle for the sperm.

The prostate gland, through which the seminal fluid must pass next, provides a highly alkaline, thin, milky fluid that contains proteins, calcium, citric acid, cholesterol, and various enzymes. The alkalinity of the secretions apparently allows sperm to move quickly through the hostile, highly acidic environment of the vagina.

The prostate is in a continual state of activity, providing both preejaculate and ejaculate fluids. It surrounds the ejaculatory ducts that partially house the semen coming from the seminal vesicles until discharge. When called for, the semen enters the *urethra,* the canal through the penis through which urine also passes. Except for a few sperm occasionally found in urine, urine and semen never use the urethra at the same time. The prostate gland, which also contains muscle fibers, contracts to help eject the semen from the penis.

Two *Cowper's glands,* pea-sized structures situated slightly below the prostate on either side of the base of the penis, operate during excitation. They secrete an alkaline fluid that lubricates the urethra and that serves to neutralize any undue acidity. This fluid, and all of the other fluids that make up semen, are transmitted from the male into the female through the penis.

A cylindrical organ composed mostly of erectile tissue, the penis hangs in front of the scrotum. Its size varies from person to person in both the flaccid and the erect states, and there is little relationship between the size of an individual's penis when it is flaccid and when it is erect. Little relationship exists between penile size and general body size, and virtually no relationship exists between the size of the penis and sexual function.*

The shaft of the penis is covered by a loose skin that is continuous with the skin over the scrotum. As erection occurs, the skin tightens, pulling the scrotum closer to the body in anticipation of orgasm. (Although orgasm can occur without erection, under conditions of anxiety, breath-holding, or suffocation, for example, the two generally go together.) Erection also pulls back the foreskin or *prepuce* (the loose skin at the head of the penis of the uncircumsized male), exposing the urethral opening.

Erections of the penis are not all due to sexual stimulation, nor does every erection result in orgasm. "Morning erections" presumably are caused by bladder tension; sensate erections, like those that may occur when a man holds a tiny infant in his lap, or even periodic erections for no known reasons are common and are not indicative of anything beyond normal functioning. Even newborn babies and young boys experience erections without physical stimulation, probably caused by nerve irritability.

Erection of the penis is controlled by nerves in the spinal cord and involves the synchronization of several reactions. While the brain can enhance or inhibit the sexual response, a man has very limited voluntary control over erection, and what control he does have is most frequently associated with reduction.

As seen in figure 4.6, the penis contains three cylindrical bodies of spongy tissue (*corpora cavernosa*) running its entire length. Friction on the surface of the penis and/or of surrounding areas, sexual thoughts, dreams, exotic odors, or exciting sensations cause impulses to be sent to the sacral area of the spinal cord, or to spinal area of the brain, activating a series of synchronized reactions. The spongy tissue becomes engorged with blood, and a contractile spasm at the base of the penis prevents the blood from escaping through the veins. These reactions are caused by inhibition of the vasoconstriction centers of the sympathetic nervous system and by excitation of the vasodilator centers of the parasympathetic system. These spinal centers, while primarily operating reflexively, are in communication with the cortical, subcortical, and medulla oblongata portions of the brain.[6] As long as there are appropriate stimulations to the penis and/or to the brain, the erection can be maintained. Painful stimulation, emotional trauma, or psychological diversion usually cause an erection to subside.

---

*This discussion is presented in recognition of childhood anxiety about penis size, which is mistakenly linked to masculinity. The size of the penis has little to do with the pleasure experienced by either the man or the woman during intercourse, or with the man's ability to impregnate the woman.

A few drops of fluid (preejaculate) may be released before orgasm, and a series of events build up to a sudden discharge of semen called *ejaculation.* Contractions in the ampulla, the seminal vesicles, and the ejaculatory ducts move the semen to the urethral tract. Then muscle spasms in the urogenital floor discharge the semen in spurts from the penis. Ejaculation is accompanied by a highly pleasurable psychophysical sensation known as *orgasm.* The force of ejaculation varies greatly, but is of little consequence in terms of pleasure or potency.

Ejaculation causes previously dilated arteries to narrow, and less blood flows to the penis than is escaping by way of the veins. Ordinarily about 50 percent of the erection is lost shortly after ejaculation.

What causes wet dreams? Two factors are the constant production of sperm that demand release and periods of abstinence from ejaculation. Sperm can be released in at least three ways: masturbation (direct or indirect), sexual intercourse, or nocturnal emission. In the sexually abstinent male, nocturnal emissions (wet dreams) must be considered a perfectly natural reflex, a safety valve for the testicles that prevents overcrowding and possible rupture. Such wet dreams may occur regularly, particularly in young men whose thoughts and fantasies turn frequently to sexually stimulating events and objects. Production of testosterone is influenced by thoughts of sex and testosterone influences sperm production. The more frequent and stimulating one's thoughts about sex, the greater the buildup of testosterone and the more rapid the process of spermatogenesis, hence, the more frequent the need for release. Wet dreams are a natural outlet for sperm buildup.

Masturbation

More common among males than females, masturbation, or self sexual stimulation, which usually leads to orgasm, is considered quite normal among youth. Recent figures indicate that about 92 percent of males masturbate prior to age twenty; the percentage for girls is somewhat lower. Boys also tend to masturbate more frequently and more openly than girls. Although the practice has probably not changed over the years, more lenient attitudes toward masturbation today have certainly reduced anxiety, conflict, and guilt about the practice. The critical question now is not whether a youngster masturbates or not, but rather what his or her own attitude is toward the practice. If masturbation substitutes for normal heterosexual development or leads to introversion, there may be some psychological problem. Physically, under normal conditions, masturbation is quite harmless, regardless of how frequently it is practiced, and should be considered part of the normal process of sexual maturation.

Self-discovery through sexual stimulation helps very young children understand their anatomy and perceive their bodies as a potential source of pleasure. These early experiences lay the basis for future acceptance of sex as desirable and pleasurable. Only when self-stimulation is given overzealous attention by parents or by others, in the form of either prohibition (Don't do that! followed by a sharp slap) or appreciation (Look at that, a real chip off the old block!), is there much danger of repercussion. In itself and in moderation, masturbation should be viewed as relatively harmless and natural.

Adolescent masturbation is also common and natural in both sexes. Significant physiological differences between the sexes tend to make the practice much more common among adolescent males than females at this stage, though the reverse might well occur later in life. The external appendage of the male is more likely to receive stimulus, direct or indirect, in daily living. Erections are commonplace, and the boy sooner or later recognizes the pleasure associated with such phenomena.

Further, the male is subject to the accumulation of sexual fluids. Practically any form of sexual stimulation, even imaginary, increases the production of spermatozoa and the subsequent flow of secretions from accessory sex glands. The tension created by this buildup must be released, and release comes with ejaculation. Increasing pressure excites the ejaculatory reflex and promotes the tendency within the boy to play with his genitals. He may do this by hand or by rubbing his thighs together or by pressure or friction against or by an object. Often accompanied by reading erotic literature, looking at pornographic pictures, or daydreaming, masturbation may be practiced alone or in groups. Homosexual masturbation in youth is relatively common and hardly indicative of homosexual tendencies. Masturbation is genital-centered, not social, and occurs in most males.

Young females masturbate less frequently than young males. The total number of ova present in the female reproductive system are there long before adolescence, and pressures of space do not occur within the ovaries. When ova begin to ripen, they do so singly or in very small numbers, and are released without accumulation. Further, without direct stimulation, the adolescent female is not likely to respond locally to petting.[7] She also exhibits no reflexive action similar to ejaculation in the male. Owing to the protected nature of the female genitalia, direct stimulation is frequently delayed, and the need or desire for masturbation occurs after the girl has gained a greater awareness of her sexual responses.

The critical concern in masturbation, therefore, is not the act itself, but the reason for it. If it is a substitute for normal social relationships, it may inhibit social development and therefore warrant attention.

Sexual Preference   The development of sexual preference involves a variety of adaptations, both biological and cultural. Sexual structure is genetically determined at conception and hormonally reinforced or altered during the early weeks of life. From birth until the onset of puberty, cultural factors play a dominant role in sex-typing. Most children experience role confusion and conflict in their choice of objects for hero worship. Probably most children exhibit "homosexual" behavior in the form of group exhibitionism, genital comparison, and puppy love for same-sexed elders. The young boy might even "fall in love" with a male hero. There is no harm in this feeling, unless the feeling is carried out in activities, such as group masturbation or strip poker, and the participant subsequently feels guilty or is caught and "labeled." Most kids play "doctor" at some time during their developmental years. If they are caught in the act by parents or neighbors, they may be punished and/or labeled (as sex fiends, for example). The social and psychological repercussions for the individual could be far-reaching. Yet the behavior itself is quite common and harmless. Getting caught and being labeled are the real problems.

Endocrine secretions influence attitudes and behavior before, during, and after puberty. Sexual urges and tensions grow more acute as puberty progresses, and the need for a clear sex-role identity increases. The identity need not lie at one extreme or the other. The behaviors of many individuals remain between the extremes of purely homosexual and purely heterosexual. Few persons are probably entirely feminine or entirely masculine in their role behaviors.

Gender identification is more complex than just genes. Kinsey claimed that men and women could range over a continuum from strong masculinity to strong femininity. Money has demonstrated the same in terms of morphology. It may be possible, then, for a woman to be born "trapped in a male body," or vice versa. It is also possible for individuals to combine in many ways. This helps to explain the wide range of body-personality types witnessed today.

Whereas many people direct their sexual activities solely toward members of the opposite sex, others prefer exclusive sexual involvement with persons of the same sex, and it would still be true today to say that there is also a considerable number of males and females "who include both homosexual and heterosexual activities in their histories. Sometimes their homosexual and heterosexual responses and contacts occur at different periods in their lives; sometimes they occur coincidentally."[8]

Homosexual behavior is not an either-or condition, and one must consider the importance of time, age, situation, and degree of involvement. When Kinsey reported that the actual incidence of homosexuality was around 40 percent in the male population,[9] he included all forms of homosexual behavior, and failed to distinguish between a behavior that is preferred and commonly practiced and many insignificant homosexual behaviors occurring among large numbers of the population. Since most young boys and girls participate in some relatively innocent sexual behaviors with members of the same sex during their developing years, it is particularly important to distinguish between homosexuality and sexual play. Labeling young children as homosexuals can be dangerous and full of repercussions for the individual.

Homosexual Behavior

There are many theories about the causes of homosexuality, ranging from culture to endocrines, to heredity, and trauma. None is entirely satisfactory. Although some endocrine dysfunction is common in men who are exclusively homosexual, evidence is generally inconclusive and may be misleading. The dysfunction could be a cause or it could be a result of the behavior.[10]

The Greeks considered everyone bisexual and worshipped the god Hermaphroditos who possessed both male and female genitalia. Male homosexuality was a cultural cornerstone in Spartan life. Boys generally slept among other young men and were taught that they owed no love to either their wives or their children. The Spartan husband spent very few hours with his wife, even on the wedding night, lest he stir up jealousy among his male lovers at the barracks. Marriage was encouraged, but only to provide warriors for the state.

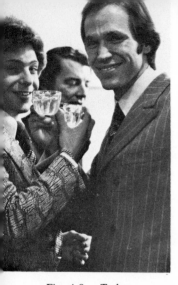

Fig. 4.8. Today homosexuals are being accepted by society. In some states homosexuals even marry.

Heredity, physique, and clothing are not valid indicators of homosexuality. Only a very small percentage of homosexuals can be readily identified by overt mannerisms or clothing.

Neither genes nor hormones determine the choice of the sex object. It is the cultural influences that teach heterosexual (or homosexual) behavior.[11]

Although estimates of homosexual involvement among the population vary greatly, it is generally believed that about 10 percent of the population is actively gay and less than half of these are exclusively homosexual. Some are married and have children.

Homosexuality appears to be more common among males than among females, although there are insufficient data on this. Female sexual behavior generally seems to have been treated with indifference. Perhaps the single most important step in acceptance of homosexuality is the American Psychiatric Association's stand: the Association no longer classifies homosexuality as an illness or a perversion.

In recent years homosexuals have increased their efforts to have their life-style accepted by society. An individual should not be discriminated against because he or she is "gay." Even though some Americans strongly object to homosexuality, our society must not prohibit homosexuals from enjoying certain rights, freedoms, and opportunities guaranteed to every citizen. For most homosexuals, their life-style appears to be one of considered choice.

Heterosexual Behavior

Most males and females prefer heterosexual relationships. Our entire family system is based on the pairing off of boys and girls to perpetuate our species. To some extent, emphasizing heterosexual behavior and marriage has been necessary: for the protection of the state (to produce soldiers), the care of aging parents, the maintenance of the family farm or business, the reduction of conflict in securing and keeping a mate, and the control of sex. Yet today, in a world fraught with population problems, with a variety of legitimate and illegitimate alternatives to marriage, one has every right to consider the questions, "Why marry?" "Why have children?" "Why settle with only one partner?" "Why push heterosexuality?"

Summary

The physiological changes each of us undergoes at puberty have been examined. This chapter has discussed at length similarities and differences between the male and female sexual systems and the behavioral phenomenon of masturbation. Understanding sexual development in adolescence may help you better understand yourself and those younger than you who are experiencing similar psychophysiological development. With this understanding you will be better equipped to empathize and to understand your peers.

Sexual preference involves a number of personal considerations. Homosexuality was discussed in this chapter under sexual preference. Because heterosexuality is more commonly associated with courtship, marriage, and family, it will be treated in chapters 10 through 12 much more extensively than it has been here.

1. Why is the pituitary gland referred to as "the master gland"?
2. List and describe the various hormones secreted by the pituitary gland that are responsible for body growth, development, and regulation.
3. Compare normal growth in adolescent males and females.
4. Describe the sexual maturation of females.
5. If you were a parent, how would you describe menstruation to your daughter?
6. How does progesterone affect the menstrual cycle?
7. What is meant by the term "premenstrual tension"? Do women experience it, or is it a theoretical fabrication?
8. Trace the path of the sperm from development to ejaculation.
9. What are the functions of testosterone?
10. Explain the importance of the prostate gland. Of Cowper's glands.
11. Discuss the pros and cons of circumcision.
12. What causes wet dreams?
13. How has the attitude toward masturbation changed over the years?
14. Why is masturbation more common in the male than the female?
15. Is homosexuality a sickness? Why or why not?
16. What physiological determinants are found among homosexuals?

Notes

1. J. J. Conger, *Adolescence and Youth* (New York: Harper & Row, 1973), p. 94.
2. J. M. Tanner, "Physical Growth," in *Carmichael's Manual of Child Psychology*, ed. P. H. Mussen, vol. 1 (New York: John Wiley & Sons, Inc., 1970), p. 94.
3. Conger, *Adolescence and Youth*, p. 112.
4. K. Dalton, "The Influence of Mother's Menstruation on Her Child," *Proceedings of the Royal Society for Medicine* 59 (1966): 1014. K. Dalton, *The Premenstrual Syndrome* (Springfield, Ill.: Charles C. Thomas, 1964).
5. J. Bardwick, *Psychology of Women: A Study of Bio-Cultural Conflicts* (New York: Harper & Row, 1971), p. 37.
6. J. L. McCary, *Human Sexuality*, 2d edition (Scarborough, Ont.: Van Nostrand Reinhold Ltd., 1973), p. 75.
7. B. A. Kogan, *Human Sexual Expression* (New York: Harcourt Brace Jovanovich, Inc., 1973), p. 20.
8. A. Kinsey, W. Pomeroy, C. Martin, and P. Gebhard, *Sexual Behavior in the Human Female* (Philadelphia: Saunders, 1953).
9. A. Kinsey, W. Pomeroy, and C. Martin, *Sexual Behavior in the Human Male* (Philadelphia: Saunders, 1948).
10. R. C. Kolodny et al., "Plasma Testosterone and Semen Analysis in Male Homosexuals," *New England Journal of Medicine* 285 (1971): 1170–74.
11. B. A. Kogan, *Human Sexual Expression* (New York: Harcourt Brace Jovanovich, Inc., 1973), pp. 297–98.

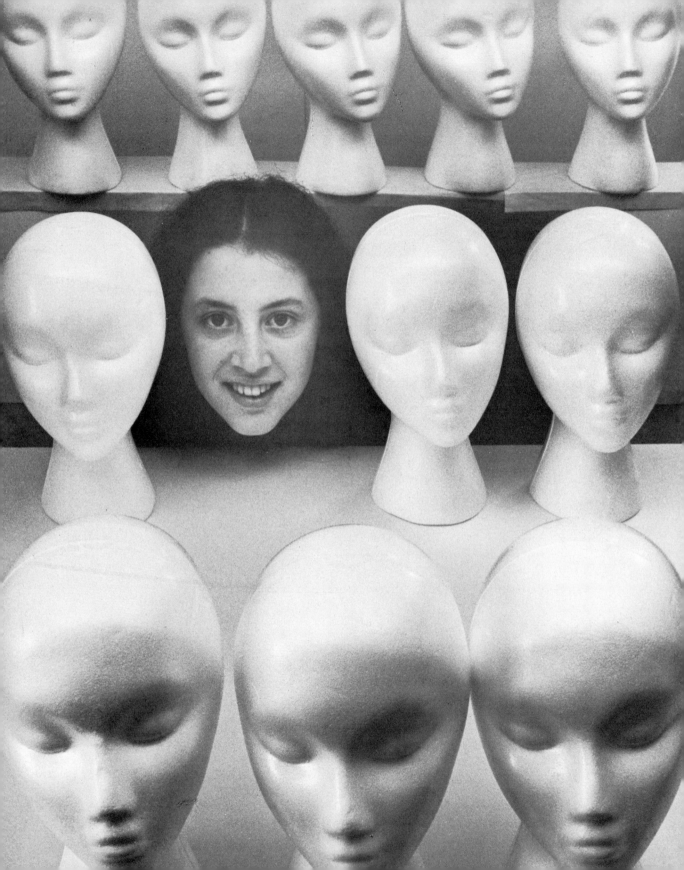

Personality and Self-Development: Indexes of Adaptation

5

In the collective life of societies, each new generation of young people has been rightly perceived as the rather fragile vessel by which the best of the past—the hard-won fruits of one's painful and slippery steps up from the primordial mists—is transmitted into the present.[1]

Caught in a whirlpool of opposing forces, both internal and external, in an age in which the self and society frequently appear to be in conflict, young persons must resolve competing ideologies and develop coping skills and life-styles strong enough to enhance their chances for attaining personal goals. The study of the methods used to accomplish these tasks is the study of humans adapting, and the consistency of individuals' adaptations reflects their psychological makeup or personality.

Although experts disagree on the theories of personality development and on the names and numbers of adaptations young persons must undertake, some consensus is evident on the latter issue. The major task is one of self-identity or ego-identification, which answers the question "Who am I?" Apparently all other developmental tasks of youth come after this.

One assumption underlies the entire process of self-identification: an individual develops through the continuous interaction between a growing, changing biological organism and its physical, psychological, and sociocultural environments. Self-identity, then, is the product of a complex series of interactions. Developmental adaptation continues throughout life, and many people never really answer the question "Who am I?"

Since adolescence is also the period of rapid biological and psychosocial change, the problem of adaptation throughout this period is complex. No wonder youth is so frequently unpredictable; the demands of adaptation are sometimes overwhelming.

Keen, cool, freaky, tough, spastic, terrific—these words have often been used to describe the impact one person makes on another. Such perceptions of individual behavior and mannerisms are commonly called personality characteristics. The so-called personality, therefore, is seen in terms of how one person rates another and how one person impresses another. This idea is confirmed in a once-popular song, which has the vocalist proclaim: "He's got personality!"

The Unique Personality

A Concept of Personality

A more accurate understanding of the human personality may be developed through the following descriptions of students confronted with test situations.

Mark typically panics. In the words of his friends, ''he seems to fall apart,'' especially at midterm and final exam time. Although adequately prepared, he seems to ''go blank,'' predictably misreads test questions, and often leaves the test room early, after throwing down his answer sheet with most of the items left unanswered.

Although she tends to worry about tests and always expects the worst, *Connie* studies hard, reads over class notes, and arrives at the examination room ''fresh as a daisy.'' She analyzes the test carefully and finishes first those test items she knows for sure. While she never thinks of herself as a bookworm, she rarely scores less than 85 percent on her tests.

Phil, the BMOC, is ''bugged'' by tests, which he views as rude interruptions of campus life. Because he knows the true value of such exams, he waits until the night before the test and then ''crams'' for several hours. He puts in just enough effort to win the ''gentleman's grade'' of C. After all, there is nothing wrong with being average or flunking a test occasionally.

In each case described, a predictable pattern of reactions to a particular situation is identified. These fairly consistent ways in which a person reacts make up the personality. Such reactions are said to reflect one's personal characteristics or dispositions, the psychological makeup of the individual.

Personality
as Adaptation

Personality includes the somewhat general, yet consistent, variations in the ways that individuals adjust or adapt to problems or perplexing situations. Common ways of adjusting or adapting include coping, solving problems, reducing tension, fulfilling needs, compromising, and being flexible.

In an explanation of human behavior, Lazarus relates the personality to these adjustive and adaptive processes.

Stable forms of adjustment can be regarded as traits of personality, in other words, characteristics of a person that make it possible to differentiate that person and his or her behavior from others in a variety of situations and occasions. We say, for example, that one individual tends to persist in striving even after suffering defeat, while another gives up.[2]

Personality can be viewed, then, as an index or measure of adaptation, without any particular value being placed on the quality of personal responses. As described, personality is merely a reflection of probable behavioral reactions. It should be emphasized, though, that one's behavior is more than a mirror of the mind or psyche. Behavior is the result of the personality's interaction with physical and social forces.

Shaping Forces
and
Self-Development

Most authorities who study personality and self-development believe that many complex forces interact continuously throughout life to shape human behavior and techniques of adaptation. However, there is no agreement over which factors, those of heredity or those of environment, are more influential.

Heredity refers to one's genetic inheritance, already present at birth and unaffected by learning or by the physical and sociocultural environment. At the time of conception each of us receives the basic potential for development and behavior. In describing this genetic inheritance, Coleman and Hammen state that

> this endowment includes potentialities not only for . . . physical structure but also for striving, thinking, feeling, and acting, and for patterns of growth and change throughout a predictable life cycle.[3]

Some evidence suggests that states of feeling, emotional expressiveness, and motivating powers of pleasure, displeasure, excitement, and depression are strongly determined by the genetic code. Relatively stable tendencies, present from birth and existing into adulthood, have also been noted. These include the tendency toward certain levels of activity, passivity, crying, nurturing or mothering in both males and females, sensitivity to specific stimuli, and adaptability. Even the human brain, with its capacity for storing data, reasoning, and learning, and its interconnection of nerve cells and pathways, represents a genetic endowment common to all humans that is yet responsible for our unique differences.

In his research William Sheldon related types of temperament to types of inherited physique or body build. Three structural components of physique or body build were identified by measuring muscle mass and fat deposits beneath the skin. Brief descriptions of Sheldon's body-build classifications (somatotypes) are as follows.[4]

- Endomorphy—Physical roundness marked by prominence of the abdomen, digestive organs or viscera, poor muscle and bone development, fatness, and softness. The extreme endomorph is somewhat circular in shape, rather short, and stocky.

- Mesomorphy—Heavy shoulders characterized by firmness, hardness, strength, and upright physique. Bones, muscles, and ligaments are highly developed, and the mesomorph's shape is described as athletic and triangular, with the base at the top.

- Ectomorphy—Slenderness identified by slight development of muscles, bones, and organs of the viscera. The ectomorph is viewed as fragile and slender, with a flat-chest and a shape described as a straight line.

Sheldon then distinguished three groups of personality characteristics or temperaments that he found correlated with the basic physiques. Each temperament—viscerotonia, somatotonia, and cerebrotonia—was marked by a general manner of behavior and certain goals in living, as illustrated in table 5.1. (It should be emphasized that correlation does not necessarily mean that body build causes a particular temperament or set of personality characteristics.)

Although one's body build is inherited, research has shown that a particular somatotype may have some physical and temperamental characteristics of the other two basic physiques. Research and personal experience have also shown that, through various physical adaptations such as dieting, exercising, and changing clothing styles, one's body build can be appreciably modified within limits.

Table 5.1 Sheldon's Correlation of Physique with Temperament and Personality Characteristics

Physique	Temperament	Personality Characteristics
Endomorphy	Viscerotonia	Easy-going, good-natured, loving, very sociable; enjoys eating, drinking, and sleeping; realistic, practical
Mesomorphy	Somatotonia	Bold, assertive, active, energetic, aggressive, present-oriented, noisy; easily tolerates fasting from food when engaged in physical activity
Ectomorphy	Cerebrotonia	Inhibited, restrained, secretive, difficult to awake in the morning, alert at night; active in thought processes, night-dreaming, and self-meditation

Fig. 5.1. Part of a person's genetic inheritance is body build. Sheldon found that physique and personality are related.

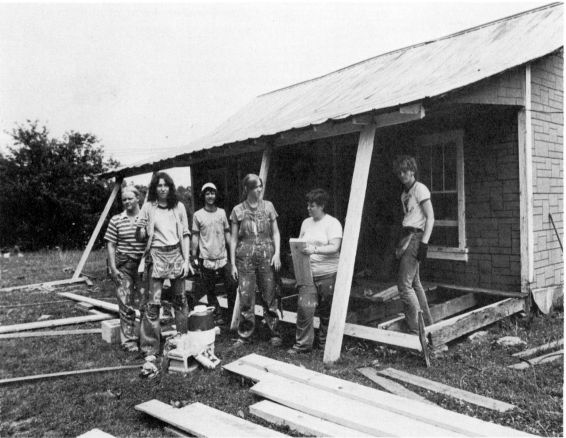

Chapter Five

The environment represents those shaping forces of our physical surroundings, together with the influences of society and culture. Factors of altitude, weather, family interactions, social class, economic status, religion, ethnic background, education, social interrelationships, childhood training, mass media, and the opportunities or restrictions in one's surroundings are quite influential in personality development, as well as in fostering specific values and beliefs.

Society itself often fosters certain personality responses by imposing specific *role expectations,* or life parts, on developing individuals. These expectations, with their accompanying scripts of anticipated behavior, are reflected in traditional and approved mannerisms associated with the roles of parent and child, student and teacher, and male and female. Until very recently, for instance, social expectations for the male generated traits of independence, assertiveness, directness, and objectivity, but severely limited displays of outward affection. Females were expected to be passive, dependent, creative, subjective, and nurturing. Although such role expectations have often produced sex-role stereotypes (behavior traditionally associated with either the male or female), they have nevertheless been powerful determinants of human reactions and responses in given situations.

In addition to imposed role expectations, the environment influences personality formation through the mechanism of *operant conditioning.* By definition, operant conditioning is a form of learning whereby correct responses are reinforced by rewards and thus become more likely to be repeated. Unrewarded or punished responses are less likely to be repeated. The application of operant conditioning is evident in those cases in which parents successfully change children's overly dependent behavior by using a series of positive reinforcement procedures. For example, first-graders who are reluctant to be separated from their parents and extremely afraid of school may receive small pieces of candy, coins, verbal praise, and family approval for attending school. The modified behavior—attendance at school—is thus supported. In schoolwork, an academic grade of A is equivalent to a reward for superior performance, whereas an F represents not only failure, but also punishment through the denial of class credit.

Another powerful yet subtle influence on personality is *modeling.* This form of learning is basically the imitation by one person of a significant other person's behavior. Parents serve as important models for children as they display various emotional responses, decision-making skills, and coping behaviors. This is especially true in the case of child abuse, a tragic national problem of immense proportions. Research now indicates that children who are abused by their parents grow up to be abusing parents themselves, apparently because they are following the parental model observed during their formative years. Peers, famous athletes, television and motion picture stars, and other celebrities also serve as models of behavior for humans both young and old.

With so many environmental and hereditary factors interacting in the developing personality, there is little wonder in the countless variations that occur in human behavior. And as the individual confronts new and challenging problem situations with a wide range of responses and adaptations, the behavior reflects an even more unique and distinct person, namely you.

Sequential
Growth of
the Personality

Freud and
Psychosexual
Growth

While modern psychologists no longer agree with some of his original ideas, Sigmund Freud was the first investigator of human behavior to view personality as a composite of dynamic, interacting, and sometimes conflicting subparts or systems. He also proposed a psychoanalytic theory of personality development. According to this once revolutionary explanation, one's personality passes through various stages of psychosexual growth between infancy and adulthood.

Freud's construct of the personality has three distinct subparts or structures—the id, the ego, and the superego—which identify various mental processes and functions. The id is the source of psychic energy (libido) expressed as basic, primitive instincts or drives. The instincts are of two major types: (1) those concerned with life and survival, and (2) those focused on death and destruction. Blind and irrational impulses from the id demand immediate satisfaction.

A second subpart of the personality, the ego, functions to satisfy the demands of the id within the realities of the external world. Through the mental processes of perceiving, thinking, and deciding, the ego redirects the id impulses so that they can be satisfied in some reasonable manner.

The third subpart, the superego, gradually evolves as the force of conscience representing moral and social values, restraints, and inhibitions. Sometimes the psychological forces of the id, ego, and superego are in conflict and thus create anxiety in the individual. When the id and superego come into conflict, the ego resorts to defensive tactics in its role as referee between the opposing forces.

According to Freudian theory, adult behavior is directly related to early parent-child relationships and to conflicts aroused in the following five stages of psychosexual development.[5]

Oral Stage   Throughout the first year of life, the infant derives pleasure from the mouth, mainly from sucking, biting, and chewing. Unfulfilled oral needs, anxiety (free-floating fear), or insecurity during this developmental stage may give rise in the adult to personality traits of dependency, passivity, greediness, and tendencies toward smoking, chewing, and talkativeness.

Anal Stage   During the second and third years of life, the infant's primary pleasure is associated with anal activities of holding and expelling fecal matter. Conflicts and fears related to toilet training may surface years later as personality traits of stubbornness, stinginess, destructiveness, and a tendency to inflict pain.

Phallic Stage   In the fourth and fifth years of life, manipulation of the sexual organs is the child's source of pleasure. The young boy normally directs his sexual feelings toward the mother, while the young girl is attracted to her father. Such a situation places the child in hostile competition with the parent of the same sex: it gives rise to the Oedipus complex in the young male, and to the Electra complex in the young female. Through repressing such sexual desires or by identifying with the parent of the same sex, the complexes are usually resolved. Complications, though, are related to the later development of homosexual tendencies, difficulty with authority figures, and rejection of appropriate sex roles.

Latency Stage From about the sixth year of life until adolescence, no significant personality changes occur. Psychological conflicts are minimized or repressed, and few fears are aroused that would adversely affect the child's behavior as an adult.

Genital Stage With the onset of puberty and the reemergence of sexual instincts, individuals' interests shift away from their own bodies, their own parents, and their own needs. The focus of their interest is adult heterosexuality and the needs of others. With the accomplishment of these developmental tasks, psychological maturity is achieved.

Departing from the influences of both Freud and the behavioral psychologists who emphasized the role of learning in personality formation, Abraham H. Maslow proposed a new concept of personality growth and development.

Maslow and the Self-Actualizing Personality

Maslow's humanistic approach recognizes the central role of personal striving and self-intention in determining the direction of one's life. In developing a theory of personality health, Maslow made several basic assumptions:[6]

- Each individual has a biologically based inner nature that is partly unchangeable.
- This inner nature is shared by all members of the human species and yet is partly unique to the individual.
- One's inner nature is either neutral or positively good, rather than necessarily evil.
- It is desirable to bring out and encourage one's inner nature rather than suppress it.
- Denial or suppression of one's inner nature results in sickness.
- The delicate inner nature is easily overcome by "habit, cultural pressure, and wrong attitudes about it."
- Even if denied, the inner nature "persists underground forever pressing for actualization," i.e., striving for personal growth and fulfillment.
- Discipline, deprivation, frustration, pain, and tragedy can be desirable experiences if they "reveal and foster and fulfill our inner nature."

Fig. 5.2. Through willing and striving, one can determine the direction of one's life, says Maslow.

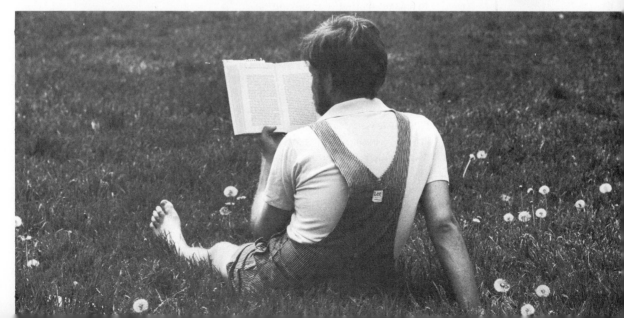

According to Maslow's theory, one's inner nature of strivings (motivations) for personal fulfillment can be achieved only when certain maintenance needs (thirst, hunger, social acceptance) are satisfied first. Thus there is a sequential order or hierarchy of needs ranging from the lower, biological ones to those of a higher, self-fulfilling nature.

Physiological needs: food, water, sleep, activity
Safety needs: avoiding threats and bodily harm; protection and self-preservation
Belongingness and love needs: affection, warmth, attachment, attention
Esteem needs: status, reputation, worthiness, prestige
Self-actualization needs: personal growth and professional accomplishment; vocational fulfillment; realization of one's capacities and talents; becoming a more organized and functioning person

Maslow maintained that personality develops in a continuing progression from lower needs to higher needs. When one level of needs is satisfied, then the next higher level can dominate one's personality and behavior. For the mature personality striving is an ongoing process to free oneself for growth-oriented behavior. On the other hand failure to progress to higher levels of need satisfaction can result in psychological illness, anxiety, despair, boredom, inability to enjoy, aimlessness, and a lack of personal identity.

Self-actualization or growth behavior is concerned with developing proficiencies and increasing personal capabilities. While it is difficult to measure self-actualization, Maslow identified some characteristics of healthy psychological growth.[7]

A clear perception of reality
Comfortable in relation to one's surroundings
Tolerant of uncertainty
Spontaneous in responsiveness
Creative
Self-accepting
Relatively independent
Able to love
Problem-centered rather than self-centered
Identified with all humankind

Additionally Maslow offers some personal and objective indexes of self-actualization or growth toward it. These include feelings of zest in living, happiness, serenity, calmness, responsibility, and confidence in handling problems. How would you rate yourself in progress toward self-actualization?

A Word of Caution

Because of the relationship between personality and mental health, researchers have proposed many theories about the nature and significance of human behavior. Although the several explanations presented here may seem to be conflicting, they are more complementary than competitive. Other complementary approaches to personality development will be illustrated later in this chapter when Erikson's theory and the processes of self-definition and self-identification are discussed.

While each explanation of personality development has its unique focus, none should be accepted as the ultimate or exclusive truth. Each theory offers some insight into the personality as a whole. The remainder of this chapter will be devoted to helping you better understand yourself and your pattern of adaptive responses to the tasks of youth.

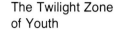

"Hiatus status" is a term frequently applied in literature to a condition of youth in general and of college students in particular. It denotes the existence of a twilight zone, a state in which the individual is neither here nor there, but in a state of suspended animation, caught in a normless existence or moratorium, bewildered and rootless. Depending to some extent on financial and living arrangements, the freshman college student in particular may experience for the first time a real feeling of independence from the family. Clearly the human relationship is changed, and the young person's first day on campus is generally perceived as a rite of passage, a landmark in the developmental process. Home is never quite the same again.

In American society the university experience is likely to bring about cross-pressure from the student's many reference groups. The family and peer groups in particular present the student with contradictory, or at least inconsistent, expectations. Sometimes the contradictions between expectations of family and peers are real; other times they are imagined. The critical fact is that, real or imagined, they result in symptoms of stress and raise real questions for the student about potential behaviors. Whereas a few months earlier the student might have enjoyed a conservative life-style within a closely knit family, in the first few weeks at a college or university he is presented with numerous opportunities, real or imagined, to engage in virtually any activity, ranging from sex to religion, from drug-taking to starvation or transcendental meditation, from athletics to pure intellectualism.

The Twilight Zone of Youth

Fig. 5.3. College students, caught in the cross-pressures between family and friends, seek comfort in various activities.

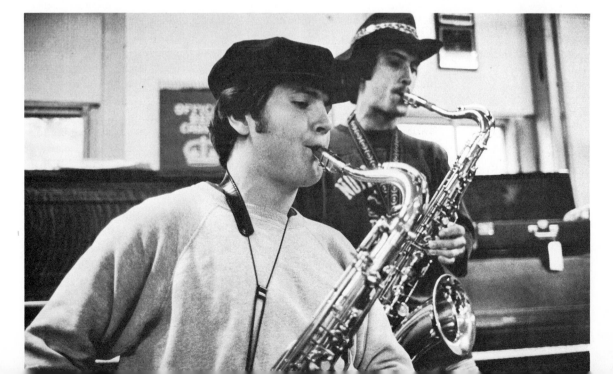

As college students tend to depend more and more on their peers, parental relationships begin to change. Peer influence increases as students progress from the freshman year through the senior year, and it is particularly strong in the social realm of fraternities, sororities, teams, clubs, and other group memberships. Various allegiances create occasional conflicts and simultaneously pull the unsuspecting individual in different directions. Cast in an environment in which other people always seem to have the answers, to be more experienced, more knowledgeable, and more confident, the student seeks comfort in any number of behaviors, ranging from complete withdrawal to overzealous participation.

College experiences can be somewhat artificial, in that cognitive development is frequently encouraged and functional maturation is inhibited. The tendency to idealize is strong. Grandiose schemes to solve the world's problems are often proposed, but frequently die untried. The college community is often a world unto itself, truly the ivory tower.

Suspended in the cross-pull of forces, the college student faces the classic tasks of growth—ego-identity, sex-role identity, independence, and vocational choice—in a setting where family, college, peer groups, and other associates continue to expect certain behaviors and accomplishments, with or without consideration for the individual student (fig. 5.4). Each group participates in the establishment of goals, norms, roles, and sanctions for the individual. Each makes demands, applies pressure, and seeks priority. Integrating the effects of these expectations—putting it all together—is complex indeed!

The Tasks of Youth: Self-Identification

Who Am I?

Although the problem of self-identity is likely to be most critical during adolescence, it neither begins nor ends there. Young children pass through a series of identities: daddy's girl, a cowboy, a Smith, a Methodist, one of Peter's gang, another Jack Nicklaus or Chris Evert, and so forth. New identities are frequent, and fantasy plays a major role in the child's daily experiences. With limited and undeveloped mental abilities, narrow time perspectives, and few critical decisions to make, most children live in well-protected worlds. This changes with adolescence.

Oddly enough, the less democratic a society, the easier the task of self-identity. In a dictatorial military state, for example, identification may be as simple as this:

> I am a Spartan boy, a young warrior. My life belongs to the State; everything I do or say is for the State. I will raise new warriors by impregnating my wife—but I will live among my warrior friends. For me, life is serving the state—and that is all that matters.

The dilemma in our own society is the range of choices available to us; the more we appreciate the variety of choice, the greater our quandary. What a paradox—the greater one's awareness of the alternatives, the greater the range of decisions one might make, as in the choice of one's vocation. The greater the number of potential choices, the less one feels that any one decision is the right decision. The greater the insecurity in this decision, the less likely one is to identify with that career choice, and the more fragile one's self-identification

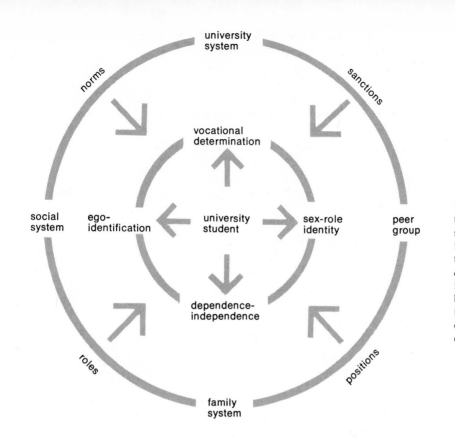

university
system

norms

sanctions

vocational
determination

social
system

ego-
identification

university
student

sex-role
identity

peer
group

dependence-
independence

roles

positions

family
system

Fig. 5.4. This classic tasks-of-youth wheel shows that the common force that creates tension is the *expectation*, real or imagined, that emanates both from within the individual and from each of the external components.

with respect to that choice. The problem is borne out by the facts—few people stick with their first jobs, many people are not really happy in the jobs they finally choose, and some people really do not identify with their work at all.

Similarly, free-choice marriages produce greater stress and more instability than arranged marriages. In cultures in which arranged marriages are the custom, the mates have little or no say about who their partners will be, and consequently their major concerns lie beyond the choice of a marriage partner. While the partners must learn to get along, the marriage and its roles have been anticipated for years, and the couple doesn't expect a twenty-one-gun salute every time they "make love." American couples, on the other hand, not only have to adjust to each other's life-style, but the partners are further plagued with such questions as "Did I really marry the right person?" "Could I have done better?" "Was I too young for marriage?" "Was I really ready for marriage?" "Should I have looked longer?" "Should I divorce and try again?" Choice creates tension. Complexity increases stress. Freedom makes self-identification difficult.

Self-identity is a lifelong search. Decisions affecting career commitments and interpersonal involvements are made daily, and all of them test one's identity, offering potential for change. Yet the problem of self-identity seems to be most acute in youth, at a time

Fig. 5.5

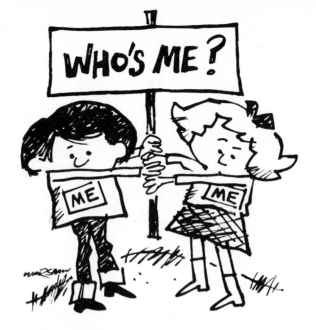

when the individual is confronted with what is virtually a physical, physiological, and cognitive revolution within himself, he must also consider how he is going to deal with the varied intellectual, social, and vocational demands of adulthood that lie directly ahead.[8]

Development of Self-Identification   How does a sense of identity develop? How does it change? According to Erik Erikson, a famous psychoanalyst, such an identity evolves gradually out of the many identifications of childhood.[9] It includes but goes beyond the sum of all earlier identifications in which the child wanted to become like, and was frequently forced to become like, the people he depended on. Although all prior, continuing, and future identifications play a part in the development of self-identity, they alone do not produce it. One needs the capacity to put together all of these parts into a coherent, consistent whole.

It is a widely held view that self-identity evolves or develops along with several other basic tasks, such as those described in Erikson's eight stages of human development illustrated in table 5.2. To the extent that an individual is able to complete the basic task at each stage successfully, that person moves on to the next task with increased self-confidence. The tasks are never really finished, but continue throughout life. Successful confrontations with basic tasks at earlier stages, however, make the resolution of later tasks easier. Thus adequacy in the development of basic trust, autonomy, initiative, and industry should help individuals define themselves in terms of function, unique characteristics, life goals, and estimations of self-worth and social acceptance. The evolution of self-identity is not an all-or-nothing proposition. Some persons achieve it relatively early in life, some later in life, and others not at all. By modifying Freud's theory of psychosexual development, Erikson emphasized the importance of mental processes in the human being's adaptations to the forces of physical and social

Table 5.2 Erikson's Eight Stages of Human Development

Stage	Developmental Phase	Basic Task	Characteristics of Psychosocial Crises
I	Infancy—oral-sensory (first year)	Basic trust vs. mistrust	Confidence originates in mother's consistent actions and care of infant's needs; mistrust develops from a sense of abandonment and deprivation.
II	Early childhood—muscular-anal (1–3 years)	Autonomy vs. shame and doubt	Expressions of independence, coupled with parental protection, surface; failure to achieve autonomy results in self-consciousness, feelings of inadequacy, and self-doubt.
III	Preschool—locomotor-genital (3–5 years)	Initiative vs. guilt	Pleasure derived from attack and conquest, self-observation, and identification with same-sex parent in work roles and adult roles; denial and inhibition give rise to guilt.
IV	Elementary school—latency (6–11 years)	Industry vs. inferiority	Desires for production, use of tools, doing things with others; nonaccomplishment results in a sense of inadequacy and mediocrity and in conformity.
V	Adolescence—puberty (12–19 years)	Identity vs. role confusion	Concern with other persons' views of oneself and with the search for continuity, values, and commitment to ideals; failure to achieve identity gives rise to role confusion and doubts about one's sexual and occupational identity.
VI	Young adulthood (20+ years)	Intimacy vs. isolation	Willingness to enter affiliations, to make self-commitments and close friendships, and to express heterosexuality; avoidance of intimacy related to fears of losing self and to developing sense of isolation and self-absorption.
VII	Middle adulthood	Generativity vs. stagnation	Capacities of teaching, guiding the next generation, producing, and creating evolve; without generativity, a feeling of personal impoverishment and nonaccomplishment develops, along with psychological nonmovement.
VIII	Late adulthood	Ego integrity vs. despair	Embraces the order and meaning of one's life, with its joys and sorrows; defends dignity of the life cycle; the sting of death is diminished; without enough time to start life anew, feelings of disgust and fear of death predominate.

reality throughout the life cycle. He redefined personality as "... a reality-oriented, continually learning, and always adapting system."[10]

As noted in table 5.2, the individual progresses through various developmental stages (the eight ages of man).[11] Each stage presents the person with a unique psychosocial crisis. The crisis or conflict is between two dynamic counterparts, one positive and the other negative. However, Erikson warns that each stage should not be seen as an achievement of goodness, completed once and for all, since "the personality is engaged with the hazards of existence continuously, even as the body's metabolism copes with decay."[12]

Therefore none of the stages is really exclusive. At times, a person may be coping with all of the tasks together. On the other hand the more successful one is in completing each task in turn, the less likely one is to return to it later.

At each stage the lasting results of a "favorable ratio" between conflicting attitudes or tasks are development of "essential strengths" of personality: self-control and willpower; direction and purpose; method and competence; devotion and fidelity; affiliation and love; production and care; and renunciation and wisdom. These personality traits tend to reemerge from generation to generation.

Variety in Self-Identification

The patterns of identity formation vary widely, and may be influenced by many forces, positive or negative, including social change itself. Persons trying to avoid the anxiety of seeking an identity, such as the youngster who identifies as the teacher's pet, may form premature and frequently unstable identities. "His sense of identity can become permanently fixed on being nothing but a good little worker or a good little helper, which may or may not be all that he could be."[13]

Some people never really achieve a self-identity. They wander aimlessly, year to year, always in a hurry, but getting nowhere. A good example of this is found in Jack Kerouac's *On the Road*.

"Whee. Sal, we gotta go and never stop going till we get there."
"Where are we going, man?"
"I don't know but we gotta go."[14]

One's self-identity, once established, is not completely fixed, though change is usually more apparent than real. The inner core (the psychological genotype) remains relatively constant; only the incidentals change, and they may or may not affect the character (or psychological phenotype). A change in job may alter a person's outer manner, for example, but probably not his central core. Also people really do not change much with age. A stubborn fool before marriage is usually the same old stubborn fool twenty years later, married or not.

Role models frequently affect the process of gaining self-identity. When the role model fails, or drastically changes course, the follower is left in either a vacuum or a quandary. There is a beautiful example of this in *Siddhartha,* Hermann Hesse's famous character novel. Having left home at a young age, turning aside a promising life as a Brahman priest, the young Siddhartha seeks wisdom through a series of great teachers, many of whom he adopts as role models and from whom he learns much. Eventually, however, he suffers in recognizing that even the greatest and wisest cannot teach him what he really needs to learn. He ponders the dilemma.

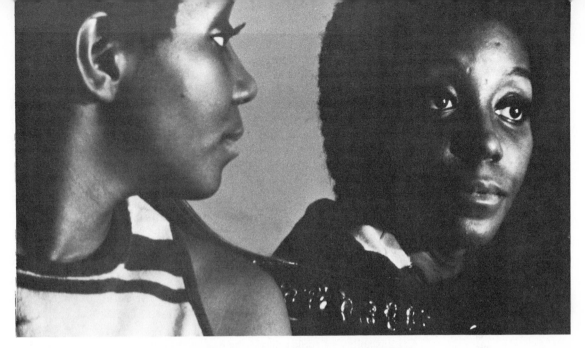

What is it you wanted to learn from teachings and teachers, and although they taught you much, what was it they could not teach you? And he thought: It was the Self, the character and nature of which I wished to learn. I wanted to rid myself of the Self, to conquer it, but I could not conquer it, I could only deceive it, could only fly from it, could only hide from it. Truly, nothing in the world has occupied my thoughts as much as the Self, this riddle, that I live, that I am one and am separated and different from anybody else, that I am Siddhartha, and about nothing in the world do I know less than about myself, about Siddhartha.[15]

The story is a good one, for Siddhartha seeks answers in many fields—religion, Yoga-Veda, Artharva-Veda, asceticism, sex and love, even business—yet finds that in all of these he avoided what he needed most.

I was afraid of myself, I was fleeing from myself. I was seeking Brahman, Atman, I wished to destroy myself, in order to find in the unknown innermost, the nucleus of all things, Atman, Life, the Divine, the Absolute. But by doing so, I lost myself on the way.[16]

There is a striking similarity between Siddhartha's quest and that of contemporary youth. The major difference often lies only in the means—Siddhartha didn't use sports, drugs, or sexual conquest as we frequently do today, but he could have.

It is almost amusing how quickly we alter images. Beer-drinking law students suddenly acquire a taste for scotch once they become practicing attorneys; cigarette-smoking undergraduate students switch to a pipe in graduate school; shy freshmen become avant-garde ''seniors'' when next year's freshmen arrive on campus; and playboys become strict fathers when their daughters reach puberty. Some people even become religious with advancing age . . . just in case! Situation obviously plays a major role.

Many young people seek self-identity through ''mind-expanding'' experiences, including the use of psychedelic drugs. Occasionally these experiences are revealing; frequently they are not. An interesting corollary to drug experiences is the actual trip, at home or abroad. Young people are frequently heard to say, ''I'm going to Europe for a year, just to lie in the sun, smoke pot, and find myself,'' or ''I'm going to bum around for a year or so and, you know, try to put it all together—get a grip on myself.'' Unfortunately, unless that person has sufficient material for the synthesis of self-identity, it is more likely that the year off will just delay the resolution of any current confusion, rather than hasten it. One must seek to find; yet even this is paradoxical. Siddhartha said:

> When someone is seeking, it happens quite easily that he sees only the thing that he is seeking; that he is unable to find anything, unable to absorb anything, because he is only thinking of the thing he is seeking, because he has a goal, because he is obsessed with his goal. Seeking means: to have a goal; but finding means: to be free, to be receptive, to have no goal.[17]

Some people never achieve self-identity. Perhaps most people never achieve identity entirely, but some don't even come close. These are lifelong adolescents who ''cannot 'find themselves,' who keep themselves loose and unattached, committed to a bachelorhood of preidentity.''[18]

The instability of adolescence is natural, claims Erikson.

> There is a ''natural'' period of uprootedness in human life: adolescence. Like a trapeze artist the young person in the middle of vigorous emotion must let go of his safe hold on childhood and reach out for a firm grasp on adulthood, dependent for a breathless interval on his training, his luck, and the reliability of the ''receiving and confirming'' adults.[19]

As in most aspects of life, the simpler the identity, the easier it is to achieve and maintain. Although it is highly unlikely that many intelligent and/or educated people ever achieve complete confidence in their self-identities during the more active phases of their lives, virtually all seek it. Perhaps it is unfortunate that we have so loudly proclaimed adolescence as *the* most critical stage in identity-seeking. ''Would some of our youth act as openly confused and confusing if they did not know they were supposed to have an identity crisis?''[20]

Inadvertently we have given the adolescent license to behave in joyous, random, abandoned disorder, and frequently we see him take full advantage of that license!

The Tasks of Youth: Sexual Identity and Sex Role

In these times of the so-called sexual revolution, the concepts of sexual identity (gender identity) and sex role (gender role) are of continuing importance. For some, there is no greater concern than what it means to be a man or a woman in today's society.

The private, inner sense or awareness of self as male or female is defined here as one's *sexual identity*. It is at the very core of your unique definition of personhood, and as a personal estimate of one's sexual nature, it becomes an anchor of emotional health or illness. On the other hand, *sex role* is the outward expression of one's sexual identity revealed in speech, mannerisms, sexual arousal and response, and interrelations, which indicates to others the degree to which one is either male or female. These definitions are based on the work of John Money and Patricia Tucker, who emphasize that sexual (gender) identity and sex (gender) role are not two different entities. Rather,

> . . . they are different aspects of the same thing, like the proverbial two sides of a coin. Your gender identity is the inward experience of your gender role; your gender role is the expression of your gender identity.[21]

Individual perceptions of sex role are being challenged today by a society that is disregarding some of the traditional gender stereotypes. Indeed, socially determined sex roles are not only changing, but merging, as more women enter the fields of politics and science and as more men actively engage in childrearing and household management. Some people perceive these changes as threats to their own sexual identities, particularly with regard to aggressiveness and assertiveness, seduction, virginity, vocational choice, marriage, parenthood, display of affection, initiation of sexual activity, and one's sexual feelings.

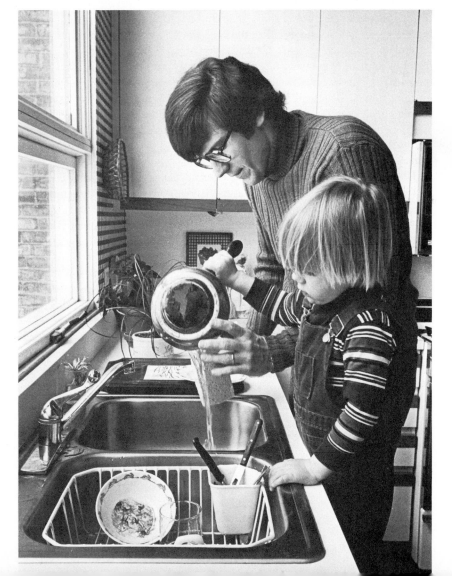

Fig. 5.7. Today, men are taking a more active part in childrearing and household management.

Even more threatening to some is the recent scientific revelation that concepts of masculinity and femininity are not necessarily absolute, permanent, and unalterably determined at birth by the sex chromosomes. Indeed, most sex differences are relative, the result of varying hormonal and socially imposed influences, and develop in stages during prenatal life, infancy, and childhood. In addition, Money and Tucker maintain that sex differences ''can be assigned as long as we allow . . . that men impregnate, and that women menstruate, gestate, and lactate.''[22] These are the only so-called biologically imperative differences between males and females.

There is an emerging consensus that the major factors in the development of sexual identity are (1) the silent effects of learning through psychological reward and punishment experiences, and (2) the experienced modifications that result from frustration, trauma, and conflict, and the attempt to resolve these conflicts.[23]

Nevertheless, sexual differences in behavior and roles, as well as in work and play, probably will always exist to some degree. It is just too difficult to change an adult's perception of maleness and femaleness once it is learned so well in early childhood. In reality, some specific sex roles do exist, and there are at present some differences between the sexes in their social roles.

As indicated in chapter 4 in the discussion of physical and chemical changes in puberty, testosterone levels in boys consistently exceed those in girls prior to puberty. At puberty, however, the young male's testosterone level increases ten to thirty times. Beginning at a much lower base, the testosterone level in the young female merely doubles. These overwhelming differences, seen in the light of all evidence linking testosterone to activity, competitiveness, and aggression, may help explain the physical aggressiveness and increased sex drive found in adolescent males.

Conversely, among females, the menstrual cycle has been shown to be related to fluctuations in psychological state, probably as a function of changing levels of various female hormones, particularly estrogen and progesterone. Since women taking the combination oral contraceptive pill do not experience as much emotional fluctuation as those taking no pill at all, one plausible hypothesis is that there is a link between personality and menstrual cycle.

Evidence exists that boys also experience psychophysical tensions due to high testosterone levels and to the accumulation of sperm. This evidence is frequently used to explain the state of excitability in males that leads to the desire for orgasm. We do know that testosterone is at a higher level in the morning than at any other time of the day and that the level varies to some extent with sexual stimulation. We also know, however, that lack of orgasm for any length of time is quite harmless. When a boy claims he ''has to have sex,'' he is technically accurate (accumulating sperm must be released) but sociologically misleading (the sperm may be released involuntarily in wet dreams or voluntarily through masturbation or petting). Sexual intercourse is hardly essential.

Sex Role and Identity in the Male   The rewards for a strongly masculine orientation in adolescence are high, but they rapidly diminish with maturity. While the assertive, well-built, independent, aggressive male (within limits, of course) is frequently considered the man of social prestige (MOSP) on campus or the big man on campus (BMOC), few vocations support that role. In fact, within contemporary American society, highly masculine vocational roles may be relatively low in social, if not financial, reward (boxer, trucker, professional wrestler, rodeo rider). The more prestigious vocations frequently combine "masculine" independence and assertiveness with "feminine" nurturance and interpersonal sensitivity, for example, physician, teacher, minister. This undoubtedly occasions turmoil in the young male, caught as he is between the more immediate image of a man of social prestige on campus and the long-range picture of a man in society. Which way should he lean? How much, and when?

Although changes in sex role are occurring today, radical departures from past expectations are not likely to become the ideal. Males and females are clearly different—anatomically and chemically or hormonally, and probably emotionally in certain instances, due to early learning from role models. The more males and females strive for sameness, the less they rely upon their innate strengths and the greater their eventual role confusion as they realize they cannot achieve satisfactorily in tasks for which they are not well suited or adequately prepared. The mind and the body are not dichotomous.

Sex Role and Identity in the Female   The female, too, is socially rewarded for maintaining a strongly feminine orientation in adolescence. As she moves away from the family, however, her independence, assertiveness, and competitiveness must increase. In some instances the pressure to adopt more "masculine" traits is relieved through marriage and the acceptance of motherhood. In other instances, marriage and motherhood only intensify the female's problem.

Perhaps we have uncovered the reason why the classic teenage marriage of the high school athlete and the campus queen is predestined to conflict. If both are

Fig. 5.8. Today, women are increasingly taking jobs and assuming responsibilities traditionally held by men. The young woman at the left is a lineman, and the girl at the right is one of the first female jockeys to compete with men in professional races.

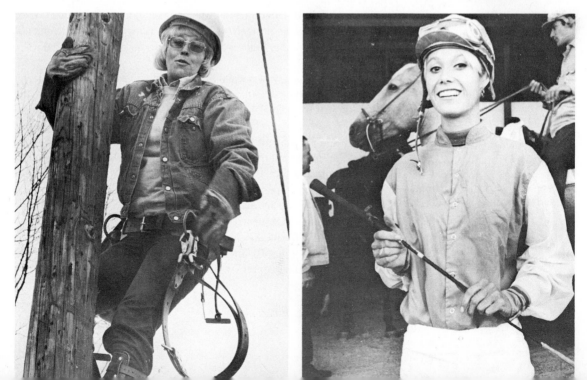

caught up in their stereotypic identities at the time of marriage, their identities will be particularly subject to challenge over time, and both will have to revise drastically their concepts of ideal self. Peer group values change with age, and the "super jock" and "plastic woman" of high school days may no longer be idealized in college. As each partner in turn realizes the need for an overhaul in identity, each may move to make the adjustment. Even if each is capable of adjusting, it is doubtful that both will be able to do so at the same time and that both will be able to cope with their own frustrations, as well as those of their partner. And even if all of these adjustments take place in harmony, who's to say that the "new" bride and the "new" groom will find each other suitable as mates? The odds are heavily against it. Of course, the odds are heavily against the success of early marriage, as will be noted in chapter 11.

Stereotypes breed their own problems, for the narrowness of their definitions is incompatible with a transient society. Both sexes undoubtedly experience great trauma in their attempts to achieve sex-role identity. The current movement toward unisex only masks the problem and delays the solution. As long as real biological differences exist between the sexes, unisex, even in role development, is somewhat artificial and frequently unrewarding.

Communes have idealized *androgyny* (a situation free of sex-role differentiation), yet none has really even approached it. Until men bear children and truly share in the early upbringing of children, androgyny is impossible. However, the development of desirable human traits such as rational thinking, objectivity, assertiveness, concern, and sensitivity is needed in both sexes.

Stereotypes, so commonly portrayed in the electronic media, increase the difficulty that young people have in establishing their own sex-role identities. Although the popular heroes at the time of this writing will undoubtedly be different from those at the time of your reading, examine the current heroes and note their stereotypic behavior. Generally the same stereotypes also will appear in books, lyrics, and even comic strips. Few "normal" lives are depicted in any medium. The norm is far too dull for entertainment; it belongs at home. Unfortunately for young people, home is never "normal" ("Other homes may be 'normal,' but not ours"), and as a consequence, many young people look to the mass media for guidance. What a tragedy!

Perhaps the greatest travesty of normal life as it is depicted in the media lies in the time distortion. At 9:05 P.M., for example, a man and a woman meet for the first time; by 9:06 P.M. they're in bed making love; and by 9:07 P.M. he's off on another mission, and she's nowhere to be seen. All perspective of time, of human interplay, and even of mystery is lost; yet people of all ages frequently confuse fiction with reality and try to adopt the behaviors they have witnessed in the realm of entertainment.

One major effect of the women's liberation movement has been to legitimize a wide range of behaviors and involvements for females. To date, this has not happened for males, and consequently many men are still trapped in stereotypic behavior as it is shown in the media. Many men still deny themselves the right to be wrong, particularly in front of women. For many men, the narrowness of the male stereotype is so stifling, oppressive, and all-consuming that they are not

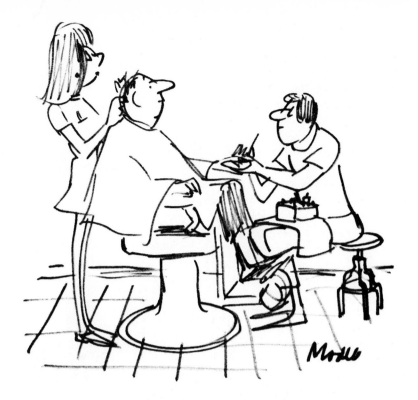

Fig. 5.9. As women have assumed employment usually carried on by men, so have men assumed traditionally female roles as shown in this cartoon.

Drawing by Modell; © 1975 The New Yorker Magazine, Inc.

free to act spontaneously in an emotional situation. And yet freedom to express oneself voluntarily is a human characteristic, a step beyond instinct, a departure from the autonomically controlled stimulus-response pattern.

The development of independence is central to any discussion of the tasks of adolescence, not only in its own right, but also because of its intimate relationship with the accomplishment of other tasks.[24]

The Tasks of Youth: Dependence and Independence

Without the achievement of some autonomy, the adolescent can hardly be expected to develop mature sexual relationships, pursue self-directed vocational interests, or develop a true sense of worth. Self-identity is possible without independence, but in its absence the evolution of a positive self-image that will stand up under pressure over time is doubtful.

Independence is a relative state and must be considered in both concrete and abstract terms. Frequently, half of the battle is feeling independent, regardless of the actual state. The sixteen-year-old who purchases a first car feels quite independent, until the payments for gasoline, insurance, repairs, and the consequent expansion of social activity catch up with him.

In our eagerness for independence we become frustrated at what we don't have, particularly money. Financial status is often assumed to be the single most important variable in the quest for independence and probably the one that is least understood. True independence is having complete control over earning and

Personality and Self-Development   133

Fig. 5.10. By not marrying until they are older, these young people will increase their chances for a successful marriage.

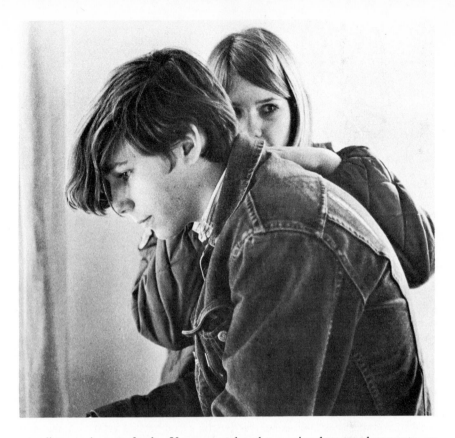

spending one's own funds. Young people who receive large endowments, or even guaranteed allowances (with or without conditions attached), may feel that they are independent, when in fact they are not, since the source of their money is entirely external to them and outside their control. Further, many young people leave home or get married early as a demonstration of their independence, only to find themselves even more dependent on their families later for shelter and emotional and/or financial support. It is unusual for a young couple to start out wanting less than they had in their own homes. What they forget is that it took their parents many years to arrive at their current position.

Young people seeking independence by means of communes, drugs, promiscuity, travel, or simply isolation find that freely chosen, nondirective behavior is frustrating, shortsighted, and brief—with very few exceptions, humans detest freeloaders. Even if virtually every other criterion for freedom is met, most of us depend on others for social support.

What we really seek, then, is not total independence, but a degree of freedom compatible with our current needs. We wish to control our own destinies. Nine times out of ten we'll do what is expected of us, or what could have been predicted for us, but we demand the right to do the unpredicted. Even if we clearly understand the dire consequences of a particular decision, we demand the freedom to make it. We demand the right to be wrong!

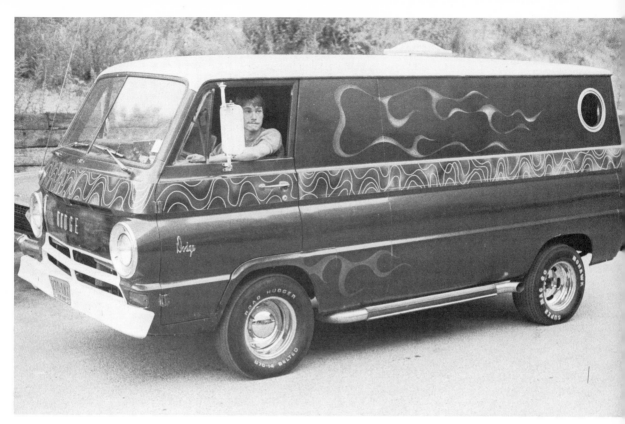

Absolute freedom destroys freedom. When the college dormitory votes to have freedom from rules about noise, it deprives its members of the freedom to have quiet for study (unless soundproofing in every room is perfect). When roommates agree on unlimited visiting privileges, they may give up their freedom of privacy, and the desire for privacy is a transient state. Freedom begets confinement when freedom becomes absolute. Absolute freedom can be stifling. What is really needed then is responsible freedom, the freedom of realistic alternatives.

Total independence is, of course, impossible. We are all dependent on air, food, space, shelter, clothing, biological rhythms, gravity, water, and myriad other life-supporting materials and conditions. We do seek, however, a level of independence, a degree of freedom compatible with our total capacities. We want to feel capable of controlling our own destinies within the general limits of our personal, ecological, and sociocultural surroundings.

Freedom depends on trust in human nature and in oneself. Only when we truly know ourselves, can truly predict ourselves, can truly control ourselves, and can truly predict happenings in our entire ecosystem can human beings enjoy a measure of independence. Independence depends on structure and our ability to work within it. What we seek, therefore, is limited—but we strive to get as close to the limits as we can!

Fig. 5.11. Making decisions and choosing alternatives are part of freedom. The independence that this young man feels in buying and revamping his own van must be accompanied by the maturity to make wise decisions about how to use the machine.

The Tasks of Youth: Vocational Choice

The youth who recognizes and accepts his destiny early, whose path is clear, whose goal is attainable, whose abilities are equal to the task, and who strives unremittingly toward his goal is fortunate indeed, and quite unusual. This may well be the case for a Prince Charles of England, or a Baby Doc Duvalier of Haiti, or a Donny Osmond of the United States, but few others fit the description. For most of us, basketball, football, the stage, and other sports and entertainment are among the few vocations that offer people opportunities to succeed quickly—people who may not even speak English or have any talent beyond their very specific field. They only have to "sell tickets" by singing, swinging, playing, hitting, running, catching, or whatever. Such routes to success are not common in industry. They are the exception!

For individuals deciding on a vocation, their early interests in and attitudes toward particular fields may change quickly. What may stimulate them today may be quite boring tomorrow. Even new inventions grow obsolete quickly, and one's reputation in a field is almost always subject to daily tests in the early years. Values change, and unless individuals completely identify with their chosen job, they are likely to doubt its real worth from time to time. Since, ideally at least, one's vocation is an extension of oneself in a productive sense, one's choice of vocation is constantly subject to the same challenges as one's self-concept. To maintain vocational integrity, therefore, one needs the same flexibility that is essential to the maintenance of one's ego-identification. The closer one identifies with the vocation itself, the tighter the fit. Such adaptation becomes a lifelong challenge!

The Tasks of Youth: Developing a Value System

The Nature of Values

Decision-making is often difficult, and actions frequently precede the development of a rationale for them. How often, for example, after having done something unusual or out of character, have you been asked "Why did you do that?" and you had to invent a reasonable response on the spot? And how often have you given a reason and then come to believe that it is a good one, that it must have really been the cause for your action? The mind is capable of wonderful shifts in perception of cause, effect, and time, particularly when such shuffling helps relieve embarrassment, anxiety, and even guilt. Ideally, though, decision-making is based on your system of values.

Value systems are odd—they keep changing. No two systems are exactly alike, and few people agree on whose values are best. But just what are values? In their simplest form, values are preferences. They are expressed in the internal choices people make when alternatives are available. However, values are hierarchical or ordered in character, ranging from simple to complex, from local to universal, and from single to multiple. Let us examine a few.

Horne has claimed that some values are universal, that is, widely held throughout the entire world.[25] He proposes that health, character, social justice, skill, art, love, knowledge, philosophy, and religion are the basic values of human living. Others have claimed that only the fight for life, the quest for knowledge, and the acceptance of something greater than the self are universal

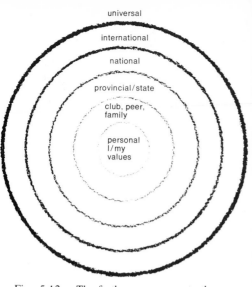

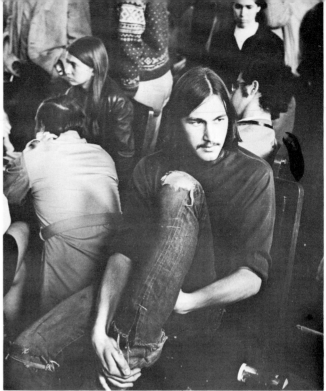

Fig. 5.12. The further one moves to the outside of the values wheel, the more stable are the values. The validity of the entire wheel, however, depends upon the *respect* one has for the values of others and the *responsibility* one holds in the personal decision-making process.

values. Undoubtedly, there are many such theories, but they are not critical for our discussion here.

If you will just accept the idea of universal values, we can place them on the rim of a broad wheel (see figure 5.12), without any confining boundary and just outside the ring of international values.

Slightly less concerned with the welfare of others are the so-called international values. These values can be defined by some of the ways in which they are expressed; peace, as in the United Nations; child nurturance, as in the United Nations Children's Fund (UNICEF); education, as in the United Nations Educational, Scientific, and Cultural Organization (UNESCO); health, as in the World Health Organization (WHO) and the Red Cross. Though agreement between nations may be strained at times, particularly during conflict, these internationally acclaimed values are common among most countries of the world.

National values form a still smaller, inner ring, differing from country to country in terms of both character and emphasis. Americans favor democracy, it's true; yet the pursuit of democracy is quite different in the United States and in Canada. Further, local issues create different hierarchies of values within these countries—in the United States, preoccupation with black-white integration; in Canada, the English-French dilemma. Although many values are the same for both North American nations, still many are different.

There are even greater differences in values as we approach the center of the wheel, viewing values at the regional, state, municipal, church, school, family, group, and individual levels. The closer we move toward the center of the wheel, the closer we get to the "I" level, and the more diverse and changeable the values become. At the individual level, for example, a person may detest all foreign languages at one minute, and then meet a fascinating foreigner the next, and suddenly develop a passionate liking for that person's language. Individuals' values can and do change quickly, depending on how deeply those values are held and at how many levels they are influenced. The greater the influence on particular values from outer rings, the less likely they are to be changed easily.

The Problem Is Change

Instability of values is common, but it is disturbing for individuals who are working toward an acceptable concept of self. "How can I know myself when my values keep changing, when new experiences give me greater insight, and greater insight gives me a better perspective?" The question is common, the answer simple. All of the "preferences" discussed so far have been relatively tangible, readily recognizable. Two new ones need to be added that are less objective: respect and responsibility.

Respect, for oneself and for others, and responsibility for one's decisions that affect others are two concepts that permeate the entire value system and provide a framework for decision-making at all levels, but, most important, at the individual level.

Respect means behaving out of consideration for oneself, but in deference to others. It includes, therefore, due respect for one's own needs and desires, as well as those of others.

Responsibility, of course, means accountability or liability for one's own actions and may be regarded as a natural partner for respect. Operationally, an individual holding these twin values of respect and responsibility is obliged, when making value decisions, to examine all available facts, seek new information, and examine the full consequences of alternative decisions.

This is not merely an expression of pragmatism (whatever works is right); values apply equally to both the ends and the means. Nor is this definition of responsiblity stated without concern for religion, or law, or family, or tradition, for all of these, and more, must be considered in making value decisions. The definition is not unrealistic, for it demands no more than the decision-maker is able to give; it simply insists that the individual fully explore the limits of the problem in making decisions of consequence.

The wider the frame of reference for a given value, that is, the farther out it is on the values wheel, the more unchangeable it is. Some people refer to these broad values as *extrinsic* values (meaning coming from without) or values determined primarily by others—values we are expected and educated to accept. Conversely, the closer we move toward the center of the wheel, toward ourselves alone, the more changeable a value becomes. This is to be expected—the farther out a value is on the wheel, the greater its impact on the entire system, in terms of both current argument and history. The outer limits are as broad as humanity, the inner circle as narrow as the self.

One can expect universal values to change slowly, if ever, and individual values to change more frequently. Individual preferences may even change daily, but these shifts usually involve only minor questions. The more important the choice, even for the individual, the less changeable it is, once it is made. Individual values are called *intrinsic*. Their strength depends entirely on how strongly we are committed to them, and it often takes a test for us to realize the extent of our commitment.

At fifteen, for example, we may feel disgust for drivers who exceed the speed limit; at sixteen, we may frown at those who don't. Obviously our commitment at fifteen to that value, abiding by traffic regulations, was not strong! On the other hand, there may be a difference between one's attitudes and one's behaviors. A white storekeeper, for example, may be prejudiced against blacks, yet not discriminate against them behaviorally in his store. In this case, the "dollar" value supersedes other, less important considerations. Similarly, young boys may say they strongly oppose masturbation, yet masturbate frequently; older men clearly may accept the practice in others, but not masturbate themselves. We find far more young people who *believe* that premarital intercourse is acceptable than who actually engage in it. Situation is obviously a factor here, but so is the complexity of the "attitude versus behavior syndrome."

One of youth's most confusing tasks is coping with the association of love and sex. Traditional American society binds the two together, even setting a schedule for their mutual development. Contemporary society questions that bond and challenges even the idea that the two need be related. Popular writers propose that young people engage in a variety of interpersonal experiences, including cohabitation with full sexual expression, if both partners agree. In his famous novel *The Harrad Experiment*[26] Rimmer invented a coed environment free from the restraints of contemporary society, one in which boys and girls shared everything from showers to beds. Sexual involvement was limited solely by the boundaries of mutual consent and responsibility. However, students were expected to study and discuss the questions of sex before experimenting with it, and they were expected to use contraceptives. The double standard did not apply, and egalitarianism was preached. Harrad, however, was fictional.

Coeducational dormitories are common on college campuses today; visiting privileges are liberal, and heterosexual cohabitation is common. Still the conflict of love and sex persists and gives rise to lively debate between generations.

In *The Sexual Wilderness* Vance Packard claimed that "boys tend to play at love when what they really want is sex; girls play at sex when what they really want is love."[27] Sex and love are treated as things, and both are used for buying and selling in the dating and mating markets. Love and sex have not always been linked, nor are they always so linked today. In the days of chivalry it was common for a knight to love his towered princess, to sing to her, crave her, suffer for her without the slightest hope that he might bed her. (One should remember, of course, that the only time a knight ever "showered" was when it rained or when he fell in the moat. This may have influenced the female's tendency to remain in the tower!) In those days marriage was for reproduction and for family maintenance only. Love was a separate value, generally reserved for someone in an

The Tasks of Youth: Resolving Love-Sex Conflicts

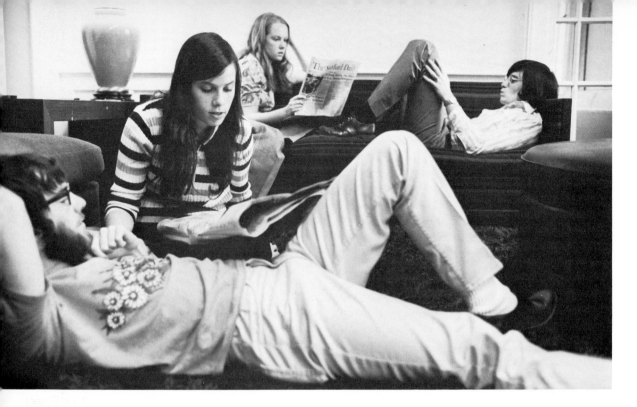

Fig. 5.13. Coed living arrangements are both popular and common at many American colleges and universities. Students feel segregated housing creates an artificial situation in that men and women are not segregated by sex in the "real" world.

exalted position, such as a princess, goddess, or beautiful person. The loved one was unattainable, and, as a consequence, sex and love were often associated with different people.

Today it is still quite common for males to dissociate love and sex, as evidenced in the *Playboy* philosophy. It is becoming increasingly common for females to do the same, though the tendency toward expectation of "strong affection" persists.[28] Sometimes affection develops quickly, when the need arises. Couples sometimes fall in love over a drink or two, make love to express their affection in a mutually satisfying way, then forget all about it the following morning.

Although today's females express less guilt over short-term sexual involvement, still they need some assurance of affection. In a way, females require some room for rationalization, some room in which to maneuver so as to calm a restless conscience. Guilt-producing behavior has a diminishing effect when it is repeated frequently. As a consequence, once a level of behavior is reached, even if it produces twinges of conscience, it will probably be repeated again and again. Such a behavioral pattern is potentially hazardous in a youth culture that revels in risk-taking behavior. It also plays havoc with the development and maintenance of a personal value system.

The peer group and its demands play a major role in the "attitude-behavior syndrome," as do the family, the church, and the social environment. Each of these might be described as a *reference group*, or as an audience of real·or imaginary persons to whom certain values are imputed.[29] These are audiences before which one tries to maintain or improve one's status. Behavioral decisions are generally made within the context of one or more reference groups.

Reexamine the schematic representation of the tasks of youth in figure 5.4 and you will see that we are caught in the middle of many reference groups, all exerting their influence, actively or passively, on our decision-making. Levine[30] believes that even in college, conformity to peer-group expectations provides the transition between dependence on parents and the attainment of personal adulthood. Although potentially the student is influenced by many groups, most studies show that parents and peers are the most important ones.[31] As the student advances through college, the peer group assumes more and more influence, particularly when it comes to questions of sexual behavior.

Teevan's study of reference groups and premarital sexual behavior involved interviews with more than 1,200 male and female college students from all geographical regions in the United States.[32] His study verified previous findings of direct correlation between personal and peer group attitudes and behaviors. More important, however, he found that students who merely perceived peers as being sexually permissive tended to be sexually permissive themselves. Students with a strong peer-group orientation tended to conform not only to the expectations of their friends, but also to the expectations, as they perceived them, of all their age-mates. This finding has serious implications for ''truth'' in advertising about student behavior in all fields. College students, as well as most human beings, tend to be swayed both by real peer group behaviors and by their anticipations of peer group behaviors. If students have unrealistic perceptions of peers' expectations or behaviors, their personal decisions about their own values and behaviors are involved. In these instances, extrinsic values clearly dominate intrinsic values and make life exceedingly difficult for innately sensitive and responsible people.

Unfortunately, few data are available on the influence of real versus anticipated peer group behavior on personal behavior. If personal decisions are based on anticipated or perceived peer group behaviors that in reality are different from actual behaviors, then decisions about personal behaviors are being made unwisely. The implications for personal decisions made in the areas of drugs, sex, and religion are obvious. We tend to generalize about others' behaviors in these fields, usually to the liberal side. Facts about actual behaviors are badly needed if ''honest'' decisions are to be made respectfully and responsibly.

Summary

Personality and self-development have been described as measures of adaptation—the dynamic and continuous process of change in response to our internal and external environments. Personality was viewed as a pattern of individual reactions, influenced by hereditary, environmental, and sociocultural forces. The theories of Freud, Maslow, and Erikson were also considered in relation to the sequential development of the unique self.

Arriving at a self-identification, accepting an appropriate sex role, solving problems of dependence and independence, making a vocational choice, developing a value system, and resolving love and sex conflicts were identified as important tasks of youth. However, these tasks are not peculiar to adolescents or young adults. As Erikson stressed, these and other basic tasks in the "eight ages of man" are of continuing concern throughout the human life cycle and require frequent adaptations in our psychological makeup. These mental adaptive responses are the focus of the next chapter.

Review Questions

1. Identify and describe the complex factors that influence one's personality.
2. Explain how the personality can be a measure or index of personal adaptation.
3. Define the terms *endomorphy, mesomorphy,* and *ectomorphy* in relation to personality or temperament.
4. Compare and contrast the theories of personality development as proposed by Freud, Maslow, and Erikson.
5. Discuss the factors that contribute to the process of self-identification.
6. Interpret the following statement: "The less democratic a society, the easier the task of self-identity."
7. How do role models affect self-identification?
8. What forces are complicating the young person's search for sex-role identification?
9. Describe the factors that played a role in determining your value system.
10. Do males and females differ significantly in what they mean by sexual involvement?

Notes

1. J. J. Conger, *Adolescence and Youth* (New York: Harper & Row, Publishers, Inc., 1973), p. 2.
2. Richard S. Lazarus, *Patterns of Adjustment,* 3d ed. (New York: McGraw-Hill Book Company, 1976), p. 17.
3. James C. Coleman and Constance L. Hammen, *Contemporary Psychology and Effective Behavior* (Glenview, Ill.: Scott, Foresman & Company, 1974), p. 46.
4. Desmond S. Cartwright, *Introduction to Personality* (Chicago: Rand McNally & Company, 1974), pp. 373–74.
5. David Krech, Richard Crutchfield, and Norman Livson, *Elements of Psychology,* 2d ed. (New York: Alfred A. Knopf, Inc., 1969), pp. 745–46.
6. Abraham H. Maslow, *Toward a Psychology of Being,* 2d ed. (Princeton, N.J.: D. Van Nostrand Company, 1968), pp. 3–4.
7. Ibid., pp. 27, 155–57.
8. Conger, *Adolescence and Youth,* p. 85.
9. Erik H. Erikson, *Identity: Youth and Crisis* (New York: W. W. Norton & Co., Inc., 1968).
10. Krech, Crutchfield, and Livson, *Elements of Psychology,* p. 752.
11. Erik H. Erikson, *Childhood and Society,* 2d ed. (New York: W. W. Norton & Co., Inc., 1963), pp. 247–74.

12. Ibid., p. 274.

13. Erik H. Erikson, "The Problem of Ego-Identification," *Journal of the American Psychoanalytical Association* 4, no. 56 (1956): 56–121.

14. Jack Kerouac, *On the Road* (New York: Viking Press, 1955), p. 238.

15. Hermann Hesse, *Siddhartha,* translated by Hilda Rosner. Copyright 1951 by New Directions Publishing Corporation. Reprinted by permission of New Directions Publishing Corporation, New York.

16. Ibid.

17. Ibid.

18. E. Douvan and J. Adelson, *The Adolescent Experience* (New York: John Wiley & Sons, Inc., 1966), p. 16.

19. Erik H. Erikson, "Identity and Uprootedness in Our Time," in *Varieties of Modern Social Theory,* ed. H. M. Ruitenbeek (New York: E. P. Dutton & Co., Inc., 1963), pp. 55–68.

20. Ibid.

21. John Money and Patricia Tucker, *Sexual Signatures* (Boston: Little, Brown & Company, 1975), p. 9.

22. Ibid., p. 230.

23. Robert J. Stoller, "Gender Identity," in *The Sexual Experience,* eds. Benjamin J. Sadock, Harold I. Kaplan, and Alfred M. Freedman (Baltimore: The Williams & Wilkins Company, 1976), p. 186.

24. Conger, *Adolescence and Youth,* p. 202.

25. H. Horne, "An Idealistic Philosophy of Education," in *Forty-First Yearbook of the National Society for the Study of Education,* pt. 1 (Chicago: University of Chicago, 1942), p. 154.

26. R. Rimmer, *The Harrad Experiment* (New York: Bantam Books, 1967).

27. Vance Packard, *The Sexual Wilderness* (New York: David McKay Company, Inc., 1968).

28. Ira L. Reiss, "Premarital Sexuality: Past, Present, & Future," in *Readings on the Family System,* ed. Ira L. Reiss (New York: Holt, Rinehart & Winston, 1972), p. 172.

29. T. Shibutani, "Reference Groups as Perspectives," *American Journal of Sociology* 60 (1955): 562–69.

30. R. Levine, "American College Experience as a Socialization Process," in *College Peer Groups,* eds. T. Newcomb and E. Wilson (Chicago: Aldine Press, 1966).

31. H. Floyd and D. Smith, "Dilemma of Youth: The Choice of Parents or Peers as a Frame of Reference for Behavior," *Journal of Marriage and the Family* 34, no. 4 (November 1972): 627–734.

32. J. J. Teevan, "Reference Groups and Premarital Sexual Behavior," *Journal of Marriage and the Family* 34, no. 2 (May 1972): 283–91.

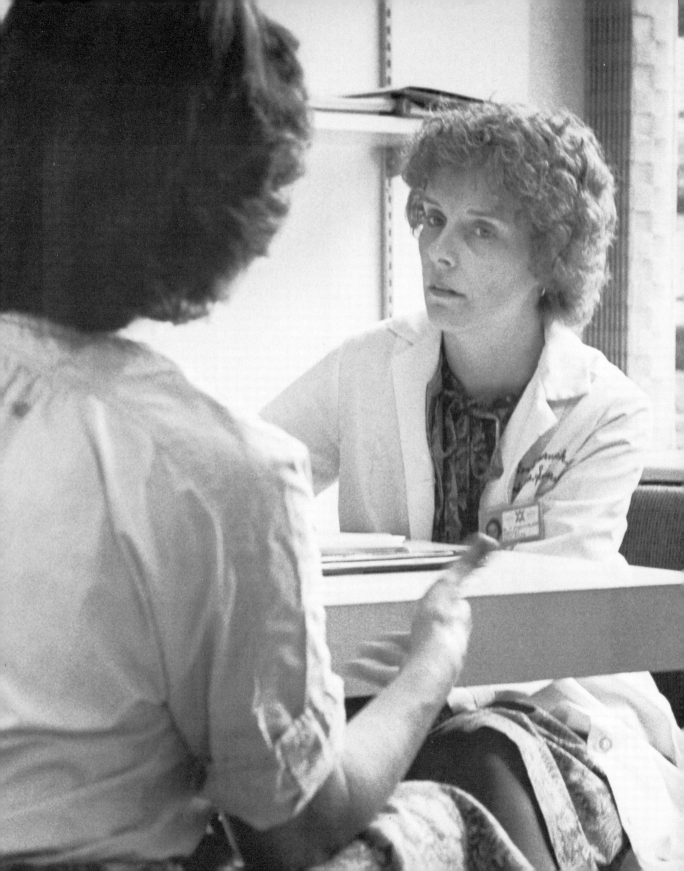

Mental Health: Successful Coping

6

The health of the mind or the psyche has been of great concern to individuals for centuries. As recorded in ancient and classical literature, the restless and troubled mind was not an uncommon condition, although it was considered mysterious and unusual. And depending on the powers attributed to the prevailing gods, the disturbed mind was judged to be either desirable or undesirable, and sometimes both!

It has been less than a century since scientists have dared to probe the depths of the mind. While many mysteries remain, most authorities now agree that nearly everyone experiences some mental trauma throughout the life cycle. It is quite normal to experience some failures, losses, pressures, disappointments, conflicts, loneliness, rejection, fear, and those many other reactions that tend to complicate life or disrupt our feelings of confidence, stability, and contentment. However, the ability to handle or cope with these problems in a manner that is satisfying to both the self and society has become a measure of one's mental health.

Despite many attempts to define mental health more precisely, it remains an elusive concept at best. Many people confuse mental health with mental illness, and you may even hear people seriously express a well-intentioned desire to stamp out mental health, as if it were a public threat. Some people claim that mental health is the absence of mental disease, although mental illness is not easily defined, and its distinguishing marks differ greatly from one culture to another. Some people believe that mental health is the complete lack of everyday challenges, tensions, and risks, or a blissful form of conformity and passivity, and still others define mental health as normal human behavior, even though normality is difficult to define without statistical measurement. In our pluralistic society, what is abnormal for one person is quite often thought of as normal for another.

Whatever it is, mental health is something we all strive for. When we speak of self-fulfillment, inner happiness, peace of mind, becoming more organized and functional, and handling problems confidently, we are really describing dimensions of mental health.

According to the National Association for Mental Health, people with good mental health have the following characteristics:[1]

1. *They feel comfortable about themselves.* Such persons are not overwhelmed by their own fears, love, anger, guilt, or worries. They estimate their abilities accurately and accept personal shortcomings.
2. *They feel right about other people.* Mentally healthy people have satisfying and lasting personal relationships. They can give love, consider others' interests, respect differences in persons, and feel responsible for their fellow human beings.
3. *They are able to meet the demands of life.* They try to solve problems as they arise, accept responsibilities, plan ahead, welcome change and new experiences, set realistic goals, think for themselves, and make independent decisions. Additionally they use their natural abilities to control their environment when possible and fit themselves to the environment when necessary.

Mental Health As Emotional Maturity

A unique interpretation of mental health has been offered by the famous psychiatrist Dr. William C. Menninger of the Menninger Foundation. He describes good mental health in terms of emotional maturity, an ideal quality or state.[2]

According to Menninger, mental health and emotional maturity are matters of degree. We all have some state of mental health, along with emotional quirks and problems, all the time. We approach "perfect mental health" only on occasion. Likewise, emotional maturity is an ideal quality, but because of the many facets of personality, we display strange combinations of degrees of maturity. We are grown up or mature in some ways and quite childish or immature in others.

Menninger has proposed several criteria of maturity that may be applied to your daily life and your relationships with others.[3] You can use them as measures of your potential emotional maturity and effectiveness.

Ability to function under difficulty Acceptance of reality depends on your ability to accept frustration (the blocking of need satisfaction) with minimal distress. Even though you can't have everything you want when you want it, you continue to work toward realizable goals and make constructive compromises in this world of difficulties and uncertainties. How well do you work when the going gets rough?

Capacity to change Though many people resist change, the only certainty in life today is change. You can remain stubborn and become irrelevant, or you can embrace new experiences for their learning and growth potential. Daily living confronts you with opportunities for adapting, solving problems in new ways, and profiting from past errors. To what extent are you flexible?

Control over tension and anxiety Many common physical complaints have their origin in emotional problems. When you feel under pressure, or are threatened or anxious about something, you sometimes have a tension headache, an upset stomach, or an aching back. Pressures of life also surface as aggression, passiveness, illogical and irrational behavior, excessive excuse-making, bluff-

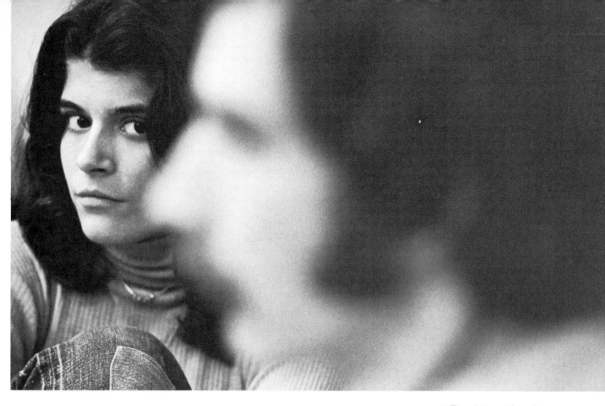

ing, and blaming others for personal faults. Are you relatively free from these symptoms, which are so often produced by tension and anxiety?

Capacity to find more satisfaction in giving than in receiving   While it is natural to delight in receiving, growing up means being on the giving end of the line more often and assuming more social responsibility. Your greatest satisfactions will likely be found in giving of yourself to your family, friends, and communities. A thought- and an energy-consuming mission for the common good is an ideal way for you to lose your own life in order to find it. Are you able to find more contentment in giving than in receiving?

Consideration of other persons   Actions reveal the nature of our current relationships, often characterized by exploitation, unhappiness, fault-finding, hate, bickering, sniping, prejudice, and superficiality. Relations can also be marked by mutual satisfaction and stimulation, respect, loyalty, sincerity, and integrity. While not often valued in the mass media, these latter qualities are vital for healthy and comfortable relationships. What improvements are needed in your relationships with your family members, friends, spouse, or roommate?

Curbing hate and guilt   When not controlled or neutralized, your instinctive tendency to hate can surface as hostility toward loved ones and associates. Anger, thoughtlessness, aggression, selfishness, cheating, and lack of involvement and concern are all too common. Sometimes your hate is turned on yourself

Fig. 6.1. Mutual satisfaction and stimulation, respect, loyalty, sincerity, and integrity are vital for healthy, comfortable personal relationships.

and frequently evolves into guilt and a need for self-punishment. With effort your hate can be directed into more constructive outlets. How do you handle the hate in your life?

Capacity to love   Each of us also has an instinct to love, that is, to care in the broadest sense and to desire to do something creative. This instinct needs expression within our families and circles of friends and also in our communities and nation. Learned first in the early experience of parent-child interaction, the ability to love and care is the only neutralizing agent for hate. What have you done recently to improve your capacity to love and care?

These criteria are not to be viewed as mental health laws. Nor do they represent a magic formula for happiness and success. Rather they are based on principles learned in clinical psychiatry. When applied to yourself, they can indicate areas of possible improvement in your attempt to become more mature and to improve your own mental health.

Achieving better mental health is not easy. Effort must be expended. But realizing that we ought to become more effective persons is the first step in getting there. How would you rate yourself in terms of emotional maturity and mental health?

Stress:
A Demand
for Adaptation

Stress is a word often used to describe an unfavorable mental state or condition. You have probably heard of people cracking under stress. You may have experienced a threatening situation yourself, such as possible loss of a scholarship, preparation for final exams, or demotion on the job. You felt stress! On occasion, your friends may have warned you to avoid stress when they said, ''Take it easy or you'll get bent out of shape!''

Contrary to popular belief, we cannot avoid stress. It is a normal state of living. Stress can even be pleasant and healthy. In fact, some stress is absolutely essential for the maintenance of human life. The real challenge of mental health then is not to avoid stress, but to deal with it without being overwhelmed by it.

The Condition
of Stress

There is within each of us a self-regulating power that tends to maintain a constant, steady level of operation or functioning despite changes in our external surroundings. For instance, one can maintain one's own body temperature while being exposed to great extremes of heat or cold. This inner state of constancy or staying power is known as *homeostasis*. When an individual is at ease, there is an equilibrium of body functioning, thought processes, emotions, and feelings. With homeostasis, we have it all together, as the saying goes.

Frequently our homeostasis or inner equilibrium is disturbed in the course of daily living and interactions with others and our environment. We may be confronted with the pressures of study, the demands of parents and professors, the frustration of an overcrowded parking lot, the delays encountered in registering, the peculiarities of a new roommate, the restrictions of a low-income budget or a gasoline shortage, the loss of a friendship, the death of a parent, or the conflict

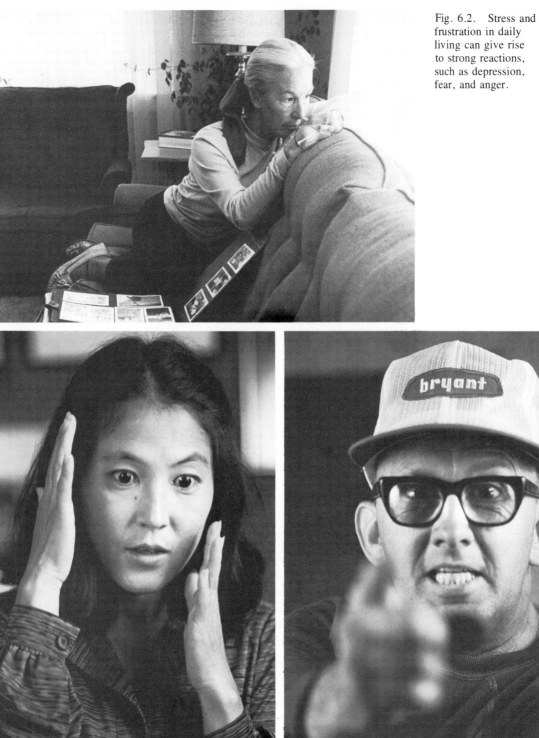

Fig. 6.2. Stress and frustration in daily living can give rise to strong reactions, such as depression, fear, and anger.

between a social affair and preparation for a midterm exam. All of these factors disturb the inner equilibrium. As a result we are in what is described as a state of stress.

An individual under stress is not at ease. To reestablish inner equilibrium or homeostasis, some action must be taken—defense, escape, attack, compromise, or compensation. Changes or adjustments must be made so that either the person better fits the immediate circumstances or the environment is altered to better meet the person's needs. Such effort and action help humans survive threats, resolve conflicts, restore fractured egos, relieve physical and mental upsets, and restore the orderly relation of physiological and psychological functions. These actions of self-preservation are known as adjustments or adaptations.

Stress, therefore, is a condition of disturbed inner equilibrium that demands some adjustment or adaptation. The methods or techniques used to adjust or adapt are called coping techniques or skills.

Bodily Reactions to Stress

Undoubtedly, you have experienced some of these common reactions to stress: sweaty palms, tense muscles, blushing, wobbly knees, pounding heart, nervousness, irritability, worry, insomnia, anxiety, reduced powers of concentration, and a queasy stomach. These are typical human emergency responses to stress.

When the stress situation is severe, the nervous system and the hormones that regulate the emergency response produce what is called the flight or fight reaction.[4] Several bodily changes that occur in the flight or fight reaction are listed in table 6.1. These changes tend to protect the threatened individual.

The body in reaction is ideally prepared to escape the perceived threat as rapidly as possible or to attack and fight the threat. All body resources are now mobilized for defense or counterattack. Of course, the strength of the emergency response depends on the perceived or experienced strength of the threat, pressure, frustration, or conflict.

In his study of disease, Hans Selye has identified the so-called stress syndrome, known as the general adaptation syndrome (GAS).[5] The syndrome, or

Table 6.1 Physical Reactions to Stress

Bodily Changes in the Flight or Fight Reaction
The heart beats faster.
Blood vessels in the stomach and intestine and along the surface of the skin constrict (become smaller).
Blood pressure increases.
Blood supply to the large muscles increases due to the dilation (increase in size) of the arteries serving the extremities of the body.
Pupils of the eyes dilate, increasing the amount of light striking the retina and thus improving visual acuity.
The adrenal glands located on top of each kidney secrete adrenaline, a hormone that frees blood sugar stored in the liver, thus making available more energy for muscular activity.
Breathing becomes faster and deeper, increasing the oxygen supply to the muscles for added energy.

combination of symptoms, represents various structural and chemical changes that have taken place in the internal organs. Some changes are evidence of body damage; others are signs of the body's adaptive reactions, the operation of its mechanisms of defense against stress.

A famous physician and physiologist, Selye defines stress as the rate of wear and tear on the body, which contributes to the aging process. He observes that regardless of the stress-producing agent—a painful body blow or a passionate kiss—the same universal, nonspecific reactions occurred to protect the threatened body and help it regain its homeostasis. The commonly occurring GAS has three stages, as described by Selye.[6]

1. *Alarm reaction*—the bodily expression of a generalized call to arms of the various defensive forces: production of adrenal and anti-inflammatory hormones and infection-fighting white blood cells; irritation of the gastrointestinal tract, with a loss of body weight.
2. *Stage of resistance*—the establishment of acquired bodily adaptation to the stressor, with the eventual return to physiological equilibrium.
3. *Stage of exhaustion*—the loss of acquired adaptation through long-term exposure to stress-producing agents, with the development of stress-related diseases and eventually with death.

Selye proposed that sometimes the body's physical adaptations were excessive or too strong for the body's own welfare. The result was not superprotection but damage to the body. Such damage is evidence of a maladaptation, as revealed in heart and blood vessel diseases, kidney disease, arthritis, allergies, and mental breakdowns, to name a few. He also concluded that during stress bodily changes can affect one's mentality and that mental stress can affect physical functions. Thus he opened the door to a better understanding of psychosomatic symptoms and diseases, subjects examined later in this chapter.

Unrelieved stress and stress that is too severe, too frequent, or too constant can be harmful to the individual. Sometimes stress overwhelms the person's ability to adjust or adapt!

Various stress-producing agents are termed *stressors*. Although most stressors are generally perceived as undesirable, and in some cases as destructive, perceptions of stress and reactions to it are individual matters. No two people react the same way to the same stressors. What is seen as harmful to one may be quite harmless or even stimulating to another.

Some stressors in the following list are inevitable events in most persons' lives, such as interrelating with others, being separated from friends, leaving school or college, finding a job, and interacting with new environments. Other stressors are not as predictable, yet seem to be common elements of reality. These would include experiencing delays, being disappointed, having accidents, and not accomplishing all of your life goals.

Physical stressors that give rise to physiological stress include strenuous and even moderate physical activity (jogging, swimming, weight lifting, tennis, and other athletic endeavors), hunger, thirst, heat, pain, cold, lack of sleep,

Sources of Stress: Stressors

bacteria, viruses, other disease-causing organisms, physical injuries, and terminal illness.

Psychological stressors that cause mental stress include pressures in the form of threats to security and integrity, frustrations, conflicts between goals or demands, military combat, loss of a friend, death of a relative, rejection, academic failure, loneliness, competition, fears, mind-altering drugs, inability to change, and boredom.

Environmental and *social stressors* include polluted air and water, noise, overpopulation, natural disasters (tornadoes, floods, fires, explosions), economic impoverishment, racial and religious prejudice, commuting to college, living in one's parents' home, social pressures to conform, restraints of law, and sexual and vocational expectations of others.

While they are frequently overlooked or even denied, there are many positive features about stress and its causative agents. The rigorous training and competition of the Olympics proved stressful to many participating athletes. Yet these stressors enabled Bruce Jenner to win a gold medal in the decathlon. Pain is interpreted as undesirable, but it usually motivates the sufferer to seek medical treatment. Fatigue brings on sleep, which refreshes the body and promotes effective mental functioning. The fear of being trapped in a burning building is beneficial if it motivates you to leave rapidly, saving your life. Even the stress generated by college life seems worthwhile if your degree and training help you get a good job. For some, the pain of childbirth and trauma of parenting seem more tolerable as their children grow in maturity, intelligence, and love. The applause and standing ovation received by a great musician or actress seem to overshadow the pre-performance stress.

In these instances, then, stress can be pleasant or healthy. Beneficial stress is termed *eustress;* unpleasant or unhealthy stress is designated *distress.*[7] Successful coping enables a person to experience a maximum of eustress with a minimum of distress.

Life Changes
and Stress

Throughout your life, you will experience many stressful situations, because living is a series of adaptations. Recent research has revealed that when adaptations requiring significant changes in life style occur close together, your chances of becoming physically or mentally ill are increased.

Investigations by Holmes and Rahe determined that even changes considered socially desirable, such as achievement, success, increased self-reliance, marriage, and birth of a new family member, could play roles in the onset of disease.[8] They concluded that stress was not necessarily related to the psychological meaning, emotion, or social desirability of life change events, but rather to the change or adaptation itself, to the seriousness of the events, and to the number of life change crises experienced.

Holmes and Rahe developed a rating scale, as seen in table 6.2, to measure common life changes that can serve as stressors. Note that numerical values have been assigned to each life event, as determined by actual survey. According to follow-up studies, it was concluded that an individual having a life change unit

Table 6.2   Social Readjustment Rating Scale

Rank	Life Event	Mean Value in Life Change Units
1	Death of spouse	100
2	Divorce	73
3	Marital separation	65
4	Jail term	63
5	Death of close family member	63
6	Personal injury or illness	53
7	Marriage	50
8	Fired at work	47
9	Marital reconciliation	45
10	Retirement	45
11	Change in health of family member	44
12	Pregnancy	40
13	Sex difficulties	39
14	Gain of new family member	39
15	Business readjustment	39
16	Change in financial state	38
17	Death of close friend	37
18	Change to different line of work	36
19	Change in number of arguments with spouse	35
20	Mortgage over $10,000	31
21	Foreclosure of mortgage or loan	30
22	Change in responsibilities at work	29
23	Son or daughter leaving home	29
24	Trouble with in-laws	29
25	Outstanding personal achievement	28
26	Wife begin or stop work	26
27	Begin or end school	26
28	Change in living conditions	25
29	Revision of personal habits	24
30	Trouble with boss	23
31	Change in work hours or conditions	20
32	Change in residence	20
33	Change in schools	20
34	Change in recreation	19
35	Change in church activities	19
36	Change in social activities	18
37	Mortgage or loan less than $10,000	17
38	Change in sleeping habits	16
39	Change in number of family get-togethers	15
40	Change in eating habits	15
41	Vacation	13
42	Christmas	12
43	Minor violations of the law	11

Source: Thomas H. Holmes and Richard H. Rahe, "The Social Readjustment Rating Scale," *Journal of Psychosomatic Research* 11 (1967): 213–IB. Reprinted with permission of Pergamon Press Ltd.

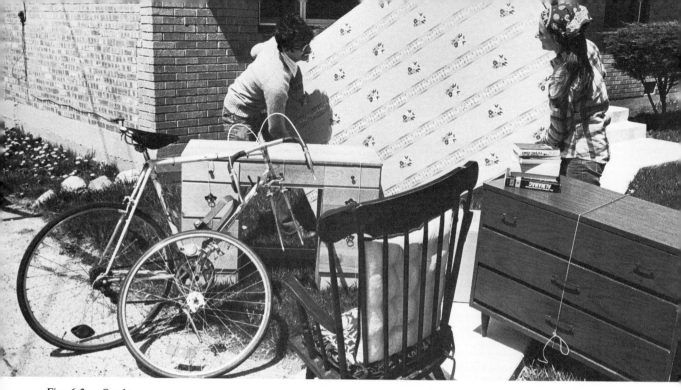

Fig. 6.3. On the Holmes and Rahe social readjustment scale, a change of residence rates 20 life change units as a source of stress.

score of more than 150 points in one year had an increased probability of becoming ill over the next two years.

Check off the life change events you have experienced over the past year, then add up the life change units assigned to each event checked. Your total score will indicate your potential for suffering stress-related illness in the near future. A score of 300 life change units or more indicates the probability of major stress. How do you rate?

Coping Skills

Methods or techniques used to adjust or adapt to the demands of stress are called *coping skills*. Some methods of coping involve changing your own personal view of the stressful situation, with a resulting change in your beliefs, strengths, weaknesses, expectations, and behavior. The emphasis here is on changing yourself. Other coping techniques focus on modifying or eliminating the stressors that are producing the distress. These techniques emphasize changing the environment, eliminating or avoiding stressors, pushing ahead despite stressful situations or resisting them. Additional actions by which the demands for adaptation are met are those that tend to protect the self from insult, devaluation, and disorganization. These latter techniques are the so-called *defense* or *ego-defense mechanisms*.

Regardless of which skill or combination of skills you use in dealing with stress, you should remember that coping is an individual matter. What is healthy and appropriate for one person may be just the opposite for another. Some coping can be unhealthy and result in severe guilt, if the person feels that important beliefs and values have been compromised too much. Coping can also be influenced by various social pressures and expectations. For example, the individual whose body is prepared to escape or attack by the flight or fight reaction often stays passively in place and faints, because both running away and open aggression are often socially unacceptable. However, the embarrassment of fainting, especially for the male, often results in additional stress.

Ideally, the decision about how to cope should be based not only on social pressures and expectations of others, but also on the range of coping alternatives available to you. There is usually more than one way of adapting, and each particular technique has a potential for success or failure. An estimate of the chances for either outcome should be made in advance.

Too often people cope without an adequate understanding of the stress-producing situation, without sufficient knowledge of self in terms of personal resources, values, and life goals, and without any consideration of the consequences of coping. For instance, certain coping methods may immediately reduce stress, but they could also prevent future accomplishment or experience by leaving the door to opportunity closed.

You may also find that weighing the possible benefits and risks of coping can be helpful. Such an evaluation might determine how much effort you are willing to expend in coping, what level of satisfaction you will find acceptable, and what degree of discomfort you are willing to endure to cope.

In an analysis of reactions to stress, Coleman and Hammen have identified several coping skills that appear to work automatically, without the need for deliberate choice and decision making.[9] These include:

Automatic Coping Skills

- Crying—a normal mechanism that relieves emotional tension and pain. Formerly viewed as acceptable behavior only for children and women, shedding tears can reduce hurt and restore physical and mental homeostasis, as many men are discovering. In situations of separation from a loved one due to death and terrible pain, it is becoming acceptable for men to cry, too.
- Talking it out—a built-in coping device that helps a person express troubling inner feelings in words. After a life-threatening crisis, such as an accident, tornado, fire, or earthquake, there is a compulsive need to share the experience with others. This process of talking-out, or catharsis, often results in relief from emotional strain and can help the individual view the stress situation more accurately.
- Laughing it off—an attempt to reveal the humorous side of traumatic life experiences. This coping skill helps keep all aspects of living in perspective and balance and acknowledges the inevitability of stress-producing situations.
- Thinking it through—a temporary mental retreat or escape into private thoughts, so as to better examine the stress situation and various stressors more carefully. This action might be seen as a salvage mission in search of meaning and significance of the hurtful failure to oneself.
- Seeking support—a desire to be with others who can offer some emotional assistance, comfort, or solace in times of personal disaster or insecurity.

- Sleep and dreams—coping mechanisms that can have a healing function. Sleep restores energy, and dreams can desensitize the individual to the reality of physical or mental trauma.

Several coping skills can be based on conscious decision-making and an objective assessment of the stressful situation. Such coping tends to deal more directly with stress than our built-in mechanisms and usually involves a deliberate change in oneself or in one's environment, or both. Moreover, these coping techniques are focused on some task or activity that either attacks the problem-causing stress directly, leads to withdrawal from the stress-producing situation, or enables the individual to achieve an acceptable compromise with the problem.[10]

Positive Attack   In dealing directly with a problem, you might decide that increased effort on your own part might reduce some frustration, so you study harder to improve academic performance, you make yourself more available to others when you feel left out or rejected, and you practice longer to make the team or attract the attention of another person. To counter loneliness and isolation, you might join with others in some group, such as a club, a service organization, or a sorority or fraternity.

Self-Management   Developing or improving personal coping resources is another effective way of dealing with stress. One such task-related skill involves the application of behavior modification strategies to improve your self-management.[11]

Coping Skills Related to Specific Tasks

1. Select a goal, some aspect of your life you want to change.
2. Record your present behavior as a reference point for evaluating progress.
3. Keep track of any changes in your behavior and the circumstances that made the desirable changes possible.
4. Change the events or circumstances that seem to foster stress by avoiding stressors, altering troublesome situations, and reducing the number of stressors to which you are particularly vulnerable.
5. Identify events or consequences that can serve as reinforcers, strengthening behaviors that tend to reward you for changing your behavior and thus making change more likely to occur.
6. Focus on the consequences of your behavior before you act, so as to reduce impulsive, unplanned actions.

Improving Communications   Another important coping skill is improving communications with other persons. Although there are several techniques for improving communications, a popular one is patterned after the principles of transactional analysis. Developed by Eric Berne[12] as therapy for emotional difficulty, transactional analysis or TA has been applied more popularly by Thomas A. Harris to improving personal interactions.[13]

According to TA, each person maintains an inner trio of Parent-Adult-Child, somewhat equivalent to Freud's superego, ego, and id. The Parent functions as a conscience in feelings, thoughts, and actions; the Adult functions as a computer and approaches the environment objectively; the Child feels, thinks, and acts in a childlike manner of a certain age.[14]

Communication proceeds smoothly and healthfully as long as verbal transactions are between complementary ego states, that is, between parent-parent, adult-adult, or child-child. Transactions between different states can also be constructive as long as the interchange is characterized as parallel, as in the case of a husband's Parent addressing his wife's Child and her Child responding to his Parent.

Communication is disrupted, however, when the Adult of one person addresses the Adult of another, but the response is more typical of a Child-to-Parent transaction. Such crossed transactions are considered to be at the root of many social difficulties. TA is analysis of behavior in terms of verbal transactions and psychological games, which can lead to more constructive living by improving communications.

Specific Coping Techniques There are additional task-related skills for coping with stress.[15, 16, 17, 18]

- Learn to relax by listening to soothing music, engaging in deep muscle relaxation after tensing your body's muscles, and quiet meditation.
- Set priorities for each day and stick to them.
- Concentrate on one task or activity at a time.
- Take up new tasks only when you have finished your current priority items.
- Manage demands from other persons by letting them know the limitations on your time and effort.
- Reduce your compliance with others, while at the same time expressing your needs and wishes in a positive way.
- Slow down, especially when you feel pressure building, by eating, walking, and speaking more slowly.
- Listen to others carefully without interruption.
- Read from books that require deep concentration.
- Plan some idleness, free time, or recreation each day, particularly during long sessions of any activity likely to induce tension and stress.
- Work off tension and anger through some physical activity, such as walking, jogging, playing tennis, dribbling a basketball, cleaning your room or apartment, or chopping wood.

Withdrawal Although many persons tend to discredit any form of withdrawal as a proper coping skill, escape and avoidance remain legitimate techniques. Admitting failure and redirecting personal efforts to more realistic goals can be a very constructive mental health measure. Some stress can only be relieved by removing yourself physically and/or mentally from the stressors. This applies equally to irritating and overly competitive persons as well as to vocational pursuits and working conditions. There is also great value in having a place for occasional retreat for contemplation or meditation at home or at school. Lose yourself for a while in a favorite book, a new experience or diversion, a concert, or a change of scene to recover your breath and balance. Then you can spring back and deal with your problems more effectively.

Compromise and Substitution   Sometimes when we cannot achieve our goals, we compromise and settle for the next best thing. We tend to accept an available or attainable substitute. In some instances goals may remain the same, but we must try alternative means for reaching the goals. Settling conflicts often succeeds only when each person agrees to mutual accommodation—the give and take displayed by each side. This is evidence of mutual adaptation. Compromising by giving in occasionally, easing up on criticism even when you know you are right, and shedding your urges for total perfection as superman or wonder woman can take you a long way toward easing stress healthfully.

   While there is no failproof formula for dealing with stress, Hans Selye's treatise "Stress without Distress" offers some useful and unique guidelines for successful coping.[19]

1. Find your own natural stress level through a process of self-analysis.
2. Select a life-style and an environment of work and friends that are in line with your preferences, satisfactions, and self-expression.
3. Practice altruistic egoism, that is, selfishly hoard the good will, respect, esteem, love, and support of your neighbors, whoever they may be.
4. Earn your neighbors' love by doing something for them. Thus you become secure in other persons' benevolence toward you and dependence on you.

Defense Coping Skills   Coping skills that primarily protect the individual from psychological hurt and disorganization are known as defense mechanisms. Though learned to some extent, defense mechanisms are often used at the habitual and unconscious levels and lead to a degree of self-deception and distortion of reality.[20] Nevertheless they help a person maintain control and self-esteem while adjusting to stress.

   By far the most common and comforting defense mechanism is *rationalization*. This coping technique provides us with socially acceptable reasons for holding an attitude or performing a behavior when the real reasons would be unacceptable to the conscience, and therefore anxiety-producing, if permitted free expression at the conscious level. The coach who ostracizes an innocent player because of his own anger, but says it is for the player's own good, is rationalizing. The young girl who has become bored with her boyfriend but feels guilty everytime she thinks of breaking off, rationalizes that for his own personal growth she must release him from their relationship and date him no longer. Rationalization does have some significant advantages!

   Projection is a common defense mechanism we use when we ascribe an undesirable thought or action of our own to another person: "I didn't get the part because the director is incapable of recognizing true talent." "I couldn't pass the course because the instructor was too difficult." In essence the blame for personal problems is shifted or projected to another person or group of individuals whose imagined faults and hostilities are responsible for your own difficulty.

   Reaction formation is described as behavior and self-expression that is exactly

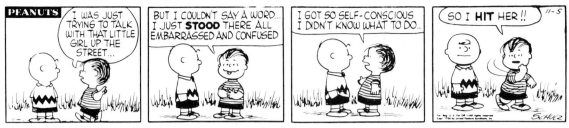

Fig. 6.4. Occasionally, in their confusion young people do or say things quite different from what they intend.

the opposite of a person's true feelings or behavior. To maintain social acceptance, the student who has just flunked an examination or feels unjustly ridiculed will suddenly begin to idolize and openly praise the instructor. In reality the student would prefer to curse the professor or thrash the "idiot," in accordance with his or her innermost desires.

Occasionally a threatened individual may reduce anxiety through *identification*. A young, aspiring actor, clearly short on talent but long on imagination, might identify with Robert Redford. Carrying it to extremes, he might adopt Redford's style of dress, speech, mannerisms, even life-style. In a sense, through identification, a person behaves and acts as if he were some other person, who is often perceived as a model. When the identification process results in the adoption of the other person's values and aims, the coping technique is referred to as *introjection*.

A primitive defense mechanism, *denial* is a clear refusal to believe that an anxiety-producing event is true. The individual actually comes to believe his own denial. For example, a young girl who has been openly rejected by her father may actually deny that he is hostile toward her and insist that he is kind and loving.

Somewhat different from denial, *repression* keeps anxiety-producing events at a subconscious level. The individual simply blots out the frightening event, for example, seeing one's father strike one's mother, by removing the perception completely from awareness. Repression is neither a refusal to remember the event nor a denial of it; it is simply the removal of the perception from consciousness by forces beyond the individual's control.

There is a subtle but important difference between denial and repression. In repression the individual has no awareness of the anxiety-producing thought (cannot recall the father's action); in denial the individual simply rejects the event (it never happened). Repression is generally considered more harmful to the individual. In Freudian psychology repression is thought to be the cause of many later disturbances; for example, a young wife's frigidity may be caused by her repression of an earlier advance made toward her by her own father. In repressing that memory, she sets up the mechanism for the later rejection of her husband.

Psychoanalysts claim that some childish behaviors of early adolescence are due to *regression*, the readoption of behaviors characteristic of an earlier phase in one's life. Sulking, thumb-sucking, and silently crying in one's bed while lying

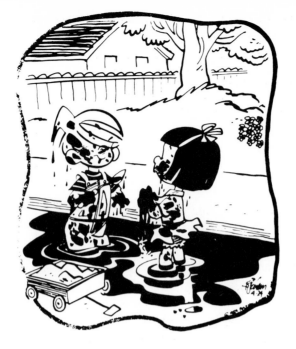

in the fetal position may be considered relatively mild examples of regression. Temper tantrums and tirades are somewhat more serious examples.

Asceticism involves denial of the instinctual drives. Young people, for example, may for a time completely mistrust enjoyment, and they may counter urgent desires with even stronger prohibitions (''I must not go out with girls because I have a strong desire to touch them. I will avoid them altogether.''). Carried to extremes, a young man might give up sleep for fear of dreaming of girls; give up most food, because eating is giving in to pleasure; and even give up company, as other people might distract him from his purpose. Such an individual constantly tests his capacity for withstanding pain.

Intellectualism may serve as indirect relief for people with anxieties in areas too delicate to be handled directly. The youth in turmoil over his sex values, for example, may argue about freedom versus responsibility, free love versus marriage, or even the nature of God!

Compensation is an attempt to emphasize or develop a desirable personal trait over an undesirable one. For example, a person who is not especially gifted in athletics may be able to excel in academic endeavors. Of course, the reverse situation would also be a form of compensation. According to Nikelly,[21] compensation is one of the best defense mechanisms for weaknesses and inferiority, as long as the form of compensation is socially desirable.

When an individual redirects or transfers socially unacceptable feelings and hostile thoughts from the actual stressor to some unrelated object or person, the defense mechanism of *displacement* is being used. Many roommates, husbands, wives, and even children have unknowingly been the innocent targets of displaced anger that originated in a conflict between employer and employee or student and teacher. As Nikelly explains:

> The reason for this transfer is that if the person behaved as he really felt toward the source of his feelings and thoughts, he may suffer undesirable consequences which may cause him to become anxious. . . . With the mechanism of displacement he can unload his unacceptable feelings on someone else . . . where the consequences may not be as severe.[22]

If all other coping mechanisms fail, one may use *fantasy* to alleviate frustration and satisfy specific goals through imaginary accomplishments. Although this temporary withdrawal from stress-producing situations can be healthy on occasion, it can all too easily evolve into maladaptation when fantasy is always substituted for real-life activities.

Realistically, fantasy and all other defense mechanisms are essential for the reduction of tension, the protection of one's feelings of adequacy, and the maintenance of emotional stability. However, their frequent and repeated use often forestalls the development of constructive, problem-solving adaptations.

To some degree each defense mechanism is related to one's having or not having enough psychic space. Psychic space is freedom to maneuver, and in interpersonal relationships we may grant it to each other or take it away. It's that intangible force that makes the weaker sex really stronger than the stronger sex, because of the weakness of the stronger sex for the weaker sex. It's that undeniable force that permits one person to lord it over another, even when the "lord" is clearly not in a position of objective advantage, such as an average but confident person who clearly dominates a person of greater talent.

When his red-faced, disheveled, teenaged daughter came creeping up the stairs an hour after curfew last week, Mr. Jones was irate and suspected that he knew what she had been doing that had kept her out so late. Also aware of the situation, Mrs. Jones managed to reach the door before her husband did, move out

Psychic Space

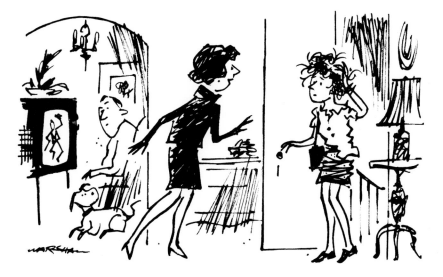

Fig. 6.6. Psychic space. Sometimes we find ourselves without "space" even in privacy or in the right place at the proper time.

quickly, and, after a quick appraisal of her daughter's state, ask, "What's the matter, dear? You don't look well. Do you have a headache?" That's giving psychic space; it gives the daughter room to maneuver, and it gives the father time to cool down. Had Mr. Jones gotten to the door first, he probably wouldn't have given her as much space! More likely, he would have left her gasping for air!

Psychic space is critical in interpersonal relationships; it makes it possible for two people to communicate meaningfully with a minimum of threat. In a father-son confrontation over drug use, for example, both parties can destroy psychic space by saying, "I don't care what you say, drugs are bad business. I don't want to hear any more about them!" or "Marijuana is illegal, and that's that!" and "You're just too old-fashioned to listen!"

The same parties could create psychic space for each other and improve their chances for meaningful dialogue through the use of less directed, less emotion-laden comments: "Son, even if it isn't ruining your health, it's certainly not adding anything interesting to you as a human being." "Didn't you ever drink before you reached the legal age, Dad?" "Dad, you're always willing to listen to both sides of a question. Will you hear mine now?" Skillfully used, psychic space can be a tool in persuading others to one's own purposes, licit or illicit!

Ineffective Coping

The person who has problems in coping effectively is often referred to as malad-justed. Yet that person's behavior is not usually different in kind from the so-called normal person's behavior. The difference is mainly in degree and is characterized by an exaggerated use of attack, withdrawal, or defense mechanisms. As Morgan and Johnston explain:

> We all project at times, but a mentally ill person will use projection as a major technique in relieving his anxiety. Again, a degree of shyness in a person is not considered too great a deviation from normal, but when this form of withdrawal intensifies so that the withdrawn person sits alone in one position, head down, never speaking and seemingly unaware of his surroundings, we recognize that his behavior is far from normal.[23]

In one sense, then, the maladjusted individual is just like you and me, only more so!

Psychological abnormality can also be described as maladaptive, since the decline in one's ability to adjust comes about in response to stress that most individuals could handle effectively and without much difficulty. People with problems in living generally display adaptive inflexibility. They lack or are incapable of using alternative methods for interrelating with others, for achieving their goals, and for coping with difficulties.[24]

Ineffective coping tends to be nonintegrative, that is, maladaptive attempts to cope with problems usually complicate them, prevent the satisfaction of one's needs, and not only make new problems but intensify old problems. A person whose coping behavior is ineffective is described as displaying personality disorganization.

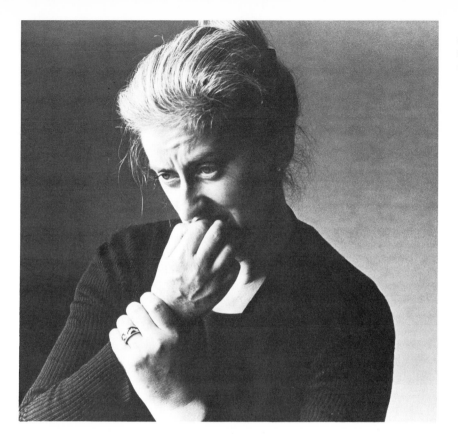

Fig. 6.7. The neurotic
overreacts to conflict
and lives in a state
of mental disruption.

The term *neurosis* is generally used in reference to minor personality disorders or less severe mental problems. Although neurotic behavior may interfere with personal effectiveness, it does not severely disable or incapacitate a person. With neurosis, the individual usually stays in touch with reality, is not likely to be hospitalized, and is not usually seen as a threat to the health and safety of the community.

Neuroses are often thought of as expressions of conflict between impulse and reality and between desires and duties that are essentially irreconcilable.[25] Of course, conflict may also exist between the individual and the environment. Most people live with conflicts and accept them as inevitable, along with the temporary upsets that pass over in time. From time to time most persons also feel lonely, afraid, inadequate, powerless, and angry. However, the neurotic person manages conflicts and troublesome emotions in ways that are considered immature. The neurotic overreacts to conflict and lives in a state of mental disruption. Reactions to conflict tend to be more severe and long-lasting than those displayed by more normal persons.

Nearly everyone has a predisposition to some neurotic behavior, as we all experience some fears, act compulsively, and feel varying degrees of depression on occasion. These symptoms especially become apparent in stressful situations, such as before and during examinations. The symptoms tend to disappear when

Minor
Mental Problems

the demand for adaptation has been met and the stress has been resolved. Neurotic traits are quite common and are no longer considered unusual. Neurotic reactions are particularly evident in humans at points of developmental transition in the life cycle; for example,

> ... when first going to school, during the changes of puberty, when a child is born, when gray hair first appears or sexual responsiveness begins to decrease, when children leave home and the nest is empty.[26]

Neuroses are often classified according to the primary symptom observed.[27] Here are some specific neurotic patterns.

Anxiety Neurosis   Feelings of overconcern and eminent dread best describe this form of neurosis. The person suffering an anxiety reaction is always uneasy, tense, and nervous, reports difficulty in sleeping and sometimes in breathing, and is often unable to concentrate. Such an individual is overwhelmed with fear! However, the fear of an anxiety neurosis is not restricted or fixed on some specific object or person. Rather, this fear is said to be free-floating, that is, the anxiety tends to shift from one person or object to another, and the apprehension is not identified with an objective source.

A specific form of anxiety reaction is *hypochondriasis,* a preoccupation with one's body and fear of presumed disease. The hypochondriac's anxiety about personal adequacy and death is displaced toward preoccupation with bodily function, staying young, and vigorous exercise. On occasion, hypochondriacs will use their symptoms to win the sympathy of others.

Hysterical Neurosis   This minor mental problem is characterized by a disorder or loss of some function caused by a person's unconscious. Originally, when such problems occurred in the female, they were blamed on a wandering uterus. Hence, the Greek name for *uterus (hystera)* was applied to this disorder. (Obviously, sexism is not of recent origin.)

One type of hysterical neurosis is *conversion reaction,* so called because an individual's voluntary nerve system and/or spinal senses are affected, causing paralysis of an arm or leg, convulsions, loss of speech, insensitivity to pain, blindness, deafness, or loss of muscular coordination. All of these physical symptoms are without organic or physical basis.

Another form of hysterical neurosis is *dissociative reaction.* In this disorder disturbing memories, thoughts, and feelings are separated from one's consciousness because they cannot be integrated easily within the personality structure. Results include loss of memory (amnesia), sleepwalking, beginning a new life without any knowledge of one's former identity, and the development of a multiple personality within the same individual—the classic Dr. Jekyll and Mr. Hyde syndrome.

Phobic Neurosis   A phobia is an overpowering fear of some specific object or situation, which a person willingly acknowledges as harmless in the light of reality. Such an irrational fear is often accompanied by fainting, fatigue, sweating, nausea, and minor body tremors. Examples of phobias include fear of enclosed places, fear of flying, fear of moving vehicles, fear of high places, and fear of certain animals, such as snakes and mice.

Obsessive-Compulsive Neurosis This neurotic reaction consists of the unwilling repetition of unwanted thoughts (obsessions) and the persistence of certain actions that the person cannot resist performing (compulsions). Individuals may be obsessed with thoughts of revenge or of killing someone, or even hear a tune repeated over and over again in one's mind. Compulsions may be observed in frequent and unnecessary handwashing, excessive bathing, or avoidance of stepping on cracks in the sidewalk.

Apparently the repetition of certain acts reduces anxiety, although the need to persist in a particular activity always remains unsatisfied. You have to keep doing it because you have to! Obsessions may be attempts to keep even more terrifying thoughts out of one's consciousness.

Depressive Neurosis Mild depressive reactions are marked by feelings of discouragement, worthlessness, sadness, and guilt. Depression may be related to the loss of a loved one through death or to separation from a cherished object. Sometimes depression occurs without any specific cause. Depressed individuals not only look and sound sad; they also slow down in their bodily movements.

More severe maladaptive behavior problems are evidence of an unbalanced and deranged condition of one's mental processes. Known as *psychoses,* these serious disturbances in thoughts, feelings, and actions are usually detrimental to the individual and quite often to other people. Sometimes psychotic persons display behavior that is self-destructive and antisocial in nature.

In contrast with the neurotic individual, the psychotic appears to have lost contact with reality. Coping ability has collapsed or is impaired to a significant degree. Hospitalization is usually required. Although the abnormal behaviors of psychotics tend to be episodic and even reversible in some instances, surfacing only in situations of acute stress, the persons involved do not often comprehend

Major Mental Problems

When to seek help for mental problems:

1. When you think you need help
2. When you experience wild mood swings
3. When a psychological problem seriously interferes with your daily life
4. When you develop unreasonable fears and guilt feelings
5. When you start isolating yourself from other persons
6. When you begin to have hallucinations
7. When you feel life is not worth living
8. When you think of yourself as inadequate and worthless
9. When your emotional responses are inappropriate to a particular situation
10. When your daily life becomes nothing more than a series of crises
11. When you feel you can't get your "stuff" together anymore

Modified from "Who Can I Turn To?" *Go To Health* (New York: Dell Publishing Co., Inc., 1972), pp. 27–34.

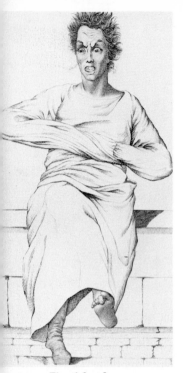

Fig. 6.8. In nineteenth-century France, severely disturbed persons were restrained in straitjackets.

the nature and seriousness of their disability. While neurotics are usually aware of their ineffective coping, psychotics are not.

Psychosis is often distinguished by symptoms not generally found in the less severe mental disorders. Among these are hallucinations (sensory perceptions without any basis in reality); severe withdrawal and regressive reactions; total apathy; inappropriate emotional responses, especially in excitement; delusions (false beliefs based upon misinterpretation of reality); and marked depression. In general, the psychotic has no apparent control over his thought processes or emotions, both of which are expressed in bizarre behavior.

Schizophrenia Among the most serious and least treatable functional psychoses—those not related to identifiable brain damage—is schizophrenia. The term itself is derived from Greek words meaning "split mind." Originally known as dementia praecox, schizophrenia is characterized by serious disturbances of thinking and behavior.

Various types of schizophrenia are distinguished by their unique symptoms.

- *Simple*—progressive withdrawal and regression, emotional flatness, deterioration of personal appearance, irresponsible behavior patterns
- *Hebephrenic*—emotional indifference, fragmented speech, smiling and frequent giggling without cause, the development of infantile behaviors in toileting, feeding, dressing, and cleanliness
- *Catatonic*—impulsiveness, poor coordination, and purposeless activities in combination with either stupor and assumption of motionless positions or excitement and frenzied activity necessitating restraint
- *Paranoid*—delusions of grandeur, persecution, and suspiciousness of others' intentions and actions

Affective Disorders These psychoses are basically disorders of mood or emotion ranging from extreme sadness and depression to extreme elation and euphoria. In one type of affective psychosis, *involutional melancholia,* the individual appears to be worried, anxious, agitated, and preoccupied with feelings of guilt and impending death. Attempts at suicide are common.

In *manic-depressive psychosis,* mood swings from elation to severe depression are common. Mania is marked by excessive motor activity, talkativeness, and irritability, while depression is identified by expressions of sadness, guilt, and hopelessness. In some cases extended periods of normal behavior separate recurring episodes of mania or depression or serve as interludes in cycles of overactivity and underactivity.

Paranoia This major psychotic disorder is characterized by delusions of persecution and grandiosity. Frequently the delusions focus on politics and religion. The paranoiac is strongly convinced that others are talking about, spying on, and plotting his harm and eventual destruction. With the enlargement of this persecution complex, the paranoid individual assumes an inflated sense of self-importance. The person imagines himself to be a high government leader, a general, a religious prophet, or even God.

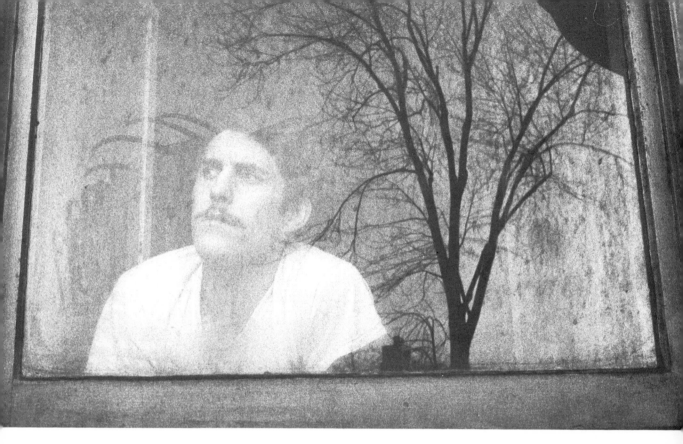

Although paranoia can occur in combination with schizophrenia, Morgan and Johnston note that the typical paranoid individual

> is well oriented as to person, place, and time, and that, outside of his special delusional system, he thinks, speaks, and acts rationally in all other areas.[28]

Personality Disorders   Disturbances related to a person's failure to acquire effective coping skills are referred to as personality disorders. Such abnormal conditions usually are not accompanied by anxiety, internal conflict, or the collapse of defense mechanisms, as seen in neuroses and psychoses. Those with personality disorders include the psychopath or sociopath who apparently lacks a conscience and engages in antisocial behavior. Persons with inadequate personalities rarely achieve social, emotional, and occupational adjustment. The passive-aggressive personality, for instance, has considerable difficulty dealing effectively with interrelationships. Alcohol and other drug dependencies are frequently regarded as personality disorders, as detailed in later chapters of this text.

Psychosomatic Disorders   As mentioned earlier, medical research has concluded that mental states can have an impact on bodily functions. This mind-body relationship is the basis for psychosomatic or psychophysiologic disorders.

Fig. 6.9.   Psychotic disturbances in thoughts, feelings, and actions are usually detrimental to the individual and often to other people.

When bodily reactions to stress are not reduced in the process of adaptation or adjustment, physical energies increase and persist. The organism remains in a high state of readiness for flight or fight. If the changes in heart action, blood vessels, blood circulation, and hormone secretion continue indefinitely, permanent physical damage can occur to tissues and organs. Psychological in origin, these psychosomatic disorders are the result of ''. . . unexpressed protective physiological reactions.''[29]

The more common psychosomatic disorders include peptic ulcers of the stomach and small intestine, inflammation of the large intestine (colitis), chronic elevation of blood pressure (essential hypertension), migraine headaches with severe pressure on one side of the head, bronchial asthma with severe wheezing and gasping for breath, and inflammation and itching of the skin.

Suicide   Suicide or self-destructive behavior has long been a taboo topic, as well as a source of curiosity, intrigue, and repulsion, for both the behavioral scientist and the lay person. For many, suicide is a crime against oneself, God, and nature. Taking one's own life is troubling and appalling to others because suicide rejects the conviction that life is worth living. Moreover, suicide challenges those who fear death and hope for a better future because it confirms ''. . . not only the suspicion that life may not be the highest good but the one that death may not be the greatest evil.''[30] Depending on one's values, suicide can be viewed as the ultimate form of escape from stressors and stress, the ultimate form of maladaptive or ineffective coping, or the ultimate expression of personal freedom.

A Leading Cause of Death   Despite the moral and social prohibition against suicide, about 30,000 Americans take their own lives each year. Currently ranked as a leading cause of death in the United States, suicide is the third most frequent cause of death among fifteen- to nineteen-year-olds and ranks second among college students. An estimated 10,000 college students in the United States attempt suicide each year, and some 1,000 succeed.[31]

Two-thirds of all suicides actually occur among persons between the ages of thirty-five and seventy-four.[32] Attempted suicides—those who try to take their own lives but fail—number approximately 300,000 per year. Although more females than males attempt suicide, males are more prone to successful self-destruction, probably because they employ methods that produce a more immediate lethal effect, that is, firearms and hanging.

During the past fifteen years the United States has witnessed a marked change in the patterns of suicide mortality. Suicide rates among males under forty-five have risen sharply but have declined in males forty-five and over. Among young women, especially those fifteen to twenty-four, the increase in suicide has been appreciably higher.[33] Although suicide has been significantly more frequent among whites than blacks, recent surveys indicate that the racial gap is narrowing, especially in urban populations.

Because of the general reluctance to admit publicly that suicide was the cause of death and because it is sometimes difficult to establish whether death was due to homicide, accident, or suicide, the true number of suicides is not known.

Myths about Suicide   To understand and perhaps prevent suicide, we should note and dismiss some popular myths about it. Kastenbaum identifies several ideas that should be laid to rest.[34]

- The person who talks about suicide rarely takes his own life.
  False! Nearly three out of four who attempt suicide give some detectable hint or message ahead of time.
- Only the poor and the rich commit suicide.
  False! Persons in every income and social bracket kill themselves.
- Suicide has simple causes that are easily established.
  False! The surface cause or explanation often has a complex underlying cause imbedded in a complex motivational system reflecting individual life values.
- Only depressed or insane people commit suicide.
  False! Though more suicides occur among those diagnosed as psychologically depressed, the potential for self-destruction is present in persons with any mental disorder, as well as in persons in a rational state of mind.
- The tendency to suicide is inherited.
  False! There is no evidence that suicide has a hereditary basis, although two persons in the same family may commit suicide.
- Suicide is related to the weather, moon phases, sunspots, or magnetic forces.
  False! No reliable trends have been detected in numerous studies. Although there may not be a direct causal relationship, Wenz believes that some temporal factors, such as seasonal ceremonies or rituals, including birthdays and Christmas celebrations, may postpone or precipitate a suicidal act.[35]
- When the suicidal patient shows improvement, the danger is over.
  False! Patients discharged from the hospital or those who stop therapy are actually in special danger. The patient has more opportunity to commit suicide and has often recovered enough energy and will to try again.
- Persons who are under a physician's care or hospitalized are not suicidal risks.
  False! Studies reveal that about half of all suicides occur among those who have received psychiatric care within six months prior to their act. Patients can and do commit suicide in hospitals.

Factors that precipitate suicide   If there are factors that commonly precipitate suicide, they are probably loneliness and hopelessness spawned by serious illness, emotional conflicts, loss of a meaningful relationship with some "significant other," guilt, and the impoverishment of life. These same conditions diminish one's self-esteem, which plays an important role in motivating self-destructive behavior.

Various theories have been advanced to explain suicide.[36] These are summarized as follows:

- Failure of the individual to become integrated into society or family life
- Willingness to sacrifice one's life because of a felt duty, allegiance to authority, or religious beliefs
- Disruption in societal regulations that have formerly governed the satisfaction of the individual's needs

- Overregulation of the individual and lack of opportunity in life experiences
- Severe mental depression induced by early childhood disappointments, emotional deprivation, and the physical or psychological absence of parents
- Existence of a death instinct that strives to ruin life and reduce it to its original inanimate matter
- Presence of an emotional constellation of dependency, aggression and hostility, guilt and anxiety

From the suicide's viewpoint, however, self-destruction may be seen as a convenient coping skill. Worden and Proctor list these possible motivations for self-destruction.[37]

- Retaliation or the wish to punish another by inducing guilt
- Reunion with someone who has already died
- Escape from an intolerable or hopeless situation
- Destruction of unbearable feelings or impulses
- Atonement for some wrong to reduce guilt feelings
- An inner need to show courage and conquest of fear of death
- A desire to be reborn or reincarnated

Regardless of the cause or causes of suicide—whether it is a wish to kill, a wish to be killed, or a wish to die—most medical authorities view suicide attempts as cries for help. Suicidal tendencies are often expressed verbally as a death wish or as an intention to destroy oneself. Sometimes personal actions suggest imminent death. Danger signals include depression, hysteria, feelings of guilt, sudden mood changes, drug dependency and alcoholism, and a history of previous attempts at taking one's own life.

Suicide Prevention To prevent suicide and thus reduce its incidence, hundreds of suicide prevention centers have been established in the United States. Such centers, often staffed by trained volunteers, maintain a twenty-four-hour telephone service for individuals who desperately need to talk with someone in a time of personal crisis. These centers sometimes function as short-term clinics and conduct research in various aspects of suicide. While prevention of suicide is not compulsory, the centers have been credited with saving many lives each year. Justification for the existence of suicide-prevention or crisis-intervention centers is based upon

> the ambivalence of most suicidal persons, the passing nature of suicidal crises, and the serious psychological trauma that suicide causes in the survivors. A further argument, however, is that many suicidal people have gifts and talents which can benefit society.[38]

While many observers believe that suicides are the result of insanity, it is apparent that self-destructive behavior is a human adaptation that reflects the increasing difficulty persons have in dealing with their problems. This is particularly true with the decline in traditional value systems and the growing complexities of our ever-changing society.

If you ever detect a potential suicide in a friend or loved one, do take the suicide's concern seriously. Do not provoke the suicide into desperate action by issuing dares; explore alternative forms of action with the individual; do not impose your value judgments on the suicide; do not agree with the suicide's reasons for considering self-destruction; and listen with sincerity. Be aware of community resources that can help the potential suicide.[39]

Although various treatments for mental disorders have been developed over the years, therapies generally represent one of the following major types: (1) psychotherapy, (2) behavioral therapy, and (3) somatic therapy.[40] While it is true that treatment for psychological problems is more effective with the minor mental disorders, some success also has been achieved in the treatment of psychoses. However, some forms of psychotic behavior appear to benefit very little from any therapy.

Appropriately applied, therapy for mental problems can be of benefit when it serves as an emotional cushion during crisis, when it provides deeper understanding of self and makes more clear one's status and circumstances, and when it removes external stressors or helps a person cope more effectively.[41] These three goals of therapy are also the general goals of counseling. Yet therapy for troubling behavior, feelings, and thoughts focuses more on the internal functioning of the individual. Counseling deals more with problems that lie outside the individual.

Treating Mental Disorders

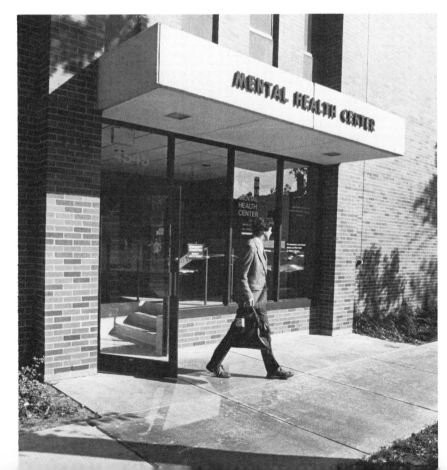

Fig. 6.10. Therapy often helps the individual weather emotional crises, cope more effectively with problems, and come to a better understanding of self.

Psychotherapy

The term *psychotherapy* can actually refer to any treatment that employs psychological rather than physical means in helping mentally disturbed persons. More accurately applied, it is those treatments that feature verbal interchange or talking between a patient and the therapist. The goals of verbal therapy are to promote deeper self-understanding, provide insights into oneself and one's personal meaning, and bring disturbed patients into closer contact with split-off elements of their mental lives. This therapy tends to analyze the self and to leave it to the patient to resynthesize or put the self back together again.[42] Verbal therapy also permits the disturbed individual to vent rage, frustration, and hate without fear of condemnation, thus releasing built-up tension.

Among the many psychotherapies is classical Freudian *psychoanalysis* with its techniques of free word association, interpretation of dreams and repressed wishes, recall of early childhood conflicts, and the establishment of a therapeutic alliance between patient and therapist. Another more common and more current practice is *psychoanalytic psychotherapy,* which emphasizes helpful supportive verbal exchange about specific internal conflicts of the patient.

Recently psychotherapy has dealt not only with inner conflicts and unconscious drives, but also with interpersonal relationships and events outside the self. Several forms of *group therapy* and *family therapy* have evolved from this new approach. An individual's problems are viewed as being rooted in relationships with others, especially family members. Thus the entire family becomes involved in treatment. Role-playing in which individuals assume different characters within the family for purposes of expression and interpretation of behaviors is sometimes used in family therapy, as are other psychotherapeutic practices.

Behavior Therapy

A major alternative to psychotherapy is *behavior therapy* or *behavior modification.* Like psychotherapy, behavior therapy seeks to change behavior, but it utilizes different techniques. As Kiernan explains, "In many respects the theory behind behavior therapy is nothing more than an extension of the learning theory. . . ."[43] Therapists teach disturbed persons to engage in less bizarre and more normal behavior, replacing behavior characteristic of ineffective coping.

Rejecting the significance of inner feelings and attitudes and discounting the concepts of ego and the unconscious, behavior therapists believe that neurotic behavior is an expression of habit. Learned at an early age, such conditions as compulsion, phobia, and depression will persist and intensify as long as these habits are rewarded and reinforced by their consequences. Therefore Kiernan recommends that

> instead of rewarding compulsive behavior with further positive reinforcements, punish it with negative reinforcement (aversive conditioning) until the habit becomes desensitized and blocked, and seeks to express itself through a substitute habit. Encourage the new habit, making sure it's a healthy one, with the very same positive reinforcement that established the undesirable habit.[44]

The therapist thus formulates methods of setting new behavioral goals and encourages and rewards new behavioral patterns.

Where to seek help for mental problems:

1. Sympathetic family members
2. Understanding and supportive friends
3. Your family doctor or religious counselor
4. Social service community organizations
5. Counseling services
6. Crisis centers, telephone hotlines
7. Community mental health centers
8. Local branch of the National Association for Mental Health
9. Outpatient hospital clinics
10. Psychologists
11. Psychiatrists

Somatic Therapy

Somatic therapy is the use of physical agents to treat mental disorders, especially severe mental illnesses, the psychoses. Perhaps the most common somatic method utilizes mood-altering drugs. The so-called *minor tranquilizers,* such as meprobamate, reduce the effects of anxiety. Chlorpromazine and reserpine are representative *major tranquilizers* that normalize and stabilize abnormal, erratic behavior and apparently reduce disturbing thought processes in the patient.

Other drugs used in somatic therapy sedate the patient, while *antidepressants* combat feelings of sadness and depression. When some patients are adequately treated with these psychotropic or mind-altering drugs, they may benefit from certain forms of psychotherapy and behavior therapy.

Other somatic therapies include the controversial and much feared shock therapy or *electroconvulsive treatment*, which is sometimes used in emergency psychotic depression, and *psychosurgery* performed on the whole, intact brain so as to cause behavioral change or reduce inner tension, conflict, and anxiety.

Nutritional treatments also may be used when foods, allergies, extreme diets, and even low blood sugar are thought to contribute to specific mental disorders.

Summary

Mental health has been described as successful coping. The mentally healthy person feels comfortable about himself, feels right about other people, and is able to meet the demands of living.

Stress-producing situations and agents known as stressors are common elements in our daily lives. Often thought of as undesirable, experiences of stress—a condition of disturbed inner equilibrium that demands some adjustment—also can be healthy and stimulating. Successful coping (dealing with stress) leads to experiences of maximum stress with minimum distress.

Various coping skills were examined, including automatic, task-related, and defensive reactions. When coping does not relieve stress, various physiological and psychological disturbances may develop. These include neuroses, psychoses, personality disorders, psychosomatic conditions, and suicide. Current therapies for mental disorders were discussed briefly.

Review Questions

1. How would you define or describe mental health?
2. What criteria could be used to evaluate emotional maturity?
3. What is stress? What causes it?
4. Define *homeostasis* and relate it to the condition of stress.
5. List some bodily reactions to stress. Why do they occur?
6. What are the three stages of Selye's general adaptation syndrome (GAS)?
7. Distinguish between *eustress* and *distress*. Give examples of each.
8. What is meant by coping?
9. How do the following categories of coping skills differ from one another: automatic, task-related, and defensive? Give five examples for each skill category.
10. How does a neurosis differ from a psychosis?
11. Define *psychosomatic disorder*. Name several psychosomatic conditions.
12. Identify several commonly held myths about suicide.
13. Compare and contrast the major therapies for mental disorders.

Readings

Brown, Barbara B. *New Mind, New Body*. New York: Bantam Books, 1975.

David, Lester. "The Many Faces of Guilt," *Family Health/Today's Health* 9, no. 7 (July 1977): 22–25.

Forem, Jack. *Transcendental Meditation*. New York: E. P. Dutton & Co., Inc., 1974.

Harmin, Merrill. *Better Than Aspirin: How To Get Rid of Emotions That Give You A Pain In The Neck*. Niles, Ill.: Argus Communications, 1976.

Pelletier, Kenneth R. "Mind as Healer, Mind as Slayer," *Psychology Today* 10, no. 9 (February 1977): 35–36, 40, 82–83.

Snyder, Solomon H. *The Troubled Mind: A Guide to Release From Distress*. New York: McGraw-Hill Book Company, 1976.

Notes

1. National Association for Mental Health, *Mental Health Is 1, 2, 3* (Arlington, Virginia: The Association, 1973).
2. William C. Menninger, "Emotional Maturity," in *A Psychiatrist For A Troubled World, Selected Papers of William C. Menninger*, ed. Bernard H. Hall (New York: The Viking Press, 1967), pp. 799–807.
3. Ibid.
4. R. A. Sternbach, as quoted by Richard S. Lazarus, *Patterns of Adjustment*, 3d ed. (New York: McGraw-Hill Book Company, 1976), p. 108.
5. Hans Selye, *The Stress of Life* (New York: McGraw-Hill Book Company, 1956), pp. 25–43.
6. Hans Selye, *The Stress of Life*, rev. ed. (New York: McGraw-Hill Book Company, 1976), pp. 36–38.
7. Hans Selye, "Secret of Coping with Stress," *U.S. News & World Report* 82, no. 11 (March 21, 1977), 51.

8. Thomas H. Holmes and Richard H. Rahe, "The Social Readjustment Rating Scale," *Journal of Psychosomatic Research* 11 (1967): 213–18.

9. James C. Coleman and Constance L. Hammen, *Contemporary Psychology and Effective Behavior* (Glenview, Illinois: Scott, Foresman & Company, 1974), pp. 128–31.

10. Ibid., pp. 131–37.

11. Robert L. Williams and James D. Long, *Toward a Self-Managed Life Style* (Boston: Houghton Mifflin Company, 1975), pp. 21–50.

12. Eric Berne, *Games People Play: The Psychology of Human Relationships* (New York: Grove Press, Inc., 1964).

13. Eric Berne, *What Do You Say After You Say Hello?* (New York: Bantam Books, Inc., 1972), pp. 11–12.

14. Thomas A. Harris, *I'm OK—You're OK* (New York: Avon Books, 1967).

15. Richard M. Suinn, "How To Break The Vicious Cycle Of Stress," *Psychology Today* 10, no. 7 (December 1976): 59–60.

16. Rolland S. Parker, *Emotional Common Sense* (New York: Harper & Row, Publishers, Inc., 1973), pp. 122–30.

17. "Cracking Under Stress," *U.S. News & World Report,* 80, no. 19 (May 10, 1976): 59–61.

18. Meyer Friedman and Ray H. Rosenman, *Type A Behavior and Your Heart* (Greenwich, Conn.: Fawcett Publications, Inc., 1974), pp. 260–66.

19. Hans Selye, "Stress without Distress," in *Psychopathology of Human Adaptation,* ed. George Serban (New York: Plenum Press, 1976), pp. 137–46.

20. Coleman and Hammen, *Contemporary Psychology and Effective Behavior,* p. 138.

21. Arthur G. Nikelly, *Mental Health for Students* (Springfield, Ill.: Charles C Thomas, Publisher, 1966), p. 97.

22. Ibid., p. 112.

23. Arthur J. Morgan and Mabyl K. Johnston, *Mental Health & Mental Illness* (Philadelphia: J. B. Lippincott Company, 1976), p. 63.

24. Theodore Millon and Renee Millon, *Abnormal Behavior and Personality* (Philadelphia: W. B. Saunders Company, 1974), p. 6.

25. Clara Claiborne Park with Leon N. Shapiro, *You Are Not Alone: Understanding and Dealing with Mental Illness* (Boston: Little, Brown & Company, 1976), p. 33.

26. Park and Shapiro, *You Are Not Alone,* pp. 33–34.

27. Morgan and Johnston, *Mental Health & Mental Illness,* pp. 89–92.

28. Ibid., p. 109.

29. Millon and Millon, *Abnormal Behavior and Personality,* p. 311.

30. Jacques Choron, *Suicide* (New York: Charles Scribner's Sons, 1972), p. 4.

31. "Campus Suicide," *Parade* (February 8, 1976): 22.

32. "Regional Variations in Mortality from Suicide," *Statistical Bulletin* (August 1973): 2.

33. "Suicide: International Comparisons," *Statistical Bulletin* (August 1972): 3–4.

34. Robert J. Kastenbaum, *Death, Society, & Human Experience* (St. Louis: The C. V. Mosby Company, 1977), pp. 288–290.

35. Friedrich V. Wenz, "Effects of Seasons and Sociological Variables on Suicidal Behavior," *Public Health Reports* 92, no. 3, (May-June 1977): 233–39.

36. Robert Kastenbaum and Ruth Aisenberg, *Psychology of Death* (New York: Springer Publishing Co., 1972), pp. 276–79.

37. J. William Worden and William Proctor, *PDA* Personal Death Awareness* (Englewood Cliffs, N.J.: Prentice-Hall, Inc., 1976), p. 165.

38. Choron, *Suicide,* p. 81.

39. Kastenbaum, *Death, Society, & Human Experience,* p. 295–96.

40. Park and Shapiro, *You Are Not Alone,* p. 52.

41. Joel Kovel, *A Complete Guide to Therapy: From Psychoanalysis To Behavior Modification* (New York: Pantheon Books, 1976), p. 47.

42. Ibid., p. 72.

43. Thomas Kiernan, *Shrinks, etc.: A Consumer's Guide to Psychotherapies* (New York: The Dial Press, 1974), p. 211.

44. Ibid., p. 215.

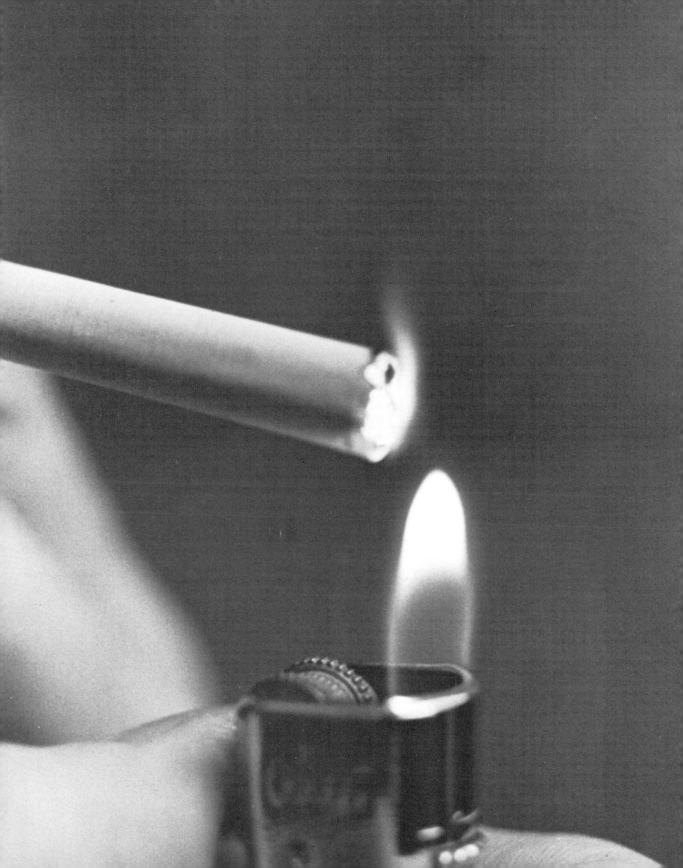

Smoking: One Hazardous Adaptation

7

Since the beginning of time, human beings have searched for substances that would not only sustain and protect them but also would act on their nervous systems to produce pleasurable sensations. Among the things that have been found to have a *psychoactive effect*—a temporary change in mood, thought, feeling, or behavior—are ethyl alcohol, hemp and cactus plants, mushrooms, poppies, and tobacco, an herb that has been smoked and sniffed for more than 400 years.

People have been attracted to these psychoactive substances because they have been useful in helping individuals adapt to an ever-changing environment. Indeed, smoking, drinking, and drug-taking have lightened the load of life; reduced tensions, anxieties, and frustrations; counteracted boredom as well as fatigue; enhanced the pleasures of the moment; and in some instances, provided an escape from the harsh realities of existence. Chemical mood and behavior modifiers have also been employed to enhance self-image, build confidence, gain approval or acceptance, and heal psychological hurts.

Use of substances for such personal gratification and temporary adaptation often carries a high price tag, such as various forms of drug-dependency, personal and social disorganization, and predisposition to serious and sometimes fatal diseases. These undesirable and health-threatening consequences of adaptive and adjustive behavior are referred to as *maladaptations*, which usually occur as the remote consequences of behavior that has an immediate beneficial effect.

Such is the case with cigarette smoking, now characterized as one of the most serious and yet preventable health problems, a major international threat, and "suicide-in-slow-motion." The dimensions of this adaptive, yet disease-producing, activity are more easily recognized when one examines the reasons for the inability to stop smoking. Horn cites two areas in which remedial action is most difficult to initiate:

1. The individual smoker who becomes "hooked" after taking 60,000 or more puffs a year on a cigarette. The minor vice of smoking—that silly little habit—has been well learned through repetitive practice. Habits well learned are hard to break!
2. Our society at large which finds itself "hooked"—burdened with a king-sized tobacco industry, a mammoth agricultural enterprise, a considerable source of governmental revenues, and a significant customer of the communications media.[1]

Although cigarette smoking is less prevalent among adults today than it was just ten years ago, the number and percentage of teenagers who smoke are increasing. Nearly a million teenagers begin smoking each year. Research indicates that the percentage of teenage girls who smoke is nearly as high as the percentage of teenage boys who smoke.

Thus, we identify sociocultural and economic factors, in addition to personal gratification, in the perpetuation of a learned, adaptive behavior that is also a primary health risk.

Prevalence of Smoking in U.S. Adults

Although cigarette smoking is a popular and widespread form of behavior, only an estimated 39 percent of adult men and 29 percent of adult women in the United States are now classified as smokers.[2] While these percentages account for nearly 47 million Americans (20 years of age or older) who consume 600 billion cigarettes each year—an annual per capita consumption of 4,000 per person of legal age—smokers make up a declining minority of the total adult population, just 34 percent. The remainder have never smoked at all or have managed to join the "unhooked generation" by reverting to nonuse.

From its introduction into Western civilization by explorers returning from the New World, smoking until recently was viewed almost exclusively as a masculine activity. Before World War I, a woman who smoked usually demeaned her femininity. During the past fifty years, however, women have gradually cast aside the moral and social stigmas attending cigarette use, and for years they have been smoking more and more like men—and dying like men. Women are not only starting to smoke at a younger age, but also are becoming heavier smokers. While some smokers eventually give up the practice, once a woman takes up smoking, she is less likely to quit than is a man. According to surveys conducted by the U.S. Department of Health, Education and Welfare, the number of men smokers dropped from 53 percent in 1964 to 39 percent in 1975, but women smokers declined from 32 percent in 1965 to only 29 percent in 1975.

It appears that attitudes toward smoking are becoming increasingly negative, even among smokers themselves.[3] More than 70 percent of smokers currently agree that smoking is harmful to their health and could lead to disease and death.

Table 7.1   Who Smokes Cigarettes? Estimated Cigarette Smokers, by Sex, in Persons 20 Years of Age or Older, United States, 1955, 1965, and 1975

Sex	Year	Total Population* (millions)	Cigarette Smokers** (millions)	% Smokers
Male	1955	50.9	26.5	52
	1965	65.8	30.0	53
	1975	66.1	25.9	39
Female	1955	53.9	13.1	24
	1965	61.2	19.7	32
	1975	72.7	21.0	29

*U.S. Department of Commerce, Bureau of the Census. Current Population Report. Estimates of the Population of the United States, by Age, Sex, and Race: 1970 to 1975. Series P-25.
**Based on national surveys in 1955, 1965, and 1975.

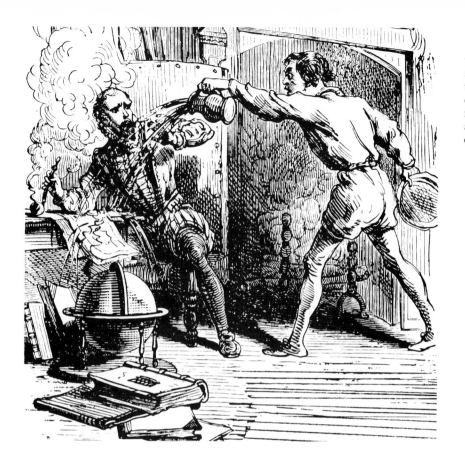

Fig. 7.1. Sir Walter Raleigh is credited with introducing pipe smoking to England in the late 1500s. As this engraving shows, some nobles found smoking a dangerous activity even then.

In addition, an estimated nine out of ten smokers would like to quit, and a large percentage of smokers think that there should be some regulation against smoking. Evidently both smokers and nonsmokers are becoming somewhat less tolerant of smoking.

Although proportionately fewer people are smoking today, the adult population of the United States has increased significantly during the past ten-year period. Therefore it should not be surprising that the total consumption of cigarettes has increased to an all-time high.

The pattern of teenage smoking stands in marked contrast with the adult usage pattern. In 1975, 20 percent of 13- to 19-year-olds smoked, an increase of 6 percent from 1965. An estimated 6 million of the 29.5 million teenagers in the United States smoked in 1975, compared with only 3.5 million out of 24.4 million in 1965. Surveys indicate that almost one million teenagers take up smoking each year. The influence of peers who smoke and the role model of smoking parents continue to attract new smokers despite the real health hazards. In fact, most teenagers who smoke regularly are from families where one or both parents smoke.

Data collected by the National Center for Health Statistics[4] and the National Clearinghouse for Smoking and Health[5] have revealed some important characteristics of smokers and former smokers. Among both men and women, the highest proportion of cigarette users was found in the age groups of 25–34 and 35–44. Beyond those age groups, the use of cigarettes declined considerably. Males and females who lived in cities and metropolitan areas outsmoked their counterparts on farms.

For men, smoking varied *inversely* with level of income and years of education—the greater their income and their years of education, the less likely they were to be smokers. In contrast, for women, smoking was more prevalent among white-collar than blue-collar workers, and among those with some college education than those with high school education only. In both adult males and females, smoking was significantly more common among those who were divorced or separated than those who were married, single, or widowed.

When additional data from these surveys were analyzed, it was found that the percentage of *former* smokers varied *directly* with education and income level for both men and women. As the educational level and family income rose, the percentage of *former* smokers increased. Could it be that anti-smoking educational programs have had some, although limited, success?

One important finding for both men and women smokers relates to the type of cigarette smoked. In 1970 more than half of the smokers interviewed reported using a cigarette with 20 or more milligrams of tar. By 1975 the percentage had dropped to only 20 percent. Also in 1970, 45 percent of smokers reportedly smoked cigarettes with nicotine levels of 1.4 mg or more. By 1975, only 18 percent reported using cigarettes with this nicotine content. According to an analysis of manufacturers' new tobacco products and media advertising, this trend to lower tar and nicotine cigarettes is continuing. Most health authorities approve of this switch away from high-tar and high-nicotine cigarettes. However, this change may be a mixed blessing. Research indicates some disturbing smoking behavior related to the new, milder brands promoted as cigarettes without apparent risk.[6]

1. The less nicotine in the cigarette smoke, the more cigarettes smoked per day.
2. Smokers tend to smoke a low-nicotine cigarette to a shorter butt, thus getting more tar, nicotine, and carbon monoxide in later puffs than that found in early puffs.
3. Some smokers tend to increase the size of each puff, thus increasing the nicotine dose per puff.
4. Some smokers shorten the interval between puffs, thus increasing the dose per minute.
5. To compensate for a drop in nicotine yield, some smokers draw the smoke deeper into their lungs or hold it there longer before exhaling.

It is evident that such behavior adaptations lessen the alleged advantages of low-tar and low-nicotine cigarettes for many smokers. Unfortunately, in such cases, less is more.

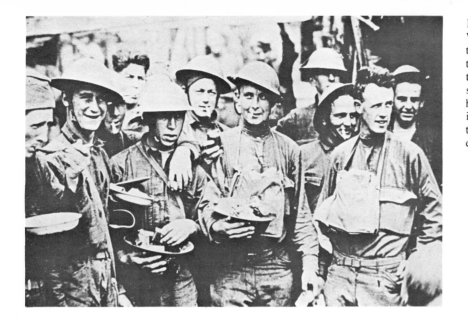

Until the invention of the cigarette manufacturing machine after the Civil War, tobacco was principally consumed in pipes and cigars and in chewing and sniffing. Once mass production of cigarettes was a reality and production costs decreased, cigarettes became readily available. Their preeminence as a tobacco form has been traced to World War I where they found the favor of the doughboys (soldiers).

Preeminence of Cigarettes As a Tobacco Form

Cigarettes have enjoyed an immense popularity because they provide the user with certain personal gratifications unobtainable in other tobacco forms. They can be smoked easily and quickly; they can be inhaled; they are readily available and relatively inexpensive; and they are socially accepted or at least tolerated.

Personal Gratification

Recently, however, the silent majority of nonsmokers has become assertive in its demands for plain, unpolluted air. Tired of being assaulted by tobacco smoke, the vocal and visible nonsmokers now proclaim that the smoker's liberty ends where their noses begin. Organized groups of nonsmokers, such as Action on Smoking and Health (ASH) and the Group Against Smokers' Pollution (GASP), together with the American Lung Association, the American Cancer Society, and professional medical and dental associations, have been successful in restricting smoking in public areas and in establishing the legal right of nonsmokers to be free of others' cigarette smoke.

The nonsmokers' liberation movement has been successful in banning cigarette commercials on television, limiting smoking in certain hospitals, lobbying for laws and regulations that require health warnings on cigarette packages and separate smoking and nonsmoking sections on commercial airlines and interstate buses, and prohibiting smoking in some elevators, indoor theaters, libraries, art galleries, museums, and dining cars of passenger trains.[7]

Smoking: One Hazardous Adaptation

| Motivational Research | Not to be overlooked as a factor in cigarette consumption are the persistent promotional activities of tobacco companies and their advertising agencies. Agencies long ago discovered through motivational research that sales could be increased if products were linked with basic human desires and drives. Not content with assertions of mildness and good taste, advertisements soon depicted smokers as models of sophistication, eternal youth, handsome ruggedness, enduring beauty, alluring sexuality, and determined individualism, and with athletic prowess sufficient to walk at least a mile for a favorite cigarette. |

| Smoking: An Adaptive Behavior | These phenomena alone do not explain why people begin and continue to smoke, especially when they frankly admit awareness of possible health hazards. Many smokers express a desire to quit, but they just cannot manage to do so. A consideration of smoking as "adaptive behavior" may illuminate the reasons and motivations involved in the use of cigarettes. |

| A Learned Behavior | Smoking is a learned behavior. No one is born a smoker, although the new baby may interact with smokers and with smoke early in infancy—often on the way home from the hospital after delivery. Curiosity and the desire to imitate adults, especially smoking parents, probably encourage many children to experiment. The initial reaction, however, is likely to be unpleasant, and usually there is no social approval forthcoming. It is not until adolescence that smoking becomes a live option for most young persons. More time is now spent away from home with peers; there is increased freedom from authority figures who often discourage or forbid smoking; needs for security and acceptance through group conformity grow; and the demand for immediate need gratification flourishes. The psychological stage for smoking has been set and is fertile enough to generate nearly one million new, young smokers each year. |

| Psychological Rewards | The search for adulthood or maturity through the act of smoking appears to be a primary factor in the initiation of cigarette use. Following the example set by many adults and parents, adolescents partake of adulthood by smoking—they feel older, more mature, and more important. Smoking may also help them to overcome feelings of uncertainty and embarrassment in situations that they find awkward. Thus, security is enhanced. There are other psychological rewards for the new smoker. Smoking may be the passport to acceptance among one's peers; it may represent freedom or independence from restrictive home life or revolt against parental authority; it may be the result of an unconscious desire to imitate esteemed smokers; it may be nothing more than a soothing and pleasurable way to counteract boredom. Because of the hand-to-mouth motions associated with lighting up, the cigarette may amount to a convenient "psychological recycling center" that provides a socially approved and refreshing activity between environmental challenges. Some people like the taste and smell of cigarettes, and a few get a kick out of watching the smoke. In essence, the cigarette provides a smoker with a readily available way to deal with a host of personal problems and needs. |

The reasons for initiating smoking are not always the same as those for continuing smoking. Original motives are replaced by powerful and irresistible factors, both psychological and biochemical.[8] These factors are most apparent in the Tomkins-Horn-Waingrow classification of experienced smokers, according to their characteristics and reasons for continuation of cigarette use.[9] The following is an interpretation of that classification.

Stimulation Smoker   This person gets a lift from smoking, a perking-up due to nicotine's transient stimulation that temporarily relieves fatigue. He uses cigarettes to get started in the morning.

Oral Gratification Smoker   Having something in one's mouth to chew on, such as a toothpick, straw, or pencil, provides great satisfaction to the oral gratification smoker. From a Freudian perspective, cigarette smoking may be seen as a satisfaction of infantile needs to suck or chew—a fixation at the oral level.

Pleasure-Relaxation Smoker   This kind of person smokes for positive feelings of contentment, achievement, victory, and satisfaction—such as upon completion of a job well done or after a delicious, mouth-watering meal. This smoker typically loves the cigarette in a quasi-romantic fashion.

Negative Effect-Management Smoker   This person smokes to cope with stressful situations and feelings of anger, fear, and anxiety. Cigarettes are escape vehicles from cares and worries. Thus, smoking represents a tension-reducing activity. When the going gets rough, cigarettes can be a crutch, a comfort, or a consolation.

Habit Smoker   A behavior pattern has been established almost involuntarily by the habit smoker. The habit smoker responds automatically to some cue—a cup of coffee, getting into a car, or nearing the vicinity of an ashtray. Once regarded as psychologically significant, smoking has become devoid of any of its former affective components.

Addicted or Dependent Smoker   An addicted or dependent smoker must have a cigarette after a certain time lapse or otherwise experience mild withdrawal symptoms—a "nicotine fit" with its uneasiness, nervousness, and anxiety. Peculiarly, the dependent smoker craves a cigarette, as in chain-smoking, first to increase positive feelings and then to decrease negative feelings. In essence the smoker satisfies a need to smoke—a physical need for more nicotine. Contrary to popular belief, research now suggests that smoking does not reduce anxiety or calm nerves.[10] Under stress, smokers consume cigarettes heavily because stress depletes the body's nicotine. Thus nicotine-deficient smokers smoke more under stress to maintain their usual nicotine level.

It should be noted that while any one smoker may have more than one reason for smoking and thus fit into two or more of the foregoing classifications, "... one reason tends to be more prominent than the others."[11]

AREN'T YOU A LITTLE OLD TO BE SMOKING?

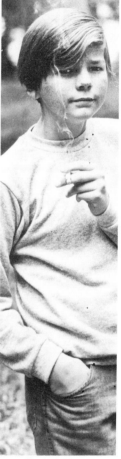

You look like you're old enough to read. And if you're old enough to read, why don't you sit down and read that pack of cigarettes. Especially the warning.

AMERICAN CANCER SOCIETY

Fig. 7.3.

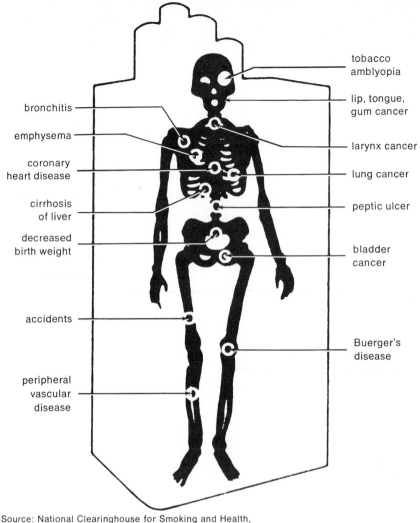

Fig. 7.4. Many diseases and conditions can be considered to be associated with smoking. Not all are causally related, but they should not be overlooked. For instance, accident rates are higher for smokers than nonsmokers. This includes fires in the home caused by the smoker who dozes off with a lighted cigarette in hand. The blood level of carbon monoxide is higher in smokers during the time they are smoking. Increasing attention is being given to the question of whether this carbon monoxide in the blood may be dulling the alertness of drivers to the point where this is a contributory factor in auto accidents.

bronchitis

emphysema

coronary heart disease

cirrhosis of liver

decreased birth weight

accidents

peripheral vascular disease

tobacco amblyopia

lip, tongue, gum cancer

larynx cancer

lung cancer

peptic ulcer

bladder cancer

Buerger's disease

Source: National Clearinghouse for Smoking and Health, United States Public Health Service

---

Smoking: Agent of Maladaptation and Disease

From a health point of view, personal gratification is acceptable for most persons as long as it does not injure the individual or cause harm to other persons. Unfortunately, smoking is now seen as a health threat to both. Smokers, nonsmokers, and even unborn children are caught up in this multifaceted problem leading to self-inflicted morbidity and premature mortality, increased health and welfare costs, added irritating effects of cigarette-induced air pollution, and the mounting threat of home, commercial, and forest fires caused by discarded cigarettes.

Components of Cigarette Smoke

The starches, proteins, sugars, and hydrocarbons of the tobacco leaf, when burned, are converted into a complex aerosol mixture of gases, uncondensed organic vapors, and particulate matter. The temperature of the smoke at the burning zone is nearly 900°C, although that which reaches the smoker's mouth is in a temperature range from 30°–50°C.

While scientists estimate the number of cigarette smoke components to be several thousand, only 1,200 have been identified to date. These components of smoke are sufficient to produce an extremely dense "respiratory environment," more concentrated than the air pollution of major urban centers.[12] The smoke from an average, nonfiltered cigarette is composed of several types of chemicals.

Gaseous Elements and Compounds   Gaseous elements and compounds, notably *nitrogen* and its oxides, *carbon dioxide, oxygen,* and *carbon monoxide,* combine with the hemoglobin in red blood cells and thereby reduce the oxygen-carrying capacity of the blood. Also isolated in the fraction of smoke from cigarettes are small amounts of toxic chemicals, particularly *acetaldehyde, acetone,* and *hydrogen cyanide.*

Particulate Matter   Particulate matter, containing tiny particles of tobacco smoke, is a respiratory tract irritant. Investigations have shown that more than 90 percent of these particles remain in the lungs of the smoker who inhales. When condensed, the particles—regarded as lung-damaging in size—form a yellow-brown sticky mass known as tobacco tar. The tar contains several *carcinogenic* (cancer-producing) *hydrocarbons,* especially *benzo(a)pyrene* and *chrysene; nitrosamines; nickel compounds; fatty acids; phenols,* which have tumor-promoting activity in addition to being toxic to the cilia; and *nicotine,* a colorless, oily compound in commercial insecticides.

Nicotine   Identified as the addictive or dependency-producing component in tobacco smoke, *nicotine* is responsible for the temporary stimulation following smoking. Nicotine initiates a series of nervous and endocrine functions that result in a release of glycogen from the liver. This causes the brief "kick" and reduction of fatigue often reported by smokers. Once absorbed into the bloodstream, nicotine is also responsible for increasing the work load of the heart and vasoconstriction (blood vessel narrowing) that in turn lowers skin temperature.

Human population studies, health surveys, animal experimentation, and clinical and autopsy studies have been the bases for the present knowledge of the health and disease effects of smoking cigarettes. Summarized here are the significant findings of these research endeavors.[13]   Research Findings

1. The risk of death is significantly higher for men (70 percent higher) and for women who smoke cigarettes than for men and women who do not. Estimates of excess deaths associated with cigarette smoking have ranged up to 300,000 deaths per year.
2. Cigarette smokers tend to die at earlier ages and to have a greater incidence of certain diseases—cancer of the lung, larynx, lip, oral cavity, esophagus, and bladder; chronic bronchitis and emphysema; diseases of the cardiovascular

Fig. 7.5.
Smoking
and disability

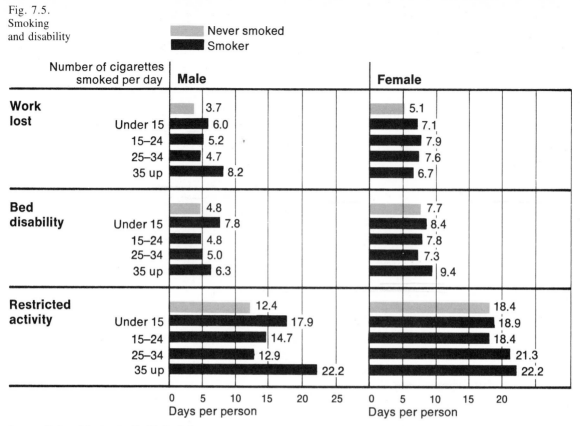

Fig. 7.5. Smoking and disability

Legend: Never smoked / Smoker

Number of cigarettes smoked per day	Male	Female
Work lost		
(Never smoked)	3.7	5.1
Under 15	6.0	7.1
15–24	5.2	7.9
25–34	4.7	7.6
35 up	8.2	6.7
Bed disability		
(Never smoked)	4.8	7.7
Under 15	7.8	8.4
15–24	4.8	7.8
25–34	5.0	7.3
35 up	6.3	9.4
Restricted activity		
(Never smoked)	12.4	18.4
Under 15	17.9	18.9
15–24	14.7	18.4
25–34	12.9	21.3
35 up	22.2	22.2

Days per person

Source: National Center for Health Statistics.
Chart shows age-adjusted number of days per person per year, 1970.

system, including coronary artery disease and atherosclerosis of the aorta; and peptic ulcer—than do those who refrain from smoking.

3. Those who smoke experience more days of disability, more days of work lost, more man-days spent ill in bed, and more chronic illnesses than do comparable nonsmokers in the population.

4. The greater the number of cigarettes smoked daily, the higher the death rate. Life expectancy among young men is reduced by an average of eight years in heavy smokers (two packs or more per day) and an average of four years in light smokers (less than a half pack per day).

5. The risks of death, disease, and disability are greater for those who start smoking at young ages.

6. Health risks are greater for those who inhale cigarette smoke than for those smokers who do not inhale smoke.

7. Maternal smoking, especially during the last two trimesters of pregnancy, has been found to contribute to a lower average birth weight of babies born to smoking than of those born to nonsmoking mothers. In addition, smoking mothers ran a higher risk of bearing stillborn children, and their infants were

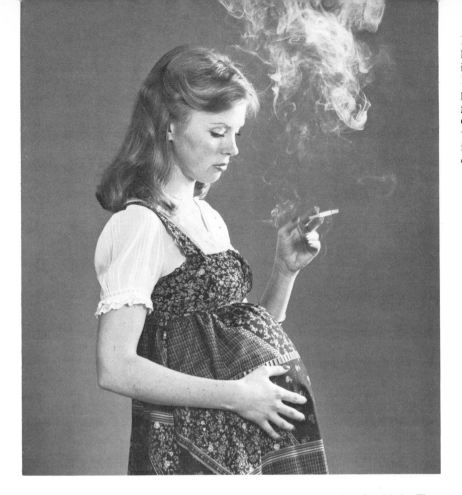

Fig. 7.6. How not to love your baby before it is born—smoke! Maternal smoking during pregnancy retards fetal growth, as shown by decreased infant birth weight and an increased incidence of prematurity defined by weight alone.

more likely to die in the last months before birth or shortly after birth. These effects may occur because carbon monoxide passes freely across the placenta and is readily bound by fetal hemoglobin, thereby decreasing the oxygen-carrying capacity of fetal blood.[14]

8. The nonsmoker exposed to an atmosphere containing tobacco smoke in a confined space may be subject to various physiological impairments (minor eye and throat irritation) and stress, discomfort, respiratory symptoms of coughing and wheezing, and allergic reactions.[15] However, persons with certain heart and lung diseases may suffer a worsening of their symptoms as a result of exposure to tobacco-smoke-filled environments.[16] Carbon monoxide levels occasionally reached in some involuntary smoking situations result in measurable cognitive and motor effects.

9. Elevated carbon monoxide levels in the blood have been shown to decrease maximal oxygen uptake in healthy people, as well as decrease the exercise tolerance of persons with heart disease.[17] Additionally, cigarette smoking tends to impair exercise performance, especially in some types of athletic events and activities involving maximal work capacity.[18]

Fig. 7.7.
Death rate of smokers
versus nonsmokers

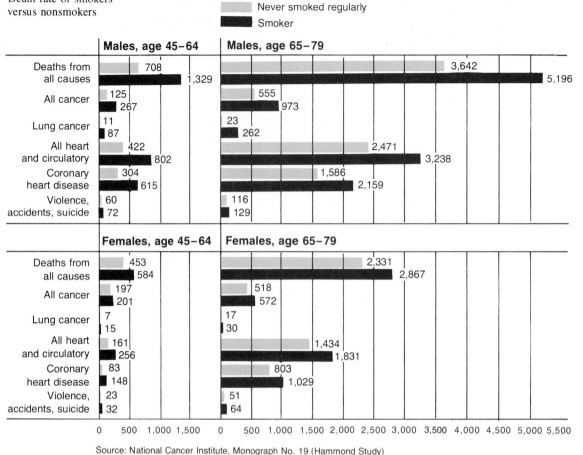

Never smoked regularly
Smoker

Source: National Cancer Institute, Monograph No. 19 (Hammond Study)

Smoking and
Cardiovascular
Diseases

Cigarette smoking is now recognized as a significant risk factor contributing to the development of specific cardiovascular diseases (heart and blood vessel diseases), namely, *coronary heart disease, atherosclerosis,* and *peripheral blood vessel disease.* The risk of death from coronary artery disease alone is nearly 70 percent greater for smokers than for nonsmokers. Recently, cigarette use has been associated with increased mortality from cerebral vascular conditions (strokes) and nonsyphilitic aortic aneurysm (ballooning of the major artery of the body).

The exact mechanisms of cigarette-related cardiovascular diseases are not fully known, but they are thought to involve nicotine and carbon monoxide as principal malefactors. Smoking may initiate a disease process by causing irreversible damage; it may provide positive support to the development of an abnormal condition; it may interfere with and thereby reduce the normal ability of an organism to cope with a disease process; or it may produce temporary conditions

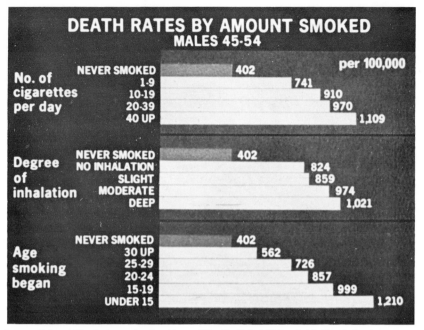

DEATH RATES BY AMOUNT SMOKED
MALES 45-54

		per 100,000
No. of cigarettes per day	NEVER SMOKED	402
	1-9	741
	10-19	910
	20-39	970
	40 UP	1,109
Degree of inhalation	NEVER SMOKED	402
	NO INHALATION	824
	SLIGHT	859
	MODERATE	974
	DEEP	1,021
Age smoking began	NEVER SMOKED	402
	30 UP	562
	25-29	726
	20-24	857
	15-19	999
	UNDER 15	1,210

Source: National Clearinghouse for Smoking and Health, United States Public Health Service

Fig. 7.8. The more one smokes, the greater is the hazard. This is called a *dose-response relationship*. The smoker's dose can be measured by how many cigarettes he smokes, how deeply he inhales, or how many years he has smoked. The person who has never smoked has the lowest death rate, and the one who has exposed himself to the greatest amount of cigarette smoke has the highest death rate.

that increase the likelihood that some critical event will occur with possibly fatal consequences, for example, a heart attack. One or more of these mechanisms may be operable independently or in conjunction with other factors often associated with cardiovascular diseases: obesity, high serum cholesterol, high blood pressure, and physical inactivity.[19]

It is an established fact that nicotine is responsible for increasing heart rate, blood pressure, cardiac output, heart contractions, and consumption of oxygen by heart muscle. Since the heart is working harder, it requires more oxygen to function in its adaptive response to smoking. But carbon monoxide from cigarette smoke tends to displace oxygen from hemoglobin (the substance in red blood cells that carries oxygen and imparts to blood its red color), thus interfering with oxygen-transport and depriving heart muscle of its needed oxygen supply. In a compensatory action of adaptation, the body produces more red blood cells, which are associated with increased clotting as the blood becomes viscous or gummy. The body is slowly starved for oxygen, particulary the brain, which is dulled. Reaction time is lengthened and may be a factor in causing auto accidents in rush hour traffic. Because of its vasoconstriction activity, nicotine can decrease peripheral blood flow, thus placing added stress on the smoker's heart.

Recent evidence suggests that absorbed nicotine and carbon monoxide contribute to the development of atherosclerosis. Cigarette smoking also may be a factor in increased platelet adhesiveness, which predisposes to blood clot formation. It is not surprising, therefore, that there are 280,000 more persons in the United States who report having a heart condition than there would be if all people had the same disease rate as those who never smoked.

Smoking: One Hazardous Adaptation

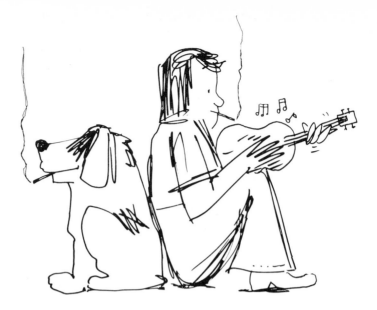

Fig. 7.9. In just three seconds, a cigarette makes your heart beat faster, shoots your blood pressure up, replaces oxygen in your blood with carbon monoxide, and leaves cancer-causing chemicals to spread through your body.

Smoking and Chronic Obstructive Pulmonary Disease

Pulmonary emphysema and *chronic bronchitis,* two diseases that until recently were infrequently reported in the population, today are reaching epidemic proportions. Often seen together in the same patient, the two diseases are jointly referred to as *chronic obstructive pulmonary disease* or COPD, which is characterized by slow, progressive interruption of the airflow within the lungs. COPD is an adaptive response to inhaled irritants and a maladaptation to smoking.

Cigarette smoking has been identified as the most important cause of COPD[20] and increases greatly the risk of dying from pulmonary emphysema and chronic bronchitis. While other factors, including hereditary predisposition, may contribute to COPD, cigarette smoking is now recognized as the major factor in the promotion of "pulmonary cripples." When COPD morbidity is considered, there are more than one million more cases in America than there would be if all people had the same disease rate as those who never smoked.

Pulmonary Emphysema

In pulmonary emphysema the *alveoli* (tiny air sacs of the lungs) lose the elasticity that ordinarily permits them to expand and contract. Air becomes trapped in the alveoli. Eventually, many of the air sacs are stretched abnormally, rupture, and are destroyed. In a vain attempt to accommodate the overstretched lungs, the chest cage enlarges, which unfortunately reduces the efficiency of the diaphragm. As this condition progresses, the ability of the lungs to exchange gases is so seriously impaired that the bloodstream becomes low in oxygen and retains carbon dioxide. Typically, the victim develops shortness of breath and an overworked heart, which speeds up to supply body cells with their oxygen requirements.

Recurring inflammation of the bronchial tubes with excessive mucus production is common in chronic bronchitis. Invariably, a persistent cough develops in an attempt to dislodge the mucus from the narrowed airways. Deep coughing and thick mucus interfere with normal breathing and reduce normal lung function.

Chemicals in inhaled cigarette smoke irritate the bronchial tubes and alveolar sacs over and over again with each puff. In time, the tissues lining the bronchi thicken, the mucus glands enlarge, and the normal cleansing system of the lungs, especially ciliary function, is impaired. The smoker is now more predisposed to respiratory infections and aggravation of existing ones than is the nonsmoker.

Persons who sustain COPD as a result of smoking often spend many years of their lives incapacitated, gasping and struggling for breath, never moving more than a few feet away from a supply of oxygen.

While the relative importance of air pollution in the development of COPD remains controversial, clearly air pollution is a less significant factor under most circumstances than cigarette smoking.

In addition to an increased risk of COPD, cigarette smokers are more frequently subject to, and require longer convalescence from, other respiratory infections than nonsmokers. Also, if they require surgery, smokers are more likely to develop postoperative respiratory complications.[21]

Fig. 7.10. The air sacs are too fine to be visible in the normal lung tissue. Lung tissue (right) of heavy smoker, showing abundance of greatly enlarged air sacs.

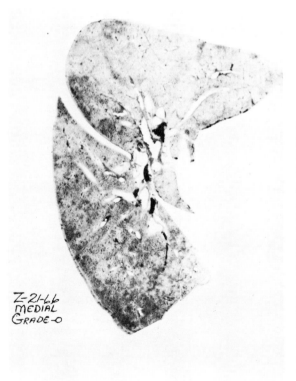
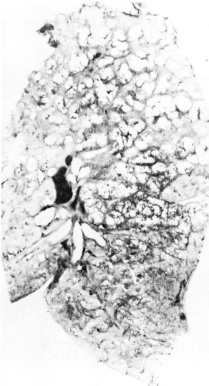

In lung cancer victims, cures are rare, and 95 out of every 100 persons who develop lung cancer will be dead within five years. In fact, the survival rate for the first year after diagnosis of lung cancer is only 25 percent.

Studies of the frequency, distribution, causes, and control of cigarette-related diseases have led an overwhelming number of scientists to conclude that *smoking is the major cause of lung cancer in men*. It is also a cause of lung cancer in women, but for a variety of possible reasons—genetic, hormonal, and differences in dose and frequency of exposure—it accounts for a smaller proportion of cases in women than in men. However, the percentage of women smokers in the United States has increased steadily in the last thirty years, and since 1955 the death rates from lung cancer in women have increased proportionately more rapidly than the rates for men.[22] Lung cancer, unfortunately, is the leading cause of cancer deaths in the United States today with a yearly toll of nearly 89,000 victims. It is estimated that the risk of death from this disease is nearly ten times greater for smokers than for those who do not use cigarettes.

This uncontrolled cellular growth or malignant neoplasm in the lungs is termed *bronchogenic carcinoma* because it arises in the lining of the bronchial tubes through which air passes inwardly to various parts of the lungs. The chances of sustaining lung cancer are enhanced with increased numbers of cigarettes smoked per day, with the duration or length of smoking, and with earlier initiation of use. The risks are reduced when smoking ceases. Apparently, cigarette smoking triggers a disease process (via the tobacco tars) in which continual repair and recovery are possible up to some "critical point." Beyond this point, the process is not reversible.

Laboratory Experiments

In laboratory experiments involving dogs, hamsters, and mice, the cancer-producing nature (carcinogenicity) of the tobacco tars, whole cigarette smoke, and filtered smoke has been demonstrated. When applied to test animals by skin

Fig. 7.11. Two thousand cigarettes, shown on the table, produced the amount of tar shown in the flask.

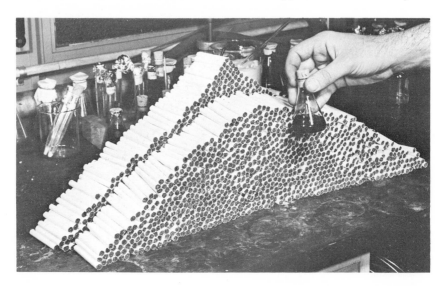

painting, tracheal installation or implantation, and inhalation, the components of cigarette smoke were capable of producing cancerous growths similar to those found in the lungs and larynx of smokers.

However, the most incriminating evidence against cigarettes has been derived from detailed autopsy studies conducted on patients who died of lung cancer in comparison with noncancer patients. Lung cancer victims were found to have increased presence of bronchial tissue changes considered by investigators to be the precursors of invasive cancer. Additional studies then compared the frequency of these cancer-related changes in the lungs of smokers and nonsmokers. In nearly every case, there was noted an increased prevalence of these cellular alterations or adaptations among smokers as compared with nonsmokers. Such changes in the lungs generally occur before cancer cells break through the basement membrane of the bronchial lining and spread throughout the lungs and to other parts of the body. These changes are: (1) *hyperplasia*, (2) *loss of ciliary function in columnar cells*, and (3) *carcinoma in situ*.[23]

Hyperplasia   An increase in the number of layers of basal cells that underlie the inner surface of the bronchial tubes was the first major effect observed. This condition was prevalent in 95 percent of heavy smokers and in 80 percent of light smokers. It was rarely found in nonsmokers. A typical reaction of surface tissue to irritation, hyperplasia probably results from the constant bombardment of tobacco smoke products that under certain conditions accumulate on the lining of the bronchial tubes.

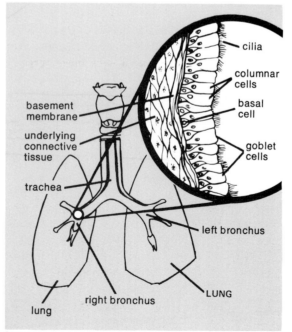

Source: National Advisory Cancer Council

Fig. 7.12.   Most lung cancers originate in the lining or epithelium of the bronchi. Normal epithelium cleanses the lungs of foreign matter, such as dust or smoke particles. Mucus, secreted onto the surface of the epithelium, traps foreign substances. Cilia, extending from the columnar cells, continually move the mucus from the bronchi, through the trachea, and into the mouth, where it is either swallowed or expectorated.

Smoking: One Hazardous Adaptation

Loss of Ciliary Function   Both particulate matter and gaseous components of cigarette smoke have been shown to retard greatly and eventually stop the sweeping movements of cilia, tiny hairlike projections extending from the surface of the columnlike cells of the bronchial tubes. Cilia sweep mucus and other debris out of the respiratory tree into the mouth where it is swallowed or expectorated. Retarded ciliary function interferes with mucus removal and permits the deposition of smoke irritants on the bronchial tube lining. The remaining columnar cells undergo a flattening and enlargement, characteristic of smokers' lung tissue.

Carcinoma in Situ   The development of disordered cells with atypical nuclei was another major change noticed in the lung tissue of smokers. This is a condition of cancer confined to the lining (epithelium) layer of the tissue. Such a phenomenon usually precedes the spreading of uncontrolled cell growth throughout the individual. Significantly, the number of cells with abnormal nuclei decreased noticeably in the bronchial lining of ex-cigarette smokers, depending upon the length of time between cessation of smoking and death. There are advantages to giving up cigarettes!

Reward vs. Risks   The preceding recital of serious health risks should be sufficient to discourage smokers from continuing their life-threatening form of adaptive behavior and to deter new smokers. But the mere presentation of facts has little effect upon all but a few smokers—those who are highly motivated to reduce their exposure to or to quit smoking entirely. Persistence in smoking might seem contradictory in this enlightened, scientific era, but it is due in part to the effectiveness of early learning reinforced thousands of times, puff after puff. As a result of so many rewarding interactions with cigarettes, smoke, and other smokers, the individual's personal values and basic attitudes about life become so ingrained and inflexible that they cannot be cast aside, even when the person recognizes and openly admits the errors of prior learning.

Other considerations play a role in maintaining the conflict between smoking behavior and possible health hazards. One, of course, is the fact that not everyone who smokes becomes ill, incapacitated, or dies. Indeed, certain of the cigarette-related diseases may require some genetic, biological, chemical, or physical factor to be operable before smoking takes its toll.

Then, too, rationalization is commonly employed to justify the smoker's action. We often hear these replies to probing inquiries: "Just one cigarette never hurt anybody." "It won't happen to me because I'm lucky." "Why should I quit since I don't feel sick?" "Why worry? They will find a cure for cancer before I die." Do any of these excuses sound familiar? Many of them are based on the remoteness, the delayed action of the possible harmful effects of smoking. If one cigarette caused serious, immediate illness or death on-the-spot, smoking would rapidly decline or become extinct.

Risk-taking, a necessary component of daily living, compounds the smoking problem. Certainly people should avoid certain risks, but sometimes risks are

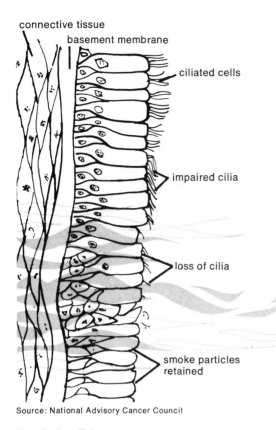

connective tissue

basement membrane

ciliated cells

impaired cilia

loss of cilia

smoke particles
retained

Source: National Advisory Cancer Council

Fig. 7.13. Tobacco smoke contains, in addition to tumor initiators and promoters, substances that affect the cleansing action of the bronchial cells, and thus indirectly influence the induction of lung cancer. These agents may impair and destroy cilia and may affect the mucus layer so that smoke particles are retained in the bronchi.

Fig. 7.14. Microscopic examination of epithelial cells frequently reveals changes in the bronchi of cigarette smokers. These changes usually precede invasive cancer, the stage at which cancer cells break through the basement membrane, spread through the lungs, and then to the rest of the body.

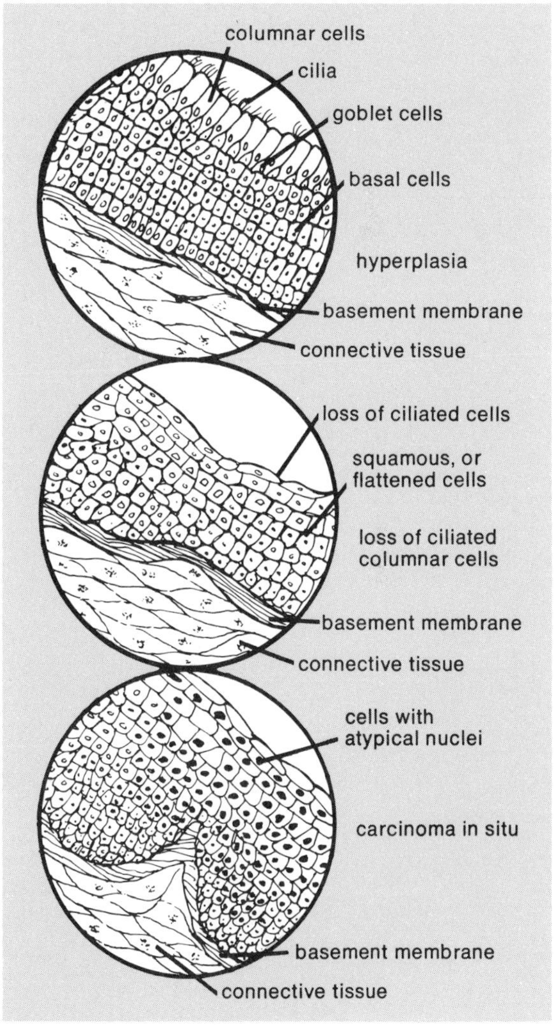

columnar cells

cilia

goblet cells

basal cells

hyperplasia

basement membrane

connective tissue

loss of ciliated cells

squamous, or flattened cells

loss of ciliated columnar cells

basement membrane

connective tissue

cells with atypical nuclei

carcinoma in situ

basement membrane

connective tissue

Source: National Advisory Cancer Council

Smoking: One Hazardous Adaptation   195

taken if they seem negligible or remote in anticipation of the possible, immediate rewards. Not to be overlooked as a further explanation for perpetuating a disease- and death-inducing adaptive behavior is the very real reluctance of individuals to acknowlege that their actions are stupid, irrational, or injurious to themselves.

Still another dimension of the cigarette problem is raised by Norman Cousins who inquires about the significance of life in an affluent society. His classic essay suggests that some smokers really do not care if their life expectancy is reduced.[24] Such dangerous indifference may reflect an insensitivity to the "fragility and preciousness of life" and may correlate with the spread of violence and our life-style of abundance. In essence, the real danger beyond smoking may be a crisis in basic human values.

| Reducing the Risks | Virtually every type of study has led scientists to conclude that increased exposure to cigarette tars, nicotine, and other smoke ingredients leads to increased health risks among the smoking population. Elimination of the exposure to cigarettes is the best and quickest way to reduce both dosage and risks. The longer persons refrain from smoking after once stopping, the more probable it is that their health condition will approach that of their nonsmoking counterparts. After ten years of nonsmoking, death rates of ex-smokers approximate those of nonsmokers. |

Many former smokers report a reduction in smoker's cough and a decrease of nasal stuffiness and discharge, and sputum production. Shortness of breath usually improves within a few weeks. In time, food tastes better, sleep is sounder, fatigue diminishes, taste in the mouth improves, and yellowish stains on teeth and fingers disappear. The economics of giving up cigarettes should not be discounted. Giving up smoking one 60-cent pack of cigarettes a day over a thirty-year period will result in a savings of more than $6,500.

Although the development of a cigarette that is absolutely safe with respect to all presently associated diseases is not likely at the present time, tobacco companies have been successful in reducing the tar and nicotine content of their products. Reconstituted tobaccos and improved filters have met with considerable acceptance by the smoking population. These measures have helped to reduce exposure to potentially harmful substances. The risk to a filter-cigarette smoker, however, still remains above that of the nonsmoker. Unfortunately, the popular 100- and 200-millimeter cigarettes increase both the dosage and risk. Moreover, the addition of menthol may improve the taste, but it does not reduce the health hazards.

While *there is no safe way to smoke*, there are some suggestions that smokers can follow if they wish to make their cigarette use less hazardous. The following recommendations are included in a Public Health Service publication entitled *If You Must Smoke*.[25]

1. *Inhale less.* Cigarette smoke that enters the lungs is the disease-causing agent in pulmonary and cardiovascular disorders. Death rates and morbidity rates

increase with the degree and frequency of inhalation. Some smokers may wish to switch to pipes or cigars, whose smoke is not usually inhaled. Having switched, they may reduce their risks of having lung cancer, COPD, and cardiovascular diseases, but they may increase their risks of developing cancer of the larynx, lip, and esophagus.

2. *Smoke fewer cigarettes.* The exposure to health risks is in direct proportion to the number of cigarettes smoked. The fewer smoked, the lower the risks. This procedure can be promoted by making a conscious effort to stretch the existing supply, by postponing smoking, by placing cigarettes in an out-of-the-way location, and by promising oneself not to smoke during a particular time of day.

3. *Take fewer puffs.* Although a smoker may not be able to reduce the total number of cigarettes used, puffing less on each one will reduce the exposure to the total dose of tars, gaseous components, and toxic chemicals inhaled. While this procedure might seem expensive in the purchase of more cigarettes, it is cheaper in the long run as expressed in personal health, working ability, and longevity.

4. *Smoke one-third down.* Regardless of the brand smoked, the major amounts of tars and nicotine are found in the last few puffs of a cigarette. Tobacco acts as a filter and screens out a portion of the tars and nicotine as they pass through it. As a consequence, smoke from the first third of a cigarette contains approximately 2 percent of the total tars and nicotine, while the last third yields nearly 50 percent. Do not smoke all the way down on cigarettes. Those extra puffs can be perilous puffs!

5. *Choose a low tar and low nicotine cigarette.* By reducing one's exposure to these constituents of cigarette smoke, health risks are likely reduced but not eliminated. No minimum levels of these substances have as yet been determined risk-free or safe. Because of governmental action and increased public interest, cigarette manufacturers now reveal the tar and nicotine content of their products. Periodically the Federal Trade Commission publishes a comparative list showing the tar and nicotine content of cigarette brands produced in the United States. Choosing a less harmful cigarette may be as easy as switching to another brand or to another version of the same brand for any other reason. In every instance, the buyer should beware!

Anything short of quitting completely is only a compromise, however. About 50 percent of successful quitters stop smoking immediately and permanently; the other 50 percent give up smoking gradually.[26] Sometimes attendance at a smoking withdrawal clinic is helpful. Stop-smoking clinics have been particularly effective, especially those conducted by the American Cancer Society, Seventh Day Adventist Five-Day Plan to Stop Smoking, SmokEnders (a commercial organization), and Smoke Watchers. Other techniques, including individual counseling and hypnosis, have proved helpful for many. Whatever the approach, some personal adaptations to a cigarette-free life will probably have to be made, especially during the crucial period immediately after quitting. There are some alternatives to lighting up "just once more."

Table 7.2 Tar and Nicotine Content of Selected Domestic Cigarettes

Brand	Type	Tar (mg)	Nicotine (mg)	Brand	Type	Tar (mg)	Nicotine (mg)
Carlton 70's	Reg.	<0.5	<0.05	Eve 120's	120 mm (HP)	15	1.0
Carlton	King, M*	1	0.1	Kent	King (HP)	15	1.0
Now	King, M (HP)	1	0.1	Saratoga	120 mm, M (HP)	15	1.0
Carlton	King	1	0.1	Viceroy	King	16	1.0
Now	King (HP)	1	0.1	DuMaurier	King (HP)	16	1.1
Iceberg 100's	100 mm, M	3	0.3	Vanguard	King	16	1.0
Lucky 100's	100 mm	3	0.3	Virginia Slims	100 mm, M	16	0.9
True	King	5	0.4	Kent	King	16	1.0
True	King, M	5	0.4	Benson & Hedges	King (HP)	16	1.0
King Sano	King, M	6	0.3	Long Johns	120 mm, M	16	1.3
Pall Mall Extra Mild	King (HP)	6	0.5	Eve	100 mm	16	1.0
King Sano	King	6	0.3	Virginia Slims	100 mm	16	0.9
Pall Mall Extra Mild	King	6	0.5	Pall Mall	100 mm, M	16	1.2
Tempo	King	7	0.5	Eve	100 mm, M	16	1.0
Kent Golden Lights	King	8	0.6	Silva Thins	100 mm, M	16	1.1
L & M Lights	King	8	0.6	Tall	120 mm, M	16	1.3
Merit	King, M	8	0.5	Saratoga	120 mm (HP)	16	1.0
Merit	King	8	0.6	American Longs	120 mm	16	1.3
Kent Golden Lights	King, M	8	0.7	L & M	King (HP)	16	0.9
American Lights	120 mm	8	0.7	Raleigh	King	16	1.1
Lucky Ten	King	9	0.6	American Longs	120 mm, M	16	1.3
Salem Long Lights	100 mm, M	9	0.7	Philip Morris International	100 mm (HP)	16	1.0
Parliament	King (HP)	10	0.6	Philip Morris International	100 mm, M (HP)	16	0.9
Benson & Hedges	Reg. (HP)	10	0.6	Tareyton	100 mm	16	1.2
American Lights	120 mm	10	0.8	Marlboro	100 mm (HP)	17	1.0
Parliament	King	10	0.6	Benson & Hedges 100's	100 mm (HP)	17	1.0
Vello	King, M	10	0.7	Benson & Hedges 100's	100 mm, M	17	1.0
Vello	King	10	0.7	Marlboro	King (HP)	17	1.0
Multifilter	King, M	11	0.7	Marlboro	100 mm	17	1.0
Vantage	King	11	0.7	Silva Thins	100 mm	17	1.3
Vantage	King, M	11	0.8	Kent	100 mm	17	1.1
Salem Lights	King, M	11	0.8	St. Moritz	100 mm	17	1.0
Doral	King, M	11	0.8	Old Gold Filters	King (HP)	17	1.2
Hi-Lite	100 mm	11	0.7	Benson & Hedges 100's	100 mm	17	1.0
Marlboro Lights	King	12	0.7	Twist	100 mm, L/M	17	1.3
Parliament	100 mm	12	0.7	Kool	King, M (HP)	17	1.3
Doral	King	12	0.8	Kool	King, M	17	1.3
Multifilter	King	12	0.8	Max	120 mm, M	17	1.3
Winston Lights	King	12	0.9	Tareyton	King	17	1.2
Fact	King, M	13	0.9	Marlboro	King	17	1.0
Vanguard	King, M	13	0.9	Benson & Hedges 100's	100 mm, M (HP)	17	1.1
True 100's	100 mm, M	13	0.8	St. Moritz	100 mm, M	17	1.1
True 100's	100 mm	13	0.8	Max	120 mm	17	1.3
Fact	King	13	0.9	L & M	100 mm	17	1.1
Marlboro	King, M	14	0.8	Newport	King, M (HP)	17	1.2
Alpine	King, M	14	0.8	Raleigh	100 mm	17	1.2
Kool Milds	King, M	14	0.9	Newport	King, M	17	1.2
Marlboro	King, M (HP)	14	0.8	Sano	Reg., NF	18	0.6
Raleigh Lights	King	14	1.0	Lark	King	18	1.1
Viceroy Extra Mild	King	14	1.0	Montclair	King, M	18	1.3
Eve 120's	120 mm, M (HP)	14	1.0	Kool	100 mm, M	18	1.3
Kool Naturals	King	14	1.0	Pall Mall	King	18	1.2
Belair	King, M	15	1.0	L & M	100 mm, M	18	1.1
Galaxy	King (HP)	15	0.9	Old Gold Filters	King	18	1.2

*Abbreviations: M, menthol; L/M, lemon/menthol; HP, hard pack; NF, nonfilter
Source: Federal Trade Commission

Brand	Type	Tar (mg)	Nicotine (mg)	Brand	Type	Tar (mg)	Nicotine (mg)
Viceroy	100 mm	18	1.3	Kool	Reg., NF, M	21	1.3
Salem	King, M*	18	1.2	More	120 mm, M	21	1.6
Belair	100 mm, M	18	1.3	Old Gold 100's	100 mm	21	1.4
Long Johns	120 mm	18	1.4	Picayune	Reg., NF	21	1.4
Chesterfield	101 mm	18	1.1	Domino	King	21	1.1
Camel Filters	King	18	1.2	Home Run	Reg., NF	22	1.5
Tall	120 mm	18	1.4	Hallmark	100 mm, M (HP)	23	1.8
L & M	King	18	1.1	Stratford	King	23	1.1
Winston	100 mm, M	18	1.2	Mapleton	King	23	1.2
Kent	100 mm	18	1.2	Hallmark	100 mm (HP)	23	1.9
Eagle 20's	King	18	1.1	English Ovals	Reg., NF	24	1.6
Eagle 20's	King, M	18	1.1	Piedmont	Reg., NF	24	1.3
Lark	100 mm	18	1.1	Raleigh	King, NF	24	1.4
Salem	100 mm, M	18	1.3	Chesterfield	Reg., NF	24	1.4
Salem	King, M (HP)	19	1.2	Lucky Strike	Reg., NF	24	1.4
Winston	King (HP)	19	1.2	Philip Morris Commander	King, NF	24	1.4
Winston	King	19	1.2	Old Gold Straights	King, NF	25	1.5
Spring 100's	100 mm, M	19	1.1	Camel	Reg., NF	25	1.6
Chesterfield	King	19	1.1	Pall Mall	King, NF	26	1.6
Pall Mall	100 mm	19	1.4	Half & Half	King	26	1.8
Oasis	King, M	19	1.1	Mapleton	Reg., NF	28	1.3
Winston	100 mm	19	1.3	Herbert Tareyton	King, NF	28	1.8
L. T. Brown	120 mm	19	1.5	Stratford	King, NF	29	1.1
L. T. Brown	120 mm, M	19	1.4	Fatima	King, NF	29	1.7
Camel	King (HP)	19	1.2	Bull Durham	King	29	1.9
Newport	100 mm, M	20	1.4	Chesterfield	King, NF	29	1.7
Old Gold Straights	Reg., NF	20	1.2	English Ovals	King, NF (HP)	30	2.1
Philip Morris	Reg., NF	20	1.1	Domino	King, NF	33	1.4
More	120 mm	21	1.5	Players	Reg., NF (HP)	34	2.5

*Abbreviations: M, menthol; L/M, lemon/menthol; HP, hard pack; NF, nonfilter
Source: Federal Trade Commission

To assist those having an impulse to light up again after once quitting, the following alternatives to smoking are suggested.[27]

Alternatives to Smoking

1. Drink many glasses of water, and sip water frequently.
2. Nibble fruit, celery, carrots, or cookies.
3. Suck candy mints or chew sugarless gum.
4. Gently chew bits of fresh ginger.
5. Bite a clove.
6. Use nicotine replacements, such as lobeline sulphate tablets, unless you have an ulcer.
7. Engage in strenuous physical activity.
8. Spend as much time as possible in no-smoking areas, such as motion picture theaters and libraries.
9. Use mouthwash after each meal.

Summary

Although the proportion of smokers has been declining, the consumption of cigarettes has reached an all-time high. National advertising has contributed greatly to the prevalence of cigarette smoking in the United States. The many different reasons why people start to smoke and continue to smoke are discussed. It is impossible to escape the fact that smoking causes numerous physiological maladaptations. Many of the disease-causing components of tobacco smoke have been identified. Cardiovascular diseases and chronic obstructive pulmonary diseases are found to be more prevalent among those who smoke than among those who do not. The incidence of lung cancer has been shown to be related to cigarette smoking. Once one begins to smoke, it usually becomes increasingly difficult to stop. Yet there is hope that a person, however slightly motivated, can stop smoking. Some suggestions are given for making cigarette use somewhat less hazardous. A few alternatives to cigarette smoking are recommended. It is very difficult to stop smoking—are you up to the challenge?

Review Questions

1. How has smoking helped man adapt to his environment?
2. Explain what is meant by "Smoking is suicide in slow motion."
3. According to health statistics, how do men and women differ in smoking habits?
4. How do cigarettes provide the smoker with personal gratifications that are not found in other tobacco forms?
5. How has motivational research increased the sale of cigarettes?
6. Explain some of the psychological rewards obtained by smoking.
7. What physiological effects does nicotine have on the body?
8. How does cigarette smoking account for the higher incidence of cardiovascular disease?
9. Show how reaction time is influenced by smoking.
10. What is pulmonary emphysema? How does it affect airflow within the lungs?
11. What are the effects of chronic bronchitis? Is this more serious than emphysema?
12. How does cigarette smoking promote the development of cancer in various parts of the body?
13. What is hyperplasia?
14. Do you think that risk-taking behavior is a valid excuse for smoking?
15. Discuss the advantages of smoking vs. nonsmoking.
16. Although there is no safe way to smoke, discuss the recommendations made to make cigarette use less hazardous.
17. Discuss the many possible alternatives to smoking.

1. Daniel Horn, "How Did Society Get into the Cigarette Mess? Why Is It So Hard to Find a Way Out?" *A Summary of the Proceedings of the World Conference on Smoking and Health* (New York: September 11–13, 1967), p. 126.

2. "Adult and Teenage Cigarette Smoking Patterns—United States," *Morbidity and Mortality Weekly Report* (May 13, 1977): 160.

3. Lucille Fisher, "National Smoking Habits and Attitudes," *American Lung Association Bulletin* (September 1977): 6–9.

4. U.S. Department of Health, Education, and Welfare, *The Facts about Smoking and Health* (Washington, D.C.: U.S. Government Printing Office, 1970) and *Facts: Smoking and Health* (Washington, D.C.: U.S. Government Printing Office, 1971).

5. Fisher, "National Smoking Habits," pp. 8–9.

6. "Less Tar, Less Nicotine: Is That Good?" *Consumer Reports* (May 1976): 275.

7. Don C. Matchan, *We Mind If You Smoke* (New York: Pyramid Books, 1977), pp. 16–22.

8. Godfrey M. Hochbaum, *Health Behavior* (Belmont, Calif.: Wadsworth Publishing Co., 1970), p. 31.

9. Silvan S. Tomkins, Director, Center for Research in Cognition and Affect, City University of New York, N.Y.; Daniel Horn, Director, and Selwyn M. Waingrow, Assistant to the Director, Public Health Service, National Clearinghouse for Smoking and Health, U.S. Department of Health, Education, and Welfare, Rockville, Md.

10. "The Chemistry of Smoking," *Time* 109 (February 21, 1977): 48.

11. Harold S. Diehl, *Tobacco and Your Health: The Smoking Controversy* (New York: McGraw-Hill Book Co., 1969), p. 137.

12. National Advisory Cancer Council, *Progress against Cancer* (Washington, D.C.: U.S. Government Printing Office, 1970), p. 49.

13. Unless otherwise indicated, summary statements have been derived from the following publications of the U.S. Department of Health, Education, and Welfare (Washington, D.C.: U.S. Government Printing Office): *The Facts about Smoking and Health,* 1968, 1970; *Smoking and Illness,* 1969; *A Physician Talks about Smoking,* 1971; *Facts: Smoking and Health,* 1971.

14. Public Health Service, Center for Disease Control, *The Health Consequences of Smoking 1975* (Washington, D.C.: U.S. Government Printing Office, 1976), pp. 5–6.

15. Public Health Service, National Clearinghouse for Smoking and Health, *The Health Consequences of Smoking: A Report to the Surgeon General* (Washington, D.C.: U.S. Government Printing Office, 1972), pp. 99–135.

16. Public Health Service, *The Health Consequences of Smoking 1975,* p. 107.

17. Ibid., p. 33.

18. Public Health Service, National Clearinghouse for Smoking and Health, *The Health Consequences of Smoking: A Report to the Surgeon General* (Washington, D.C.: U.S. Government Printing Office, 1973), pp. 239–49.

19. Public Health Service, National Clearinghouse for Smoking and Health, *The Health Consequences of Smoking: A Report to the Surgeon General* (Washington, D.C.: U.S. Government Printing Office, 1971), pp. 4–5.

20. National Heart and Lung Institute, *Respiratory Diseases: A Task Force Report on Problems, Research Approaches, Needs* (Washington, D.C.: U.S. Government Printing Office, 1973), pp. 48–49.

21. Public Health Service, *The Health Consequences of Smoking 1975,* p. 61.

22. Ibid., p. 5.

23. National Advisory Cancer Council, *Progress against Cancer,* pp. 47–48.

24. Norman Cousins, "The Danger beyond Smoking," *Saturday Review,* 25 January 1964, p. 22. *Saturday Review* was one of the first national publications to withhold acceptance of cigarette advertising.

25. Public Health Service, National Clearinghouse for Smoking and Health, *If You Must Smoke* (Washington, D.C.: U.S. Government Printing Office, 1970).

26. American Cancer Society, *Danger* (New York: The Society, 1971).

27. American Cancer Society, *If You Want to Give Up Cigarettes* (New York: The Society, 1970).

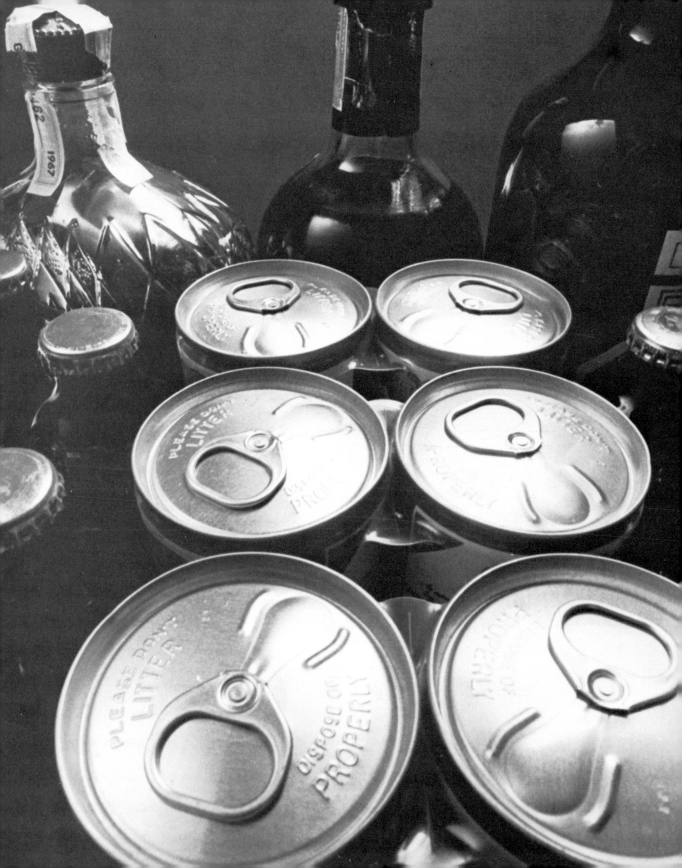

Drinking: Bottled Promises, Canned Problems

8

- *Drinking is okay, but getting smashed and kicking in walls is not okay. Social norms say it is not only okay to get smashed; you're supposed to. That's just not intelligent or sensible.*
- *I see a number of kids drink until they black out at night and then start drinking again in the morning. We're so used to it being a normal part of life that we don't recognize the alcoholic.*
- *Everybody is driving you to "Come on drink, drink." But you also do it because you want to get drunk, and at the particular moment it is socially acceptable to get plastered out of your mind.*
- *Getting drunk isn't just socially acceptable here—it's encouraged.*

These comments have been taken from various college articles written on alcohol use and abuse and campus life.[1] The views expressed are evidence that today's drinking population probably understands alcohol—the drink-drug—and its effects no better than people did twenty centuries ago. Unfortunately, these comments also reveal that the American drinking culture not only allows but encourages relief and escape drinking, the use of alcohol for tension-reduction and tranquilization. In addition, we seem to give status to the person who can drink large amounts of alcohol and to laugh at the individual who gets drunk. These drinking attitudes, in combination with heavy consumption of alcoholic beverages, are the underlying factors of alcohol abuse.

Alcohol and the Drinking Society

Beverage alcohol has been used by many people for centuries. Having originated spontaneously in nearly every culture, the phenomenon of drinking persists because individuals like the effect it produces. Unlike cigarette smoking and marijuana puffing, the use of alcoholic beverages has been an established custom in America for more than three hundred years. Most people consider alcohol as a social beverage; few recognize it as a drug with drug-abuse potential.

Part of our social fabric, drinking has been viewed as a source of desirable, temporary mood-modification and conviviality on the one hand, and as a significant factor in personal and social disorganization, disease, and immorality on the other. These contradictory effects have given rise to an ambivalent attitude toward alcohol use. Thus, while most Americans are "wet," that is, they are

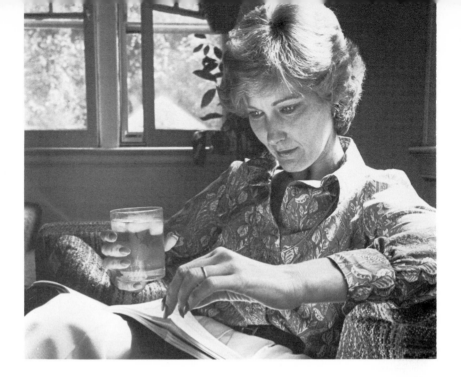

Fig. 8.1. The drink
this woman is having
represents a very
small part of the more
than $21 billion spent
on alcoholic beverages
each year by individuals
and nonprofit
institutions.

drinkers, many of these same persons think "dry"—they feel guilty to some degree and are quite apprehensive about the pleasure derived from alcohol.

Approximately 112 million Americans partake of alcoholic beverages to some extent.[2] These persons make up almost 70 percent of the adult population in the United States. Furthermore, an even larger proportion of alcohol users is consistently found in the younger age groups, with campus surveys reporting that 71 to 96 percent of college students drink.

Each year in the United States drinkers consume a nationwide per capita average of 2.6 gallons of absolute (water-free) alcohol—nearly 28 gallons of beer, 2.25 gallons of wine, and 2.58 gallons of distilled spirits.[3] The annual price tag for such a monumental thirst is approximately $21 billion, or nearly 3 percent of all personal consumption expenditures.

Presently, all states provide for the legal sale and consumption of beverage alcohol. However, definite restrictions controlling manufacture and the time, place, occasion, and qualifications for drinking persist. Two illegal activities—moonshining (illicit production of distilled spirits) and bootlegging (secret and unlawful transportation and sale of beverage alcohol)—also persist and are not confined to the hills of Appalachia.

Historical and Cultural Aspects

Alcohol has not been inconsequential in our national history and commands a rather significant place in our modern life. For example:

1. During the colonial period, many a Yankee fortune was based on the manufacture of rum from supplies of West Indian molasses and the trading of that rum for slaves in Africa.

2. The first rebellion to confront the infant American federal republic was the Whiskey Rebellion in 1794.
3. Early attempts to promote temperance and moderation in the use of beverage alcohol evolved slowly into the legally mandated abstinence movement and culminated in the "noble experiment" of national prohibition from 1920 to 1933.[4]
4. The only amendment to the United States Constitution that has ever been repealed was the Eighteenth (prohibition) Amendment, repealed by the Twenty-first Amendment in 1933.
5. Performing artists generate a mystical alcoholic appeal through their tranquilized manner, their proclamation of "how sweet it is," and their lovable imitation of intoxicated persons.
6. Modern drama, novels, television plays, and films frequently deal with some aspect of alcohol use or abuse.
7. Newly constructed ships are launched with champagne, not with soft drinks, cigarette smoke-rings, or marijuana puffing.
8. When a modern woman puts on one of her fancy dresses in the late afternoon or early evening, she often refers to it as a cocktail dress.

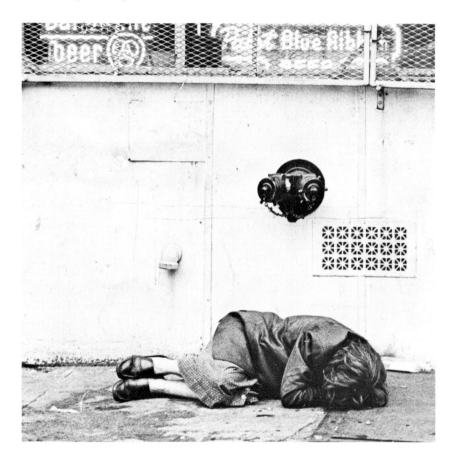

Fig. 8.2. Society must learn to see alcohol abuse as a health problem. For example, Illinois recently passed a law stating that drunks picked up by the police are to be taken to a hospital for care, not to the police station to be locked up.

Additionally, one might consider the numerous breweries that sponsor broadcasts and telecasts of sporting events; the vast acreage of farmlands devoted to the growing of grains, hops, and grapes; and the complex of commercial enterprises concerned with the manufacture, distribution, and sale of beverage alcohol. Alcohol has had and will continue to have a king-size role in our drinking society.

Attitudes
Toward
Drinking

One fact seems of paramount importance. For a variety of reasons and with a measure of moderation, a majority of people in America use alcohol. A significant minority refrains from drinking. But there is strong disagreement about the use and nonuse of alcohol. Such conflict between the closely coexisting value structures of *abstinence* and *permissiveness* generates a good deal of confusion and mixed feelings regarding alcoholic beverages and their effects upon human behavior and society.

There is no consensus on the goodness or badness of drinking. There is no standard of moderation or agreement as to what constitutes responsible drinking. There are no strict controls for social use of alcohol or against abuse of alcohol. In a society marked with such *cultural ambivalence,* many alcohol-related problems, including alcoholism, are likely to exist.[5] The contrasting and often contradictory nature of our attitudes and practices regarding alcohol become apparent in several areas:

1. The different moralities of alcohol use as reflected in different religious denominations. "Drinking is evil." "Alcohol is a gift of God."
2. The varying reactions of individuals to inebriation. These range from horror and contempt to admiration and hilarity.
3. The conflict over the major focus in alcohol education. Shall it be on abstinence, moderation, or alcoholism?
4. The crazy-quilt pattern of governmental laws and college regulations—many of them unenforceable—regarding purchase and consumption of alcohol. Although twenty states have lowered the legal drinking age to eighteen, six states require an individual to be nineteen years old in order to purchase distilled spirits. The remaining twenty-four states have maintained the drinking age for hard liquor at twenty-one. It is somewhat odd that a person is considered an adult in all respects at age eighteen, except for the legal purchase and public consumption of distilled alcoholic beverages.
5. The confusion as to the nature of alcoholism. It is variously described as a disease, a lack of will power, a form of self-indulgence, a basic personality defect, a personal health problem, and a sociolegal problem.
6. The difficulty in reducing public intoxication. The standard procedure of arrest, jailing, and release, followed soon by the rearrest, jailing, and release of the same person (the "revolving door routine") does not appear to reduce the incidence of public intoxication or alcoholism. Such punitive measures will not give way to medical treatment and rehabilitation until society perceives chronic alcoholism as a *health problem* and as a *drug problem* and begins to treat it as such.[6]

Therefore, in our ambivalent, drinking society, everyone "does his or her own thing" with regard to beverage alcohol. Unfortunately, our highly prized diversities may actually thwart the development of an environment less conducive to the abnormal, self-destructive, and antisocial use of alcohol.

National surveys conducted throughout the United States have revealed that the use of alcohol is *typical* behavior for both men and women, whereas abstinence and heavy drinking for escape purposes only are *atypical*.[7] However, when the respondents were classified according to the amount, frequency, and variability of drinking, abstainers, former drinkers, and infrequent drinkers together constituted 43 percent of the total population that was sampled.

Profile of the Drinker

While the proportion of women who drink has increased significantly since World War II, the level of drinking is still higher among men and younger adults than among women and senior citizens. Use of beverage alcohol also varies according to the position of the individual in society, with proportionately more abstainers at the lower social levels. Drinking behavior, according to the surveys, is most likely to occur among persons in the following categories: men and women under fifty years of age, of higher social status; professional and semiprofessional people; technical workers and management officials; college graduates; single men; residents of suburban cities and towns; those whose fathers were foreign-born; and those whose parents drink or approve of it.

Categories of Drinking Behavior

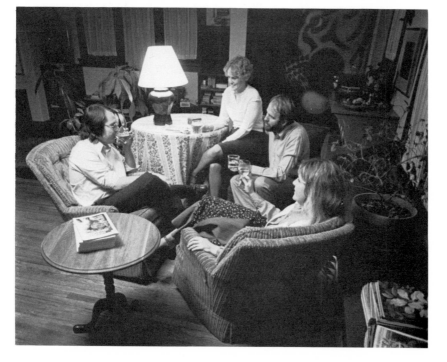

Fig. 8.3. Light social drinking is popular and socially sanctioned in the United States.

When *heavy drinkers* (those who drank every day with five or more drinks per occasion at least once in a while, or about once weekly with usually five or more drinks per occasion) were compared with all other drinkers in the sample population, some major demographic differences were noted. Among drinkers, those most likely to be *heavy drinkers* are men ages forty-five to forty-nine; operatives and service workers; men who completed high school but did not finish college; single, divorced, or separated men and women; residents of the largest cities; and those without any religious affiliation. It should be noted, however, that heavy drinking per se was not related to problem drinking. It was the combination of heavy drinking with nonsocially-oriented reasons for alcohol use that most likely resulted in personal and social disorganization.

A careful analysis of the above data suggests that drinking may be more of a *sociological and anthropological variable* than a psychological one. Furthermore, it was found that among many individuals there is a high turnover rate in drinking or nondrinking status. Also revealed was a strong relationship between drinking and cigarette smoking, especially among women. For certain individuals, drinking and smoking may serve similar functions.

Patterns of Alcohol Use

In a drinking society several patterns of alcohol use are generally evident.[8] Together with associated problems, five different patterns have been identified.

Nondrinking Pattern Nondrinkers are those who never drink with the exception of consuming communion wine in religious ceremonies. About 30 percent of the population fit into this group, many of whom are subtly discriminated against by drinkers at social functions. Some abstainers cannot tolerate the drinking practices of alcohol users and develop hostility and aggressiveness toward them.

Social Drinking Pattern Social drinkers are distinguished by their control over the quantity and rate of ingestion and by their ability to choose whether to engage in such social activity. A substantial proportion of alcohol users, social drinkers, encompass a range of drinking behavior—light, moderate, and heavy. They reject drinking by certain persons in various circumstances as inappropriate, and they themselves are subject to peer-group sanction and laws and ordinances against antisocial behavior resulting from alcohol use.

Episodic Excessive Drinking Pattern The use of alcoholic beverages sometimes exceeds social norms and results in intoxication. For the drinker following this pattern, such occasional episodes of excessive drinking do not become more frequent and apparently do not result in severe social problems, although intoxication increases the drinker's risk of accidents and arrests for drunkenness.

Progressive Excessive Drinking Pattern In the progressive excessive drinking group, persons typically drink to excess when given a drinking opportunity. In time, drinking episodes become more frequent, and periods of intoxication lengthen. Physical disorders, deterioration of social relationships, and difficulties with law enforcement agencies become apparent. Although some control over the frequency and quantity of alcohol use is retained, individuals in this group will develop alcohol dependency unless the pattern is interrupted.

Chronic Alcoholic Drinking Pattern   Chronic alcoholics no longer confine their use of alcohol to social occasions. They have developed a drug dependency in which control over the quantity and frequency of drinking is lost. A return to controlled drinking is not considered possible by most authorities. Continued alcohol abuse is marked by severe physical disabilities, impaired social and economic relations, and sometimes frequent acts of public intoxication.

It is important not to view these drinking patterns as progressive steps from nonuse to alcohol dependency. They merely represent groups of individuals in most communities. Clearly, some of these drinking patterns are more socially acceptable and less personally destructive than others. But when alcohol controls the drinker, risks to health and to society itself multiply rapidly.

For many people, there will probably always be the need for an *adaptive mechanism*—a means of altering man's inner being in relation to his surroundings, his environment. Alcohol serves that function well.

Personal and Social Uses of Alcohol

Drinking is here to stay and likely will not be ejected by our drinking society. By definition, drinking is the consumption of beverages containing ethyl alcohol. Within a sociological interpretation, drinking is described as a particular group's customary way of ingesting beverage alcohol.[9] Such a custom is learned by other members of that group and is perpetuated by the group because drinking serves to facilitate association, to promote interpersonal activity, and to enhance feelings of camaraderie and solidarity. The pleasure derived from drinking is primarily reciprocal, that is, drinking by one of the group brings satisfaction to the other drinkers. Alcohol is seen as the "social lubricant" in which the conscience is dissolved and rigid inhibitions are lowered. For Americans, this social drinking is the common way of imbibing alcoholic beverages.

Social Drinking

Ritualistic use of alcohol is seen in religious ceremonies wherein wine is sacred and drinking is an act of communion. Other cultural ceremonies—celebrating birth, birthdays, engagement, marriage, anniversaries, good fortune, sometimes even death—are also traditionally celebrated with alcoholic beverages.

Ritualistic Drinking

For some, alcohol is an essential part of one's dietary intake, a complement to certain foods or, like cooking wine, a basic ingredient in special food dishes. When alcohol is served along with meals and integrated with routines of family living, the risks of excessive use and intoxication are considerably diminished.

Dietary Drinking

Of course, drinking is often used to satisfy personal needs rather than social or expressive ones. Alcohol can produce a *tranquilizing effect* that reduces tension and anxiety. Perhaps this explains why small doses of beverage alcohol are being

Alcohol as a Tranquilizer

served in increasing numbers of hospitals and rest homes. Stressful situations are more easily tolerated; irritations of everyday living seem to diminish; and relaxation is often promoted. Furthermore, drinking may provide a pleasant and safe way to *feel high or powerful* with one's peers. Thoughts of power, aggression, sexual conquest, and being strong and influential increase regularly with drinking among men.[10] Perhaps having occasional feelings of power is safer than spending time trying to be stronger and more important than others. As such, there is power in positive drinking. In contrast, recently studied females apparently sip to *enhance their sense of womanliness,* with heavy drinking offering to some a "... temporary escape from sex role conflict."[11]

However, while recognizing that alcohol relaxes individuals, temporarily frees them from their inner selves, brightens the world and heightens pleasures, Chafetz contends that even more practical (though not readily understandable) reasons are responsible for the widespread and continuous use of beverage alcohol.[12] He asserts that alcohol has been the most popular and readily available agent for temporarily *increasing awareness* and psychic stimulation, resulting in variations in thought processes, ideas, and activities. Allowing for liquor's ability to induce increased unawareness, he nevertheless views the temporary relaxation provided by alcohol as promoting an enlarged "life scope" and the creation of exhilaration and new enthusiasms. As such, beverage alcohol has played an integral role in the human struggle for survival and in mental evolution of the human being.

Unfortunately, millions of drinkers use alcohol to produce *unawareness* (narcosis) exclusively. They do not wish to return to reality but seek a hiding place from the world in a bottle. Frequent drinking for narcosis only is the type that often leads to alcohol dependency and reduced life expectancy.

Thus, alcohol can serve a variety of personal and social uses. Some of these are more adaptive than others.

| Alcoholic Beverages | The term "alcohol" is used to describe a chemical compound, ethyl alcohol. It is a thin, clear, colorless fluid with a mild, aromatic odor and pungent taste. It is capable of being mixed with water in all proportions, is diffusible through body membranes, and is the essential and characteristic ingredient of beverage alcohol. |

The ethyl alcohol contained in beverages is derived from certain grains and fruits by *fermentation.* In this natural chemical process, yeast cells act on the sugar content of the grain or fruit juice and convert the sugar to carbon dioxide and alcohol. Rarely does one consume pure alcohol. Ingestion is accomplished in the form of beverages generally classified as either wines, beers, or distilled spirits.

Wine

Wine is most often made from the juice of grapes and has an alcohol content of 10 to 14 percent. Sometimes plain alcohol or brandy is added to wines to increase the alcohol content to as high as 24 percent. The result is a fortified wine, such as sherry, vermouth, and the aperitifs.

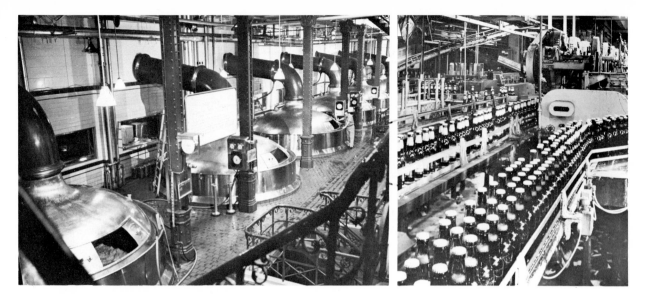

Fig. 8.4. (left) A mixture of brewing grains and water, called *wort,* is boiled prior to fermentation in these 15,500-gallon copper brew kettles. Hops, which give beer its distinctive taste and aroma, are added during the boiling process. The bottling and packing process (right) is the end of the production line and is almost totally automatic.

Beers, including both the regular and the newer light varieties, are derived from cereal grains—barley, rye, corn, and wheat. The process of beermaking is referred to as brewing and includes mashing (the conversion of cereal broth starch to sugar), fermentation, and storage. The resulting product contains from 3 to 6 percent alcohol by volume. The clarified fluid is then carbonated and bottled or canned. Besides water and alcohol, beer contains minute substances called *congeners*. Dextrins, maltose, certain soluble minerals and vitamins, organic acids, salts, and carbon dioxide are common congeners.

Beer

Whiskey, vodka, gin, and brandy are distilled spirits and are made from fermented mixtures of cereal grains or fruits that are heated in a still. (Rum is derived from molasses.) Because alcohol has a lower boiling point than that of other substances in the fermented mixture, ethyl alcohol boils off first. Its vapors are cooled and condensed. These distilled fluids have a relatively high alcohol content along with some water and flavoring ingredients. The alcohol content of such distilled beverages, ranging from 40 to 50 percent by volume, is indicated by the term *proof.* Proof is twice the percentage of alcohol by volume. Thus, a whiskey labeled 90-proof contains 45 percent alcohol by volume.

Distilled Spirits

Each type of alcoholic beverage differs as to alcohol content. Nevertheless, a typical serving of any one beverage contains approximately the same amount of

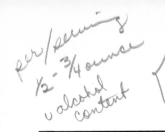

alcohol as does a typical serving of any other alcoholic beverage, though in varying concentrations. The amount of alcohol per serving ranges from just under one-half ounce to three-fourths of an ounce. In most cases, it approximates 0.6 ounce.

Alcohol Within the Body

Once the beverage is swallowed and conveyed to the stomach, the process of *absorption* begins. Unlike other foods, alcohol requires no digestion and diffuses readily through the walls of the gastrointestinal tract where tiny blood vessels pick up the alcohol. About one-fifth of the total alcohol consumed is absorbed in the stomach. The major site of absorption, however, is in the small intestine. A number of factors can influence the absorption.

Factors that Influence Absorption

Concentration of Alcohol   The greater the concentration of alcohol in a beverage, the more rapid will be the rate of absorption. Given the same quantity of alcoholic beverages, two ounces of whiskey will produce a higher blood-alcohol level than two ounces of beer. Blood-alcohol level is the ratio of alcohol present in the blood to the total volume of blood, expressed as a percent.

Amount of Alcohol   The more alcohol ingested at any one time, the longer the absorption period will be.

Rate of Drinking   Rapid ingestion through gulping a drink will likely result in an elevated blood-alcohol level. Drinking in small, divided amounts prevents high concentrations of alcohol because less is available for absorption.

Amount of Food in the Stomach   The presence of food in the stomach delays the absorption of alcohol. Diluted by the food contents, alcohol is retained for a longer period in that body organ where absorption occurs more slowly than in the small intestine.

Body Weight   The more a person weighs, the lower will be the blood-alcohol level. Heavier persons have more body fluids in which the alcohol is diluted.

Body Chemistry   Unique patterns of body functioning may determine individual reactions to alcohol. Anger, fear, stress, nausea, and the condition of stomach tissues have been identified as factors affecting the emptying time of the stomach.

Drinking History   In drinkers with a long history of consumption, the phenomenon of tolerance may be operable so that more alcohol is required to produce a "high" than in inexperienced drinkers.[13]

Distribution and Oxidation of Alcohol

Having diffused through the capillary walls of the small blood vessels in the intestines, the alcohol is now circulated to all parts of the body. Eventually, it is distributed evenly in the body's fluids and cells, achieving a concentration pro-

Table 8.1 Quantity of Serving, Percent Alcohol by Volume, and Quantity of Alcohol per Serving of Various Alcoholic Beverages

Beverage	Quantity of Serving	Percent Alcohol by Volume	Quantity of Alcohol per Serving
Beer	12.0 oz.	4	0.48 oz.
Beer	12.0 oz.	6	0.72 oz.
Table Wine	5.0 oz.	12	0.60 oz.
Sherry	3.0 oz.	20	0.60 oz.
Highball	1.5 oz.	40	0.60 oz.
Highball	1.5 oz.	50	0.75 oz.
Cocktail	1.5 oz.	40	0.60 oz.
Cocktail	1.5 oz.	50	0.75 oz.

Source: Charles R. Carroll, *Alcohol: Use, Nonuse, and Abuse,* second edition, Wm. C. Brown Company Publishers, Dubuque, Iowa, 1975, p. 35. Reprinted with permission of the author and publisher.

portionate to the water content and blood supply of the organ or tissues in question. The *distribution* of alcohol continues a general dilution process begun when the beverage was consumed. Regardless of the original alcohol concentration, the blood-alcohol level rarely exceeds a concentration of 0.60 percent. The moderate drinker's blood-alcohol level approximates a few hundredths of 1 percent.

Most of the alcohol ingested, absorbed, and distributed—more than 90 percent—is combined with oxygen. This process of *oxidation* results in the formation of water and carbon dioxide and the production of heat and energy. First, ethyl alcohol is converted into acetaldehyde in the liver where an enzyme functions as a catalyst in the chemical reaction. Immediately thereafter, the acetaldehyde, a toxic substance, is oxidized to acetic acid in a process occurring both within the liver and in other organs. Authorities disagree as to the site of the third phase of oxidation, in which acetic acid is changed to water and carbon dioxide, the process yielding about seven calories of energy per gram of alcohol.

While the rate of alcohol oxidation varies from person to person due to size of the liver, enzyme activity, diseases of the liver, and certain drug reactions, the average rate of disposition is estimated to be one-third ounce of pure ethyl alcohol or two-thirds to three-fourths of an ounce of whiskey per hour. Moreover, this rate is fairly constant for each person, and no practical way of significantly increasing the oxidation rate has been developed. Researchers do report, however, that intravenous doses of fructose—a fruit sugar—cause a rapid lowering of the blood-alcohol level in intoxicated patients.[14]

The most dramatic consequences of alcohol use pertain to *mood and behavior modification.* Such alterations of feelings and conduct are due to the action of alcohol on the central nervous system, specifically the brain, and are in direct proportion to the *blood-alcohol level* or *blood-alcohol concentration (BAC).*

Effects of Alcohol

Drinking: Bottled Promises, Canned Problems

Table 8.2 Relationship Between Type and Amount of Alcoholic Beverages Consumed and the Estimated Potential Blood-Alcohol Concentration

Alcoholic Beverages	Alcohol Content (%)	Normal Measures Dispensed	Estimated Potential Blood-Alcohol Concentration in One Hour*		
			One Drink	Two Drinks	Three Drinks
			Body Weight 100 140 180 220 (% w/v)	Body Weight 100 140 180 220 (% w/v)	Body Weight 100 140 180 220 (% w/v)
Beer					
Ale	5%	12-oz. Btl.	0.05 0.04 0.03 0.02	0.08 0.06 0.05 0.05	0.11 0.09 0.08 0.07
Malt Beverage	7%	12-oz. Btl.	0.06 0.05 0.04 0.03	0.09 0.07 0.06 0.05	0.15 0.12 0.09 0.08
Regular Beer	4%	12-oz. Btl.	0.04 0.03 0.02 0.02	0.07 0.05 0.04 0.03	0.10 0.08 0.06 0.05
Wines					
Fortified: (Port, Muscatel, etc.)	18%	3-oz. Gls.	0.04 0.03 0.02 0.02	0.07 0.05 0.04 0.03	0.10 0.08 0.06 0.05
Natural: Red/White Champagne	12%	3-oz. Gls.	0.03 0.03 0.02 0.02	0.06 0.05 0.04 0.03	0.08 0.06 0.04 0.04
Cider (Hard)	10%	6-oz. Gls.	0.05 0.04 0.03 0.02	0.08 0.06 0.05 0.05	0.11 0.09 0.08 0.07
Liqueurs					
Strong: Sweet, Syrupy	40%	1-oz. Gls.	0.03 0.03 0.02 0.02	0.07 0.05 0.04 0.03	0.08 0.06 0.05 0.05
Medium: Fruit Brandies	25%	2-oz. Gls.	0.04 0.03 0.02 0.02	0.08 0.06 0.04 0.04	0.10 0.08 0.06 0.06
Distilled Spirits					
Brandy; Cognac; Rum; Scotch; Vodka; Whiskey	45%	1-oz. Gls.	0.04 0.03 0.02 0.02	0.07 0.05 0.04 0.03	0.09 0.07 0.06 0.05
Mixed Drinks & Cocktails					
Strong: Martini; Manhattan	30%	3½-oz. Gls.	0.08 0.06 0.04 0.04	0.15 0.12 0.09 0.08	0.22 0.16 0.12 0.10
Medium: Old Fashioned; Daiquiri; Alexander	15%	4-oz. Gls.	0.05 0.04 0.03 0.02	0.08 0.06 0.05 0.05	0.11 0.09 0.08 0.07
Light: Highball; Sweet & Sour Mixes; Tonics	7%	8-oz. Gls.	0.05 0.04 0.03 0.02	0.08 0.06 0.05 0.04	0.12 0.09 0.07 0.06

*For each hour additional subtract 0.015% w/v from the number shown.
Source: U.S. Department of Transportation, National Highway Traffic Safety Administration.
Adapted from "Alcohol & the Impaired Driver" (AMA)

Most drinkers who have a relatively low BAC from 0.01 percent to 0.03 percent (the result of one or two servings of alcoholic beverages) will experience only mild effects, such as slight changes in feeling, heightening of existing moods, and minimal impairment of mental function. Definite impairment begins in a zone ranging from 0.03 percent to just below 0.10 percent. As the BAC increases, the degree of mental inefficiency increases. Feelings of relaxation and sedation are experienced, and the control of voluntary muscles declines in the performance of fine motor skills. These changes are manifestations of alcohol's *progressive, depressant action* on the brain.

Functional impairment increases rapidly and more noticeably after the BAC reaches 0.10 percent and takes several forms: decreased inhibitions, less efficient vision and hearing, slurring of speech, difficulty in performing gross motor skills, deterioration of judgment, and a general feeling of euphoria. Studies reveal that with a BAC between 0.10 percent and 0.15 percent, about 65 percent of drinkers display definite signs of physical and mental impairment. When the BAC increases to 0.20 percent, nearly all drinkers display profound and obvious signs of intoxication—difficulty in walking and speaking and irresponsible and often antisocial behavior; they are intoxicated! Intoxication can be defined as a temporary state of apparent malfunctioning or mental chaos that results from the presence of alcohol in the central nervous system. Alcohol is being consumed faster than it can be oxidized in the body. As the brain becomes more anesthetized, the drinker has difficulty maintaining an upright position, experiences dulled perception and minimal comprehension, and finally loses consciousness. If the BAC exceeds 0.60 percent, the drinker's brain becomes so depressed that breathing and heartbeat cease and death results.

Because the mood or mind-set of the consumer, along with the psychological atmosphere of drinking, will likely influence the drinker's responses to alcohol, estimating the degree of impairment by observation has proved very unreliable. Therefore, chemical tests for an objective evaluation of intoxication have been developed and involve the determination of alcohol levels in the blood and the breath. The tests are based on the constant proportion between alcohol concentrations in blood and in the breath. Several breathalyzer instruments are available, namely, the *alcometer*, *drunkometer, intoximeter*, and especially the *breathalyzer*. The latter has been used increasingly by law enforcement agencies to identify drunken drivers.

Other body parts and functions can be influenced directly or indirectly by alcohol. The short-term effects include the following:

1. Accumulation of fat in the liver—a direct toxic effect of frequent alcohol consumption and now considered the forerunner of or predisposing factor in other liver diseases associated with long-term alcohol use, such as alcoholic hepatitis and alcoholic cirrhosis.
2. Increased production of urine, due to the effect of alcohol on the pituitary gland.
3. Temporary increase in heartbeat and blood pressure, and in some males with an abnormal blood condition an increase in blood fats.

Effects of Alcohol on the Brain

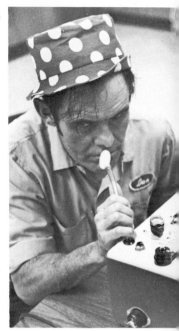

Fig. 8.5. The breathalyzer, developed by Dr. Robert F. Borkenstein of the Center for Studies of Law in Action, Indiana University, is one method used by police to determine whether a driver is legally intoxicated. The results of such tests are admissible in court.

Effects of Alcohol on Other Body Parts and Functions

4. Dilation of peripheral blood vessels, which leads to a loss of body heat while producing a feeling of added warmth.
5. Increased production of gastric juices that may help in the digestion of food.
6. Shifting of water from within the body's cells to the spaces between the cells, which may account for the sensation of thirst.
7. Production of the temporary but acute distress of the hangover, which is possibly related to the toxic congeners (contaminants that add color, aroma, and flavor) in beverage alcohol, the type of food eaten and the liquor consumed, emotional influences, and physical factors, especially fatigue. As Chafetz notes,

> heavy doses of alcohol so put our brain to sleep that we do not recognize and respond to the signals telling us that our nerves and muscles are exhausted. We push ourselves beyond our points of endurance because we have anesthetized the protective warning systems in our brains.[15]

Consequently, the nausea, gastritis, headache, and anxiety we experience are painful reminders of disrupted body functions that could not be felt while we were overdosed with alcohol.

Prolonged, heavy consumption of alcoholic beverages can result in more tragic consequences.[16]

1. Brain disorders, marked by either short-term or prolonged psychoses
2. Inflammation of the liver, or alcoholic hepatitis
3. Alcoholic cirrhosis, one of the severest disorders suffered by alcohol abusers, characterized by the shriveling and hardening of the liver with fibrous tissue that impairs liver function
4. Irritation and inflammation of the stomach lining
5. Various heart disorders
6. Muscle weakness
7. Disturbed function of the endocrine glands
8. Serious malnutrition
9. Conditions of tolerance, physical dependence, and psychological dependence, as described in detail in the chapter on drug-taking behavior

In addition, research has revealed two other health problems associated with heavy use of alcohol: (1) the excessive use of alcohol, especially in combination with tobacco, has been implicated in the development of cancers of the mouth, throat, esophagus, liver, and pancreas;[17] and (2) heavy drinking during pregnancy can adversely affect the offspring of alcohol-abusing mothers.[18] Children of alcoholic mothers not only have been born dependent or addicted to alcohol, but also have exhibited the Fetal Alcohol Syndrome (FAS). This syndrome is a group of abnormalities including physical deformities of the ribs and of the bones of the face and impaired learning abilities.

It should also be noted that due to the *potentiation effect* of certain drugs, the multiplied drug effect of using tranquilizers and antihistamines in combination with alcohol may be extremely hazardous and even fatal, as in the case of barbiturates or sleeping pills.

Although recent studies suggest that a substantial excess in early mortality exists among frequent heavy drinkers and those with a high number of drinking-related problems,

> the nonexcessive use of alcohol does not appear to adversely affect the overall mortality rate or the mortality from a specific major cause of death, coronary heart disease. In fact, the mortality of drinkers is lower than that of abstainers and ex-drinkers.[19]

As the *Second Special Report on Alcohol and Health* concludes, the devastating problems associated with the use of alcohol all relate to excessive use, not moderation—to misuse, not to responsible use. Moderation appears to be the key. Moderate consumption of alcohol is generally not harmful. In some cases, such as among the elderly, it may have beneficial physical, social, or psychological effects. The only question is "What is moderate or responsible drinking?" ???
What is your definition of moderate drinking?

Problem drinking refers to alcohol consumption that results in damage to the drinker, the drinker's family, or the drinker's community. Included among problem drinkers are not only the alcoholics but also those who drive after excessive drinking and cause accidents, those who engage in drinking to become intoxicated, and those who drink when such imbibing is contraindicated by some medical condition. Some problem drinkers even engage in the "sport" of competitive ingestion to determine who can hold more.

Problem Drinking: Personal and Social Aspects

For the person involved, immoderate drinking can result in intoxication, death or injury by accident, loss of a job, disruption of family life, quarreling and fighting, and certain deficiency and metabolic diseases often associated with excessive drinking. Dependence on alcohol as a psychological crutch to hide or mask problems of everyday living is particularly hazardous, especially for young persons. Young people dependent on alcohol may never develop and practice decision-making skills for coping with the perplexities and disappointments of reality. Furthermore, some evidence indicates that alcohol—not marijuana—is the first mood modifier used by a high percentage of people who later become drug addicts.[20]

Effects of Problem Drinking on the Individual

While the relationship between alcohol and various social problems cannot be explained as a direct cause-and-effect phenomenon, that such problems may be the aftermath of excessive drinking is a fact.

Effects of Problem Drinking on Society

The Cost to Industry Consider the cost to industry alone, for problem drinkers typically continue working during most of their developing alcoholism, making up about 3 percent of the normal work force.[21] Both quality and quantity of work performance decline, accidents occur more frequently, absenteeism increases, experienced and trained personnel are sometimes discharged, and relationships with fellow workers and especially supervisors generally deteriorate, affecting the work of everyone involved.

ten terrific hangover cures.

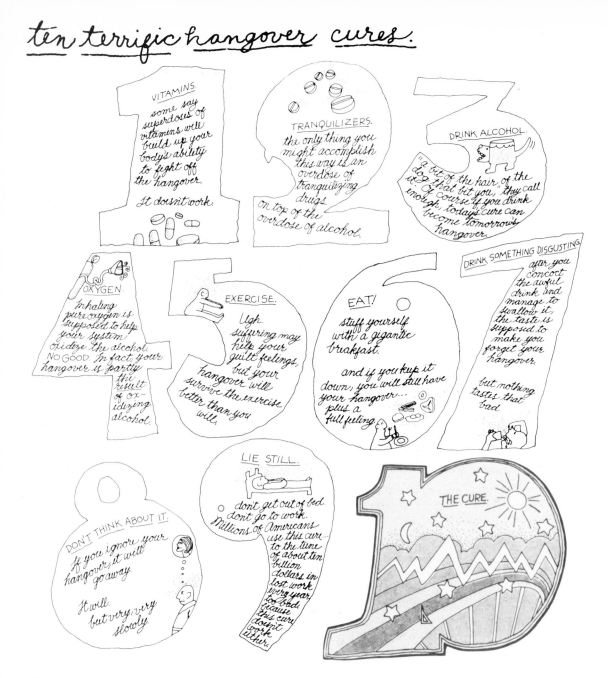

1 VITAMINS
some say superdoses of vitamins will build up your body's ability to fight off the hangover.

It doesn't work.

2 TRANQUILIZERS.
the only thing you might accomplish this way is an overdose of tranquilizing drugs on top of the overdose of alcohol.

3 DRINK ALCOHOL.
"a bit of the hair of the dog that bit you," they call it. Of course if you drink enough, today's cure can become tomorrow's hangover.

4 OXYGEN.
inhaling pure oxygen is supposed to help your system oxidize the alcohol. NO GOOD. In fact your hangover is partly the result of oxidizing alcohol.

5 EXERCISE.
Ugh. suffering may help your guilt feelings, but your hangover will survive the exercise better than you will.

6 EAT!
stuff yourself with a gigantic breakfast.

and if you keep it down, you will still have your hangover... plus a full feeling.

7 DRINK SOMETHING DISGUSTING.
after you concoct the awful drink and manage to swallow it, the taste is supposed to make you forget your hangover.

but nothing tastes that bad.

8 DON'T THINK ABOUT IT.
If you ignore your hangover, it will go away.

It will, but very, very slowly.

9 LIE STILL.
don't get out of bed. don't go to work. Millions of Americans use this cure... to the tune of about ten billion dollars in lost work every year, too bad, because this cure doesn't work either.

10 THE CURE.

Fig. 8.6. Hangover cures have been sought by drinkers throughout history. Sometimes the cure chosen was worse than the ailment. If the excessive drinker cannot rely on the healing powers of time, prevention is the only other practical cure.

The Toll on Family Life, Health, and Law Enforcement   The toll on human resources is greater still in terms of family life, health problems, and law enforcement activities. Nearly 36 million Americans can be regarded as caught in the web of alcohol abuse—unhappy marriages, broken homes, desertion, divorce, impoverished families, and deprived, displaced, and abused children. Problem drinking interferes with the normal role of spouse or parent and often adversely affects the sexual life of the marriage partners. Quite often the strained relationship ends in divorce and fracturing of the family unit. Estimates of general hospital patients with alcohol problems range from 10 to 50 percent; nearly half of the tuberculosis patients requiring long-term hospitalization are alcoholics. Many municipal court cases are alcohol related, and some police departments spend from one-fourth to one-third of their time and energies in the apprehension and arrest of individuals who are publicly intoxicated.

In addition, an association with alcohol has been found in 64 percent of all murders, in 41 percent of all assaults, in 34 percent of all forcible rapes, and in one-third of all suicides. The economic cost of alcohol misuse in America, in terms of lost production, health and medical expenses, motor vehicle accidents, alcohol treatment programs and research, social welfare, and criminal justice has been estimated conservatively at $25 billion annually.[22]

Problem Drinking and Automobile Accidents   The magnitude of problem drinking in relation to automobile safety and traffic offenses has become widely known. It is commonly recognized that many of those who drink and drive do not display the obvious signs of intoxication, and yet they are under the influence of alcohol. Slightly impaired judgment, false sense of security, slower reaction time, narrowed peripheral vision, lessening of depth perception, reduction of cue-taking, inflated ego, and undue expansion of aggression all take their toll on the driver's ability. Also subtly affected at moderate BACs are those time-sharing capabilities and various complex decision-reaction processes involved in operating a motor vehicle.[23] Consequently, the focus of traffic safety programs has been the "social drinker." Now, however, it is held that:

> The use of alcohol by drivers on the highways, particularly the *continued, excessive use of alcohol by problem drinkers,* is the single most important highway safety issue today.[24]

Drinking drivers and pedestrians are responsible for about half of all traffic deaths and injuries with a yearly toll of more than 25,000 fatalities. Most of these fatal accidents are caused not by the social drinker but by drivers who drink to great excess—an excess rarely attained by the social drinker.

These problem drinkers have BACs 50 to 100 percent higher than the 0.10 percent level. This level (0.10 percent) has been set as indicative of intoxication by the National Highway Traffic Safety Administration. The same level also has been adopted by most states as legal evidence of driving under the influence of alcohol.

The individual with a BAC of 0.10 percent is six to seven times more likely to cause an auto accident than is a nondrinker. With a 0.15 percent BAC the person

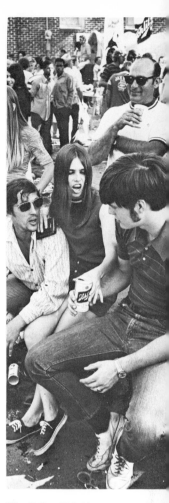

Fig. 8.7. Drinking, especially beer and wine, has once again become a popular activity for American youth. Some recent statistics show that alcohol is replacing the milder drugs, such as marijuana, as the preferred mood modifier for many young people. There is also an alarming increase in the number of teenage alcoholics in the United States.

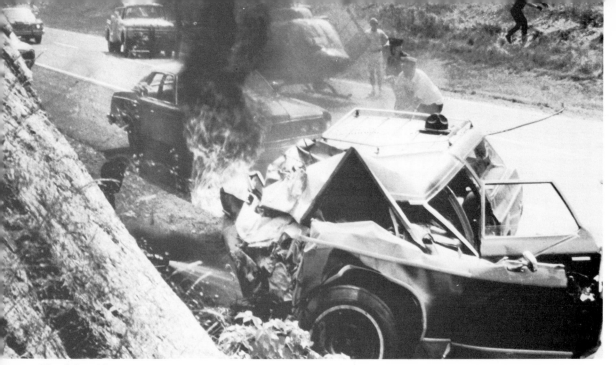

Fig. 8.8. About half of all traffic deaths and injuries are caused by drinking drivers and pedestrians.

is twenty-five times more likely to have a collision than is a nondrinker. In achieving such BACs the amount of alcohol consumed is considerable.

To reach a concentration of 0.15 percent, for example, within two hours after eating, a 160 pound man would have to drink ten one-ounce drinks of 86 proof whiskey, all to be consumed in one hour. The same drinker would reach the same state of intoxication with one-third less quantity, if taken on an empty stomach. . . . That's a lot of drinking.[25]

Faced with an ever-increasing array of countermeasures—implied consent laws, breath tests, tighter licensing and probation procedures, more effective law enforcement, and mandatory rehabilitation schools for those convicted of driving while intoxicated—the drinking driver's party is coming to an end.

Alcoholism: Nature and Prevalence

Perhaps the most extreme form of problem drinking is that of alcoholism, now considered a complex illness—a *psychosocial, physiological disorder* and a type of *drug dependence*. Alcoholism involves more than heavy drinking. It is generally described as long-term, repeated, uncontrolled, compulsive, and excessive use of alcoholic beverages that significantly impairs the drinker's health and interpersonal relationships. The chief characteristic of this disease is the drinker's inability to control either the beginning of drinking or its termination once it has started.

As a health problem, alcoholism ranks as the fourth most serious concern in the United States, exceeded only by heart disease, cancer, and mental illness. It is estimated that there are more than ten million American alcoholics, proof that:

Alcohol is not only our most extensively used and abused mind-altering drug but by far the *hardest* drug known to man. The abuse we call alcoholism proves this. . . . [26]

These alcoholics affect millions of other family members, employers, fellow workers, and even taxpayers. While alcoholism is no respecter of race, color, creed, sex, ethnic group, marital status, geographical location, or socioeconomic status, various studies reveal some intriguing facts about this illness.

1. There are more reported male alcoholics than female alcoholics, because many of the latter are hidden more easily from public view. As more and more females enter the work world outside the home, their drinking problems will more likely be detected. Unfortunately, the woman who does become an alcohol abuser is forced by society to carry a double burden.

   She is tagged with the moral stigma of alcoholism, and is doubly stigmatized because it has always been considered unladylike—the object of unforgiving scorn and disgust—for a woman to be drunk.[27]

2. Alcoholics in the past most often have tended to be thirty-five to fifty-five years old. However, an alarming increase in an adolescent-onset form of alcoholism has been noted recently. Furthermore, current statistics indicate that males in their late teens and early twenties actually have the highest incidence of alcohol-related problems and problem drinking behaviors.
3. Many alcoholics display neurotic tendencies, feelings of alienation, and the inability to tolerate frustration.
4. Highest rates of alcoholism in America prevail among persons of Irish and Anglo-Saxon backgrounds. The incidence is also particularly high among American Indians and Alaskan Eskimos; among the latter the illness has reached epidemic proportions. Lowest rates occur among Italian-Americans, Chinese-Americans, Jews, Lutherans, and Episcopalians.
5. Alcoholism rates tend to be higher in urban and industrial areas.
6. Rates of problem drinking are highest among persons who are separated, single, and divorced, and among those with no religious affiliation.
7. Less than 5 percent of all alcoholics are found on skid row. Most manage to hold jobs and maintain homes where they are sheltered by a spouse and children. The stereotyped image of the alcoholic as the skid row inebriated bum often deludes the "respectable" alcoholic and his family into minimizing the seriousness of his own problem drinking.[28] In reality, alcoholism is an illness that can occur in all walks of life. No one is immune to alcohol abuse!

Without alcohol, there would be no alcoholics. However, most persons who use beverage alcohol do not develop into problem drinkers. Therefore, while alcohol is a necessary factor in alcoholism, it is not the sole causative agent. Additionally, alcoholism does not result from drinking a particular alcoholic beverage; it is not an allergic manifestation nor is it inherited; and the disorder is not due to a well-defined "alcoholic personality."[29]

Alcoholism:
Causes, Signs,
and Symptoms

Alcoholics display such varying backgrounds and characteristics, and so many possible causative factors have been proposed that some authorities believe many alcoholisms must exist rather than a single disorder. While psychopathology may be dominant in the development of alcoholism, other aspects are also considered by researchers. Those factors most frequently cited in the causation of alcoholism are classified as physical, psychological, or social.

Physical
Factors

The abnormal response of the alcoholic to ingested alcohol may be determined by physical factors that interfere with alcohol metabolism in the body. A nutritional deficiency may result in an unusual craving for alcohol; an inherited susceptibility or predisposition, adversely affected by ingested alcohol, may be responsible for the tendency of alcoholism to occur in certain families; a malfunction of the endocrine system (the several ductless glands that act through their hormonal secretions to maintain a balance in the body's activities) may be the basis for alcoholism, the effect of hormonal imbalance.

Another physiological theory suggests that, in alcoholics, a defect in the metabolism of acetaldehyde produces addictive substances, precursors of opiate alkaloids. Such a phenomenon could serve as the common physiological basis to all types of drug addiction. Recent neurobiological research has linked alcoholism in laboratory animals with chemical changes in the brain. Perhaps alcoholism is due to some quirk in body chemistry.

Psychological
Factors

Among various theories about psychological factors is the common belief that alcoholism is the consequence of some disorder in emotions, personality, or behavior. Early environmental factors give rise to these disorders as well as to the development of adult drinking practices.

Although no single type of alcoholic personality exists, characteristics often observed in alcoholics include immaturity, impulsiveness, dependency, hostility, low self-esteem, self-punishing and self-destructive behavior, little tolerance for anxiety and frustration, feelings of loneliness and isolation, depressiveness, and compulsiveness. Many of these traits are related to childhood rejection, a lack of security, loving care, and supportive and constructive parental guidance, and the presence of friction and antagonism between mother and father. As an adult, the drinker uses alcohol to escape such painful feelings.

Another possible predisposition is seen in the child who is overprotected, overindulged, or overdisciplined. Such an individual never learns to postpone gratification of his desires or needs or to engage in effective problem-solving techniques. In adulthood, these persons may use alcohol to relieve tensions and anxieties when immediate gratification is not possible in normal interaction or experience.

Psychoanalytic theories are based on three general suppositions, any one of which may be the causative factor in alcoholism. According to the Freudian view, alcoholism results from unconscious tendencies, such as self-destruction, oral fixation, and latent homosexuality. The Adlerian view contends that alcoholism is indicative of a struggle for power by producing exaggerated feelings of importance and self-worth. Another viewpoint perceives the development of

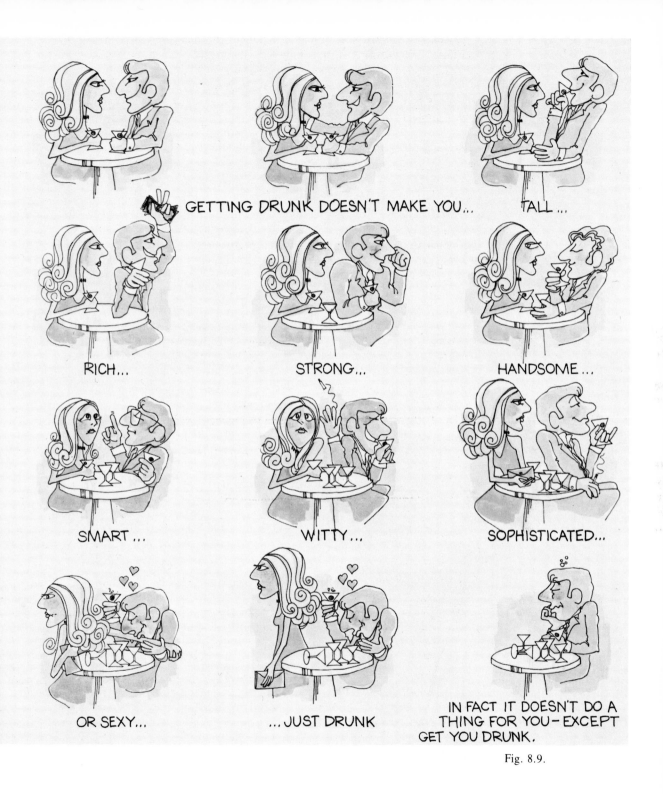

GETTING DRUNK DOESN'T MAKE YOU... TALL...

RICH...

STRONG...

HANDSOME...

SMART...

WITTY...

SOPHISTICATED...

OR SEXY...

...JUST DRUNK

IN FACT IT DOESN'T DO A THING FOR YOU — EXCEPT GET YOU DRUNK.

Fig. 8.9.

alcoholism as a response to internal conflict between dependency drives and aggressive impulses.

The learning and reinforcement theory explains alcoholism in terms of a reflex response to some stimulus. A person soon learns that the use of alcohol reduces tension or feelings of frustration and replaces unpleasantness with feelings of well-being and euphoria. Learning theory also suggests that children who see parents using alcohol to solve or escape from daily problems will themselves adopt such drinking habits. In addition, children who are served ''kiddie cocktails'' may be subtly encouraged to drink to gain adult approval and learn that alcohol is only a social beverage, rather than a dangerous drug.

Sociological Factors

Many authorities cite the anxiety-reducing capacity of alcohol as the primary reason for its near universal use and value. If a culture functions so as to create inner tensions, deprivations, or acute needs for mood modification, the incidence of heavy, escape drinking may be influenced. The existence of ambivalent attitudes and conflicting values regarding alcohol often leads to general confusion as to what constitutes acceptable drinking behavior. Unwittingly, our culture may be encouraging alcoholism by accepting ''relief drinking,'' by promoting drinking unrelated to family activities and mealtime, by enshrining alcohol use as a status symbol, and by tolerating and accepting intoxication as funny or manly.

According to some behaviorists, when society permits a large gap to develop between goals or expectations and the means for achieving them, many people express their alienation through retreatism and rebellion, as represented in alcoholism.

Fig. 8.10.

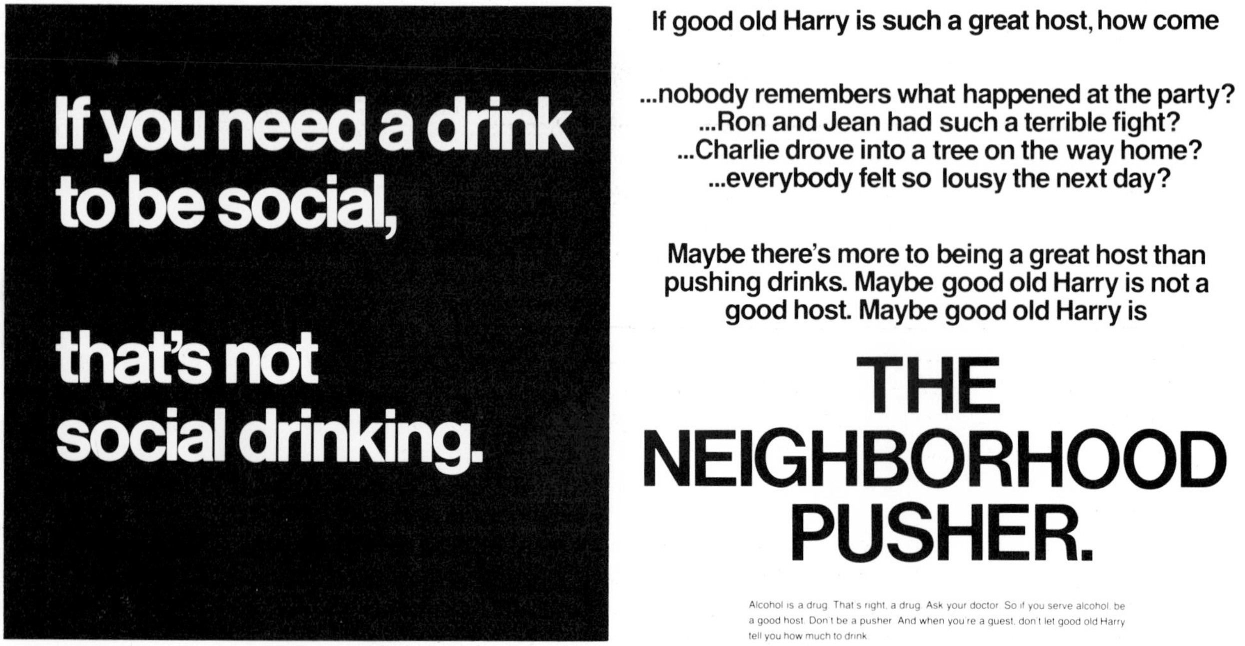

If you need a drink to be social, that's not social drinking.

If good old Harry is such a great host, how come

...nobody remembers what happened at the party?
...Ron and Jean had such a terrible fight?
...Charlie drove into a tree on the way home?
...everybody felt so lousy the next day?

Maybe there's more to being a great host than pushing drinks. Maybe good old Harry is not a good host. Maybe good old Harry is

THE NEIGHBORHOOD PUSHER.

Alcohol is a drug. That's right, a drug. Ask your doctor. So if you serve alcohol, be a good host. Don't be a pusher. And when you're a guest, don't let good old Harry tell you how much to drink.

Although the causes of alcoholism are complex and remain somewhat obscure, the signs and symptoms are generally better known.[30] Unfortunately, these signs and symptoms of developing alcoholism are often denied or effectively hidden from others by the sneaky drinker who drinks on the sly. Early warning signals are: an exceedingly pleasant response to alcohol; the need for increased intake to produce the same effect (*tolerance*); and the experience of alcohol-induced amnesia, the *blackout*. Very soon the use of alcohol deviates drastically from social drinking, and the drug effects of euphoria become the singular reason for consumption. Eventually, the alcoholic is preoccupied with procuring a source of alcohol and begins to drink alone, inventing occasions for imbibing if none exists. Intake increases rapidly as guzzling becomes the norm. Sometimes the drinker is unable to abstain. More often, the alcohol abuser cannot control drinking once it is begun. A *physiological need* for alcohol has developed and if denied an additional dose, the alcoholic will sustain *withdrawal symptoms* of *delirium tremens*—involuntary shaking of the body or convulsions, restlessness, mental confusion, and hallucinations of a terrifying nature. Now, the alcoholic craves booze!

A series of physical, mental, and social changes now occurs in the alcohol-dependent individual. These may include nervous and gastrointestinal disorders, cirrhosis of the liver, malnutrition, the overuse of defense mechanisms to justify drinking, and a general deterioration in interpersonal relationships. Chain-drinking and extended "benders" are characteristic of this phase of the illness. After a number of years, the alcoholic drinks to live and lives to drink. Completely oriented around alcohol, the individual displays aspects of the chronic phase, such as complete ethical breakdown, unreasonable fears, delirium tremens, reverse tolerance, and loss of motor coordination. The medical complications may be so severe that either institutionalization or death occurs unless there is some form of intervention.

Not every alcoholic experiences all of the foregoing signs and symptoms. Moreover, the order in which the abnormal behaviors occur displays great variation. However, the type of alcoholism most prevalent in America consists of psychological dependence, tissue tolerance, physical dependence, loss of control over drinking, and withdrawal symptoms.[31] These characteristics of drug dependency are discussed in detail in the chapter on drug-taking behavior.

Signs and Symptoms

Modern therapies for alcoholism include various physical, psychological, and social measures. Recovery from the effects of withdrawal from alcohol can be facilitated by the *use of drugs,* especially minor tranquilizers. After *detoxification* or "drying-out" has been completed, reserpine and chlorpromazine are again used to reduce tension and lessen the alcoholic's psychological dependence on alcohol.

Because many chronic alcoholics are malnourished, attention must be given to *diet therapy* and to the administration of vitamins. Specific disease entities, such as cirrhosis of the liver and disorders of the nervous system, require special medical therapies. After *medical treatment* of infections and organic disorders,

Alcoholism: Treatment and Rehabilitation

physicians sometimes employ *deterrent drugs* for those alcoholics who cannot refrain from drinking once they leave a treatment center. One such drug is *Antabuse*, which interferes with alcohol oxidation and prolongs the presence of toxic acetaldehyde in the body. If alcohol is consumed, the patient experiences a series of severe physical effects—nausea, vomiting, piercing headaches, rapid heartbeat, flushing of the skin, and hyperventilation. Forewarned of the consequences of drinking, the alcoholic usually responds with abstinence and willingness to continue therapy.[32] Another treatment involves the *aversion method* in which closely supervised patients are given modified alcoholic beverages that induce illness upon ingestion. After prolonged use this technique produces illness whenever the alcoholic contemplates drinking.

In *psychotherapy* (purposeful conversation between a counselor and patient) there is an attempt to help the alcoholic modify attitudes and behavior in order to live more effectively. Such a process involves intense self-analysis and self-acceptance. Other forms of psychotherapy that seek to reveal basic tensions and hidden fears are the self-expressive *psychodrama* and *group therapy* with its feature of mutual support.

One of the more successful approaches in recovery from alcoholism is *Alcoholics Anonymous* (AA), a fellowship of problem drinkers who want help in maintaining sobriety. Voluntary membership involves an emotional commitment that the alcoholic is powerless over the control of alcohol and that only a power greater than self can restore soundness of mind. Patterned closely after AA are the *Al-Anon Family Groups* for spouses of recovered and recovering alcoholics, and *Alateen* groups for children of AA members.

The therapies just described are offered through many individuals and groups in a variety of facilities. There are enlightened physicians; alcohol information centers; pastoral counseling programs in churches; general hospitals that offer

Fig. 8.11. Group psychotherapy provides a supportive atmosphere in which the alcoholic can work out his drinking problems.

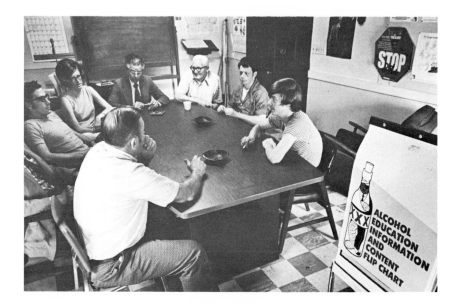

emergency services, inpatient care, and outpatient care through alcoholism clinics; mental hospitals that provide residential care; and halfway houses where recovered alcoholics receive semicustodial care while adjusting to independent living after institutionalization. Experience has indicated that when treatment and rehabilitation services are coordinated within an industrial-based alcoholism program, recovery rates approach the 70 percent level.[33]

Alcoholism—it's everybody's problem. Whether nonuser, moderate drinker, or alcoholic, everyone is directly or indirectly affected by alcohol abuse. Whether alcoholism is perceived as a personal threat or not and whether drinking is viewed as good or bad, the most important thing to remember is that "... caution is still the best thing to mix with liquor."[34]

For Those Who Drink

Moderate drinking is usually descriptive of social drinking, but the limits or propriety are likely to vary from one group to another. However, most "alcohologists" agree that acceptable drinking is governed by the nature and extent of the drinker's responsibilities. Since everyone has some responsibilities in this complex age—either to oneself, to one's family, or to other members of society—moderate drinking implies *limitation* of alcohol use. But it is not just how much one drinks, but rather how one drinks that typically differentiates between acceptable and unacceptable behavior following alcohol use. Therefore the following suggestions are offered for those who wish to preserve alcohol use as a nondestructive part of social functions, to avoid the mental chaos of intoxication, and to minimize the risks of tragic alcoholism.[35]

1. Integrate alcohol use with leisure activities, eating, and social functions.
2. Conduct drinking among friends or within the family setting.
3. Pace your consumption of alcohol by sipping drinks and becoming involved in conversation. Take your second drink no sooner than one hour after the first.
4. Avoid drinking on an empty stomach. Eat ice cream, meat, eggs, or cheese or drink milk or cream before ingesting alcohol.
5. Restrict your drinks, even on special occasions.
6. Dilute distilled spirits with water so as to retard alcohol absorption; always use plenty of ice cubes.
7. Drink in well-lighted, quiet places. Dark and noisy places produce tenseness, which in turn may give rise to overdrinking.
8. On occasion, find some substitute for alcoholic beverages at traditional drinking times.
9. Deliberately avoid beverage alcohol when confronted with problems.
10. As a host, always provide a nonalcoholic alternative for abstainers and recovered alcoholics, and gracefully signal the end to drinking by serving food and coffee at the appropriate time.
11. Watch carefully your personal drinking pattern for early signs and symptoms of problem drinking. Remember, if you need a drink to be social, that's not social drinking!

Drinking Myths[36]

One of the factors contributing to alcohol abuse is the prevalence of fables, falsehoods, folklore, fibs, fantasy, fiction, fabrications, frauds, and fallacies about alcohol, drinking, and alcoholism. This section on modern alcohol mythology is our effort to strip away the confusion concerning alcohol use and abuse and thus remove the mystique and undeserved status that surrounds the ''drink-drug,'' the number one drug problem in North America.

Myth
''Most alcoholics are skid row bums.''

Fact
Only 3 to 5 percent are. Most alcoholics are married, employed, regular people who live in relatively nice neighborhoods.

Myth
''Most skid row bums are alcoholic.''

Fact
Not so! A recent study found that less than half the derelicts on skid row had any drinking problem at all.

Myth
''Very few women become alcoholic.''

Fact
During the 1950s, there were five or six alcoholic men reported for every one woman. Now, the ratio is about three to one with some physicians reporting nearly equal numbers of men and women patients.

Myth
''Most alcoholic people are middle-aged or older.''

Fact
Although alcoholism is often manifest between thirty and fifty-five years of age, research has found that the highest proportion of drinking problems is actually among men in their early twenties. The second highest incidence occurs among men in their forties and fifties.

Myth
''You're not alcoholic unless you drink a pint a day.''

Fact
There is no simple rule. Experts have concluded that how much one drinks may be far less important than when, how, and why one drinks. However, if you drink a lot of beer or wine or distilled spirits, you still drink a lot!

Myth
''The drunk tank is a good cure for alcoholics.''

Fact
Alcoholism is an illness. We do not jail people for other illnesses such as epilepsy, cancer, or tuberculosis. Why do we continue to do so for alcoholism?

Myth
''The really serious problem in our society is drug abuse.''

Fact
Right on! And our number one drug problem is alcohol abuse. About 300,000 Americans are addicted to heroin, but nearly 9,000,000 are dependent on alcohol.

Myth
''Alcohol is a stimulant.''

Fact
Initially acting as a temporary irritant of the mouth and throat, alcohol is about as good a stimulant as ether. Alcohol eventually acts to depress or slow down the central nervous system. The loud talking and bizarre actions that often follow alcohol ingestion are really part of a ''pseudostimulation,'' the result of a loss of inhibitions as alcohol depresses brain function.

Myth
''The person who can hold his liquor will never become an alcoholic.''

Fact
Don't envy the person who can drink everybody else under the table. Such an individual may never feel the need to exercise caution and thus may tend to drink indiscriminately. In addition, the person who can hold so much liquor is developing a tolerance for alcohol. Tolerance is a polite word that describes drug dependency.

Myth
''People get drunk or sick from switching drinks.''

Fact
Switching from vodka to beer to bourbon to wine does not make much difference, really. What usually causes an adverse reaction to alcohol is the total amount consumed when a person drinks.

Myth
''You are safe as long as it's only beer.''

Fact
Sure thing! Just like it's only Scotch or gin. Actually, one beer or one glass of wine is about equal to one average highball in alcohol content. The effect of beer might be a little slower, but you can get just as drunk

on beer and become as much of an alcoholic on beer as on wine or hard liquor.

Myth
"Getting drunk is funny."

Fact
Maybe in the old Charlie Chaplin movies but not in real life. Drunkenness is no funnier than any other illness or incapacity.

Myth
"A good host never lets a guest's glass get empty."

Fact
There's nothing hospitable about pushing alcohol or any other drug. A good host doesn't want his guests to get drunk or sick. He wants them to have a good time and remember it the next day.

Myth
"People are friendlier when they're drunk."

Fact
Maybe so. But they're also more hostile, more dangerous, more criminal, and more suicidal. Half of all murders and one-third of all suicides are alcohol related.

Myth
"If parents don't drink, their children won't drink."

Fact
True, much of the time. But the highest incidence of alcoholism occurs among offspring of parents who are either teetotalers or alcoholics. Perhaps the extremism of the parents' attitude is an important contributing factor.

Myth
"It's rude to refuse a drink."

Fact
Nonsense! Refusing a drink is no more rude than refusing a piece of cake. What is rude is trying to push a drink on someone who doesn't want it or shouldn't have it.

Myth
"Alcohol warms the body."

Fact
Beverage alcohol may impart a sensation of warmth in the body by creating surface heat. However, as the blood courses near the skin's surface, a heat loss actually occurs and body temperature is lowered.

Myth
"Thank God my kid's only on alcohol and not on drugs."

Fact
If your kid is hooked on drinking alcohol, he's hooked on drugs. Alcohol is one of the hardest drugs known.

Myth
"A few drinks can help you unwind and relax."

Fact
Very true. But if you use alcohol like a medicine, it's time to see a doctor.

Myth
"Mixing your drinks causes hangovers."

Fact
The major cause of hangovers is drinking too much. Period!

Summary

Consideration has been given to a drinking society that still considers alcohol as a social beverage rather than as a social drug. Ambivalence has been responsible for complicating the many problems that society must face as a consequence of not only approving but encouraging the use of ethyl alcohol. An overview of the nature of alcoholic beverages, the effects of alcohol on human health, and the personal and social aspects of problem drinking has been presented.

Emphasis has been placed on alcoholism because this form of problem drinking affects not only the ten million alcoholics but also millions of family members and society in general. In a society in which the majority prefers to drink, perhaps the promotion of responsible alcohol use is the best preventive to alcohol abuse.

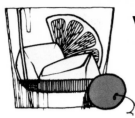

you've got to know when to say when

NATIONAL INSTITUTE ON ALCOHOL ABUSE AND ALCOHOLISM. NATIONAL INSTITUTE OF MENTAL HEALTH. U.S. DEPARTMENT OF HEALTH, EDUCATION, AND WELFARE   PO 1973 11 506-138

Fig. 8.12.

Review Questions

1. Discuss the contradictory attitudes that have given rise to an ambivalent attitude toward alcohol.
2. Describe how alcohol is an integral part of our life-style and customs in North America.
3. Do you think it ethical that the United States impose controls or standards of moderation on alcohol consumption in order to reduce alcohol-related problems?
4. In light of the many alcohol-related problems, do you think that alcohol should be prohibited again? Explain your answer.
5. If the United States chose to prohibit the sale of alcohol, what effect do you think this would have?
6. If from a medical viewpoint alcohol is such a harmful drug, why is it sold legally?
7. What possible reasons might we attribute to the increase of alcohol consumption by women since World War II?
8. Can you distinguish between heavy drinking and problem drinking?
9. Do you think that drinking is more of a social custom than a psychological habit?
10. Describe the various stages of drinking patterns.
11. Describe the process of fermentation; of distillation. How do they differ?
12. What factors can significantly influence the rate of alcohol absorption?
13. What are the short-term effects of alcohol consumption on the body? The long-term effects?
14. Do you believe our traffic laws are strict enough to handle the drinking or intoxicated driver? Explain.
15. Why is alcoholism such a complex illness?
16. Discuss the physical, psychological, and social factors that are frequently cited in the causation of alcoholism.
17. What is Antabuse? How is it used in the treatment of alcoholism?
18. How does Alcoholics Anonymous attempt to rehabilitate the alcoholic?
19. Is there such a thing as the proper way to drink?

Notes

1. National Institute on Alcohol Abuse and Alcoholism, *The Whole College Catalog about Drinking* (Washington, D.C.: U.S. Government Printing Office, 1976), p. 1.

2. Mark Keller and Carol Gurioli, *Statistics on Consumption of Alcohol and on Alcoholism* (New Brunswick, N.J.: Journal of Studies on Alcohol, Inc., 1976), p. 4.

3. Ibid., p. 5.

4. Charles E. Goshen, *Drinks, Drugs, and Do-Gooders* (New York: The Free Press, 1973).

5. For a detailed analysis of alcohol-related problems, the reader is directed to the report of the Cooperative Commission on the Study of Alcoholism prepared by Thomas F. A. Plaut, *Alcohol Problems: A Report to the Nation* (New York: Oxford University Press, 1967).

6. Joel Fort, *Alcohol: Our Biggest Drug Problem* (New York: McGraw-Hill Book Company, 1973), p. 138.

7. Don Cahalan, Ira H. Cisin, and Helen M. Crossley, *American Drinking Practices: A National Study of Drinking Behavior and Attitudes* (New Brunswick, N.J.: Rutgers Center of Alcohol Studies, 1969), p. 199.

8. Jay N. Cross, *Guide to the Community Control of Alcoholism* (New York: The American Public Health Association, 1968), pp. 38–41.

9. Selden D. Bacon, "Alcoholics Do Not Drink," *Annals of the American Academy of Political and Social Science,* 1958, pp. 55–64.

10. David C. McClelland, "The Power of Positive Drinking," *Psychology Today,* January 1971, pp. 40–41, 78–79.

11. Sharon C. Wilsnack, "Femininity by the Bottle," *Psychology Today,* April 1973, p. 43.

12. Morris E. Chafetz, *Liquor: The Servant of Man* (Boston: Little, Brown and Co., 1965), pp. 150–74.

13. U.S. Department of Health, Education, and Welfare, *Alcohol and Alcoholism: Problems, Programs and Progress* (Washington, D.C.: U.S. Government Printing Office, 1972), pp. 4–5.

14. "Fructose Used Clinically to Lower Alcohol Level," *Alcohol & Health Notes,* May 1973, p. 5.

15. Morris E. Chafetz, *Why Drinking Can Be Good for You* (New York: Stein & Day, 1976), p. 48.

16. National Institute on Alcohol Abuse and Alcoholism, *Alcohol and Health,* pp. 45–59.

17. National Institute on Alcohol Abuse and Alcoholism, *Alcohol and Health: New Knowledge* (Washington, D.C.: U.S. Government Printing Office, 1974), p. 86.

18. Ibid., pp. 61–66.

19. Ibid., p. xi.

20. "Alcohol First Drug Used," *American Medical News,* 17 April 1972, p. 16.

21. Harrison Trice, "Alcoholism and the Work World: Prevention in a New Light," in *World Dialogue on Alcohol and Drug Dependence,* ed. Elizabeth D. Whitney (Boston: Beacon Press, 1970), p. 223.

22. "The Economic Cost of Alcohol Misuse," *Alcohol Health and Research World,* Winter 1974 / 75, pp. 19–20.

23. Charles G. Keiper, *Effects of Moderate Blood Alcohol Levels on Driver Alertness* (Washington, D.C.: U.S. Government Printing Office, 1973), p. iv.

24. National Highway Traffic Safety Administration, *The Alcohol Safety Countermeasures Program* (Washington, D.C.: U.S. Government Printing Office, 1971), p. 2.

25. National Highway Traffic Safety Administration, *Alcohol Safety,* p. 4.

26. Fort, *Alcohol,* p. 103.

27. *An Emerging Issue: The Female Alcoholic* (Miami, Fla.: Health Communications, Inc., 1977), p. 8.

28. *Psychodynamics of Chronic Alcoholism* (Nutley, N.J.: Roche Laboratories, 1970).

29. American Medical Association, *Manual on Alcoholism* (Chicago: The Association, 1973), pp. 10–11.

30. For an enlightening view of alcoholism, the reader is referred to William L. Keaton, *Understanding Alcoholism* (Lansing, Mich.: Alcoholism Program, Michigan Department of Public Health, 1966).

31. E. M. Jellinek, *The Disease Concept of Alcoholism* (New Brunswick, N.J.: Hillhouse Press, 1960), pp. 35–38.

32. Marvin A. Block, *Alcohol and Alcoholism: Drinking and Dependence* (Belmont, Calif.: Wadsworth Publishing Co., Inc., 1970), p. 41.

33. Health Services and Mental Health Administration, *HSMHA Supervisors' Guide on Alcohol Abuse* (Washington, D.C.: U.S. Government Printing Office, 1973), p. 1.

34. National Association of Blue Shield Plans, *The Alcoholic American,* rev. ed. (Chicago, 1972).

35. Some of these items have been modified from a list originally prepared by the National Association of Blue Shield Plans.

36. Adapted from *Drinking Myths,* a publication of Operation Threshold by the United States Jaycees Foundation, with a grant from the National Institute on Alcohol Abuse and Alcoholism.

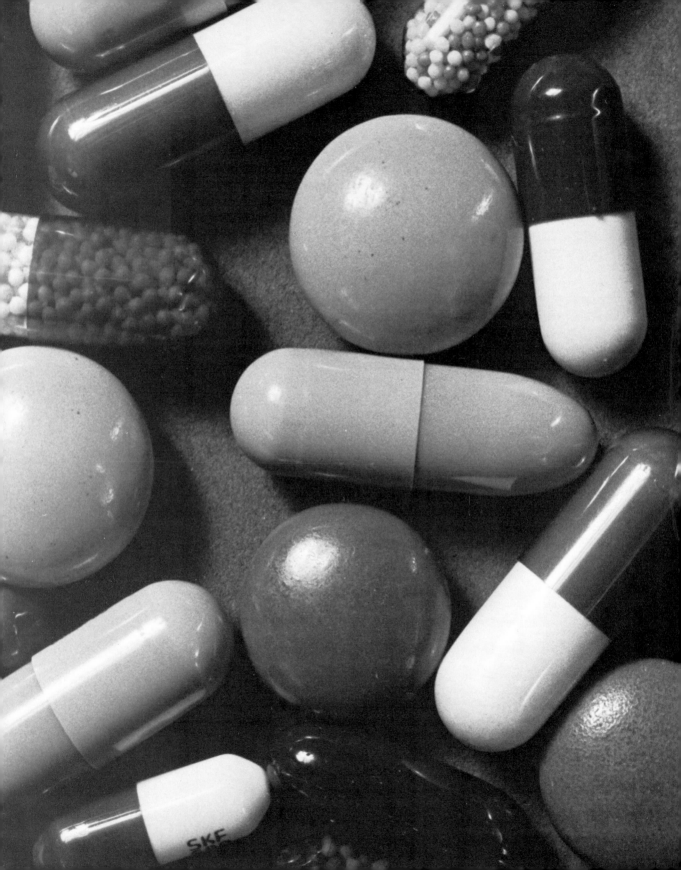

Drug-Taking Behavior: Search or Symptom?

9

Until recently, smoking and drinking were rarely perceived as drug-taking behaviors. After all, tobacco and beverage alcohol have been widely advertised, legally purchased, and socially accepted and indulged in by millions of people.

Nevertheless, the nicotine in tobacco, the ethyl alcohol in beer, wine, and distilled spirits, and the caffeine in coffee and tea are all drugs, according to a commonly accepted definition: a drug is "... any substance that by its chemical nature alters structure or function in the living organism."[1] Such a definition includes practically all foreign materials as drugs—even foods, vitamins, hormones, plants, snake venoms, air pollutants, and pesticides.

In a more limited sense, though, the medical profession would consider as drugs *those substances intended for use in the diagnosis, cure, treatment, or prevention of disease, or in the relief of pain or discomfort*. It should be emphasized, however, that "... while all medicines contain drugs, not all drugs are medicines."[2]

Many wonders of modern medical practice are based upon *chemotherapy*, the use of drugs in treating and preventing disease and in preserving health status. Vaccines and toxoids have been effective in the prevention of major communicable diseases, such as polio, smallpox, diphtheria, tetanus, and measles. Bacterial infections have been conquered in large measure by the antibiotic drugs. Epilepsy and diabetes have been appreciably controlled by Dilantin and insulin, respectively. Anesthetics have provided the patient a relatively painless experience, not only in surgery but also in the dentist's chair. Giant strides have been made in treating the mentally ill with antidepressant drugs and tranquilizers. Prescription drugs, available only with a physician's order, and over-the-counter, nonprescription drugs have been most successful in alleviating a multitude of human ailments when used responsibly. Ideally, drugs should be taken for their intended purposes, according to directions, in the appropriate amount, frequency, strength, or manner, and—in the case of prescribed drugs—under the supervision of a physician.

Drugs and Chemotherapy

Unfortunately, some individuals consume drugs in excess of recommended dosages. They double the number of capsules to be taken or they reduce by one half the standard time interval between doses. Others take prescribed medications without professional consultation or offer their own medicines to others, such as

Drug Misuse and Abuse

the parent who gives the remaining portion of a prescribed drug to his or her child because the child's symptoms resemble those of the parent's former ailment. These are examples of *drug misuse*. Furthermore, these instances testify to that great belief, originally nourished in childhood, that whatever can be swallowed just has to be good or produces a pleasant effect.

In contrast to drug misuse is the phenomenon of *drug abuse*—the deliberate use of chemical substances for reasons other than their intended purposes, use that can result in damage to personal health. Since drug abuse has become the focus of public concern and governmental action, it has been identified almost exclusively with the *psychoactive* or *psychotropic drugs* that have their primary effect on the human mind.

Psychoactive Drugs

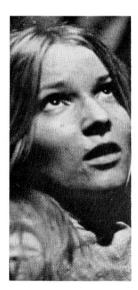

Psychoactive drugs chemically alter one's mood, feelings, consciousness, perceptions, and behavior. Included as mind-affecting drugs are those chemicals classified as sedatives, stimulants, hallucinogens, narcotics, tranquilizers, and volatile substances. Several specific psychoactive drugs already are integrated into the life-style of many people who daily consume coffee, tea, beer, cola drinks, cocktails, cigarettes, aspirin, and various sleep-enhancing and alertness-promoting preparations. Some of the psychoactive drugs, such as morphine, the barbiturates, and the antidepressants, have legitimate medical uses. However, because all the mind-affecting drugs have the ability to modify mood and behavior, they have a high potential not only for misuse but also for abuse in the human quest for pleasure or escape.

Psychoactive drugs are part of the "pharmacological revolution."[3] Powerful chemicals are now widely used by healthy people for social convenience, pleasure, and personal happiness. No longer are drugs employed exclusively for the improvement of health or the reduction of mental illness. Drugs are being used increasingly for nonmedical purposes, for nonmedical adaptations. Although the body has no current need for them in restoring health, these drugs give the user a strong sense of pleasure by activating the brain's pleasure centers. Thus, they may also be referred to as "sensual drugs."[4]

The wide availability of mood-modifying chemicals and the desire for instant pleasure and relief are major factors behind the epidemic of psychoactive drug abuse. But an even more subtle force may be at work here. The fact that many drugs do have beneficial effects has given many individuals the notion that pills will solve all human problems. Believing that happiness has become a universal expectation today, Carstairs fears that psychoactive drugs are being used to eliminate those painful realities of daily life that formerly served as "spurs for human progress."[5] With the abolition of unhappiness seemingly assured through drug use, some perplexing questions arise.

1. What is likely to occur in a society when the circumstances giving rise to unhappiness remain, while the unhappy person is only temporarily altered or pacified?
2. What will happen when unhappiness is viewed as a negative and totally unnecessary emotion?

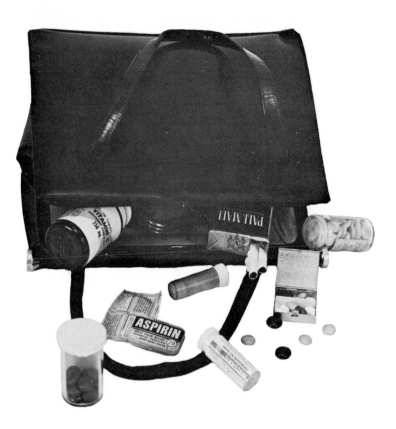

Fig. 9.1. Many people include aspirin, other over-the-counter drugs, prescription drugs, cigarettes, cola drinks, alcoholic beverages, and coffee as part of their daily life-style. A look into the average medicine cabinet or a woman's purse is evidence that a drug-oriented culture exists.

It is apparent that three major dimensions of psychoactive drug abuse merit our consideration. The problem can be studied from medical, social, and legal aspects.

Major Dimensions

Medical Aspect   The persistent use of drugs by a healthy person for a nonmedical purpose without supervision by a physician can result in significant impairment of health status and functional ability. Such drug use is actually a greater danger to a healthy person, because brain control mechanisms that determine the functional operation of the body are thrown out of balance.[6] From a historical perspective the danger of major drug disasters becomes substantial only when drugs that act on the central nervous system escape from medical control and fall into the hands of laypersons.[7]

Social Aspect   The social aspect of drug abuse refers to the view taken by the "larger society" or "the establishment," which deems as either acceptable or unacceptable the particular drug being used, the behavioral effects of drug use, and the impact of such behavior on the social order and its supporting public services. While increasing numbers of people smoke marijuana, the prevailing social order still perceives pot-puffing as a major social threat. As the National Commission on Marijuana and Drug Abuse observes:

> Use of the drug is linked with idleness, lack of motivation, hedonism and sexual promiscuity. Many see the drug as fostering a counter-culture which conflicts with basic moral precepts as well as with the operating functions of our society. The "dropping out" or rejection of the established value system is viewed with alarm. Marihuana becomes more than a drug; it becomes a symbol of the rejection of cherished values.[8]

Of course, the social and economic aspects of heroin addiction loom as even larger problems. The losers are not only the addicts themselves and their families, but also society as a whole, which eventually pays the price for heroin-related crimes and increased law enforcement.[9] Current estimates suggest that drug abuse in general costs nearly $17 billion annually.[10]

Legal Aspect   The legal aspect of drug abuse refers to society's rejection of specific drugs and their behavioral effects and the translation of this rejection into laws or governmental regulations. Such laws are intended to protect persons from the perceived or real hazards of drug abuse and to prevent disorder in a society

Fig. 9.2. Physical and psychological dependence characterize drug abuse. An addict's most important concern is how to get and pay for the next "fix." Soaring burglary and petty theft rates are partly due to addicts stealing to support $50 to $100 a day habits. These addicts have just had a heroin "fix" in a "shooting gallery" (a safe place to buy and inject heroin).

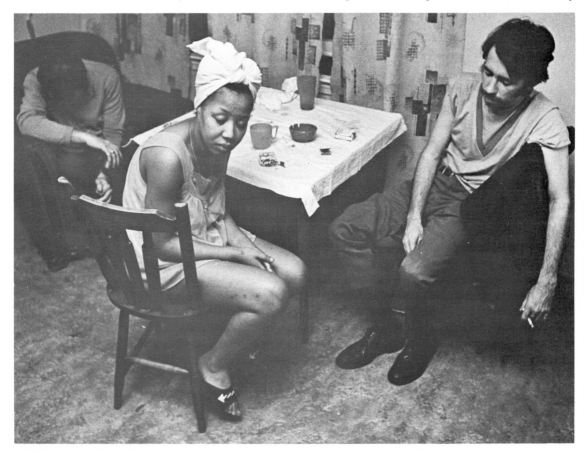

threatened by increasing lawlessness. Reflecting this attitude is the statement of one governmental agency:

> When a drug has both a harmful and a beneficial potential, governments appropriately attempt to direct the manner in which that drug is to be used in order to protect the individual and society.[11]

While such a policy expresses a philosophy of prohibition, it nevertheless is firmly held by many persons in today's society. Such individuals must be nearing the emotional boiling point as they watch the gradual decriminalization of the possession of marijuana for personal use. Just as perplexing though is the growing recognition that many users of illicit drugs suffer no ill effects. As one observer notes,

> the realization that significant numbers of users of legal substances may suffer ill effects at the same time that many users of prohibited substances have no problems with their use, has strained our national capacity to deal rationally with the fundamental social policy issues involved.[12]

Benefits to be derived from the misuse or abuse of drugs are generally expressed in the expectation of a pleasurable experience or a reduction of a negative, frustrating condition. These benefits must be weighed against the very real disadvantages, risks, and even maladaptations that can attend drug-taking behavior. Of special interest are the following health hazards.

Delay in Proper Medical Treatment   Frequent unsupervised use of drugs for a health problem may so effectively mask the symptoms of a disorder or disease that the person believes the condition has been controlled or cured. Therefore, the individual may not seek medical attention early. When such a disorder finally comes to a physician's attention, often little can be done to remedy the problem that has progressed under the protective cover of drugs.

Reduction in Personal, Problem-Solving Effectiveness   The use of drugs often makes the consumer feel better for a while. However, the underlying causes motivating drug use remain. The ability to utilize other problem-solving techniques, particularly in interpersonal relationships and self-identity crises, is often impaired, or the techniques may never even be attempted. This is especially true if one is under the influence of certain drugs, such as ethyl alcohol or barbiturates.

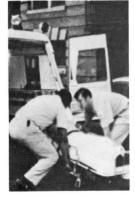

Creation of Additional Health Problems   Drug misuse or abuse sometimes involves an overdose (which can be fatal), an allergic reaction with unpleasant side effects, or the combination of two or more drugs used together that can multiply the drugs' effect and result in death. It is also well known that any drug used by a pregnant woman, especially during the first three months of pregnancy, can have detrimental effects on the developing embryo or fetus.[13] For a more complete picture, add to this list of problems such things as possible psychotic experiences, personality disintegration, hallucinations, and illusions.

Use of Adulterated Drugs   When an individual buys "street drugs," the purchaser does not always get what is bargained for. Increasingly, drugs are being mixed or "cut" with cheaper, inferior, or often more hazardous substances—the process of adulteration. Not infrequently, drugs capable of producing a physical dependency are added to marijuana. The subtle purpose is to create a steady customer who will eventually need the "hidden drug" in order to function. Poisons, insecticides, animal tranquilizers, oregano, catnip, milk sugar, and quinine are also used to cut or stretch the original substance in terms of quantity. Depending upon what the adulterating chemical is, the drug user incurs a high risk of having an unanticipated drug experience, sometimes a toxic reaction, and the possibility of being treated by medical personnel who lack information about the true nature or composition of the consumed drug.

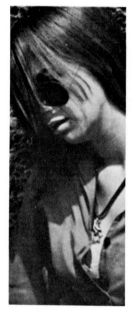

Development of Drug Dependence   A state of psychological or physical need, or both, drug dependence can occur in the individual who uses psychoactive drugs periodically or on a continuous basis. (Because of the difficulty in distinguishing among the various interpretations of the word *addiction,* the World Health Organization has proposed substitution of the phrase *drug dependence.*)[14] Although not everyone who uses mood and behavior modifiers develops a drug dependency, such a condition is a distinct possibility. The most extreme form of drug dependence is characterized by physical dependence, psychological dependence, the development of tolerance, and withdrawal sickness and mental trauma upon termination of drug use.[15] Few people—even those who are themselves dependent on some drug—consider these phenomena advantageous or beneficial. Fortunately, not all these problems occur in each instance of drug dependency. Some drugs carry the potential for psychological dependence only, while others carry the penalty of physical dependence too.

An individual who becomes *psychologically dependent* on a particular drug has a strong desire to repeat the use of that drug either intermittently or continuously for emotional reasons. Although the body does not require the drug, the person has a strong craving for it to maintain drug-induced pleasure, tension-reduction, or dulling of reality. When drug-seeking becomes compulsive and a regular behavioral pattern, psychological dependence has reached its peak intensity. Deprived of the drug, the user will experience a period of readjustment, accompanied by some degree of anxiety, irritability, and restlessness. No physical complications follow the discontinuance of drug usage.

With the repeated use of some drugs, a condition known as *tolerance* develops. In time, the body's cells become accustomed to a certain level of a drug and continued intake of the same dose has diminishing effects. Consequently, the dosage must be increased to achieve the desired effects. The onset of tolerance may be rapid or gradual, depending upon the drug used. Although tolerance can accompany psychological dependence upon a drug without the occurrence of physical dependence, increased dosages are more often seen in conjunction with the latter condition.

From a personal and social perspective, the most hazardous aspect of drug abuse is that of *physical dependence.* Over a period of several weeks or months,

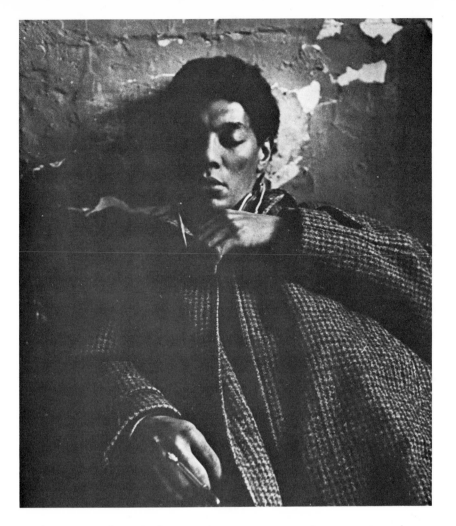

Fig. 9.3. An overdose of drugs is one of the addict's greatest problems. This young man was found with the heroin needle still stuck in his hand, but unlike many addicts, he did not die.

continuous use of certain drugs produces temporary and compensatory changes in the body's nervous system. Such changes in cellular functioning permit the nerves to work in their accustomed fashion in the presence of the foreign drug. Now, however, the cells need the drug to operate normally. In essence, physical dependence is a physiological state of adaptation to a drug.

If the drug is removed abruptly, normal cell function is disturbed, resulting in hyperexcitability or overactivity of the nervous system. Such cellular over-activity is expressed in nausea, vomiting, convulsions, and hallucinations. Collectively, these signs and symptoms are referred to as *withdrawal sickness* or the *abstinence syndrome*. Although the process of withdrawal can be painful, and in some instances results in death, it nevertheless permits the nerve cells to return to their predrugged state and reduces the level of tolerance that has developed. With increasing frequency, multiple drug dependency is being reported. In such cases, the individual goes through withdrawal from each drug abused.

Fig. 9.4. Drug addicts often end in hospital emergency rooms because they have taken an overdose, or they may end in psychiatric hospitals because their emotional and mental states have been adversely affected by a drug.

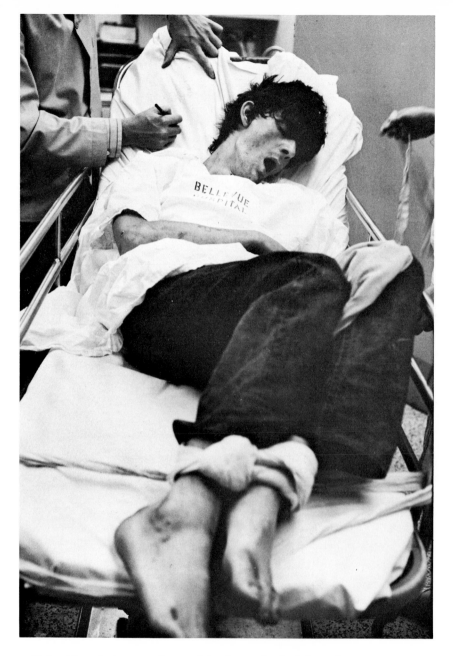

Not evident during actual use of the drug, physical dependence becomes apparent only upon termination of drug use. As a consequence, some individuals, particularly those dependent on heroin, persist in their abuse of drugs to avoid the abstinence syndrome. The money required to engage in this form of preventive medicine can amount to huge sums, often obtained through criminal acts.

Health risks of drug misuse and abuse are frequently discounted, though, and entirely rejected, especially by young persons. Such puzzling behavior may be better understood when viewed within the following set of circumstances.

The "generation gap" between younger and older addicts
Peer group acceptance of drug use as normal behavior
The "gamelike" approach to life with no future orientation
The drug effects themselves, which reduce fear or anxiety.[16]

These explanations are helpful in an analysis of the current epidemic of drug abuse. But they in turn raise some questions: Why is drug use considered by some as "normal" behavior? Why do so many people have a "gamelike" approach to life?

Some claim that drug abuse is based in the historical search for pleasure and the relief of pain. Behavioral scientists, however, increasingly see the phenomenon as having deeper social roots. Fort claims that drug abuse and other problems, including alcoholism, compulsive gambling, sexual difficulties, insomnia, and depression, originate in ". . . man's alienation from a society that incessantly tries to beat down his individuality and nonconformity."[17] It is possible, then, that drug-taking behavior represents an effort to adapt or adjust to a variety of environmental challenges. Sometimes these adaptations or changes may be beneficial to either the person or society or both. On occasion, these adaptations may have undesirable consequences, personally or socially or both. Drug-dependency, toxic reactions, drug-induced psychotic experiences and reduced personal effectiveness might even be considered as maladaptations to drug use—drug use that went wrong.

Although any drug is taken for some immediate benefit or advantage, it is quite likely that a combination of several predisposing and interrelated factors causes the illegal and nonmedical use of drugs. General, familial, societal, and personality factors, acting in concert, all have been cited as propelling individuals into drug abuse.[18] Indeed, studies concerning the prediction of marijuana use based on earlier behavior, personality, belief, and attitude indicators revealed these characteristics of users.[19]

- Tended to be adolescents and young adults who smoked marijuana during critical stages in their personality development and while developing intellectual and psychosocial skills
- Placed lower value on achievement and higher value on independence
- Tended to be more alienated and critical, more tolerant of deviance, less religious, less influenced by parents than by friends; had lower grade point averages
- Displayed a greater degree of impulsiveness; less sensitive to the feelings of others, but at the same time more sociable, talkative, and outgoing than nonusers
- Tended to be nonconformists
- Experienced a lack of closeness in family ties

The promised benefits of taking drugs are familiar. They include a change in pace or mood, relief from tension and boredom, a pick-up to combat fatigue, the promotion of sleep, or just plain fun. Such benefits also are frequently cited in the appeals of television commercials, as is well known even by preschoolers.[20] The invitation to drug use comes at an early age. It is now generally agreed that

> drug promotion on television tends to encourage favorable attitudes towards drug use through exaggerated claims and through failure to point out the need to exercise appropriate caution in drug taking.[21]

Although a causal link between drug advertising and drug abuse has not been established, it is assumed that such ads do influence the heavier use of drugs among the general public.

Pleasurable Aspects   The varieties of drug-derived fun or pleasure are many. There can be experiences of inner peace, tranquility, joyous delight, relaxation, serenity; kaleidoscopic perceptions; surges of exhilaration; heightened and prolonged physical sensations; and a gut-feeling somewhat comparable to orgasmic response. The universality of these pleasurable appeals has been acknowledged by one renowned authority who observed:

> Simple pleasure . . . is frequently offered as the general explanation for most current drug use. . . . But the desire for certain kinds of psychological gratification or release is not peculiar to the drug user or to our generations. It is an old and universal theme of human history. Man has always sought gratifications of the kind afforded by the psychotropic drugs.[22]

Utilitarian Aspects   People turn to drugs for other reasons, too. Utilitarian aspects are frequently recognized. Amphetamines can help students stay awake all night and cram for a test. They have even been used on occasion to improve physical performance. Some attribute aphrodisiac properties to marijuana and claim they are more easily aroused sexually and that sexual performance is enhanced under the influence of pot. It should be noted that there is absolutely no scientific evidence supporting the belief that marijuana has any physical aphrodisiac effect. However, the socially communicated belief in such aphrodisiac qualities is likely to have psychological substantiation. "The placebo effect is at its most powerful when supported by myth."[23] On the other hand, the passivity of the drug experience may help others to avoid the potential humiliation of an unwanted or undesirable sexual confrontation or even the necessity of any sexual activity.[24] LSD use has been related to desires for greater insight, personal understanding, awareness of unconscious thoughts, and creativity. Some have turned to drugs to forget the past and present, to keep going, to keep from going crazy or to keep from committing suicide.

Curiosity   Curiosity is quite sufficient to propel some individuals into the arena of drug experimentation. Promises of profound and unpredictable effects have enticed hundreds of thousands to explore and experience the world of the inner self. The much publicized high priests and gurus, aided by sensational accounts of drug-happenings in the news media and the lyrics of "acid rock," have raised

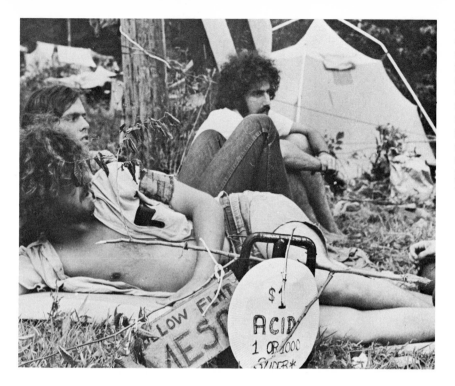

Fig. 9.5. The easy availability of drugs at rock festivals in the late sixties and early seventies was only one reason for increased drug use. Personality factors also determined whether drugs would become part of a person's life-style.

the hopes and aspirations of many with the psychedelic gospel of world salvation.

Social Aspects   And yet, most of the psychoactive chemicals are used initially as social drugs, instruments that help people better enjoy the company of others. "They are part of the social scene."[25] Their adoption is related to their ability to enrich social intercourse; their diffusion to others is often a form of social exchange, a learning phenomenon, or a rite of passage. In recreational settings, the power of peer influence is considerable. Drug-taking becomes symbolic of group-identification. Coparticipation in an activity that is both clandestine and illegal often fosters a common bond of conspiracy that further cements interrelationships. In a less dramatic manner, it can be said that ". . . emergent use often becomes a part of the young person's integration into a social subculture in which drug use is one part."[26]

As the drug abuse epidemic began in the late 1960s, the pleasurable, utilitarian, and social aspects were generally overlooked. Drug-taking by young persons was viewed as adolescent rebellion or as a "chemical copout" used by long-haired freaks when the "going got rough." To be sure, parents were outraged when their children engaged in illegal and health-endangering activities. But the concern and reaction stemmed perhaps as much from the establishment's realization that its children were challenging and in certain instances repudiating those values so dearly cherished by the older generation.[27] Organized religion, patriotism,

Rebellion
Against
Establishment

the sanctity of marriage and premarital chastity, the accumulation of wealth, the right and competence of parents, schools, and government to lead and make decisions for everyone became the targets of those espousing a "hang-loose" ethic.[28] Research now confirms that rebelliousness among children and adolescents is one of the best predictors of future marijuana use.

Drugs for Every Ailment

Indeed, it was a rebellion! But the rebellion proceeded in general according to a plan originated by and unwittingly sponsored and advertised by the establishment. The achievement of instant relief through medication and promises of a happy ending to every problem are not creations of the youth culture. The older generation has set an example with its overflowing medicine cabinets, the suggestion that for every ailment there is a drug to cure it, and the basic denial of the fact that anxiety, worry, and depression are sometimes normal feelings for human beings as they struggle with their environment.[29]

In a sense, the "teachers" have been most effective; the "students" have learned their lessons well. Increasingly and with few exceptions, both subscribe to the idea that existence without drugs is impossible. Such devoted reliance upon chemical mood modifiers may even be symptomatic of what Farber labels the "Age of the Disordered Will." We have become enslaved by willing what cannot be willed—sleep, rapid reading, simultaneous orgasm, creativity, spontaneity, and the enjoyment of old age. Drugs merely provide a temporary ". . . illusion of healing the split between the will and its refractory object."[30]

Changes and Conflicts in Society

It is true that the increased use of drugs has been related to their increased availability. But analysts also cite rapid changes and conflicts in society as contributing factors to the continuing illegal and nonmedical use of drugs. Those most frequently mentioned follow.

1. The irrelevancy of the past with its structure, order, and controlling institutions of neighborhood, community, and church
2. The unpredictability of the future in terms of international peace, national survival, employment needs, economic stability, and place of residence
3. Changes in family life with less emphasis on permanence of relationship, marital fidelity, and on the modeling, discipline, counseling, and educational functions of parenting
4. Confusion as to appropriate adult roles, responsibilities, and value systems coupled with the extension of the social and economic dependence of adolescence
5. Decline of the "work ethic," the need to achieve, the belief in self-restraint, accompanied by increased leisure time
6. A communications explosion that provides more information than one can absorb and whose commercial messages carry a theme of self-indulgence
7. The loss of privacy, the sense of community, and the ability to influence social institutions, especially bureaucracy
8. An increase in permissiveness, normlessness, and individualism manifest in the philosophy of freedom to do "one's own thing"

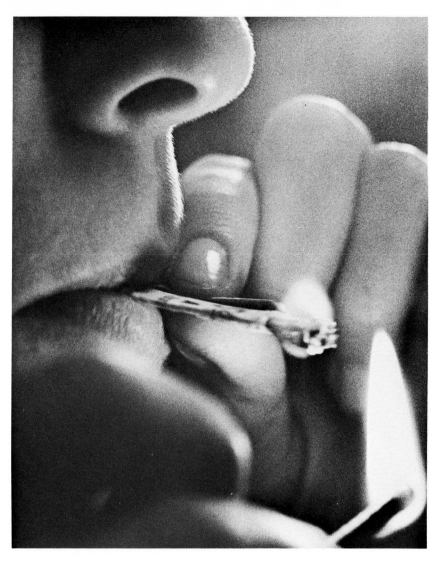

Fig. 9.6. A folded matchbook cover helps this girl smoke a marijuana cigarette down to the end. Both alcohol and marijuana are psychoactive drugs; one is legal and the other is not. The prohibition of alcohol failed, and the prohibition of marijuana is not working either.

9. Environmental deprivations, particularly those of ghetto life and Appalachia, including poor housing, high rates of disease, chronic unemployment, inadequate nutrition and education, and family disorganization
10. Loss of confidence in and a growing disrespect for law among the general population
11. Success increasingly measured in material terms, but for many the lack of opportunity for achieving success by legitimate means
12. Proliferation of superficial relationships and the ascendency of rationality at the expense of feelings and the life of emotions

Confronted thus by a confusing future certain to be marked by change and conflict; overwhelmed by the many options of life-style and career choices;

struggling with questions of self-identity and self-worth; frequently not taken seriously; reared in a permissive society and yet somewhat alienated from it; distrustful of conventions seen as hypocritical, impersonal, and dishonest; and encouraged and affluent enough to exercise a measure of independence, the individual is likely to respond *adaptively* to such crises.[31] The most frequent options are (1) constructive or destructive rebellion, (2) regression and personality disintegration, (3) passive acceptance or passive withdrawal, and (4) fixation on the immediate experience.

Drug-Taking and Adaptive Behavior

The necessity for continuing adaptation and accommodation is thus realized. And drug-taking figures prominently in both accompanying and sometimes facilitating such adaptive responses. For example, research has revealed a close association between the rise of drugs in the late 1960s and the adherence to an antiestablishment "hang-loose" ethic.[32] This relationship has already been discussed (p. 243). Opposition to the traditional, established order was demonstrated by participation in "happenings" and mass protests on campus, reading of underground newspapers, antagonism to the educational system, opposition to the Vietnam war and the draft, the expectation of great satisfaction in future life from recreational activities, and approval of premarital intercourse. Within this context, drug usage, particularly marijuana, became a means of expressing freedom from society and rebellion against the unfair restrictions of that society.

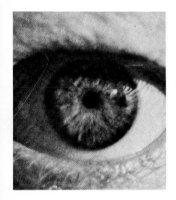

Personality Problems For the individual with personality problems, drugs sometimes offer a way to cope with immaturity, low self-esteem, chronic depression, brooding restlessness, narcissism, preoccupation with issues of identity and autonomy, and difficulties in forming interpersonal relationships. Such psychopathology frequently identifies those individuals who are especially prone to drug dependence.[33] More commonly, though, drug abuse is seen as a temporary solution to or retreat from problems of academic pressure, family discord, and environmental harshness.

Escape to World of Inner Self Others, estranged from society in general, escape or withdraw to the world of the inner self. Surrounded by ugliness, confusion, and people who cannot be trusted or believed, the person undertakes a search for beauty, meaning, and truth—a search for God within. Self-encounter with its intensity of feelings and emotions is highly prized. Drugs might provide the ticket for such an adventure. The promised rewards are self-knowledge and self-experience.

Focus on the Here and Now If the experience of the self reigns supreme, so also does the experience of the present. Without a meaningful past and unwilling to plan for an unknown and uncontrollable future, the modern person tends to focus on the here and now. Deferring gratification and working for some distant reward become counterproductive. The immediate experience is cherished; it is the only thing that matters; it is the only thing that can be grasped and held on to. The now experience is the hallmark of the now generation. Hedonism has ascended its throne. Enjoy yourself; it's later than you think! Have your pleasure; pay for it later! Maybe, if you are lucky, there won't be a later! If one lives for the experience of the moment,

> . . . Then anything that maximizes the experience—the sensations, the action—is good and true and beautiful. Drugs. Mysticism. Eastern religions. All have a primary emphasis on increasing one's capacity for experiencing.[34]

Many, of course, adapt in other ways and do not abuse drugs. They opt to change society or the environment within the system rather than change themselves. Others, perhaps the majority, perceive no need to adapt, being content with their own status and that of society. However, drug-taking, enlisted in the service of human adaptation, has assumed a significant role in the lives of millions of Americans.

Patterns and Trends in Drug Use

In an analysis of the current drug scene, several general patterns and trends of use and abuse may be noted.[35, 36, 37, 38]

Contrary to popular belief, not all drug abusers are at the same level of involvement with drugs. The following distinctions should be made for all populations:

1. The *experimenters*—those who have tried drugs only a few times, usually out of curiosity. They do not plan to continue the use of drugs.
2. The *occasional users*—those who use drugs infrequently. They confine their irregular use to special social settings or events when drugs are consumed in a somewhat recreational manner.
3. The *moderate users*—those who use drugs with some regularity. However, they do not let drugs become the single, most important factor in their lives.
4. The *chronic users*—those who regularly use drugs, often in large amounts, and frequently develop a drug dependency. A relatively small proportion of all drug users, they tend to see drugs as the central focus of their lives.

Despite major government efforts and the massive expenditure of funds to combat nonmedical use of drugs, drug abuse in the United States is increasing rapidly and among younger age groups.

No longer confined to the inner cities, to the counterculture, or to those opposed to the establishment, all forms of drug abuse have now spread to middle-sized cities, smaller towns, and even rural areas. Although much of the concern and most of the countermeasures have focused on narcotics and marijuana, significant numbers of both adults and young people now report nonmedical experience with stimulants, tranquilizers, sedatives, and over-the-counter drugs.

Heroin After a decline in the availability of heroin in the early 1970s, it has now become more available, cheaper in price, and purer in form. Users are more likely to overdose with purer heroin, since they are accustomed to having the drug cut or diluted with other substances. The greatest concentrations of heroin use and addiction appear to be in the cities of the West Coast.[39]

Sedatives   Along with high consumption of beverage alcohol, a *massive increase in the use of strong sedatives* has been recorded. The use of physician-prescribed barbiturates, especially by middle-aged patients, and the abuse of barbiturates and tranquilizers among young people have skyrocketed. Drug overdoses of Valium and Librium (tranquilizers) are routinely observed in hospital emergency rooms. Instances of multiple sedative abuse, resulting in a form of drug dependency known as *sedativism,* are reported with alarming frequency.

Marijuana   Since the early 1970s, there has been a marked increase in the social use of marijuana. It is estimated that more than thirty-five million Americans have used marijuana at least once, with 25 percent of young adults (eighteen to twenty-five years of age) currently using the substance. Users now come from a broad cross section of youths who are proving that pot-puffing may well become an enduring cultural pattern in the United States. Largely confined to the young, experimentation with marijuana and its continuing use become increasingly less common among those past the age of twenty-five.

Stimulants   Although physicians have sharply restricted the use of amphetamines, there is considerable social and private use of these stimulant drugs, often diverted from legitimate sources by the "respectable pushers."[40] An estimated 200 million doses of amphetamines, barbiturates, narcotics, and tranquilizers are diverted from legal channels annually by doctors, pharmacists, and other health professionals. Cocaine, another central nervous system stimulant, is fast becoming the drug of choice among young adults of the middle class, and those who can afford it. Often associated in the media with the rich and glamorous, it is the most expensive drug in terms of the cost-per-minute ratio.

Hallucinogens   The recent past has witnessed a spectacular increase in the use of powerful hallucinogens, the hallucination-producing, mind-expanding drugs. A decline in the use of LSD, the first and most notorious psychedelic drug to hit the American scene in the 1960s, has been observed. However, other natural and synthetic hallucinogens are used widely in the illicit market,[44] including DMT, STP, MDA, PMA, TMA, and PCP, a powerful veterinary anesthetic with effects similar to LSD. Often referred to as angel dust, hog, goon, superjoint, and love drug, PCP is a terror of a drug, responsible for numerous irrational and violent actions in users.

Drug-Oriented Society

There is no doubt that a drug-oriented society exists in America. Continued development of new mood-modifying chemicals has become the dedicated enterprise of reputable pharmaceutical companies as well as of illegal laboratories and street-corner pharmacologists.[42] These endeavors, whether seen as cause or effect, lead many to predict a continuation of the already extensive phenomena of drug use and abuse.

Drug abuse is linked to drug use. The problem of abuse is likely to be slowed only by reduced availability of specific psychoactive substances and other drugs within legitimate and medical channels. And this situation is not likely to be a

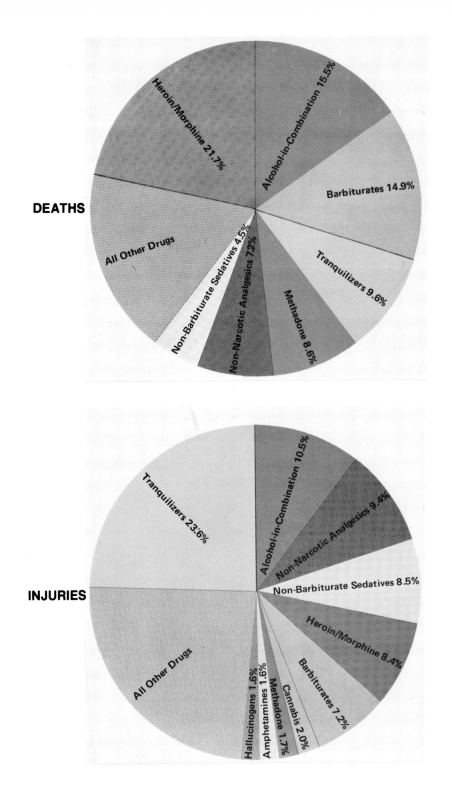

Fig. 9.7. Drug-related deaths and injuries. These pie charts are based on reports from medical examiners and hospital emergency rooms in twenty-four large U.S. metropolitan areas participating in the Drug Abuse Warning Network (DAWN).

DEATHS

Heroin/Morphine 21.7%
Alcohol-in-Combination 15.5%
Barbiturates 14.9%
Tranquilizers 9.6%
Methadone 8.6%
Non-Narcotic Analgesics 7.2%
Non-Barbiturate Sedatives 4.5%
All Other Drugs

INJURIES

Tranquilizers 23.6%
Alcohol-in-Combination 10.5%
Non-Narcotic Analgesics 9.4%
Non-Barbiturate Sedatives 8.5%
Heroin/Morphine 8.4%
Barbiturates 7.2%
Cannabis 2.0%
Methadone 1.7%
Amphetamines 1.6%
Hallucinogens 1.6%
All Other Drugs

result of prohibition. Rather, it will be more probable when and if the public at large reduces its consumption of drugs, such as alcohol, tobacco, and psychoactives. It is only when many persons change their consumption habits that per capita consumption can be reduced.[43] And consumption will not likely be curtailed unless a major change in public attitudes occurs—attitudes about handling problems, about the function of drugs, and about life in general.

Is our current reliance on drugs for nonmedical purposes a *search* for pleasure, stimulation, meaning, and escape, or a *symptom* of unmet needs, inner sickness, alienation, and social deprivation? Perhaps it is both, or neither! What do you think?

Drugs and Their Effect

Psychoactive drugs change the way we think, feel, and act because they produce functional or pathological changes in the central nervous system of the human.[44] However, the wide range of drug effects seen in the same person from time to time and in different persons is related to many factors. Among these are the following:

1. The chemical makeup of the drug itself, including possible contaminants
2. The quantity of the drug consumed, the dose
3. The duration of drug use
4. The method or route of drug administration, that is, by mouth, injection, or inhalation
5. The metabolic fate of the drug in terms of its deactivation or elimination from the body.

Two additional factors also influence the effects of drugs, particularly the hallucinogens. These are the "mind set" of the user and the environmental setting in which a drug is used. Unique qualities of personality, attitudes toward a particular drug, expectations of certain effects, and basic motivations for drug use all help determine the behavior resulting from drug intake. In addition, the mood of coparticipants and the presence or absence of controls or restrictions will likely have an impact on the behavioral effects.

Sedatives

Many drugs that depress or slow down the central nervous system are available. Referred to as sedatives, "downers," or depressants, these drugs are used medically to reduce nervousness and anxiety, to induce sleep if pain is absent, and to control convulsions, as seen in epilepsy.[45]

Derived from barbituric acid, the *barbiturates* are the largest group of sedatives. Other drugs that have sedating effects include the minor tranquilizers, bromides, methaqualone, paraldehyde, chloral hydrate, and the anticholinergics, such as atropine and scopolamine.

Among the most widely used and abused psychoactive drugs are sleeping pills containing barbiturates. Classified according to the duration of their sedative or hypnotic action, the barbiturates range from rapid-acting Pentothal, to moderately fast-acting Nembutal and Seconal, to the slow-acting Luminal (phenobarbital). These drugs act upon the brain and interfere with the transmission of nerve impulses. In small doses, they relieve tension and reduce anxiety in normal and neurotic individuals, without lowering sensory perception, reactivity to the environment, and alertness below safe levels.[46] In larger doses they produce drowsiness and sleep and can depress the brain centers that control breathing. Therapeutically they are employed in cases of insomnia, in certain psychosomatic conditions, and in mental disturbances when suppression of excitement is desirable. Some barbiturates are used for preanesthetic sedation.

Although often prescribed for sleeplessness, barbiturates, like alcohol, interfere with rapid eye movement (REM) sleep, the dreaming state of sleep. When prolonged use is discontinued, intense and frequent REM sleep occurs in a rebound fashion, often resulting in terrifying nightmares. The user then starts retaking sleeping pills to cure the poor sleeping condition.[47]

Tense, anxious persons and insomniacs often become dependent on barbiturates. Sometimes these depressants are used in conjunction with stimulating amphetamines to create a pleasant mood-elevating effect or to induce sleep after experiencing the amphetamine "jag." Increasing use results in rapid tolerance and both psychological and physical dependence. Excessive intake may produce a state of intoxication often mistaken for drunkenness, hallucinations, coma, and even death due to accidental or intentional overdose or sudden withdrawal from the drug. Marked by restless agitation, convulsions, confused thoughts, tremors, muscle cramps, nausea, and intense anxiety, the abstinence syndrome can constitute an acute medical emergency, more severe than withdrawal from heroin.

Less than lethal doses of alcohol and barbiturates taken together can be fatal. This occurs because these drugs—both depressants—act as *synergists* and are additive in their effects. Barbiturates when taken with narcotics, anesthetics, and tranquilizers may also produce exaggerated, and sometimes fatal reactions, with each drug acting to intensify the other's actions. Vital functions of breathing and heart action are depressed to the point where they cease.

Stimulants

Drugs that increase central nervous system activity and induce a temporary sense of well-being, self-confidence, and alertness are known as stimulants. Among these drugs are cocaine and the various amphetamines, including "speed." The caffeine in coffee, tea, and cola drinks and the nicotine in tobacco products are also mild stimulants.

Cocaine　Derived from the coca bush, cocaine is a short-acting yet powerful stimulant. Because it tends to reduce mucous membrane swelling and enlarges nasal and bronchial passages, cocaine was a common ingredient in patent (nonprescription) medicines during the nineteenth century and a commonly misused substance.

Enjoying a renaissance on the drug scene, cocaine is either inhaled or injected intravenously. The "high" is a short-lived sensation of extreme physical and mental power with increased psychomotor activity and the abolition of the sense of hunger and fatigue.[48] Hallucinations occur, and paranoid delusions that result from prolonged use often trigger compulsive, violent antisocial acts. Such behavior was largely responsible for the descriptive term, *dope fiend*.

Fig. 9.8. Illicit forms of cocaine are either inhaled ("snorted") or injected into the body after mixing the crystalline powder with heroin. Although cocaine is pharmacologically a stimulant—it stimulates the central nervous system—the U.S. government, for legal purposes, classifies it as a narcotic.

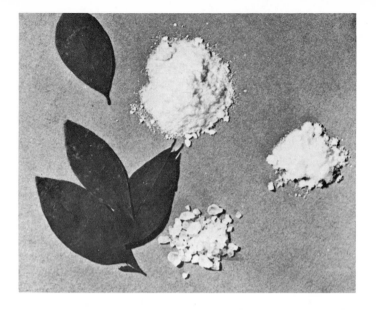

Chronic use results in nausea, digestive disorders, weight loss, insomnia, skin abscesses, and occasional convulsions. Prolonged sniffing may also perforate the septum of the nose. Overdoses can cause death from stoppage of heart and lung functions. Death sometimes occurs even when cocaine is snorted rather than injected, despite all the street lore to the contrary. Although tolerance and physical dependence do not develop, marked psychic dependence results. When the effects of cocaine diminish, severe mental depressions occur, impelling continued use.

Amphetamines Popularly termed pep pills or "uppers," the amphetamines stimulate certain areas of the nervous system that control blood pressure, heart, breathing, and metabolic rate, all of which are increased. Appetite is markedly decreased, and fatigue is effectively, though artificially, masked. The senses are hyperalert and the body is in a general state of stress. Such effects might last from three to four hours after swallowing the drug.

The three major amphetamines are Benzedrine (amphetamine), Dexedrine (dextroamphetamine), and Methedrine (methamphetamine). They are of medical usefulness only in a few conditions, such as overwhelming episodes of sleep during normal waking hours, depression, and in the treatment of hyperkinetic (hyperactive) children. Their use in the management of obesity—they have an appetite-suppressant effect—has been sharply curtailed, except for short-term weight control.

Amphetamines are a favorite of those who wish to exert themselves beyond their physiological limits. Truck drivers, students, and some athletes often fall into this category of abuse. Such sporadic use rarely leads to difficulties. However, taking larger amounts on a continuing basis to keep going, to feel high, to counteract depression, and to deal with problems of living and emotional inadequacies typically leads to drug dependency. Tolerance increases rapidly, and the person becomes psychologically dependent on the drug in a few weeks. Because amphetamine-induced power, self-confidence, and artificial exhilaration are so pleasant, and because of the fear of experiencing severe fatigue and depression following discontinuance, the abusers, even though they may stop for a while, normally revert to continued abuse.

A relatively new form of amphetamine abuse surfaced in the late 1960s when massive-dose intravenous injections of methamphetamine ("meth" or "speed") hit the drug scene. The sudden impact of "speed" is often felt before the needle is removed from the arm. Users compare this "rush" feeling to an electric shock, to being splashed in the face with ice water, or to a feeling of intense pleasure similar to a complete body orgasm.[49] Also experienced are an awareness of thinking more rapidly, a feeling of more efficient thought and action, and a heightened euphoria. Some even report enhanced sexual performance.

However, rapid mood changes and frightening illusions and hallucinations tend to mar the speed user's sense of cleverness and self-confidence. Intense hyperactivity may lead to aggressive behavior. Paranoid reactions or amphetamine psychoses sometimes develop as do "freak-outs," drug experiences that involve loss of control over thought processes. When, after a period of continuous injection, the use of methamphetamine is terminated, the "speed-freak" experiences symptoms of "crashing" or coming down from speed. There is an overpowering desire to sleep, extreme depression, anxiety, and irritability. Sometimes behavior is violent or suicidal.

Continued speed use may result in malnutrition, dehydration, skin abscesses, and hepatitis and tetanus, the penalties for using a dirty needle. With moderate doses there is little evidence of physical dependence, though there is no widespread agreement on this. Death from overdose is uncommon. The slogan "Speed Kills" more approximately describes the death of the personality or the spirit of the user who is in a limbo, neither physically dead nor psychologically alive.

Drugs that produce hallucinations (experiences of nonexistent sensations) are termed hallucinogens. These chemicals elicit changes in sensation, thinking, self-awareness, and emotions. They also can bring on illusions (misinterpretations of sensation) and delusions (false beliefs). Frequently called psychedelics because of their mind-manifesting or mind-expanding qualities, the hallucinogens include LSD, marijuana, mescaline (from the peyote cactus), psilocybin (from the Mexican mushroom), morning-glory seeds, nutmeg seeds, jimson weed, and such mod-sounding synthetic drugs as DMT, DET, STP (not the oil additive), MDA, PMA, and PCP. Two of these deserve more detailed examination: LSD, the prototype and one of the most powerful hallucinogens, and marijuana, the one most frequently used socially.

Lysergic Acid Diethylamide A partially synthetic ergot derivative, LSD or "acid" has the curious property of inducing strong and bizarre mental reactions and distortions of the physical senses. After ingestion of only minute quantities,

Hallucinogens

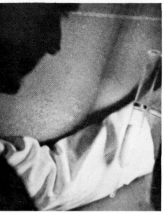

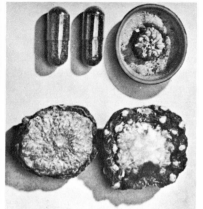

Peyote cactus, buttons, and ground buttons

Psilocybe mushrooms

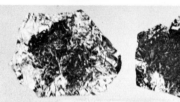

HALLUCINOGENS

Fig. 9.9.
The manufacture and use of almost all hallucinogens is prohibited in the U.S., except for approved research.

DMT (dimethyl-tryptamine) on tobacco and parsley leaves

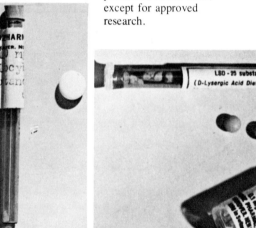

Legitimate dosage forms of psilocybin

Legitimate dosage forms of lysergic acid diethylamide (LSD)

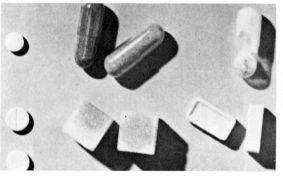

Illicit dosage forms of lysergic acid diethylamide

commonly reported physical effects include enlarged pupils, increased heart rate and blood pressure, "goose pimples," flushing of facial skin, increased body temperature, chills, and elevated blood-sugar levels. Although regular use of LSD does not result in withdrawal sickness, tolerance and psychological dependency can occur.

Psychological effects are less predictable and are determined considerably by personality factors of the user and the general setting in which the "trip" or drug experience is made. Changes tend to occur in sensation and perception, emotionality, and thought processes, and they are demonstrated in the following types of psychological experiences.[50]

1. The impression of possessing lucid thought that permits problems to be seen from a novel perspective
2. Change and intensification in sensory impressions, especially vision, in which one sensation may be translated into another, e.g., sounds may be seen; smells may be felt. Such phenomena are called *synesthesias*.
3. Distortion in the sense of time
4. Emergence of suppressed thoughts and past incidents into the consciousness of the present
5. The temporary psychedelic peak, characterized by a sense of unity with the world, deeply felt joy, love and peace, religious awareness, and keen insight into reality
6. Varying degrees of tension, anxiety, fear, unpleasant illusions, depression, and despair, all descriptive of the "bad trip" or a "bummer"
7. The "freak-out" or adverse psychotic reaction marked by negative feelings of terror and panic, loss of emotional control, paranoid delusions, hallucinations, and a sense of meaninglessness

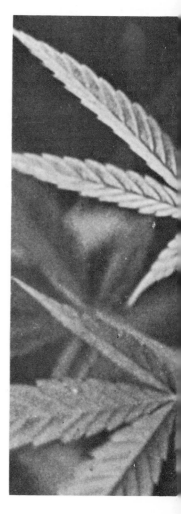

Whether LSD or any other powerful hallucinogen can cause permanent mental illness in normal persons is still an open question, as is the possibility of LSD-induced birth defects and chromosomal breaks. Scientists take opposite views on such matters. Subjectivity also clouds certain issues. Claims that LSD use heightens creative thought and skills have not been supported adequately by scientific investigation. Arguments contending that LSD is truly consciousness-expanding have been countered by those who cite the consciousness-constricting attributes shown in some users.

However, there is no doubt as to the real dangers associated with the use of LSD. There can be a terrifying panic, a fear of losing one's mind that sometimes precipitates suicide, an occasional "flashback" (a recurrence of certain features of the LSD experience, occurring days and months after the last dose and without apparent cause), and accidental death. Because the LSD user sometimes develops feelings of invulnerability, attempts have been made to walk in front of moving automobiles and to fly out high windows.

Marijuana   One of the least powerful hallucinogens, marijuana is derived from the Indian hemp plant, *Cannabis sativa*. Its leaves and flowering tops are dried, then crushed into small fragments that are rolled into cigarettes ("joints" or "reefers") and smoked. Usually inhaled deeply into the lungs, cannabis smoke is held there for an extended time to increase absorption. Marijuana may be smoked in pipes or eaten along with other foods.

The dark brown resin collected from the tops of potent cannabis plants is known as hashish or "hash." It is often several times stronger than the usual variety of marijuana, because it contains more THC (tetrahydrocannabinol), considered the basic active ingredient in both of these hallucinogenic substances. The THC content of hashish is from 5 to 12 percent, although hashish oil may have a THC concentration of 40 to 50 percent. Marijuana samples ordinarily available in the United States have a THC content of between 1 and 2 percent.

Although marijuana use evokes highly individual experiences, low social doses (one or two joints) usually produce a mild high characterized by

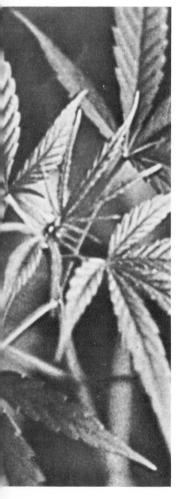

> an increased sense of well-being, initial restlessness and hilarity, followed by a dreamy, carefree state of relaxation, alteration of sensory perceptions including expansion of space and time, and a more vivid sense of touch, sight, smell, taste, and sound; a feeling of hunger, especially a craving of sweets; and subtle changes in thought formation and expression. To an unknowing observer, an individual in this state of consciousness would not appear noticeably different from his normal state.[51]

Higher doses elicit the same general reactions but in a more intensified form. At very high dose-levels, experiences similar to the LSD trip occur. Distortions of body image, loss of personal identification, sensory and mental illusions, fantasies, and hallucinations are frequently reported. Such psychic disorientation may be interpreted as either pleasant or unpleasant by the individual. In some instances, especially among inexperienced users, reactions to marijuana intoxication can bring on anxiety, depression, fatigue, dizziness, nausea, and incoordination. Feelings of panic may result when altered mental states cause the pot-puffer to fear that loss of identity and self-control may not end, and that loss of mind or death is imminent. Temporary paranoid feelings are also common in users.

In human subjects, the acute physiological effects include temporary increases in pulse rate and blood pressure, reddening of the whites of the eyes, coughing due to irritation of the smoke, and dryness of the mouth and throat. As intoxication occurs, decreased sensitivity to pain and overestimation of elapsed time are reported. Decision-making, short-term memory, and motor skills are adversely affected with maximum impairment likely within the first hour after inhalation. However, major effects may last several hours, while milder ones endure for half a day or longer. Death from an overdose is apparently extremely rare and difficult to confirm.[52]

While experimenters and occasional users stand little chance of developing psychological dependence, it can and does occur with regular use. Tolerance to cannabis—diminished response to a given repeated dose—has been substantiated as developing with prolonged utilization. Although physical dependence has been demonstrated in research studies with extremely heavy use, the withdrawal syndrome is rarely reported by physicians.

As for the issue of marijuana smoking and automobile driving, there is ample evidence that "... marihuana use at typical social levels definitely impairs driving ability and related skills...."[53] Unfortunately, as marijuana use becomes

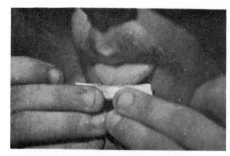

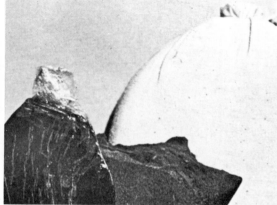

Hashish

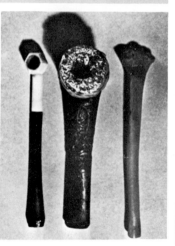

MARIJUANA

Fig. 9.10. Current scientific information indicates that marijuana may be a dangerous drug. Researchers are still exploring its short- and long-term effects.

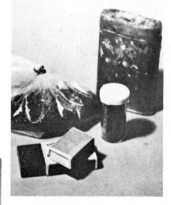

Retail forms of marijuana

Kilo bricks of marijuana

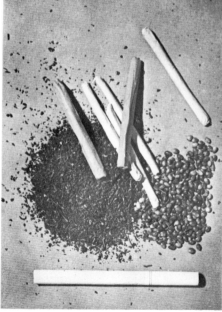

Makeshift marijuana pipes

Manicured marijuana cigarettes and seeds

more popular, it is likely that more users will risk driving while ''high.'' In addition,

> Marihuana use in combination with alcohol is also quite common and the risk of the two drugs used in combination may well be greater than that posed by either substance alone.[54]

By no means should marijuana be considered safe and harmless! Impairment in lung functioning, possibly leading to changes similar to those found in heavy cigarette smokers, has been detected. Although evidence is still fragmentary and incomplete, several adverse effects remain a possibility, including (1) impairment of the body's natural defense system against disease; (2) chromosomal alterations; (3) basic changes in cell function; (4) impairment of endocrine gland functioning, specifically a reduction in testosterone, the male sex hormone; and (5) brain damage.

While some of marijuana's properties are undesirable for most medicinal purposes, cannabis has shown promising therapeutic uses in the treatment of glaucoma (elevated pressure within the eyeball), in the reduction of nausea and vomiting among cancer patients receiving chemotherapy, and possibly in the treatment of asthma.[55]

The myth that marijuana use ultimately leads to taking heroin or some other illegal drug should be dispelled. As one observer notes:

> There is nothing inherent in the pharmacologic properties of marijuana which leads to the use of more dangerous drugs. . . . The fact that many heroin addicts have smoked marijuana does not establish a causal relationship, especially in view of the overwhelming majority of marijuana smokers who never use heroin.[56]

Escalation of drug use into polydrug (many drug) abuse is more closely related to personality and situational factors. While drug-use surveys typically find that the use of any drug is statistically associated with the use of all other drugs, the development of a dependence on or regular use of an illegal drug other than marijuana is relatively rare among college students. If any one drug is associated with the use of other drugs, it is either alcohol or tobacco, though the use of marijuana frequently precedes the use of stimulants, sedatives, and opiates.[57]

Narcotics
Drugs that relieve pain and also induce sleep are classified as narcotics. They originate from or are similar in effect to products of the opium plant, *Papaver somniferum*. Among the various narcotic drugs are *opium* (the dried juice of the unripe oriental poppy pod), *morphine* (the chief active ingredient in opium), and *heroin* (a drug synthesized from morphine). *Codeine*, another opium derivative, and the synthetic drugs *methadone* and *Demerol* are narcotics too.

Narcotics are produced in a variety of tablets, capsules, injections, cough syrups, rectal suppositories, and illegally in a gummy solid or a powdered form. All of the narcotics, including morphine, an important analgesic, and codeine, a component of some cough medicines, exert a depressant effect on the central nervous system. In addition, their persistent and prolonged use typically results in psychological and physical dependence. Because of its resultant intense

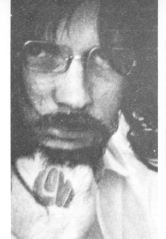

Dosage and
illicit forms
of morphine

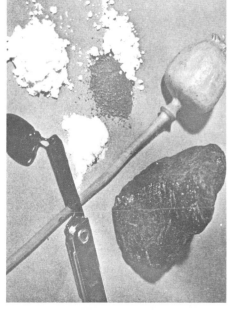

Forms of heroin

NARCOTICS

Fig. 9.11. To solve
the problem of drug
abuse, people must
educate themselves to
the potent nature of the
common drugs of abuse,
such as narcotics.

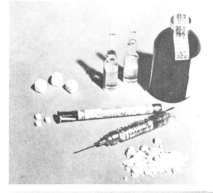

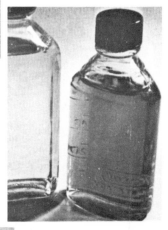

Exempt narcotics,
cough syrup
with codeine
and paregoric

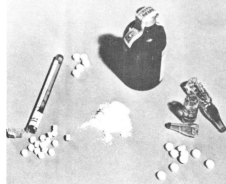

Dosage and
illicit forms
of codeine

Opium poppy and derivatives,
crude and smoking opium,
codeine, heroin, morphine

Drug-Taking Behavior: Search or Symptom?

euphoria and long effects, heroin has become the most popular narcotic drug of abuse.

The manufacture and importation of *heroin* have been outlawed in the United States where heroin is no longer used medically. Nevertheless, a vast, illegal heroin smuggling business of international proportions supplies the needs for more than an estimated 600,000 Americans who are now dependent on the drug. Adulterated or cut with milk sugar or quinine, illegally procured heroin is usually mixed into a liquid solution and administered intravenously (''mainlining''). It can also be injected just under the skin (''skin popping'') or sniffed.

Shortly after injection, the user feels a tingling sensation often interpreted as a sexual orgasm. Common reactions include a reddening of the face and constriction of the pupils of the eyes. Emotionally there is a feeling that everything is fine. Tensions are reduced; worries disappear; the rough edges of reality are dulled. Eventually, a period of stuporous inactivity (the ''nod'') follows in which splendorous daydreams occur. Such pleasurable effects last from three to six hours.

After several weeks of daily use, tolerance builds and an overpowering craving for heroin develops. Now the dosage and frequency of use must be increased. The user has become physically dependent. Body responses and processes are changed so that continued use of the drug is required to prevent the onset of withdrawal symptoms.

The heroin-dependent individual soon has but two concerns: fear of running out of the drug and fear of running out of accessible veins. Because cross-tolerance or cross-dependence is common among the opiate narcotics, an injection of any other narcotic in sufficient dose is capable of eliminating withdrawal sickness associated with heroin when the heroin supply is exhausted.

Within eight to twelve hours after the last dose is taken, withdrawal symptoms appear if another ''fix'' or injection of heroin is not procured. Perspiration, tremors, chills, diarrhea, nausea, and sharp abdominal and leg cramps are sustained and become progressively worse for two or three days, after which they

Fig. 9.12. Often addicts who use contaminated needles share their equipment with others. As a result, many addicts contract hepatitis, tetanus, infections, and abscesses.

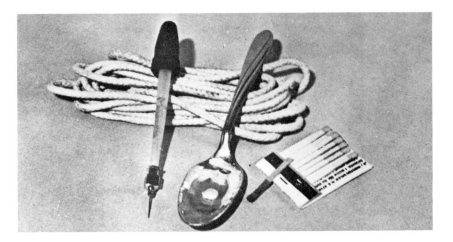

subside. In about a week the heroin abuser is free of withdrawal symptoms, but minor depression and insomnia may persist for several months. Although the withdrawal process is painful, death from withdrawal occurs only in extreme cases. What is perhaps more life-threatening is the increasing phenomenon of heroin overdose resulting in death, and death resulting from allergic or hypersensitive reactions to impurities added to cut the heroin dose and from direct toxic effects of the drug itself. Contaminated injections also pose hazards in terms of blood poisoning and viral hepatitis.

Chemicals that evaporate rapidly are known as volatile substances. When their fumes are inhaled, a state of intoxication or dreamlike high closely resembling drunkenness often results. Nausea, dizziness, slurred speech, shakiness, uncoordinated actions, double vision, and muscle spasms frequently accompany the sniffing of these drugs. The use of these substances has been associated primarily with teenagers and preadolescents.

Volatile Substances

The volatile substances are generally divided into three major groups, all of which are potentially hazardous to users.

Commercial Solvents Commercial solvents, such as toluene, xylene, benzene, naphtha, acetone, and carbon tetrachloride, are components of various commercial products, such as model airplane glue, plastic cement, paint thinner, gasoline, cleaning fluids, nail polish remover, and cigarette lighter fluid.

Aerosols In many household and commercial aerosol sprays are propellant gases that contain chlorinated or fluorinated hydrocarbons. These propellants are often abused. They are found in such products as insecticides, deodorants, glass chillers, and hair sprays.

Anesthetics Chloroform, ether, and nitrous oxide (laughing gas) have been misused in recent years. Nitrous oxide is available commercially as a tracer gas to detect pipe leaks, as a whipped-cream propellant, and to reduce pre-ignition in racing cars.

Generally, the shared hazard of all these volatile chemicals is one of intoxication, with its impairment of judgment and motor functioning. Acute intoxication

Table 9.1 Toxic Effects of Some Volatile Substances

Substance	Toxic Property
Carbon tetrachloride	Irreversible kidney and liver damage
Gasoline, naphtha in high concentrations	Heart complications, bone marrow depression
Toluene	Kidney irritant
Aerosols	Freezing and contraction of the larynx, induction of heart stoppage
Chloroform in high concentrations, trichlorethylene	Liver damage

may be relatively short—a matter of several minutes—or it may last up to an hour, depending upon the substance used and dosage. Analogous to clinical anesthesia, the high may be marked by delirium, impulsive behavior, sedation, hallucinations, and delusions. Fatal accidents have occurred, too, usually due to suffocation or oxygen deprivation. Specific substances exert toxic effects that are summarized in table 9.1.

Treatment and Rehabilitation

Because the use of drugs sometimes results in diseases or conditions of maladaptation, treatment and rehabilitation procedures have been devised to help individuals with drug problems. National and state governments have established centers and programs to treat drug-dependent persons, particularly those who have become involved with heroin. Community-based mental health centers and free clinics in some instances provide hospitalization, emergency medical treatment for detoxification and withdrawal processes, and outpatient services including post-release counseling. Job retraining, job placement, and legal services are often provided as general rehabilitation measures.[58]

For those seeking assistance in solving drug-related problems, twenty-four-hour telephone "hot lines," drop-in centers, and coffee houses have been instituted for consultation, referral, or conversation about concerns of daily life or the future. Psychotherapy between a medical specialist and a patient, and self-help therapeutic residential communities of former drug dependents have assumed increasing importance. Structured living arrangements patterned after Synanon, Daytop Village, and the initial efforts of Phoenix House provide group-centered psychotherapy for those who are dependent on drugs but are trying to quit.

Although somewhat controversial, methadone maintenance programs have increased markedly in recent years. Methadone, a synthetic narcotic drug, is used as a form of medically supervised "legalized addiction." Used originally to ease the pain of heroin withdrawal, it is now being administered as an inexpensive, long-acting substitute for heroin. Taken by mouth in tablet form or mixed with orange juice, methadone is procured at a medical clinic and taken day after day, year after year. As long as methadone is taken once each day, there is no craving for heroin. The euphoric "high" or "rush" of heroin is eliminated as is the occurrence of withdrawal sickness from heroin. Fortunately, tolerance to methadone does not seem to occur and dosages become stabilized.

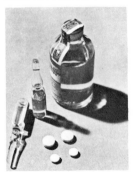

Fig. 9.13. Dosage forms of methadone

Although dependent on methadone, the patient is able to resume a more normal life. Freed from the hassle of finding an expensive fix, the dangers of infection, the incapacity of the high and nod, and the sickness of heroin withdrawal, the methadone patient is more receptive to rehabilitation services. Normal interrelationships and vocational endeavors can be resumed because "he neither acts like an addict nor thinks of himself as an addict."[59]

While the ultimate goal of methadone maintenance treatment is eventual withdrawal from methadone and elimination of dependence on any drug, for some individuals maintenance may continue for months or years. Consequently, critics claim that methadone does not cure drug dependence but merely transfers dependence from one drug to another.

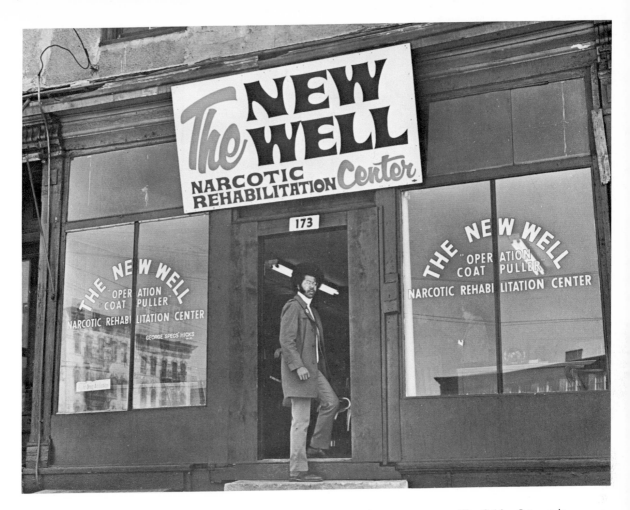

The experimental use of *narcotic antagonists* presents still another treatment for heroin dependence. Drugs, such as cyclazocine and Naltrexone, chemically block heroin from having any effect on the person. While the narcotic antagonists do not reduce the craving for heroin, they do prevent any injection of heroin from having physical effects. Eventually, the individuals learn

Fig. 9.14. Interest in helping drug abusers has increased the number of community drug rehabilitation centers and 24-hour telephone hot lines for young people having trouble with drugs.

> that heroin does not give pleasurable effects, and all of the behaviors associated with its use will become less likely to occur. . . . When this occurs, perhaps the regular use of the antagonist can be stopped.[60]

Other treatment approaches include drug-free services that focus on group or individual psychotherapy, vocational and social counseling, family counseling, vocational training, and education.

Presently there are no specialized methods for treating dependence on drugs other than opiates and alcohol. There is no chemotherapy, such as methadone maintenance, for treating abuse of amphetamines, barbiturates, and hallucinogens. Emergency treatment and counseling, forms of crisis intervention, can be

CONTROLLED SUBSTANCES: USES AND EFFECTS

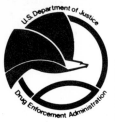

Fig. 9.15. The extent to which a drug is controlled by the federal government depends on its potential for abuse, its value as a currently accepted medicine, and the degree to which its abuse may lead to psychological or physical dependence. (From *Drugs of Abuse*, Drug Enforcement Administration, U.S. Department of Justice.)

†Designated a narcotic under the Controlled Substances Act.
‡Designated a depressant under the Controlled Substances Act.

	Drugs	Often Prescribed Brand Names	Medical Uses	Dependence Physical	
Narcotics	Opium	Dover's Powder, Paregoric	Analgesic, antidiarrheal	High	
	Morphine	Morphine	Analgesic	High	
	Codeine	Codeine	Analgesic, antitussive	Moderate	
	Heroin	None	None	High	
	Meperidine (Pethidine)	Demerol, Pethadol	Analgesic	High	
	Methadone	Dolophine, Methadone, Methadose	Analgesic, heroin substitute	High	
	Other Narcotics	Dilaudid, Leritine, Numorphan, Percodan	Analgesic, antidiarrheal, antitussive	High	
Depressants	Chloral Hydrate	Noctec, Somnos	Hypnotic	Moderate	
	Barbiturates	Amytal, Butisol, Nembutal, Phenobarbital, Seconal, Tuinal	Anesthetic, anti-convulsant, sedation, sleep	High	
	Glutethimide	Doriden	Sedation, sleep	High	
	Methaqualone	Optimil, Parest, Quaalude, Somnafac, Sopor	Sedation, sleep	High	
	Tranquilizers	Equanil, Librium, Miltown Serax, Tranxene, Valium	Anti-anxiety, muscle relaxant, sedation	Moderate	
	Other Depressants	Clonopin, Dalmane, Dormate, Noludar, Placydil, Valmid	Anti-anxiety, sedation, sleep	Possible	
Stimulants	Cocaine†	Cocaine	Local anesthetic	Possible	
	Amphetamines	Benzedrine, Biphetamine, Desoxyn, Dexedrine	Hyperkinesis, narcolepsy, weight control	Possible	
	Phenmetrazine	Preludin	Weight control	Possible	
	Methylphenidate	Ritalin	Hyperkinesis	Possible	
	Other Stimulants	Bacarate, Cylert, Didrex, Ionamin, Plegine, Pondimin, Pre-Sate, Sanorex, Voranil	Weight control	Possible	
Hallucinogens	LSD	None	None	None	
	Mescaline	None	None	None	
	Psilocybin-Psilocyn	None	None	None	
	MDA	None	None	None	
	PCP‡	Sernylan	Veterinary anesthetic	None	
	Other Hallucinogens	None	None	None	
Cannabis	Marihuana Hashish Hashish Oil	None	None	Degree unknown	

Potential: Psychological	Tolerance	Duration of Effects (in hours)	Usual Methods of Administration	Possible Effects	Effects of Overdose	Withdrawal Syndrome
High	Yes	3 to 6	Oral, smoked			
High	Yes	3 to 6	Injected, smoked			
Moderate	Yes	3 to 6	Oral, injected	Euphoria, drowsiness, respiratory depression, constricted pupils, nausea	Slow and shallow breathing, clammy skin, convulsions, coma, possible death	Watery eyes, runny nose, yawning, loss of appetite, irritability, tremors, panic, chills and sweating, cramps, nausea
High	Yes	3 to 6	Injected, sniffed			
High	Yes	3 to 6	Oral, injected			
High	Yes	12 to 24	Oral, injected			
High	Yes	3 to 6	Oral, injected			
Moderate	Probable	5 to 8	Oral			
High	Yes	1 to 16	Oral, injected			
High	Yes	4 to 8	Oral	Slurred speech, disorientation, drunken behavior without odor of alcohol	Shallow respiration, cold and clammy skin, dilated pupils, weak and rapid pulse, coma, possible death	Anxiety, insomnia, tremors, delirium, convulsions, possible death
High	Yes	4 to 8	Oral			
Moderate	Yes	4 to 8	Oral			
Possible	Yes	4 to 8	Oral			
High	Yes	2	Injected, sniffed			
High	Yes	2 to 4	Oral, injected	Increased alertness, excitation, euphoria, dilated pupils, increased pulse rate and blood pressure, insomnia, loss of appetite	Agitation, increase in body temperature, hallucinations, convulsions, possible death	Apathy, long periods of sleep, irritability, depression, disorientation
High	Yes	2 to 4	Oral			
High	Yes	2 to 4	Oral			
Possible	Yes	2 to 4	Oral			
Degree unknown	Yes	Variable	Oral			
Degree unknown	Yes	Variable	Oral, injected			
Degree unknown	Yes	Variable	Oral	Illusions and hallucinations (with exception of MDA); poor perception of time and distance	Longer, more intense "trip" episodes, psychosis, possible death	Withdrawal syndrome not reported
Degree unknown	Yes	Variable	Oral, injected, sniffed			
Degree unknown	Yes	Variable	Oral, injected, smoked			
Degree unknown	Yes	Variable	Oral, injected, sniffed			
Moderate	Yes	2 to 4	Oral, smoked	Euphoria, relaxed inhibitions, increased appetite, disoriented behavior	Fatigue, paranoia, possible psychosis	Insomnia, hyperactivity, and decreased appetite reported in a limited number of individuals

provided to counter adverse reactions resulting from nonopiate drug abuse. Such intervention provides relief for immediate drug-related problems, but as a long-range solution, it is severely limited in terms of follow-up supervision or even contact with patients.

Legal Controls

The social response to drug abuse has been manifest largely in numerous laws and regulations to reduce the availability of drugs to the general public and to penalize drug abusers. In the United States federal law provides for controls on the manufacture, distribution, and possession of dangerous drugs, including heroin and other narcotics, hallucinogens, marijuana, and the stimulants and sedatives. Such controls vary according to a drug's potential for abuse and its medical application. Pharmaceutical houses, processors, suppliers, and dispensers must keep accurate records of receipts and outflow. Limitations have also been placed on the filling and refilling of prescriptions for controlled drugs that have medical uses.[61]

However, drug laws, especially those pertaining to the possession of marijuana for personal use, are in a state of change. The movement to decriminalize possession of small amounts of marijuana—from 25 grams up to 100 grams in certain states—is gaining momentum. Already, several states have eased penalties for possessing pot by reducing the offense from a felony to a misdemeanor. Relatively small fines are assessed, rather than severe prison sentences as in other states.[62] Congress is expected to follow the trend toward decriminalization in the future.

In discussing the pros and cons of changing laws regarding marijuana use, it is important to distinguish between *decriminalization* and *legalization*.

Reduction of the penalties for simple possession of small amounts of marihuana, making it a civil offense with a fine rather than a jail sentence, seems to have been an effective and appropriate approach in many states. The offender receives a citation and no permanent criminal record. We have seen in the past where criminal penalties resulted in otherwise law-abiding young people spending time in prison and incurring permanent damage to their careers and to their ability to enter professions. This causes far greater harm to their lives than any effect the drug would have had, and the penalties are counterproductive.

Legalization of marihuana, rather than decriminalization, would be totally inappropriate and would only serve to encourage the use of the drug when we seek to deter it, and it would open the door to a broad-scale commercialization.[63]

In one sense, heroin and other so-called hard drugs have been decriminalized unofficially on the federal level. Now the emphasis in law enforcement agencies is on penalizing the dealer and drug trafficker rather than the small-time user.

Nevertheless, penalties vary considerably from one jurisdiction to another. Until agreement is reached nationally to reduce illegal consumption of drugs, the laws will be sporadically enforced and contradictory. Many foreign nations impose much stiffer penalties for drug violations, including months of pretrial confinement, life imprisonment, heavy fines, and permanent expulsion from the country. Check out the drug laws of those nations that you will be visiting. You may save yourself from a painful adaptation—to a foreign jail!

Readers are advised to investigate state laws regarding illegal drug use. Sometimes these laws carry penalties that differ considerably from the national laws. Ask your course instructor or confer with local law enforcement officials for accurate information on these matters.

Prospects for the Future

What will it be? A future without any drugs is unlikely. But will there be more or less drug abuse? The need for human adaptation will continue, but will new maladaptations develop because of drug-taking behavior?

Increased abuse of sedatives and hallucinogens could mean a quieter, calmer, less active, and less competitive society. This could result in a less productive society but possibly a happier one. If stimulants gain even wider acceptance, we may see an even more frenzied rat race in the quest for higher performance or achievement. But who will win?

As 1984 approaches, mood modification via drugs might provide the primary coping mechanism, offering occasional retreats from and isolated comfort in a world threatened by war, pollution, hunger, racial strife, economic depression, and generally lowered standards of living. Relief would be just a swallow away, or maybe an injection or inhalation away.

Will parents react in horror and dismay when their children experiment with new drugs or some old ones? They may opt for stronger laws with tougher penalties, or they could pressure for decriminalization of simple possession of nonmedical drugs. Some might even encourage their children to adopt responsible use patterns of marijuana and other drugs in controlled social settings.

Medical or Licensing Models?

We could move into a medical model of control in which certain drugs, including marijuana, could be obtained with a doctor's prescription; or a licensing model in which certain drugs would be sold essentially the same way that alcohol is sold—by a reputable dealer, assuring relative purity and standard potency of the drug and meeting other regulatory conditions.[64]

Wider availability of drugs might increase the number of psychologically troubled people or drug deviates who could pose physical or economic threats to society. How many drug-dependent individuals can a society support and still prosper? These persons may be tolerated as the price to pay for our general drug-oriented life. Or they could become the true social outcasts of the future, consigned to custodial care in some institution or prison. They might even inhabit the concentration camps of the future.

Limited Availability

A more limited availability of drugs would require a change in public attitudes toward all psychoactive substances, including those now legally procured. The belief that there is a drug to cure every ill or discomfort would have to diminish. Patients would have to make fewer demands of their physicians for chemical aids to induce sleep or relieve tension. Stricter law enforcement aimed at suppliers and big volume dealers would also limit availability.[65]

Permissive Use   Since none of the present restrictions has stemmed the tide of drug abuse, some radical approaches may be applied in the future.[66] One proposal would decriminalize the use of heroin on a worldwide basis, thus undercutting the profits of drug trafficking. Another involves perfecting a way to use heroin without becoming addicted. Complete legalization of all drugs without criminal or civil penalties is yet another alternative. Would such permissive use of hard drugs increase the dimensions of our drug abuse problems? Would our nation be prepared to finance such an expensive drug habit if millions of people became dependent on heroin?

Alternative
Methods
of Adaptation

Less potentially hazardous means of escape will have to be found in a future of less drug abuse. The use of fantasy as a means of withdrawing temporarily from unpleasantness or of enhancing self-image will have to be rediscovered by the entertainment media, which provide little relief from life's everyday burdens at present.

> In the past this escape was often provided by motion pictures or the theater. No longer. Today movies and plays caricature life or depict its most unpleasant aspects, dwell on self-destructive sexual behavior, wallow in violence, or emphasize angry confrontation.[67]

Believe it or not, loving, relating, and "turning on" without drugs are possible. Such processes, though, might require a more active and vigorous adaptation than most are accustomed to making. When confronted with some challenge, the individual typically becomes frustrated and then passively changes his life-style or mental state to accommodate the new situation. Sometimes maladaptations of anxiety, depression, and disease or other forms of incapacitation and inefficiency result. Emphasis might more profitably be placed on directing those dissatisfactions and discontent into more positive, self-fulfilling responses. As one observer notes:

> My favorite quotation is from George Bernard Shaw: "The reasonable man adjusts to society; the unreasonable man forces society to adjust to him. Therefore, all progress depends on unreasonable men." That's the message I try to get across.[68]

Whether you picture yourself as the "reasonable" or "unreasonable" person, nonchemical alternatives for various levels of experience—from the sensory to the spiritual—do exist and are becoming available in ever more appealing and relevant ways. Glasser recently has formulated the concept of *positive addiction*—behavior that develops the character and the body and strengthens a person to overcome negative addiction and lead a more integrated and rewarding life.[69] He claims that a positive addiction is anything a person chooses to do as long as it is noncompetitive, freely chosen, engaged in about one hour each day, easily accomplished without much mental effort, individually oriented and not dependent on others, valuable in some way to the participant, open to measurement of improvement, and undertaken without self-criticism. Glasser identifies meditation as the most popular way to achieve a positive addiction and running as the hardest but surest way.

Individual activities to replace, reduce, or prevent drug abuse[70]

American Indian crafts
Animal shelter volunteer work
Applique
Apprenticeship with local
    professional or craftsperson
Auto/motorcycle maintenance
Babysitting
Basketweaving
Batiking
Beachcombing
Beadwork
Bicycling
Big Sister/Brother volunteer work
Birdwatching
Bonsai
Bookbinding
Boxing
Calligraphy
Candlemaking
Carpentry
Cartooning
Cinematography
Collages/assemblages
Copper enameling
Diary of inner thoughts
Dioramas
Dollmaking
Dried flowers
Drum lessons
Eggery
Electronics
Errand-running for elderly
Ethnic dancing
Flower arranging
Fossil hunting
Freeform crocheting

Gardening/farming
Glassblowing
Gourmet/ethnic cooking
Greeting card designing
Guitar lessons
Gymnastics
Hatmaking
Hatha yoga
Heraldry
Herb gardening/drying
Hiking
Historical preservation volunteer
    work
Historical research of
    neighborhood
Home repairing
Horseback riding
Ikebana
Inkle weaving
Journalism
Kitemaking
Lacemaking
Leatherworking
Legislative change organization
    volunteer work
Linoleum/wood and vegetable
    carving relief printing
Macrame
Martial arts (judo, karate, aikido)
Meditation
Miniaturemaking
Mobilemaking
Modern dancing
Mosaics
Natural foods cooking
Needlepoint canvas designing

Origami
Pantomime
Papermaking
Papier-mâché
Pen pal correspondence (in
    U.S.A. and foreign)
Photography
Political campaign work
Pottery/ceramics
Primitive instruments
    (construction and playing)
Psychodrama (supervised)
Puppetry
Quilling
Quilting
Recycling center volunteer work
Rubbings
Sailing
Sandalmaking
Sandcasting
Scrimshaw
Scuba diving
Sensory awareness training
Silkscreening
Silver/gold/copper smithing
Soft sculpture
Spelunking
Terrarium/ecolarium building
Theater groups
Track and field sports
Tutoring
Voice lessons
Weaving
Wilderness camping
Wire sculpture
Wood carving

If more usual activities do not capture your imagination or provide you with a sense of personal worth and growth, try skydiving; well-run group therapy sessions; encounter groups; confidence training; community action in positive social change, such as ecological and consumer lobbying, and political action; nongraded instruction in art, music, and family life education; courses in the meaning of life; the study of morality; and exposure to nonchemical methods of spiritual development as found in applied mysticism and yogic techniques.[71]

What will your drug future be?

Summary

Drug use and drug abuse are themes developed in this chapter. Psychoactive drugs that primarily affect the human mind are useful in the treatment of mental illness. However, such substances are now widely used by healthy people for social convenience, pleasure, and personal happiness. The use of mind-affecting drugs presents some very real risks to personal health. One of these risks is drug dependence, characterized by physical and psychological dependence, the development of tolerance, and withdrawal sickness when drug use is discontinued.

Several reasons for the sudden increase in the use of psychoactive drugs have been presented. Frequently, the reasons are evidence of adaptation to environmental challenges. Perhaps drug abuse today is a personal search for new experiences or a symptom of some underlying need or disease process.

Also examined in this chapter were the major groups of psychoactive drugs and their possible effects. Particular attention was given to the sedatives, stimulants, hallucinogens, narcotics, and volatile substances. Treatment and rehabilitation aspects of the drug scene were reviewed for modern drug countermeasures, including the current popularity of methadone maintenance programs.

Finally, several nonchemical alternatives to drug use were suggested for the reader's thoughtful consideration.

Review Questions

1. How has chemotherapy been instrumental in treating and preventing disease and in preserving health status?
2. Differentiate between drug abuse and drug misuse.
3. Explain the difference between physical dependence and psychological dependence.
4. What is withdrawal sickness? What causes it?
5. Discuss some of the theories behind drug-taking behavior. Which one do you believe is correct?
6. What will you tell your children about drugs and drug use?
7. If you were a schoolteacher, in what grade would you implement a drug unit? Why? What important aspects would you emphasize?
8. Do you view the increase in drug abuse and misuse as a threat to our society in the future?
9. Are there ways of reaching altered states of consciousness other than through drugs? Are we beginning to see such a trend?
10. What important factors are responsible for the effects a drug will have on an individual?
11. Do you believe the marijuana laws should be changed? Do you think marijuana should be legalized? Why or why not?
12. Knowing that marijuana is illegal, would you allow your children to smoke it?

13. Compare the effects of alcohol with those of marijuana. Which do you feel is more harmful? Why?

14. List and describe the various forms of narcotics.

15. Why is heroin considered an extremely dangerous drug?

16. It has been said that governments have no legal authority to prohibit people from taking drugs. Do you agree or disagree with this statement? Defend your position.

17. If all drugs were legally sold, what effect would this have on our nation?

18. What are the various types of treatment and rehabilitation available to drug users? Are they effective?

19. What is a narcotic antagonist?

20. Do you think that drug misuse and abuse will gradually decline? If not, where are we headed in the future?

Notes

1. Walter Modell, "Mass Drug Catastrophes and the Roles of Science and Technology," *Science,* 21 April 1967, p. 346.
2. Committee on Drugs of the American School Health Association and the Pharmaceutical Manufacturers Association, *Teaching about Drugs* (Kent, Ohio: American School Health Association, 1970), p. xii.
3. Oakley S. Ray, *Drugs, Society, and Human Behavior* (St. Louis: C. V. Mosby Co., 1972), pp. 4–5.
4. Hardin B. Jones and Helen C. Jones, *Sensual Drugs: Deprivation and Rehabilitation of the Mind* (Cambridge: Cambridge University Press, 1977), p. 2.
5. George M. Carstairs, "A Land of Lotus-Eaters?" *American Journal of Psychiatry* 125 (May 1969): 1580.
6. Jones and Jones, *Sensual Drugs,* pp. 29–30.
7. Modell, "Mass Drug Catastrophes," p. 350.
8. National Commission on Marihuana and Drug Abuse, *Marihuana: A Signal of Misunderstanding* (Washington, D.C.: U.S. Government Printing Office, 1972), pp. 8–9.
9. Donald Phares, "The Simple Economics of Heroin and Organizing Public Policy," *Journal of Drug Issues* 3 (Spring 1973): 186–99.
10. "Drugs: A $17-Billion-A-Year Habit That U.S. Can't Break," *U.S. News & World Report,* 10 May 1976, p. 25.
11. Special Action Office for Drug Abuse Prevention, *Q & A, Special Action Office Answers the Most Frequently Asked Questions about Drug Abuse* (Washington, D.C.: U.S. Government Printing Office, 1972), p. 8.
12. Robert L. DuPont, "Foreword to the Sixth Annual Report," *Marihuana and Health,* National Institute on Drug Abuse (Washington, D.C.: U.S. Government Printing Office, 1977), p. vi.
13. Michael Newton, "On Popping Pills and Potions During Pregnancy," *Family Health/Today's Health,* May 1977, pp. 20, 22.
14. N. B. Eddy, H. Halbach, H. Isbell, and M. H. Seevers, "Drug Dependence: Its Significance and Characteristics," *Bulletin of the World Health Organization* 32 (May 1965): 721–33.
15. Definitions of terms related to drug dependence are based upon a publication of the National Institute of Mental Health, *What Will Happen If . . .* (Washington, D.C.: U.S. Government Printing Office, 1972), pp. 2–6.
16. Louise Richards and John H. Langer, *Drug-Taking in Youth* (Washington, D.C.: U.S. Government Printing Office, 1971), p. 20.
17. Joel Fort, as profiled by Edwin Kiester, Jr., "The Man from Help," *Human Behavior,* August 1973, p. 56.
18. Donald B. Louria, *Overcoming Drugs: A Program for Action* (New York: Bantam Books, 1972), p. 17.
19. National Institute on Drug Abuse, *Marihuana and Health:* Sixth Annual Report (Washington, D.C.: U.S. Government Printing Office, 1977), pp. 1, 10–11.
20. Helen A. Nowlis, *Drugs on the College Campus* (Garden City, N.Y.: Doubleday & Co., 1969), p. 22.
21. Barry Peterson, Judith Kuriansky, Carolyn Konheim, et al, "Television Advertising and Drug Use," *American Journal of Public Health* 66 (October 1976): 978.

22. Commission of Inquiry into the Non-Medical Use of Drugs, *Interim Report* (Ottawa: Queen's Printer for Canada, 1970), pp. 155–56.

23. John A. Ewing, "Students, Sex, and Marijuana," *Medical Aspects of Human Sexuality* (February 1972): 113.

24. Donald B. Louria, *The Drug Scene* (New York: Bantam Books, 1970), pp. 32–33.

25. Richard H. Blum, "Motivations for Student Drug Use" (Paper delivered at the National Association of Student Personnel Administrators Drug Education Conference, Washington, D.C., November 1966, and printed in a *Drug Education Booklet* prepared by students of Vanderbilt University, Nashville, Tennessee, 1971), p. 1.

26. National Institute on Drug Abuse, *Marihuana and Health,* p. 11.

27. Carstairs, "Land of Lotus-Eaters?" p. 1578.

28. Edward A. Suchman, "The 'Hang-Loose' Ethic and the Spirit of Drug Use," *Journal of Health and Social Behavior,* June 1968, pp. 146–55.

29. Ewing, "Students, Sex, and Marijuana," p. 115.

30. Leslie H. Farber, "Ours Is the Addicted Society," *New York Times Magazine,* 11 December 1966. Reprinted in Douglas Matheson and Meredith Davison, *The Behavioral Effects of Drugs* (New York: Holt, Rinehart & Winston, 1972), p. 19.

31. Stanley H. King, "Youth in Rebellion: Through Time and Societies," *Resource Book for Drug Abuse Education,* 2d ed. (Washington, D.C.: U.S. Government Printing Office, 1972), p. 12.

32. Suchman, " 'Hang-Loose' Ethic," pp. 146–55.

33. Richards and Langer, *Drug-Taking in Youth,* pp. 20–22.

34. Ray, *Drugs, Society, and Human Behavior,* p. 10.

35. National Institute on Drug Abuse, *Marihuana and Health,* pp. 5–10.

36. "Heroin Addiction Highest in West Coast Cities: NIDA," *The U.S. Journal of Drug and Alcohol Dependence* 1 (August 1977): 1–2.

37. "Drugs: A $17-Billion-A-Year Habit," pp. 25–26.

38. "Trends: Drug Abuse," *Promoting Community Health—1976* (Washington, D.C.: U.S. Government Printing Office, 1976), pp. 13–14.

39. "Heroin Use Spreads To Small Towns," *The Nation's Health,* May 1976, p. 4.

40. Gary Thatcher, "The Respectable Pushers," *Drug Enforcement* 4 (February 1977): 26–35.

41. *A Guide of Drug Information: Do You Know the Facts about Drugs?* (Miami, Fla.: Health Communications, Inc., 1977), pp. 25–27.

42. Richard H. Blum, "Drugs and America's Destiny: Trends and Predictions," *Resource Book for Drug Abuse Education,* 2d ed. (Washington, D.C.: U.S. Government Printing Office, 1972), p. 21.

43. Reginald G. Smart and Diane Fejer, "Recent Trends in Illicit Drug Use Among Adolescents," *Canada's Mental Health,* supp. no. 68 (May-August 1971).

44. Unless otherwise noted, this summary section on drugs and their effects is based on publications of the U.S. Department of Health, Education, and Welfare (National Clearinghouse for Drug Abuse Information), and the U.S. Department of Justice (Bureau of Narcotics & Dangerous Drugs):

    National Clearinghouse for Drug Abuse Information, *Marihuana: Some Questions and Answers* (Washington, D.C.: U.S. Government Printing Office, 1970).

    National Clearinghouse for Drug Abuse Information, *Drug Abuse: Some Questions and Answers; Narcotics: Some Questions and Answers; Sedatives: Some Questions and Answers; Stimulants: Some Questions and Answers; Their Drug Laws Are a Whole Lot Tougher Than Ours; Volatile Substances: Some Questions and Answers* (Washington, D.C.: U.S. Government Printing Office, 1971).

    National Clearinghouse for Drug Abuse Information, *Methaqualone; MDA* (Washington, D.C.: U.S. Government Printing Office, 1973).

    National Clearinghouse for Drug Abuse Information, *Amphetamine; The Deliberate Inhalation of Volatile Substances* (Washington, D.C.: U.S. Government Printing Office, 1974).

    National Clearinghouse for Drug Abuse Information, *Heroin* (Washington, D.C.: U.S. Government Printing Office, 1975).

    A Guide of Drug Information: Do You Know the Facts about Drugs? (Miami, Fla.: Health Communications, Inc., 1977).

    National Institute on Drug Abuse, *Cocaine: 1977* (Washington, D.C.: U.S. Government Printing Office, 1977).

45. Arthur Grollman and Evelyn F. Grollman, *Pharmacology and Therapeutics,* 7th ed. (Philadelphia: Lea & Febiger, 1970), p. 159.

46. American Medical Association Council on Drugs, *AMA Drug Evaluations,* 1st ed. (Chicago: American Medical Association, 1971), p. 213.

47. *A Guide of Drug Information,* p. 16.

48. Grollman and Grollman, *Pharmacology and Therapeutics*, p. 406.

49. Carole Cox and Reginald G. Smart, *The Nature and Extent of Speed Use in North America* (Toronto: Addiction Research Foundation, 1970), p. 2.

50. Commission of Inquiry into the Non-Medical Use of Drugs, *Interim Report*.

51. National Commission on Marihuana and Drug Abuse, *Marihuana: A Signal of Misunderstanding*, p. 56.

52. *Marihuana and Health*, second annual report to Congress from the Secretary of Health, Education, and Welfare (Washington, D.C.: U.S. Government Printing Office, 1972), p. 13.

53. National Institute on Drug Abuse, *Marihuana and Health*, p. 23.

54. Ibid., p. 24.

55. National Institute on Drug Abuse, *Marihuana and Health: Fifth Annual Report* (Washington, D.C.: U.S. Government Printing Office, 1976), pp. 8–9.

56. George Chun, "Marijuana: A Realistic Approach," *California Medicine*, April 1971, p. 11.

57. Robert Carr, "What Marijuana Does (and Doesn't Do)," *Human Behavior* 7 (January 1978): 22.

58. Special Action Office for Drug Abuse Prevention, *Community Action for Drug Abuse Prevention* (Washington, D.C.: Executive Office of the President, 1973), pp. 10–11.

59. Edward M. Brecher and *Consumer Reports* editors, *Licit and Illicit Drugs* (Mount Vernon, N.Y.: Consumers Union, 1972), p. 161.

60. Ray, *Drugs, Society, and Human Behavior*, p. 208.

61. Public Law 91–513, An Act of the U.S. Congress, *Comprehensive Drug Abuse Prevention and Control Act of 1970*, 91st Congress, October 27, 1970 and amendments of July 1, 1971.

62. Michael Satchell, "Our Changing Marijuana Laws," *Parade*, 11 December 1977), p. 16.

63. Peter G. Bourne, "Dr. Bourne on the Marihuana Issue," *Drug Enforcement* 4 (August 1977): 3.

64. John Kaplan, *Marijuana: The New Prohibition* (New York: World Publishing Co., 1970), pp. 347–50.

65. Phares, "The Simple Economics of Heroin and Organizing Public Policy."

66. "Drugs: A $17-Billion-A-Year Habit," p. 26.

67. Louria, *Overcoming Drugs*, p. 16.

68. Fort, "The Man from Help," p. 58.

69. William Glasser, *Positive Addiction* (New York: Harper & Row, Publishers, Inc., 1976).

70. National Institute on Drug Abuse, *Alternatives* (Washington, D.C.: U.S. Government Printing Office, 1976), pp. 6–7.

71. Allan Y. Cohen, "Alternatives to Drug Use: A Model of Causes and Mandates," *Resource Book for Drug Abuse Education*, 2d ed. (Washington, D.C.: U.S. Government Printing Office, 1972), p. 84.

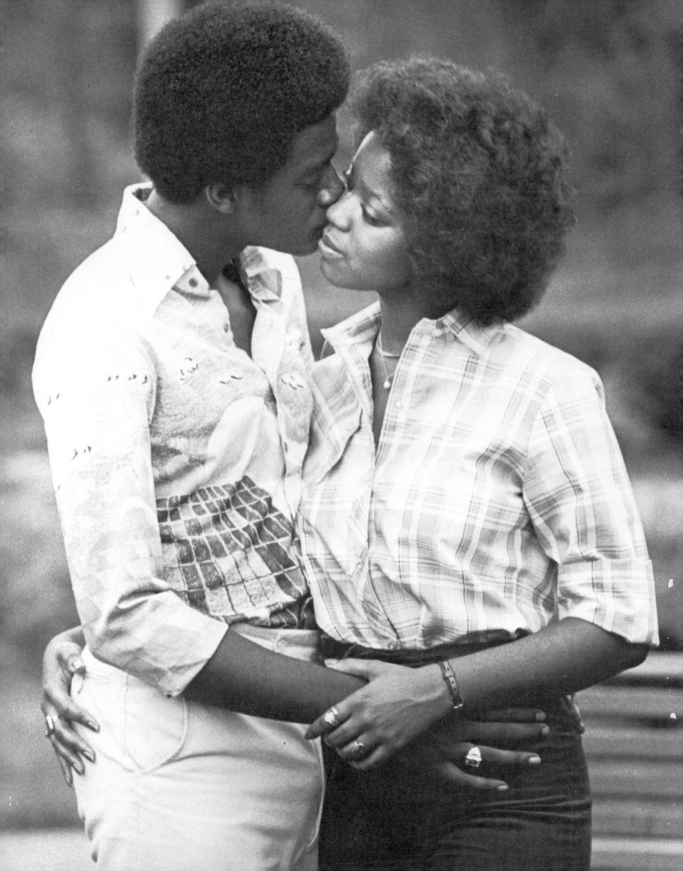

Courtship: An Institution?

10

At a time when many young people are coping with decisions about use of to-bacco, alcohol, and drugs, they are faced with another major adaptation. Rela-tionships leading to courtship begin to develop, and young adults start consider-ing questions requiring meaningful and lifelong decisions.

In his book *The Family System in America,* Ira Reiss[1] operationally defined the courtship system as interactions between young unmarried people and/or their parental kin for the purpose of mate selection. In contemporary society that defi-nition must be expanded to include unmarried, but searching, and previously married persons of all ages. Further, although traditionally courtship leads to marriage, we must recognize that today a number of courtships begin, continue, and end without anyone's intending to marry. In short, many people date and even court each other for long periods of time without marrying. For some, courtship is a lifelong affair. The courtship institution has adapted to this pattern, and therefore, we cannot automatically assume that marriage always follows courtship.

Motivation for courtship may be primarily biological among humans, but the process is strictly governed by an elaborate set of rules and practices. It is a system developed by man to provide for the upbringing of children. In contempo-rary America the explicit condemnation of sexual promiscuity is testimony to society's intention that no new societal members be born without two responsible parents sharing in the process. Through a series of steps, each carefully designed to insure "progression," our elaborate courtship system demands an ever in-creasing commitment by both partners as they approach sexual intimacy. Al-though not everyone accepts this system and its consequences (indeed some never marry, many have children regardless of marital status, and others divorce and remarry frequently in spite of children), still courtship plays a dominant role in American life, and merits considerable attention. It all begins with dating.

Primarily a western culture phenomenon, dating became popular well back in the early years of frontier society. Belief in individual effort in the struggle for survi-val and in the development of free enterprise, competition, and rivalry also en-couraged the growth of a relatively free courtship system. Many migrants were "individuals," adventurous people of high motivation and independence. They roamed across the continent in search of futures, clearly free of any parental, religious, or even civic controls. One could only expect them to continue this

Dating

pattern in both their selection of a mate and their upbringing of new generations. The emphasis was on choice and the freedom to exercise it.

The custom of bundling in the eighteenth century permitted unmarried couples to court in beds equipped with separating boards, which were not always effective. In this way, guardians protected the morality of youth, while providing them a measure of independence in their selection of marital partners. Support for this practice was strong throughout ensuing generations, testimony to the fact that pressure to marry was strong. Even mothers who had experienced bundling and undoubtedly knew that it very often led to sexual involvement, supported the practice of bundling against the outrage of the clergy.

One argument for bundling was that it preserved heat by permitting couples to huddle close together under a common blanket. Couples bundled on buggy rides as well as in bedrooms.

A young man who traveled great distances to visit a girl's home in the cold of winter could hardly be expected to return home the same night. Houses were relatively crude, and heating was expensive. Hence, the couple was permitted to share a bed and blanket, to bundle, for the night, so that they might have a chance to talk and get to know each other.[2]

In time, with new migrants from various backgrounds coming to North America, courtship customs changed, although the emphasis on choice remained great, and the provision of privacy continued. By the beginning of the twentieth century, courtship had become almost a ritual. With the coming of the automobile, privacy between young people was almost assured.

Premarital sexual involvement was probably always popular in frontier North America. The Groton, Massachusetts, Church records show that more than one third of all of its brides from 1761 through 1775 were confessed nonvirgins at the time of their marriage.[3] Further, "sparking" and "spooning," common practices in those days, bear a strong resemblance to "necking" and "petting" today, and one can conjecture with confidence that "woopitching" in the nineteenth century was much akin to "making out" in the twentieth.

"Going steady," so disfavored throughout the 1940s and 1950s, is no longer frowned upon, and young people are relatively free to date as they please. The incidence of premarital coitus has not changed much since World War II, although attitudes toward it are more liberal. A double standard persists, however, and merits attention.

The Double Standard

A double standard is two sets of rules governing the same behaviors. Traditionally, the sexual behavior of males and females has been governed by different standards: boys are expected to be forward, aggressive, dominant, and sexually experienced; girls are expected to be shy, defensive, supportive, and sexually naive.

Such a double standard is particularly powerful in a society like ours that makes marriage the desirable life-style. It gives males one tremendous advantage over females, the advantage of age. For any number of reasons, including maturity, financial stability, and vocational development, males have tended to marry

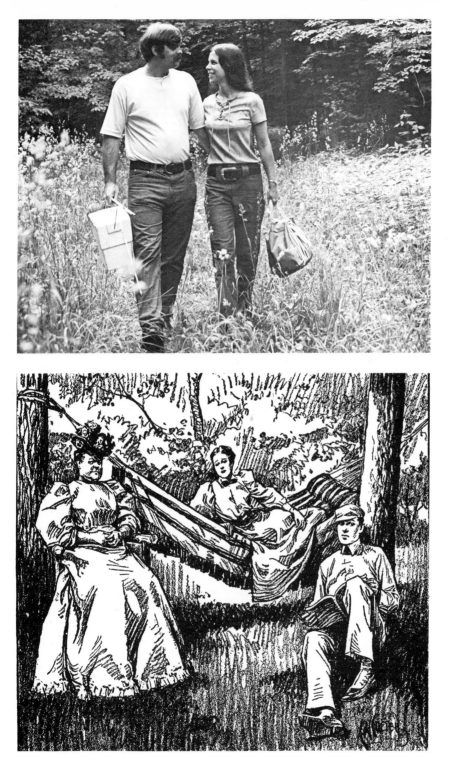

Fig. 10.1. This young married couple probably began their relationship with a first date that meant nothing more to either of them than seeing a movie or going to a party. At some point dating slipped into courtship, and they independently and jointly made a commitment to share their lives.

Fig. 10.2. Courting in the late 19th century usually was a three-way situation. The disapproving glare of the ever-present chaperon often was enough to destroy even the most romantic of young men and women.

Fig. 10.3. In our culture it is customary for males to marry younger females. As a result, the older the male the greater the number of females available to him; conversely, the older the female the fewer potential mates.

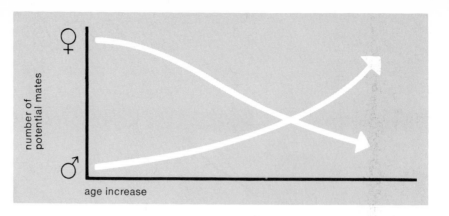

considerably later than females and to marry younger women. The advantage of this practice for the male is that as his age increases, so does his field of potential mates; as the female ages, her chances of marrying diminish. It is not uncommon for a fifty-year-old male to marry a twenty- or thirty-year-old female. The reverse is unusual.

Even in dating, this practice leads to unequal pressures on the male and female. A female college freshman, for example, has a large field of potential suitors, particularly among upper-class males, who invariably await the incoming classes with "great expectations." As she advances through her sophomore, junior, and senior years, however, her mate potential diminishes markedly. On the other hand, the mate potential of the entering male freshman increases with each passing year. From the shy, insecure boy, who believes that girls his age would rather go with older males and that most of his peers are more knowledgeable, experienced, and mature than he (hence girls would probably prefer to date them rather than him), he gradually evolves into a suave, confident senior, willing and waiting to squire freshman girls around campus. His position alone gives him status.

Sex As Bargaining Power (The Principle of Least Interest)

Unequal advantages in the marriage market, coupled with our natural and almost universal feelings of insecurity in dealing with sex in general and with the opposite sex in particular, give sex a tremendous bargaining power. Few people are really open about human sexuality, and most people feel somewhat inadequate in describing their true feelings, assuming they understand their own feelings, to a potential partner. This can and usually does lead to uncomfortable situations, as in the following case:

After three months of regular dating, Rosemary began to detect a certain apathy in John. It was nothing really obvious, but a subtle indifference. Previously when she had perceived any waning interest, she "encouraged" him toward greater sexual involvement, and he always responded ardently, at least for awhile. The problem now was that the next step involved intercourse.

Rosemary really liked John—she hadn't dated much, and his gentle but knowing ways led her into a new world of expression. Although she felt guilty petting at first, she soon forgot these inhibitions—until a new standard was sought. And John was a great one for establishing new standards! Somehow she got the impression that perhaps he wasn't all that experienced, but with John it was difficult to tell. He never talked about his past, and since she was so inexperienced herself, she was never quite certain which one of them was really responsible for those "awkward" moments.

One recognizes in this case not only the potential for using sex as a bargaining power to keep the relationship going, but also the *principle of least interest*. In any interpersonal relationship, the party with the least interest, or the least to lose, has a subtle advantage and can use that advantage to gain what he or she wants. Although the principle of least interest has implications for many types of behavior, none is more painful than that of the social variety.

An immature male dating a popular coed, for example, finds himself almost automatically at extreme disadvantage. Not only can he not fulfill the role as he perceives it, but also his feelings of insecurity may lead him to hypersensitivity and overreaction. Afraid of rejection, he is frequently rejected, but not for the usual reasons. In the following case Paul found reason to regret his inability simply to "be himself."

A little shy, and clearly inexperienced, Paul nevertheless saw himself as a "desirable" freshman. Popular in high school, he faced an awkward social climate in college—he was aware that most of his potential dates would prefer partners enrolled in the upper years. As a consequence, from the moment that he finally procured a date with the very popular Joanna, he began to feel somewhat insecure. He knew that she dated frequently and for the most part with older boys. He also had a preconceived notion of how upperclassmen behaved on dates, and he was pretty inexperienced. What a dilemma!

The entire evening proved disastrous. Not only did he drink more than usual, but he either couldn't stop talking or couldn't start—conversation was nonexistent, and he blamed himself. On the way home he knew he had to prove his "experience" so Joanna wouldn't consider him totally uninteresting. Without conversation, the radio turned up high, he pulled into a vacant laneway and became aggressive. She rebuffed him and asked to be taken home. Unfortunately, again little was said.

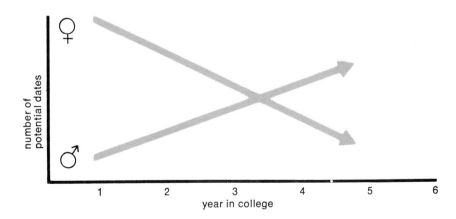

Fig. 10.4. As a male progresses through school, his opportunities to date increase; conversely, the opportunities for a female diminish. The judicious use of sex may provide equal bargaining power for some females, superior power for others.

The next morning Joanna told her roommate, "He's a really nice guy, I think, but he was so unnatural; almost as though he was trying to be someone else. It's really too bad because he has so much going for himself, if he'd just relax."

Paul told his roommate, "I was so damn uptight trying to impress her that I really blew it."

He never called her again, although he wanted to.

Regular dating between two people used to be called "going steady," and people who were going steady usually got married. The relationship between the two might best be described by reviewing Broderick's double-funnel theory of courtship.

The double-funnel idea holds that in our culture marriage can be seen as the final step in a funnel of *commitments*. We begin with a very casual commitment to have a coffee together and end with a commitment to spend a lifetime together. The other funnel is that of *intimacy*. It covers a range of behaviors from casual handholding to a full and continuing sexual relationship.

In general, the male is expected to move the relationship through the intimacy funnel, and the female is responsible for guiding developments in the commitment funnel. Reciprocally, the female is generally expected to control the pace of developing intimacy, while the male regulates successive commitments.

Depending on their values and state of readiness, couples may proceed quickly or slowly down either funnel. They could get married without ever moving past necking in the intimacy funnel; conversely, they could develop a full sexual relationship without progressing beyond steady dating in the commitment funnel. True to the funnel analogy, movement down the funnel toward greater intimacy or greater commitment is always easier than movement back up to a previously established level. For example, it is difficult for a couple that has advanced to the intimacy of breast-petting to revert to necking, and maintain this less intimate practice. It would be easier to terminate the relationship.

There are strong pressures to match important advances in one funnel with corresponding movements in the other. For example, if a couple passes from the level of light petting to heavy petting, the female is likely to press for increased assurances that the relationship is important to the male, that he loves her, and that they are committed to each other to some degree. Similarly, a male who has committed himself to a female is likely to believe that he should press for greater intimacy, that it is expected of him.

> Once a serious relationship gets started it takes little or no effort to get more and more involved but it takes an act of will to hold the line and it is often quite painful to extricate oneself altogether. Thus, if this view of North American courtship is at all accurate, we slip and slide into marriage—sometimes joyfully with great peace of mind and mutual satisfaction, and sometimes fearfully with a helpless sense of being caught in a trap we can't escape. But sooner or later almost all of us do in fact reach the bottom of both funnels and so are joined in matrimony.[4]

Unfortunately, progression down the double funnels does not always lead to marriage, as evidenced by the high incidence of nonmarital coitus common among college students and the lack of real commitment in their relationships.

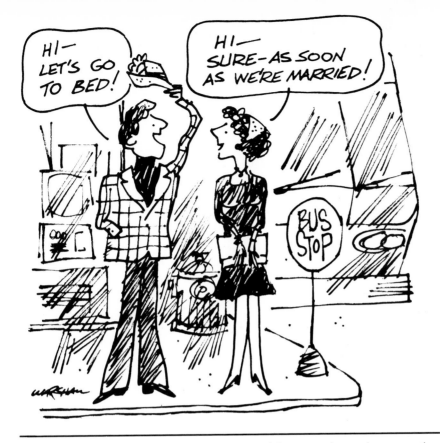

Fig. 10.5. The double funnel

Premarital Sex

Perhaps no single behavior is more prone to misinterpretation and exaggeration than human sexual involvement—premarital, marital, extramarital, nonmarital, and even historical. The most prevalent myth in contemporary North American society is that of sexual revolution—the mass arrival at a sexual freedom that allows males and females of all ages to become more sexually involved with each other, regardless of their marital or family status.

If we go back one hundred years, we can quickly dispel at least part of the myth, and no one can do it more cogently than Ira Reiss.

The recent shift toward less guilt and more sexual freedom among college coeds is clearly indicated in the study by Bell and Chaskes.[5] They compared data on college females for the years 1958 and 1968. The samples were comparable with respect to university attended, age, religion of students, and occupational status of parents. There was some increase in the percentage of girls engaging in premarital coitus while dating (10 percent to 23 percent), but of greater importance was the marked reduction in feelings of guilt at having "gone too far."

A quick review of the Luckey and Nass data[6] on international comparisons reveals North American conservatism in premarital sex behavior. Luckey and Nass compared American college students enrolled in twenty-one United States colleges with students at one university each in Canada, England, Germany, and Norway.

Premarital Sexuality: Past, Present & Future

One of our most prevalent myths is that in past centuries the typical form of courtship was that of two virgins meeting, falling in love, and doing very little with each other sexually. They then married, learned about sex together in the marital bed, and remained faithful to each other until death separated them. I am certain that some couples did have exactly that type of experience and I would go even further and grant that this happens in some cases today. But the key point is that I am sure it was never the common pattern for the majority of Americans. The evidence for this exists in large part in historical records. We know, for example, that in Massachusetts at a well-known church in the last part of the eighteenth century one in every three women who married confessed fornication to her minister. The major reason for making such a confession would be that the woman was pregnant and if she did not make that confession at her marriage, the baby could not be baptized. Many other girls who were nonvirginal but not pregnant would likely not confess fornication to their minister. This was the time of bundling in New England custom. It is probable that much

of the pregnancy occurred after engagement. Engagements in those days were very seldom broken and thus were more akin to actual marriage. In any case it seems clear that at the time of the formal marriage, the sexual innocence of many couples was questionable.

The Double Standard

If we look at male nonvirginity, the picture becomes even more extreme. Certainly the history of the western frontier was not one of male virginity. In fact it was quite the contrary. The western frontier was settled largely by males and this male-dominated society had a heavy reliance on prostitution. The very term "red light district" comes from the custom of girls in prostitution houses leaving a red lantern in the window so that the cowboys riding into town would know "where the action was." "Gunsmoke" notwithstanding, dance hall girls did more than dance. In the typical case the upstairs rooms were where the girls would entice the customers to take them and then collect a suitable fee for the sexual services rendered.

To further show the mythical quality of our view of the past, let us briefly look back at the 1870s and the women's liberation movement of that time. In New York City we find Victoria Claflin and her sister, "Tennessee," setting up a brokerage business as well as other ventures, including a weekly newspaper. Commodore Vanderbilt took to them favorably and helped considerably in getting them established. Victoria was a left-wing feminist who favored free love. She believed that a woman should live with a man if she loved him and leave him when she no longer loved him. She practiced what she preached and had more than one man living with her in New York City. The more conservative feminists like Harriet Beecher Stowe and Catherine Beecher attacked Victoria regularly and Victoria was annoyed by their statements. The brother of the Beecher sisters, the Reverend Henry Ward Beecher, lived in New York and was one of America's most famous ministers. Victoria tried to persuade the Reverend Beecher to prevail on his sisters to be less critical, but to no avail. Finally she learned that while she was having an affair with Mr. Tilton, Mrs. Tilton was having an affair with the Reverend Beecher. She threatened to reveal the adultery in her weekly newspaper if the Beecher girls were not quieted. Either due to inability or lack of effort, the Reverend Beecher did not succeed in quieting his sisters' criticisms of Victoria. True to her word, Victoria publicized the adulterous affair of the Reverend Beecher and Mrs. Tilton in her weekly newspaper on

Tennessee Claflin

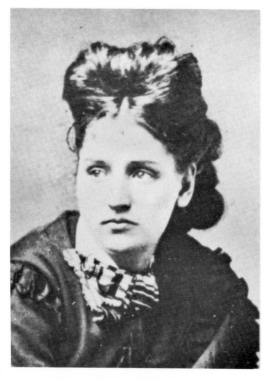

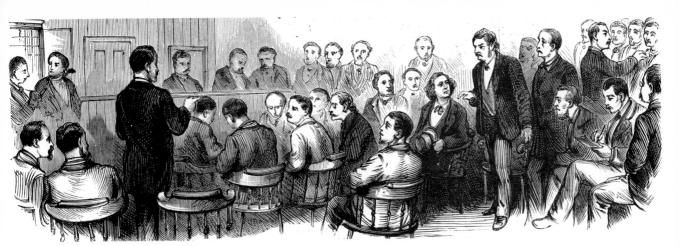

November 2, 1872. Adultery was against the law and a trial ensued. The character of the age was revealed in the outcome of the trial. During the events that followed, the Reverend Beecher was acquitted by a hung jury of the charge of adultery and Mrs. Tilton was charged by a church committee of "indefensible conduct" with the Reverend Beecher. The Victorian era of 100 years ago was surely not an era of the single

Elizabeth Tilton

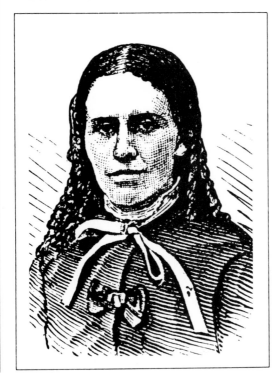

Fig. 10.6. Theodore Tilton is arraigned on a charge of libel.

standard of abstinence. The Beecher-Tilton scandal displayed the nineteenth century's orthodox double standard with its granting of greater sexual privileges to males. Once again the data fail to support the virginal view of our historical past.

One final example that illustrates the sexual orientation of the nineteenth century is afforded by the Philadelphia World's Fair of 1876. The aspect of that fair that echoed around the country was the introduction of the first vulcanized rubber condom for males. This condom was on display at the Fair and created a great deal of interest. Previous to that time condoms were made out of animal skins and a vulcanized rubber condom was a notable advance. But in a culture that was largely practicing abstinence, this contraceptive advance would hardly have received so much notice. However, in a society where prostitution was rampant and where people were concerned with avoiding venereal disease and unwanted pregnancy, such an advance was important. It was about this same time that the diaphragm and the pessary cap were invented. A few decades later, by the time of World War I, knowledge of these contraceptive techniques had spread widely among the wealthier and better educated classes and did create an impact of major importance on their sexual behavior. I will speak of this impact very shortly.

Not only is it mistaken to think of earlier generations of Americans as people who mostly entered marriage virginally, but this view would be erroneous for virtually any society. I have examined the historical and cross-cultural record rather closely and have found no society, at any time in history, in which the majority of even one generation of its males remained virginal on reaching physical maturity—say age twenty or so. This is not an argument against a single standard of abstinence, it is rather a statement of the fact that no society has been able to achieve abstinence for both sexes unless they sanctioned either child marriage or very youthful matings. It is not difficult to understand why no society has been able to produce a generation of virginal males. The reason is very likely that since males are in power in almost all societies, it is unlikely that they would structure that societal system so as to deny themselves access to sexual pleasures before marriage. The major change in premarital sexuality throughout history has been in the partners of men. Such partners have at times come from groups such as slaves, prostitutes, lower-class females, or the girl next door. The basic shift in the partners of men in the twentieth century is toward a majority of the women and away from small select groups. In earlier centuries cultures utilized other categories of females and smaller groups of females as the sex partners for males. There have been historical periods wherein women have been temporarily liberated sexually—for example, the Elizabethan period. But the situation in twentieth-century America is different in some key respects. First, in past times the sexual liberalization was of a small group, the ruling class or the aristocracy. Such a change then affected only a small proportion of the total female population; and such changes were not as long lived as the current sexual liberalization of women in America. Also the sexual liberalization was often in extramarital sex and not in premarital sex.

General Trends

According to our best information the majority of American women have been entering marriage nonvirginal for over fifty years. Kinsey's findings indicated that about half the women born in the 1900–1910 decade were nonvirginal at marriage. This proportion rose only slightly until the late 1960s but since then it seems to have risen rapidly. Sometime around the first world war the proportion of nonvirginal women doubled from about 25 to 50 percent and during the late 1960s the proportion probably has risen from about 50 percent to 70 or 75 percent. In the fifty years from World War I to the late 1960s, the predominant change was not in the proportion of women nonvirginal but rather the attitudes of women and men toward premarital sexuality. During that half century, guilt feelings were reduced, the public discussion of sex increased radically, probably the number of partners increased, and the closeness to marriage required for coitus to be acceptable decreased. For males, other changes were occurring. Males were becoming more discriminate; they were beginning to feel that sex with someone they felt affection for, person-centered sex, was much to be preferred to body-centered coitus. The male partners were shifting from the prostitute and the lower-class female to the girl next door. One of the most dramatic decreases that has constantly evidenced itself during the twentieth century is the rapid decline in the proportion of males, particularly college-educated males, who have experienced intercourse with a prostitute. That proportion today is probably only a small percentage.

The basic change then during the past centuries has been from an orthodox double standard ethic of premarital sexuality, which allowed males to copulate but which condemned their partners as "bad" women, to a more modified version of the double standard in which women are allowed to have premarital coitus but not quite with the abandon of men. Of course, this is an oversimplification and with almost 210 million Americans there are many variations in standards. There are those who are fully equalitarian in a permissive direction and also those who are equalitarian in a restrictive direction, and there still are those who are orthodox double standard. But the overall shift is toward less dominance of the sexual scene by males. This by no means indicates full equality of the sexes but rather a lessening of inequality.

Theodore Tilton

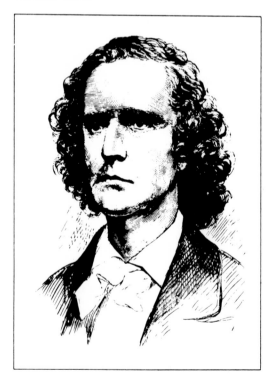

Chapter Ten

Full equality in the sexual sphere is not possible today given the different priorities of family and occupational roles that males and females have. This is a point that present-day Women's Liberation adherents have often made. Regardless of whether one agrees with all the beliefs of Women's Liberation, this particular point seems sociologically well established. If females think that getting married and starting a family is their first priority in life and place occupational ambitions secondary to this, then they will view sex in terms of these goals. This means that they will consider whether copulating with a boy will waste time in their search for a mate; whether this boy will tell others what happened and thus hurt their chances of getting married; whether having intercourse will make a boy more seriously committed to marriage or less; and so forth. These concerns are nowhere near as potent to a male, for he is not so strongly oriented toward marriage as his primary life goal. In the middle class his primary goal will be an occupational career and having premarital intercourse is not very likely to matter one way or the other in terms of that goal. Surely men today are oriented toward marriage but the immediate pressures felt by such a marriage goal are considerably less than those felt by females. A male is not that concerned with the time wasted in an affair, nor is he so worried about the impact of the word getting around that he is having an affair. In fact, in many circles news of such an affair might enhance his image as an exciting date or a romantic interest for females.*

*Adapted from Ira L. Reiss, "Premarital Sexuality: Past, Present & Future," in his book *Readings on the Family System*. Holt, Rinehart & Winston, 1972, pp. 167–189. Reprinted with permission.

The results indicate that North Americans tend to be more conservative in sexual behavior than Europeans and that women of all nationalities are more conservative than men. The percentage of students reporting premarital coital experiences ranged from 35 percent for Canadian females to 63 percent for the English, and from 53 percent for German males to 75 percent for the English.

"Little or no real evidence of change in coital incidence in recent decades" was the opinion of many noted sociologists throughout the 1960s. A number of more recent investigations suggest that such is no longer the case. There are indications of significant changes during the past few years, though the evidence is of questionable validity.

A 1972 national survey by the President's Commission on Population found that 46 percent of all unmarried women in the United States had engaged in sexual intercourse by age nineteen. About 60 percent of the respondents had limited themselves to one partner, however, with half that number expressing intentions to marry the partner in question.[7] The incidence of promiscuous or indiscriminate sexual behavior in American women was found to be quite low.

Recent studies by Packard[8] and *Playboy*[9] have indicated a clear increase in premarital sexual activity, particularly among college women. The sampling techniques in both studies were highly suspect, however, and one might well question the validity of the data. Even at face value, the figures are hardly indicative of any revolution—for males, age twenty-one, the incidence figures ranged from 58 to 82 percent; for females, from 43 to 56 percent. Further, particularly for females, the prerequisite for coitus is "strong affection," preferably with a commitment of at least "love." Promiscuity does not appear to have increased significantly in either sex.

An increase in premarital sexual relations should hardly be unexpected, however, when one realizes that societies opposed to premarital relations are in the minority. In the *Encyclopedia of Sexual Behavior*, Ehrmann[10] reported that

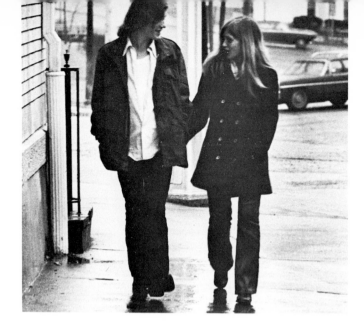

Fig. 10.7. Youth in North America are moving toward a single standard of sexual behavior. Less guilt over premarital sex is evident, and a level of commitment is increasingly demanded by *both* sexes.

70 percent of 158 societies investigated were tolerant of premarital sexual intercourse. (In most instances, however, both parties were to be single; adultery was strongly frowned upon.) Probably the most publicized tolerant society is the Trobriand Islanders, off the coast of New Guinea. Sex is seen by them as a logical extension of personality; it is natural for youngsters to be sexually active. The children take sex for granted, and it is expected that every individual will be involved in a number of affairs prior to marriage. Again, both adult-child and adulterous liaisons are discouraged.[11]

In the vast majority of the societies studied, males are viewed as being more aggressive and more active sexually than females. In cultures where women are encouraged to be free in their sexual expression, they are in fact as open and active as men. "Cultures in which there is approval of women's having orgasms produce women who have orgasms. Cultures withholding such approval produce women who are incapable of orgasm."[12]

The obvious increase in sexual awareness and demand in the American female has placed some strain on American males. For many men, their psychic space has been invaded to the point where they are afraid even to appear experienced, lest they be asked to prove their mettle. Honesty and openness may yet take their place in male heterosexual relationships! Health service units have reported an upsurge in the incidence of male impotence, however. This is not surprising, since male sexual ability is somewhat psychically controlled, at least in terms of arousal. If fear, anxiety, or even excess exuberance is present, the development and maintenance of an erection is threatened. Once again, perhaps it is the male who needs liberating from his own exaggerated ego-expectations. Performance standards have almost universally been forced upon him (usually by other men), with little or no call being made for anything beyond passive involvement on the part of the female. Perhaps "co-sexuality" should be the call of the future.

Chapter Ten

Our American dating system is elaborately designed to provide youth with freedom to select mates on the basis of mutual attraction. We permit great freedom and prolonged privacy, even in the living room of the couple's homes. Parents would never consider spying on their sons or daughters. How could they, when they teach that love is a justification for behavior, and that self-reliance is important in making decisions; when they believe that such values are essential for the development of a healthy sexual attitude on the part of young people? How, in the face of all this freedom, readily accessible contraception, sex manuals, and erotic cinema, do we still have such a high percentage of virgins at first marriage?

> The answer to this question resides in good measure in the basic emphasis by females, and increasingly also by males, on person-centered coitus. Such coitus stresses the value of close ties to another person and thus puts limits on casual coitus and imposes difficulties in locating proper sex partners.[13]

And yet the values are neither clear nor consistent. Still we have the eternal conflict of love and sex, of lasting versus ephemeral encounters, and of purely physical versus total relationships.

W. J. Goode[14] claims that North American youth are placed on a marriage conveyor belt early in life. The system impresses on them the duties and rewards of assuming appropriate sex roles, and it carries them through a series of stages that prepare them for the roles of husbands and wives and possible parenthood. Young children quickly grasp the idea that marriage is the only proper adult state, and that although bachelorhood is tolerated, it is but a single level above spinsterhood at the lower end of the scale of life-styles.

Do We Really Have Free Choice in Whom We Marry?

Table 10.1 Homogamy in Mate Selection, Class A Predictors

Factor	Comments
Race	Probably the strongest single factor, tends to recline on third generation
Religion	Still a strong factor, particularly among orthodox and fundamentalist groups
Class	Males have a much greater freedom—girls rarely marry "down."
Propinquity Residential Occupational	Neighbors marry! Lawyers do marry their secretaries, professors their assistants.
Age	Although age of first marriage is lower for both sexes, girls still marry older boys.
Education	Intelligence may be the same, but the boy usually has a more advanced degree or status.

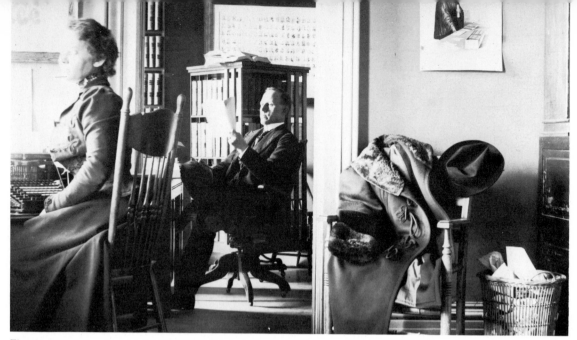

Fig. 10.8. "It's just the nearness of you." Now, as always, neighbors tend to marry neighbors, and bosses tend to marry their secretaries.

Given the concept of free choice in mate selection and belief in the myth that Cupid knows no boundaries in where he may shoot his arrows, one must question why there is such a high level of predictability in who marries whom. In fact, like tends to marry like (homogamy), and the distance they travel to find each other is frequently not very great. The "rule of homogamy" is virtually universal, and deserves our consideration.

The strongest factor in mate selection is race. Interracial marriages are rare, particularly where racial features are apparent, as in black-white or Caucasian-Oriental matchings. Well under 1 percent of all North American marriages involve interracial couples. The larger the multiracial groups that reside within a given country, however, and the farther they are spread out, the more likely they are to be assimilated as a group within their adopted culture, and the more likely they are to marry among themselves. Similarly, the fewer the number of potential "same-race" mates living within a given area, the greater the likelihood of inter-racial marriage. Such is to be expected if the conveyor belt analogy is at all appropriate.

The same holds true for religion: the stronger the conviction and the greater the concentration of adherents to a particular religion within a given area, the lower the incidence of interreligious marriage.

Like marries like in terms of money and education too, as a rule. Some interchange does go on, to be sure, but in most cases a bargaining factor is evident. A wealthy boy may marry a poor girl if she is beautiful, or a wealthy girl might marry a poor boy if he has attained a high level of education. Usually, mate selection is subconscious, and one must recognize instantly that a wealthy white girl is not likely to be attracted to a lower-class white boy under normal conditions, for it is unlikely that they would ever meet in the first place.

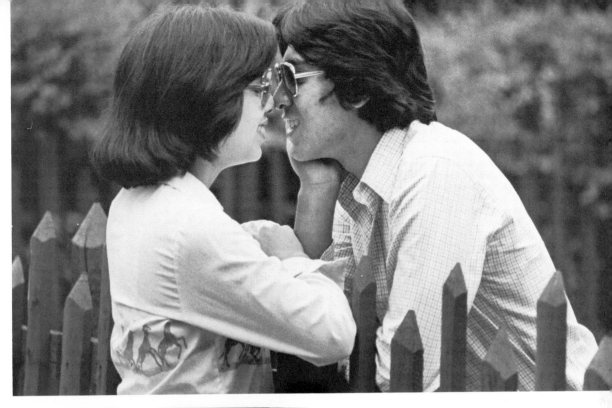

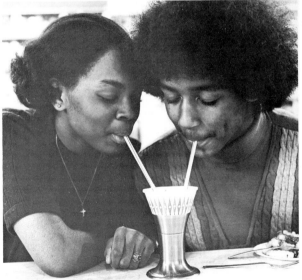

Fig. 10.9. Although interracial marriages have become more common in recent years, the majority of people still tend to marry within their own racial or cultural groups.

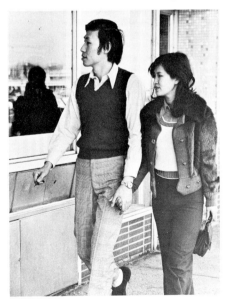

Where differences do exist (hypergamy), the boy generally has the greater advantage. It is far more acceptable for the male than for the female to "marry down" in social, educational, or occupational class. True to our double standard, the male can elevate the female in status through such a marriage. In terms of age, the boy is usually older; in terms of education, he usually has the more advanced degree; and in terms of occupational status, he usually has the higher position, as is the case when the dentist marries his assistant, the lawyer his secretary, or the professor his graduate assistant.

People also tend to marry neighbors, even in today's transient society. Fiances may travel a lot, but when they apply for a marriage license, chances are their respective addresses won't be very far apart.

Such data frequently offend young people in the marriage market, for the facts throw cold water on their romanticism. Freedom of choice really does exist; it is simply limited by cultural bias and a preference for characteristics similar to those of one's own inheritance and upbringing.

Summary

We have examined the courtship institution as it developed in history and as it exists today in North America. The evolution of dating and mating patterns was discussed, and the double standard identified. Most important, we have studied courtship apart from marriage. It now behooves us to look at marriage—and at the various alternatives to it.

Review Questions

1. Why did dating become popular in the early years of North American colonization?
2. What is bundling? How would such a custom be received today?
3. What is the double standard? How are women usually at a disadvantage because of it?
4. Discuss the principle of least interest. Do you think that this is a valid principle? Explain.
5. React to Broderick's double-funnel theory of courtship. Do you agree or disagree with this theory?
6. Why was the introduction of the rubber condom such a remarkable breakthrough in the late nineteenth century?
7. From a sexual standpoint, is full equality between males and females possible today? Why or why not?
8. How has the increase in female sexual awareness affected the male in our society?
9. Does our society accept alternatives to marriage?
10. Do we really have free choice in whom we marry? What factors influence this choice?

1. Ira L. Reiss, *The Family System in America* (New York: Holt, Rinehart & Winston, 1971).

2. Ibid.

3. A. Calhoun, *A Social History of the American Family* (New York: Barnes & Noble, 1945), p. 133. The letters C.F., for Confessed Fornication, were inscribed in the church ledger after the names of these girls. The girls were probably pregnant; if they didn't confess their ''sin'' before giving birth, the baby could never be baptized. The incidence of fornication may well have been higher, since girls who were not pregnant might not have confessed.

4. Carlfred B. Broderick, ''Going Steady: The Beginning of the End,'' in *Teenage Marriage and Divorce,* eds. S. Farber and R. Wilson (San Francisco: Diablo Press, 1967), pp. 21–24.

5. R. Bell and J. Chaskes, ''Premarital Sexual Experience Among Co-Eds, 1958 and 1968,'' *Journal of Marriage and the Family* 32, no. 1 (1970): 81–84.

6. E. Luckey and G. Nass, ''A Comparison of Sexual Attitudes and Behavior in an International Sample,'' *Journal of Marriage and the Family* 31, no. 2 (1969): 364–79.

7. M. Zelnik and J. Kantner, *Survey of Female Adolescent Sexual Behavior Conducted for the Commission on Population* (Washington, D.C.: 1972).

8. V. Packard, *The Sexual Wilderness: The Contemporary Upheaval in Male-Female Relationships* (New York: Pocket Books, 1970).

9. *Playboy,* 1971.

10. W. Ehrmann, ''Premarital Sexual Intercourse,'' in *The Encyclopedia of Sexual Behavior,* vol. 2, eds. A. Ellis and A. Abarbanel (New York: Hawthorne Books, 1961).

11. B. Malinowski, *The Sexual Life of Savages in Midwestern Melanesia,* 2 vols. (New York: Harcourt, Brace & Co., 1929).

12. P. Kronhausen and E. Kronhausen, *The Sexually Responsive Woman* (New York: Ballantine, 1965).

13. I. Reiss, *Readings on the Family System* (New York: Holt, Rinehart & Winston, 1972).

14. W. J. Goode, *World Revolution and Family Patterns* (New York: The Free Press, 1963).

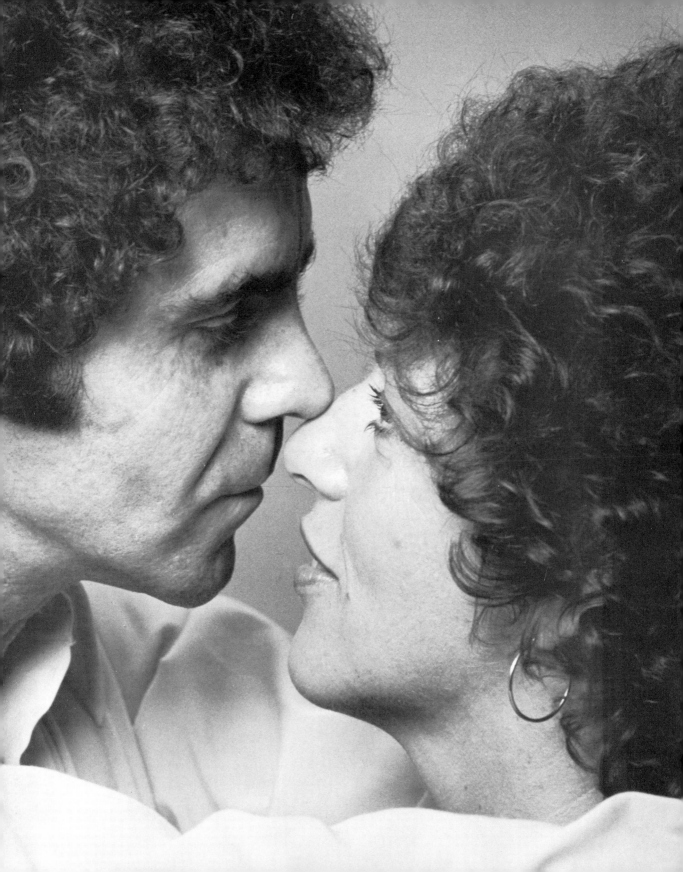

Marriage and Sexual Expression: How Close Is the Fit?

11

The last fifty years have apparently changed the marriage relation from a permanent and lifelong state to a union existing for the pleasure of the parties. The change thus swiftly wrought is so revolutionary, involving the very foundations of human society that we must believe it to be the result not of any temporary conditions. [1]

Note how current the above conclusion is, and yet it was made over eighty years ago in a chapter entitled "The Family Destroyed." The theme of impending disaster for the institution of marriage has been a popular one for a long time! In spite of all predictions, however, the marriage institution continues to survive. In fact, it's thriving in the '70s with less than 4 percent of the population never marrying. Marriage rates throughout North America have increased steadily during the past twenty years.

The divorce rate has also increased rather dramatically in recent years, as has the average length of marriage decreased. More liberal divorce laws and a greater acceptance of divorce in society have undoubtedly contributed to these rates. Remarriage rates are high, however, and divorced people remarry faster than those widowed and more easily than those never married. This holds for practically every age level. The never married person typically has the least likelihood of marrying at almost any age, the widowed a somewhat greater chance, and the divorced person the greatest. [2]

Marriage as an institution fulfills certain needs in society. As the needs change, so does the institution. Marriage advocates today, for example, are seeking a change in the qualitative aspects of marriage. There is a growing interest in restructuring both the mate selection process and the style of married life itself. Alternative marital living styles are discussed in the mass media, and many writers argue that experimentation in sex and marriage is needed to break away from the limitations of monogamy.

Group marriages are more popular in literature than in practice. The trend appears to be more toward group sex than group marriage, but even here there is some question about how popular it really is.

We shall examine many forms of marriage, old and new, including monogamous, contract, group, and common law marriage, as well as communal living, extramarital affairs, and swinging. We shall see that each practice is not so much the development of a new institution as an adaptation of the old—marriage.

In 1976 there were 2,134,248 marriages and 1,077,000 divorces in the United States, a ratio of 2 to 1. Second, even third, marriages are common among Americans.

The universal purposes of marriage as an institution generally include the legitimization, nurturance, and socialization of children, the regulation of sex, and the development of an economic arrangement that makes one member of the partnership primarily responsible for providing revenue while the other provides the household. In virtually all human societies legitimization and nurturance of children are of primary concern, and elaborate customs have been developed to insure both.

Contemporary North Americans' ready access to means of contraception, clear tendency toward later marriage, and childless or smaller families, with subsequent independence and emphasis upon instant pleasure have markedly reduced the importance of legitimization and child nurturance in marriage. At the same time, these factors have greatly increased the recreational role of human sexual activity, both in and out of marriage. Human sexual response has become a topic of primary interest in itself, apart from its purely reproductive value.

Human Sexual Response

Thanks to the active participation of 694 subjects, 312 men and 382 women ranging in age from 18 to 89 years, and the diligent clinical work of Masters and Johnson,[3] we now have a reasonably clear understanding of how humans respond to sexual stimuli. Four phases of response are common to both sexes: (1) excitement, (2) plateau, (3) orgasmic, and (4) resolution.

North Americans use the term "making love" to cover everything from totally indiscriminate intercourse between two people to the most meaningful, responsible, emotion-filled love sharing of a mature couple. "Making love" refers to the biological act; "sharing love" implies far more. When making love, one may well care only for oneself and one's own sexual pleasure. Love sharing, on the other hand, implies giving and receiving love in a mutual endeavor to fulfill both partners' needs, psychological as well as physical, to the greatest possible extent.

Although it is unlikely, particularly among inexperienced partners, that all four phases in the sexual cycle will be experienced in perfect harmony by both parties, still, procreation aside, the purpose of lovemaking is to share pleasure. Both psychologically and biologically this sharing requires a mutual awareness of and consideration for each other. Response varies enormously, even within the same person. The nature and sequence of the sexual phases are quite predictable; the mystery in the encounter is provided by the variety in both intensity and timing of the relationships between the two people. We shall examine these phases in sequence.

Excitement Phase

The pattern of physiological changes in both sexes during the excitement phase is the same; the degree of response varies. As excitement heightens, blood pressure, pulse rate, and breathing rate increase. Voluntary and involuntary muscles contract.

As his level of arousal intensifies, the male's penis begins to stiffen. Engorgement with blood (*vasocongestion*) of the corpus cavernosum, increased sensitivity of nipples, penis, and scrotum, and the buildup of tension in the muscles of the abdomen all add to the male's preparation for orgasm.

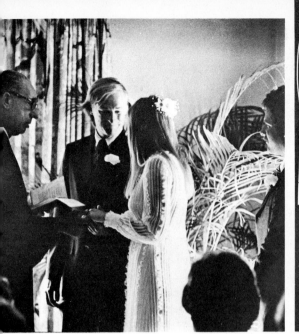

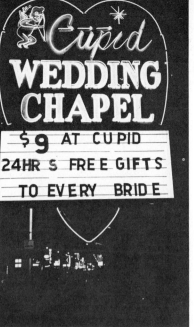

Fig. 11.1. Modern marriages are performed in churches, on shipboard, in airplanes, atop flagpoles, on mountain tops, in airborne balloons—virtually anywhere you can think of.

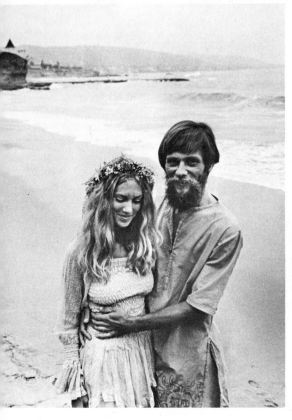

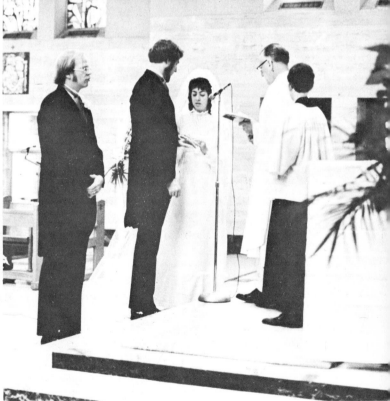

Though generally slower to respond, the female's clitoris hardens during excitement. This small organ, which lies just above the opening from the urinary bladder, is usually hooded by skin called the prepuce. Upon excitation, the clitoris extends out from under this hood. Vaginal fluid may be secreted, while the inner two thirds of the vagina lengthens in preparation for intercourse. During this phase the nipples frequently become erect, particularly when stimulated directly, and a sex flush (a pink rash) may appear around the rib cage and breasts.

Plateau Phase

The buildup of blood in the veins of the genital area continues in the female, and the sex flush may spread to the abdomen during the plateau phase. The labia minora become quite red. The clitoris usually withdraws under the prepuce hood at this stage, a sign that stimulation has been successful. Continued specific stimulation of the clitoris is then no longer advised, the indirect stimulation of coital thrust providing a continuing source of excitement.

Although the conscientious male undoubtedly experiences a plateau phase, it is probably best described by the word "restraint." Engorgement brings about an increase of 50 to 100 percent in the size of the penis. Sex tension continues to build, and it may take a conscious effort on his part to delay orgasm. However, sex researchers agree that a conscious delay of orgasm by the male will help increase the intensity of his orgasm later.

Orgasmic Phase

With the exception of the male's ejaculation of semen, orgasm for male and female is basically the same. Both experience deep contractions of the muscles of the genital area, and pulse rate, blood pressure, and rapid breathing reach a peak in both. Blood engorging the penis and the vagina is forced out of the veins by orgasmic contractions, creating the pleasant sensation of orgasm.

All of the fluids making up the semen ejaculated by the male during orgasm are forced by contraction from the epididymis, the vas deferens, the seminal vesicles, and prostate gland into the urethra. The semen, about a teaspoonful, leaves the penis in spurts, ejected by contractions of the perineal muscle. At this point the male has no voluntary control over the contractions that lead to ejaculation.

Differences in sexual response are greater between individuals than between males and females. The intensity and duration of orgasmic contractions vary within the individual, depending upon a host of biophysiological and psychosocial factors operating at any given time.

Resolution Phase

With the loss of vasocongestion in the female, the sex flush disappears and muscular tension subsides slowly. Detumescence in the male is rapid after orgasm, signaled by the immediate loss of almost 50 percent of erection. The male enters a refractory period, during which he is unable to have another orgasm. He must rest before he responds to further stimulation with another erection. Some young adult males, however, are capable of more frequent arousal.

The female is capable of having another orgasm soon after the first. In fact, she may experience several orgasms in a row. This is not common in the male.

Probably the differences between the sexes in relation to sexual arousal are less than those among members of the same sex. The sex drive in women is basically as powerful as that in men, although they tend to respond to different types of sexual stimulation. Years of inhibition and restraint make it difficult for some women to really "let go," even at the moment of orgasm. And yet the more reckless and uninhibited her response at the peak of sexual excitement (within limits, of course) the more pleased most men are.[4] Conversely, the more open the man is in expressing his pleasure, the happier most women are.

Whether he likes it or not, the burden of directing a couple's sexual activity still falls primarily to the man. Further, he is expected to be confident, even if he is inexperienced. These are among the fixed roles in male-female relationships in our society that we are trying to overcome. "The disparity between expectations on the one hand and experience on the other, together with the faulty sex education that both husband and wife may have received, frequently paves the way for emotional stress that may eventually manifest itself in any of a variety of sexual problems."[5]

Sexually inexperienced young people about to enter marriage should acquire as much accurate information about sexual relations as they can. Although entering marriage with only academic information will probably make the couple's early experiences more mechanical than spontaneous, their confidence at least will be greater than if they had no knowledge; their ability to cope with early failure should be greater as well, since both can share in the responsibility. Confidence on the part of both partners, confidence that things will go well, at least in the long run, will enhance the couple's chances for sexual success in marriage. As open communication about sex is firmly established between the husband and wife, each can help the other toward greater sexual fulfillment.

Mystery is a great asset in lovemaking. Sensuous odors, seminudity, coy gestures, variations in setting and approach, and teasing not only help both partners approach immediate readiness, but also serve as reminders (fantasies) in the future, when personal contact may not be immediately possible. Boredom has no place in the bedroom, or any other place where two people who care about each other are together! Certainly some monotony is inevitable, particularly when spontaneity becomes difficult, but even planned romance can be exciting, if the partners are enthusiastic and willing to make it that way.

Some advice is in order about several popular sexual myths. Although most marriage manuals have stressed direct clitoral stimulation as a means of exciting the female, it may have the opposite effect. Most marriage manuals are written by men, claimed Dr. Lise Fortier of Quebec, when questioned on this point at the Canadian First National Conference on Family Planning in 1972. She denied the supposed benefits of clitoral stimulation, particularly during the plateau phase, when it may, in fact, be both irritating and painful to the woman.

Nor does the size of a man's genitals have much to do with pleasure during sexual intercourse, for either sex. Penile size is of little importance in stimulating the female, since most of the female's pleasure derives from friction in the lower one third of the vagina. Penile size also has nothing to do with the man's ability to impregnate the woman. Similarly, since the vagina is relatively elastic, it is unlikely that any penis will be too large, if the female is given enough stimulation and time to produce adequate lubrication.

Finally, Dr. B. A. Kogan maintains that no distinction is possible between vaginal and clitoral orgasm. "The whole notion of a vaginal orgasm separate from a clitoral orgasm is biologically impossible and, therefore, utterly invalid. And to consider clitoral orgasm immature and vaginal orgasm mature is sense-less."[6]

We have considered human sexual response primarily from a physiological viewpoint, without regard to marital status or social circumstance of the partners. Let us now return to the study of marriage.

Forms of Marriage

Even today, marriage takes many forms throughout the world, ranging from casual to formal, monogamous to polygynous, arranged to free choice, legal to common law, religious to civil, tacit agreement to contractual arrangement; even homosexual marriages are possible. How have so many arrangements come to be? Why have so few survived? What lies ahead?

Let's examine one society that survived for almost fifty years in spite of great external pressure to destroy it—a society in North America that ran completely contrary to the ideals of monogamy.

Complex Marriage

The Perfectionists of the Oneida community (1841-1888) in New York accepted neither monogamy nor polygamy, but developed a system of complex marriage in which every man was married to every woman in the community. The accepted monogamous pattern of one man being married to one woman was looked upon by the Perfectionists as a sign of selfishness. All men should love all women; all women should love all men. Not to do so was to be imperfect.

On the other hand sex was rigidly controlled within the Oneida community. Only selected members were permitted to breed children to insure superior parentage, and all sexual encounters had to be prearranged through an elder in the community. Such a third-party arrangement provided a safeguard against monopolization and also made it possible for one party to refuse the request of another without undue embarrassment. Refusal was quite in order if love did not exist mutually in the hearts of the potential mates at the time of the request. However, all members were encouraged to love all others, and persistent refusal would be noted in the "mutual criticism" sessions.[7]

Since sexual relations were encouraged rather than discouraged in Oneida, some form of contraception was essential. Coitus reservatus, a technique in which the couple engaged in prolonged sexual intercourse, but the male restrained from orgasm, was used. Needless to say some training was essential for young boys, and this was provided by older women who were past the childbearing years. This arrangement had its advantages, as it provided a legitimate sexual outlet for less desirable females.

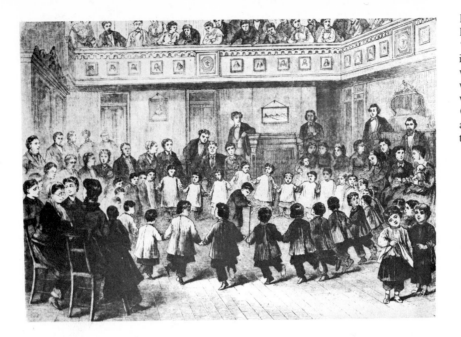

Fig. 11.2. The Oneida
Perfectionists practiced
"complex marriage"
in which every man
was married to every
woman and every
woman to every man.
Children belonged to
and were raised by
the community.

Monogamy is still the practice of choice in American society, and though mate selection patterns run the gamut from arranged, through influenced, to free choice, monogamous marriage itself is, and always has been, universally accepted. Some people like marriage so well they try it again, following the death or divorce of their spouses, or again and again in a practice somewhat euphemistically referred to as serial monogamy.

Although a person may undertake many marriages over a lifetime, legally one may be married to only one spouse at a time. Historically, the family pattern in America has been dominated by the father. He provided the sole financial support for the family and made the major family decisions. The woman did not work outside the home. She was a homemaker, meaning she cared for the feeding and other basic needs of the family members. This family pattern, so prevalent in history, is known as the *patriarchal family.*

Recent years have witnessed a significant change in this traditional family pattern. There has been a movement to an egalitarian marriage relationship. The father's role varies, but he is no longer the all-dominating factor. The mother has become more involved in activities outside the home. Increasingly women with children still at home are working in regular employment. For many, it is a matter of personal fulfillment to have a career. In other instances it is a financial necessity.

Children are cared for in a number of ways. Many are placed in day-care centers or nurseries. Sometimes the father is able to adjust his work schedule to help care for the children.

One of the greatest threats to contemporary monogamy is our almost fanatical emphasis upon individual happiness and instant pleasure. Self-actualization,

Monogamous
Marriage

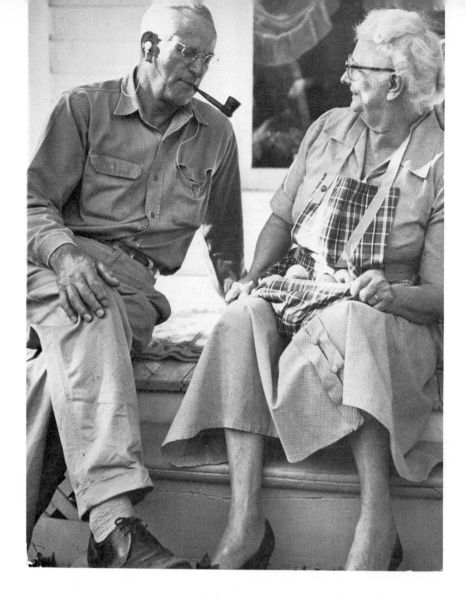

Fig. 11.3. Monogamy is still the practice of choice in American society. While some people change partners repeatedly, many others spend their lifetimes with a single spouse.

self-fulfillment, and self-awareness are some of the terms commonly used to describe the goals sought by each mate. Since the avowed purpose of monogamous marriage is "happiness through love," and since virtually any relationship of this type is not likely to continue to yield the same intense feeling year after year, far more may be expected of monogamous marriage than it can possibly bear. In fact, most marriages probably carry too heavy an emotional dependency burden.

Perhaps no other major nations have given as prominent a position to love as we Americans have. Only North Americans have assumed love to be so essential for marriage.[8] Our subjective appraisal of love tends to be urgent. Love is now. The fact that we may have loved for thirty years, through illness and health, poverty and wealth, is incidental if the question arises, "Am I really in love right now?" How many cannot say, "I could love you more" or "I could have more love if I were elsewhere"? Perhaps we even fantasize where that elsewhere might be, and with whom. Elsewhere is like the grass on the other side of the fence; it's always more appealing, yet only rarely does it meet full expectation when tested over time. Perhaps that is why so many divorced people divorce again, and again, and again. Defined subjectively, love is without limits.

In view of these strains upon monogamous marriage, expanded sexual relationships, extramarital or otherwise, can hardly be unexpected. They serve as safety valves, as logical alternatives for all the tensions of a highly intimate, emotionally overloaded relationship from which far too much is expected.

Some people reduce the risks of marriage through the use of marriage contracts—legal documents clearly defining mutual obligations, such as financial arrangements, child custody, and social responsibilities. These contracts are frequently arranged on a renewable basis and serve as insurance in case of marital breakdown. A number of popular authors have proposed that all marriages start on a trial, contractual basis, and that no children be created during this period. Only after the trial period is over and the real marriage is entered into should conception be considered.

"Do you, Mary, and Anne, and Beverly, and Ruth, take these men...,"[9]   Group Marriage

A relatively small number of North Americans have engaged in group marriages. Although no society in history has ever accepted group marriage as the norm, current trends are toward its increasing acceptance.

Group marriage, as opposed to mate-swapping or swinging, attempts to involve all parties, including the children. Total commitment is sought and on a long-term, if not permanent, basis. Unfortunately little data are available, although some studies are currently underway.

In their nationwide search for functioning multilateral marriages, Larry and Joan Constantine[10] gained the cooperation of ten "families" in the United States. Their estimation of the prevalence of such arrangements in the United States was "possibly fewer than a hundred, and certainly fewer than a thousand." Nevertheless, interest in and speculation about innovations in marriage and family relations is considerable, and since a sample of ten units is hardly sufficient for general conclusions, the following discussion is limited to the sample that was actually studied.

Although the expressed justifications for the group marriages were generally ideological, no consistent picture emerged. In all fairness to the subjects, however, their reasons for joining in a multilateral relationship were almost completely unique to the individuals and to their marriages. Most groups sought constructive interaction and felt a pressure to grow. This pressure to grow is consistent with the nearly universal orientation toward self-actualization and self-realization found among group marriage participants.

Children within the group marriages readily adjusted to the new family structure and apparently benefited from it, although it is still far too early to estimate the long-term effects. The form is so new and so heterogeneous in nature that long-range predictions are impossible. If history continues to repeat itself, group marriages are not likely to endure very long.

Swinging

Clearly an outgrowth of the dramatic changes that have taken place in the status of women, particularly in their sexual status, "swinging," or short-term mate-swapping, has grown in popularity. Kinsey, Masters and Johnson, Ellis, and others have exposed the fact that women experience sexual desire, probably every bit as strongly as men. Further, they have indicated that this desire is most appropriately satisfied through orgasm in sexual intercourse. These changes in attitude, coupled with advanced techniques in contraception, have led to more widespread acceptance of sex for recreation as well as for procreation. The current idea that female sexuality is legitimate and gratifying, the abundance of literature preaching "Any Woman Can," and the multiplicity of opportunities for private encounters provided by current life-styles make it quite predictable that women are now more likely to seek sexual adventures outside of marriage. Equality in sex is only one aspect of the whole egalitarian movement.

Of the various ways for husbands and wives to engage in extramarital sexual encounters, mate-swapping ranks as one of the least threatening to marriage and the most compatible with monogamy. Denfeld and Gordon's review[11] of the swinging club and magazine market cited over fifty nationally sold publications. Rather elaborate sets of rules are applied among swingers. The most common rules are those prohibiting one member of a couple from attending a group meeting without the other, reserving pregnancy for the duly married couple, guarding children from any knowledge of their parents' swinging, protecting their positions in the community through discretion, and making swinging an adjunct to marriage rather than an alternative.

Fig. 11.4. Mate swapping, called "swinging," is a current American sexual phenomenon. Swingers say swapping mates is beneficial to a marriage. Special magazines for swingers extoll the virtues but fail to adequately cover the problems when the mates are not equally committed to swinging as a valid life-style.

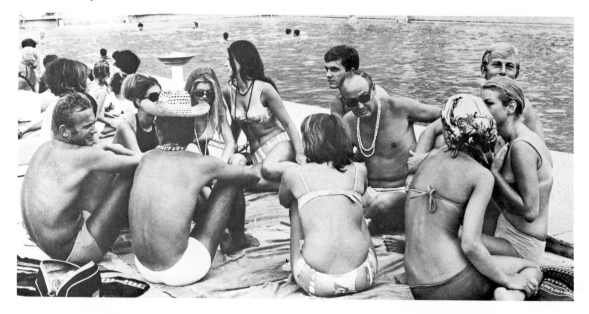

The fact that neither major newspapers nor local lawmakers have said much about swinging leads one to believe it is not much of a social problem. It is not sufficiently popular or dangerous to create much stir beyond local gossip.[12]

Communal living is the inevitable adjunct of the new Counter Culture, the highest affirmation of its basic seriousness and redemptive qualities, the ultimate commitment to it. It is also something far more: It is a search for an alternative to the existing social structure, a search precipitated by young revolutionaries questioning society's basic values.[13]

Communes

In this discussion of communal living, we shall be referring only to those situations in which many people live together for common benefit over extended periods of time, with intentions of integrating with the group and adopting common goals. Excluded, then, are short-term liaisons of both sexes who simply share living quarters and expenses for mutual benefit while living virtually independent lives.

In their anthropological investigations of West Coast communes, Berger and his colleagues[14] distinguished between urban and rural communes, and between what they called "creedal" and "noncreedal" communes. Urban communes, they found, were easy to start but hard to sustain; all that was required was a rented house and a group of willing people. Such communes tend to be fluid in membership and represent little real commitment on the part of participants. Life-style changes may be miniscule for these communards; they may not even alter their old social commitments. Failure of participants to break away from independent life-styles weakens the city commune and tends to shorten its life.

Rural communes, on the other hand, generally involve a commitment to a life-style that is entirely group-oriented and frequently agricultural. Members invest labor, money, and emotion in their group undertaking to establish independence; they may or may not establish rules and an authority structure, depending to some extent on how many members are involved. Certainly group meetings are frequent, and one would expect that group cohesion provides the unifying force.

Creedal communes are usually organized around a doctrine or creed to which members are either required to adhere or eventually expected to adhere. Jesus Freaks or communards devoted to crusading for self-proclaimed messiahs make up creedal groups. They usually have sacred books or central figures to whom they owe allegiance, if not veneration. Initiation rituals are common and recruitment campaigns are vigorous; creedal authority prevails, and members tend to be quite young.

Communards in general prefer open, candid relationships. They want to own as few possessions as possible and consume as little as possible. They strive to live in harmony with nature. Most commune members live for the present, and are given to following impulse more than calculation. They prefer egalitarianism to authoritative hierarchies, and they would rather share than hoard or even experience private feelings.

As in any system, however, freedom breeds its own problems. Tasks must be done, and independence soon depends upon structure—the vegetables must be

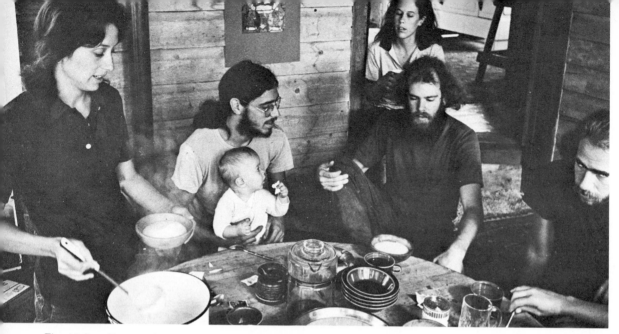

Fig. 11.5. Communal
life in America
takes many forms.

picked on time, the goats milked regularly, the meals cooked for mutual consumption, and the dishes washed for further use. Money must be garnered for rent, mortgage, or equipment; taxes must be paid; buildings must be maintained. As Berger points out, the hip-communal value system "may be regarded as an adaptive response to circumstances rather than a transcendence of them."[15]

Most of the customs of a society relate to childrearing, and women usually assume the major role in this activity, particularly during the early months. Even in communes in which natural childbirth is encouraged and the father assists in the delivery, and in which all children belong to the family but are encouraged to be free, parents face the continual dilemmas of discipline and guidance. Yet, even in childrearing, most communes "if faced with a choice between training the next generation of communards and training children to be free, would opt for the latter."[16]

Communes vary greatly in both nature and function; yet contrary to popular belief, one conservative element is almost universal. Stable communes tend toward sexual monogamy. Berger maintains that the norm against excessive sexual access runs deep and that violation of the norm within a commune, in spite of ideology, may cause deep tensions.[17]

Incest is probably the longest standing, most universally accepted taboo. It is particularly prominent among communards, who see the group as a family and thereby refrain from polygamous sexual involvements, at least within the group, that might be viewed as incestuous. This practice provides an interesting contrast to the tendency in contemporary North American society toward polymorphous sexual perversity, and yet it is entirely consistent with the counterculture ideology. Fascinating, though, is the obvious disdain for marriage as a legal institution among communards and yet their strict adherence to one of the universal purposes of marriage, namely, the control of sexual behavior. Contrast the communards' attitudes, then, with those of our "normal" society, which insists on the legality of a marriage but treats with obvious disdain the other demands of marriage as an institution.

Marriage is a structure designed by man to perform certain functions. An adaptable institution, marriage changes with the demands placed upon it. Yet it survives, and probably always will in all its various forms, both legal and extralegal, contractual and consensual. However, the challenges of the next few decades will probably shake marriage to its very roots, particularly if the function of reproduction is removed from it. Certainly, parenthood will remain optional (the myth that "parenthood is fun" is already dead). Childrearing may become government-controlled, with parents forced to accept special training for their roles. In fact, with advanced reproductive techniques, parents well may provide nurturance and socialization only. Biogeneticists would mechanically produce eugenically sound children, and human parents would raise them.

Marriages will undoubtedly adapt to new social customs. Interreligious and interracial marriages will increase as intercontinental travel increases; serial monogamy will increase as divorces or dissolutions of marriage become easier and faster to obtain; and the law will begin to accept new forms of marriage. With egalitarianism, both sexes will share in the costs of courtship, and courtship will be the testing ground for couples who are prematched by computer sorting techniques. In fact, courtship will probably lead to an institutionalized trial marriage, a contracted relationship lasting a specific period of time, but renewable. Should natural parentage be desired or permitted, a long-term contract would become essential. An increasing number of future marriages, however, are not likely to involve children.

With the emphasis on choice, the double standard for aging males and females will have to be resolved. This may prove simple up to a point: middle-aged women might accept the responsibility of educating young men in the mysteries of sex. If such a practice became fashionable, as it already is in some European countries, women could remain sexually active throughout their middle years, while middle-aged males continued to court younger women. With advancing age, however, it is to be hoped that males and females of like age would grow more compatible and develop contractual arrangements to maintain one-to-one relationships throughout their lives.

Colleague or weekend marriages will probably proliferate as egalitarianism encourages marriage between partners who have equally strong commitments to different vocational pursuits. They may well work, teach, research, and live in separate areas of the country, agreeing to meet on weekends for socializing, companionship, and sex.[18]

Age of first marriage will continue to increase for both sexes, and the pressure to marry will diminish. As nonmarital sexual involvements receive increasing approval, spinsterhood will join bachelorhood as an acceptable life-style. People who worry about such things will be able to assume that both spinsters and bachelors have access to sexual relationships when they want them. With the

Marriage: What Lies Ahead?

increase in so-called human relations clubs and singles' encounter groups, intimate relationships for short or long periods of time will be available for the price of admission.

Homosexuality will probably increase in the short run, as people adjust to the new heterosexual freedoms, but then it will level off or subside somewhat. Homosexual marriages will be legalized, though active proselyting is not likely to be permitted.

Man adapts to changing circumstances, and frequently reacts strongly. One might expect a return to conservative monogamy by the new counter-cultures, with the pursuit of holiness replacing the pursuit of hedonism as a goal. Should this happen, social structure, including organized religion, education, and marriage, will undoubtedly make a comeback. History does tend to repeat itself!

While the media daily inform us of the supposedly important events of our lives—in politics, economics, war—still the private and seemingly humdrum processes of the family continue to dominate much of our attention and concern.

Extramarital Relations

Sexual exclusiveness is the ideal in American monogamous marriages. In practice over one-half of American husbands and one-quarter of their wives become involved in extramarital relations at one time or another, depending to a large extent on how unhappy they are at the time in their own marriages. Unless separation or divorce proceedings are already active, such adulterous encounters are generally infrequent and clandestine. If the encounter does not threaten an existing marriage, people tend to ignore it, recognizing its immorality but realizing its relative safety, provided it is kept quiet.

Extramarital sex has long been a common practice, though rarely a formally acceptable one. Strict taboos against adultery are held in over 80 percent of the 148 societies analyzed by Murdoch;[19] it was only allowed freely in about 1 percent. In North America today adultery is prohibited and considered far more serious than fornication or premarital coitus, although the practice persists.

North American society protects the institution of marriage by invoking negative sanctions in almost direct proportion to the seriousness of the threat posed by a given practice. Fornication between consenting partners who practice contraception is of little threat to the family; if one of the partners is married, the threat is greater. The marriage is increasingly threatened when both partners are married, one or both partners have children, contraception is not practiced, the partners meet frequently, the partners spend weekends together or vacation together, and so forth. Little is said about an occasional extramarital encounter, particularly if discretion prevails; much is said about an open breach in a marriage that involves children.

Summary

We have examined marriage in this chapter, as well as some alternatives to it. In the next chapter we shall move on to the family, assuming that the next step after marriage on the ladder of sexual involvement and commitment is reproduction.

1. How has the function of marriage changed in the last century?

2. Describe each of Masters and Johnson's four phases of the sexual cycle.

3. Do you think monogamy will last into the twenty-first century? What other forms of marriage might become more commonplace?

4. With today's emphasis on instant pleasure and gratification, are we expecting monogamous marriage to offer us more than it can produce?

5. How important is fidelity in marriage today?

6. What possible reasons are there for entering into a group marriage?

7. Why is the practice of swinging considered one of the least threatening to the marital institution?

8. Distinguish between the various types of communal living.

9. Discuss some of the apparent problems of living in a commune.

10. Do you think a breakthrough in genetic manipulation (cloning, test-tube children) will affect marriage as an institution?

Notes

1. C. Thwing and C. Thwing, *The Family: An Historical and Social Study* (Boston: Lee & Shepherd, 1887). p. 36.

2. I. Reiss, *The Family System in America* (New York: Holt, Rinehart & Winston, Inc., 1971), pp. 280–308.

3. W. Masters and V. Johnson, *Human Sexual Response* (Boston: Little, Brown & Co., 1966).

4. K. Mozes, "The Technique of Wooing," *Sexology,* 1959, pp. 756–60.

5. J. McCary, *Human Sexuality,* 2d ed. (New York: D. Van Nostrand Co., 1973), p. 147.

6. Benjamin A. Kogan, *Human Sexual Expression* (New York: Harcourt Brace Jovanovich, 1973), p. 105.

7. W. Kephart, *The Family, Society, and the Individual,* 2d ed. (Boston: Houghton Mifflin Co., 1966), pp. 170–72.

8. W. J. Goode, *World Revolution and Family Patterns* (New York: The Free Press, 1963), p. 8.

9. Robert Rimmer, "Do you, Mary, and Anne, and Beverly, and Ruth, take these men . . .," a conversation with Robert Rimmer, in *Psychology Today,* January 1972, pp. 57–82.

10. Lawrence Constantine and Joan Constantine, "The Group Marriage" in *The Nuclear Family in Crisis: The Search for an Alternative,* ed. M. Gordon (New York: Harper & Row, 1972), pp. 204–22.

11. D. Denfeld and M. Gordon, "Mate Swapping: The Family That Swings Together Clings Together," in *Family in Transition,* eds. A. Skolnick and J. Skolnick (Boston: Little, Brown & Co., 1971), pp. 463–75.

12. For additional information see D. Denfeld and M. Gordon, "The Sociology of Mate Swapping," *Journal of Sex Research* 6, no. 2 (May 1971): 85–100.

13. G. Fonzi, "The New Arrangement," in *The Nuclear Family in Crisis: The Search for an Alternative,* ed. M. Gordon (New York: Harper & Row, 1972), p. 180.

14. B. Berger, B. Hackett, and R. Millar, "The Communal Family," in *The N.C.F.R. Non-Traditional Family Forms in the 1970s* (Minneapolis: NCFR Press, 1972), pp. 51–60.

15. Ibid., p. 53.

16. Ibid., p. 54.

17. Ibid.

18. H. Coulton, *Sex After the Sexual Revolution* (New York: Association Press, 1972).

19. G. P. Murdoch, *Social Structure* (New York: Macmillan Co., 1949), pp. 24–25.

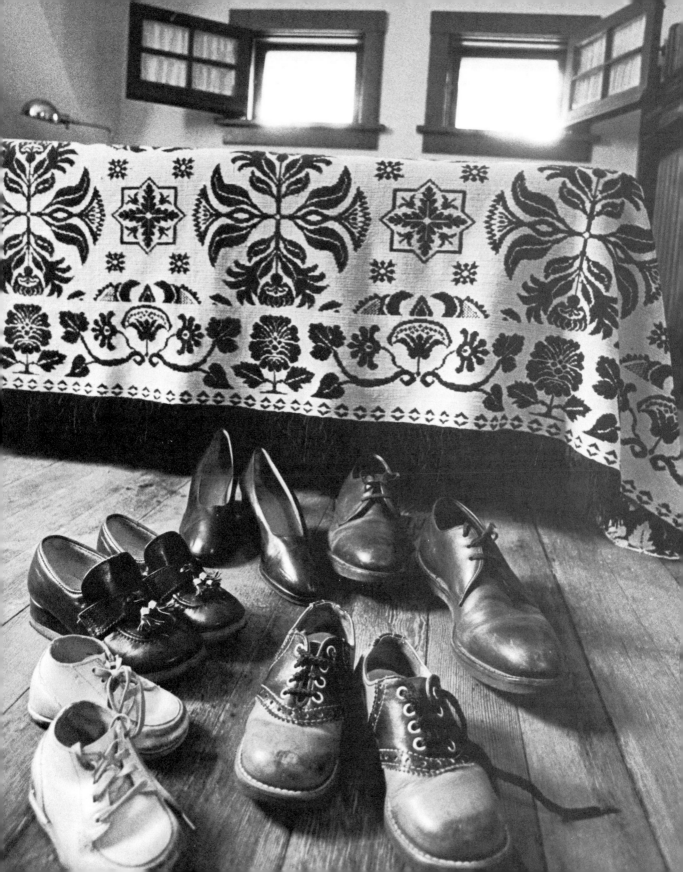

The Family: If, As, and When

12

Ah Woe, Ah Me

1. *In Trinidad, there lived a family*
   With much confusion as you will see
   There was a mama and a papa
   And a son who was young
   Who wanted to marry—have a wife of his own
   Chorus: Ah woe, ah me, shame and scandal on the family (Repeat)
2. *He found a young girl who suited him nice*
   He went to his papa to ask his advice
   His papa said "Son, I got to say no,
   The girl is your sister but your mama don't know"
   Ah woe, ah me, shame and scandal on the family (Repeat)
3. *The weeks went by and the boy looked around*
   Soon the best cook on the island he found
   He went to his papa to name the day
   His papa looked at him and to him he did say
   "You can't-a-marry that girl, I got to say No,
   The girl is your sister but your mama don't know"
   Ah woe, ah me, shame and scandal on the family (Repeat)
4. *The years went by and he wished he was dead*
   He had seventeen girls and still wasn't wed
   When he went to his papa, papa'd always say "No,
   These girls are your sisters but your mama don't know"
   Ah woe, ah me, shame and scandal on the family (Repeat)
5. *So he went to his mama and he bowed his head*
   And he told his mama what his papa had said
   His mama said "Son, Go man Go,
   Your papa ain't your papa, but your papa don't know."
   Trinidadian ballad of unknown origin

The family, too, has a need to adapt. Its purposes, roles, and functions all change over time as demands shift with societal pressures. The extended farm family gives way to the more mobile nuclear unit so essential for the city. Education moves from home to school, religion to church, transportation to mechanization, homemaking to technology, work to leisure. Family planning is now reality, and the quality of children is of greater concern than the number produced. Science has invaded the home and demanded new adaptations. We are challenged, and we respond. But the critical question is how we respond.

309

newly married pair
expectant parents
parenthood—first child
the crowded years
the early school years
the adolescent school years
the launching years
the home without children
the aging years

Fertility and Infertility

Most couples purposely trying to conceive a child are successful relatively quickly. About 30 percent will succeed in the first month, about 60 percent in the first six months, and about 75 percent within one full year. About 30 percent of all married couples, however, experience some difficulty. In some instances, conception occurs, but miscarriage always follows. Approximately one couple in ten is never able to have children and is said to be sterile. Reasons for sterility are many and complex. In about 30 percent of the cases the problem lies entirely in the male. In other cases, the fault is with the female or with both partners.

A low sperm count, less than 200 million per ejaculate, or even the absence of active sperm are problems occasionally found in men who otherwise may be perfectly healthy and enjoy active sex lives. When the sperm count is simply too low, sperm from many ejaculates can sometimes be collected, pooled, frozen, and stored for a few months. The semen is then thawed and concentrated by centrifugation. By means of artificial insemination the semen can be given to the wife at her anticipated time of ovulation. The optimal waiting period between ejaculations to achieve maximum sperm count appears to be about 48 hours.

There are many reasons for female sterility, such as congenital anatomical defects: imperfectly developed fallopian tubes, an inverted uterus, a missing organ (possibly even the vagina), or blocked fallopian tubes. Women sometimes produce antibodies, making them immune to sperm and incapable of conception.[1] The age of a woman is also a significant factor; her natural fertility steadily decreases after her early twenties.

Female infertility frequently can be treated. Where kinked or blocked fallopian tubes are suspected, a Rubin's test is used in diagnosis. Gas is forced through the tubes to measure the clearance, and an obstructed tube can often be reopened.

Vaginal acidity is sometimes high enough to kill the sperm. In such situations, a precoital douche with an alkaline solution may help. Sperm viability following intromission into the vagina can be tested by examining mucus scraped from the cervix several hours after intercourse (Huhner's test). The vitality and number of sperm can be determined as a guide in estimating the chance that they will penetrate into the uterus and ultimately travel up the fallopian tubes.

Since various psychological and physiological responses can influence the quality of chemical secretions, the linings of the vagina and the uterus should also be tested. Many of the complications detected are treatable.

In recent years there has been a persistent and dramatic, though gradual, reduction in size of the family. An increasing tendency toward higher education for women and a decline in early marriages jointly delay the date of first conception and eventually the number of children born. As more and more women develop careers, fewer and fewer of them wish to raise large families. In fact many couples may wish to have no children at all. Today that choice is available.

It takes a viable sperm, a healthy ovum, and a suitable environment for conception to take place. Any serious deficiency in one or more of these requirements effectively prevents it. When the deficiency is intentionally created, it works against conception and is therefore termed *contraception.* Unlike *birth control,* which includes contraceptive techniques as well as practices such as abortion, contraception refers only to control over conception or prevention of the creation of a viable zygote.

There are techniques currently available that, when used properly, can reduce the probability of pregnancy to zero. Although some techniques depend directly upon the individual situation, still the range for selection is sufficient to cater to almost any needs. We shall examine the more common methods of contraception, from the least promising nonmethod of chance to the most effective method short of abstinence, namely sterilization.

The theoretical effectiveness of any contraceptive is clearly different from its effectiveness in actual use. Theoretically, for example, the condom makes an effective contraceptive. In fact, however, it has proven to be unreliable. The average failure rates for each of the methods discussed here are based upon data from women of all classes who are within the reproductive age range, have normal fertility, and experience an annual frequency of at least 100 acts of sexual intercourse.

The figures employed (for example, 50 percent) refer to the number of pregnancies during a year, not to the number of women who became pregnant. Fifty women out of 100 do not have to get pregnant for there to be 50 pregnancies in a year, since several women could have more than one pregnancy in a twelvemonth period. For the determination of any percentage concerning failure rates, a pregnancy is counted as soon as it can be diagnosed and remains recorded regardless of outcome, whether or not a live birth results. For purposes of comparison, if no contraceptive technique is employed and the normal conditions for potential pregnancy are met, the expected pregnancy rate for the year is 80 percent.

To gain widespread acceptance, any form of contraception must be safe, effective, reversible, and relatively easy to use. No contraceptive will be popular that causes anxiety for the user, either because of its nature, as in self-administered injections, or its side effects, as in testicular shrinkage. When it comes to sex, the human ego is fragile—any threat to body image or function is studiously avoided by most people, either consciously or subconsciously.

The often-used riddle, "What happens to women who rely on rhythm? They become mothers!" raises the question of whether the rhythm method is in fact any better than chance alone. The rhythm method involves avoidance of sexual

Conception
Control

Contraceptive
Methods

Rhythm

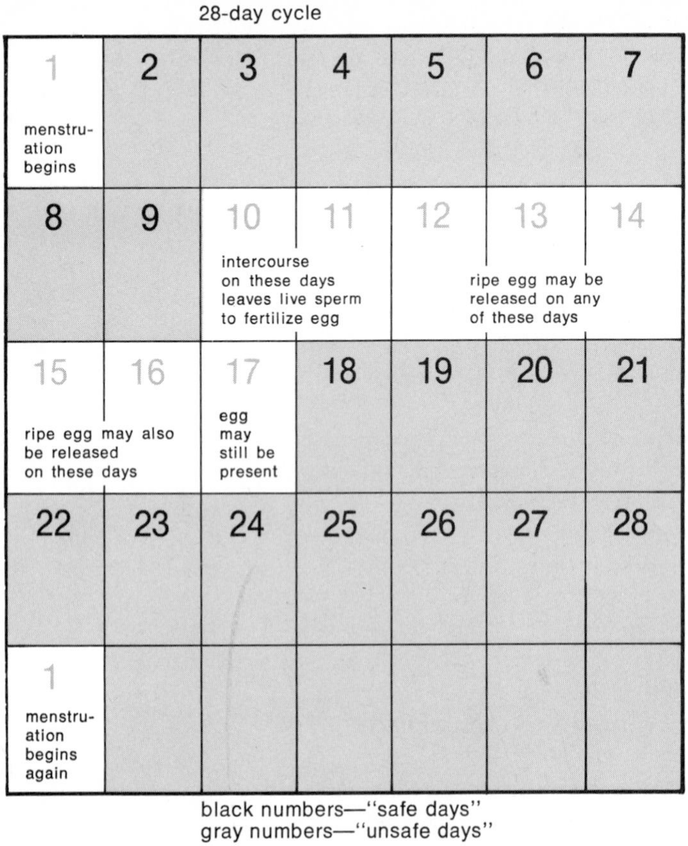

28-day cycle

1 menstru-ation begins	2	3	4	5	6	7
8	9	10 intercourse on these days leaves live sperm to fertilize egg	11	12 ripe egg may be released on any of these days	13	14
15 ripe egg may also be released on these days	16	17 egg may still be present	18	19	20	21
22	23	24	25	26	27	28
1 menstru-ation begins again						

black numbers—"safe days"
gray numbers—"unsafe days"

Table 12.1 The Contraceptive Continuum

Technique	Expected Number Pregnancies Among 1,000 Users During Any One Year
Pill { combination sequential mini	0–10 10–20 30–40
IUD	30
Condom	180
Diaphragm	210
Rhythm	270
Chemicals, foams, jellies	300
No protection	800

Fig. 12.2. The 28-day-cycle rhythm method of birth control, showing safe days and unsafe days.

intercourse during that part of the menstrual cycle during which the female is fertile. Its effectiveness is based upon the determination of ovulation date, the knowledge that neither sperm nor ova are viable for much more than forty-eight hours, and abstention from sexual intercourse during the prime fertility period. Since ovulation occurs fourteen days before the first day of bleeding, this fact can help predict the ovulation date for women whose menstruation cycles are regular. Thus a 25-day cycle means ovulation on day 11, a 29-day cycle means ovulation on day 15, and so on. Unfortunately, not all women have regular cycles. In fact, few single or childless women do.

Progesterone, secreted from the corpus luteum, causes an increase in basal metabolism and a rise in body temperature at the time of ovulation. A record of basal body temperature (BBT) can be used to identify periods of fertility. BBT should be taken early in the morning after a sleep of six hours or more. A specially designed rhythm (or ovulation, or basal) thermometer is used, which records from 96°–100° F and is calibrated in units of 0.1° for ease of reading. The log that is produced from the recordings should look something like the one shown in figure 12.2.

Unfortunately, illness, stress, or unusual bodily reactions may create temperature changes that could be mistaken for the anticipated ovulatory indicators.

Also, should a woman fail to ovulate in a given cycle, no rise will occur. A great deal of experience and a history of recordings are essential for the effective use of the rhythm method, yet it can be effective. The World Health Organization reported in 1968 that pregnancy rates averaged only 1.1 percent per year for women using BBT under supervision, a rate comparable to that of a highly effective intrauterine device.

A saliva-litmus test is currently on trial as a potential detector of chemical changes that occur in the woman's saliva just before ovulation. A piece of pretreated paper is sucked each day. Only when ovulation is imminent, does it turn blue. The developers of this product claim it provides at least a forty-eight hour warning. The test is still under investigation. The rhythm method is most effective when the woman's menstrual cycle is regular and when abstinence is possible. It is quite ineffective otherwise.

Perhaps the first contraceptive technique ever employed by man, and still popular among adolescents, is *coitus interruptus,* which requires that the man withdraw his penis from the woman's vagina prior to ejaculation. Any success experienced through using this method depends on a thorough understanding of the process of ejaculation and no small amount of good fortune. All semen must be kept well away from the vulva, and even then there may be a problem. A clear, lubricant fluid is often secreted during excitement, usually prior to and often quite separate from ejaculation, and this may contain spermatozoa. Although the number of sperm present in this fluid is usually inadequate for fertilization, still some chance of pregnancy exists.

Coitus Interruptus (Withdrawal)

Commonly used by young single couples who deplore the unnaturalness of condoms or have unpremeditated intercourse in the heat of passion, this technique is generally ineffective. Used by highly experienced couples, it can prove satisfactory, although the reported use is not high.

The logical extension of coitus interruptus, namely *coitus reservatus,* is not a common technique. Popular in the nineteenth century Oneida community, the technique involves male restraint from orgasm throughout prolonged intercourse. The female may or may not achieve orgasm, which of course doesn't matter in terms of conception, but the male must not have orgasm. The couple may continue intercourse for long periods of time if the male avoids climax. Few males can or wish to exercise such restraint.

Several chemicals are currently available that, although harmless to normal body tissue, are capable of paralyzing, if not destroying, the spermatozoa. These chemicals are used in compounds that serve three functions: (1) act as carriers for the active ingredient, the spermicide; (2) spread completely over all vaginal and cervical surfaces; and (3) create a mechanical barrier beyond which sperm cannot swim. These compounds include creams, jellies, aerosol foams, foaming tablets, foam-producing powders, liquids, and suppositories.

Chemicals

Most spermicides are inserted into the vagina with an applicator several minutes (up to fifteen) before coitus. This gives the agent time to spread sufficiently for maximum effectiveness. These compounds should be inserted immediately

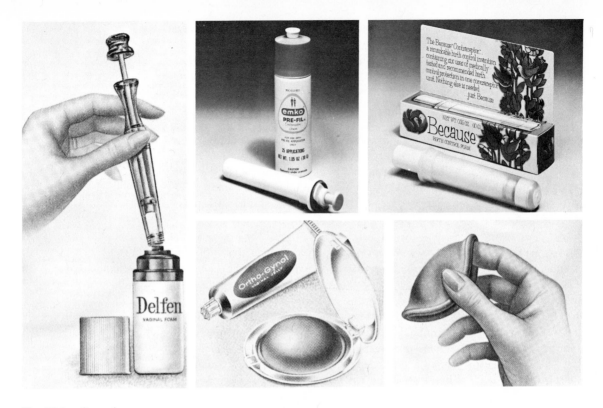

Fig. 12.3. Several kinds of contraceptive foams with applicators are shown. Also shown are a diaphragm in container, vaginal jelly for lubrication, and indication of how to insert the diaphragm.

prior to sexual intercourse. Application of the compounds too far in advance causes them to liquefy due to body temperature, thus negating their effectiveness.

Although chemicals can be valuable even when used alone, their effectiveness is increased markedly when combined with other contraceptives, particularly a mechanical agent, such as the diaphragm or condom.

Use of vaginal chemical methods cannot be separated entirely from the sex act, since timing is critical. Spermicides must be used just prior to coitus, and application tends to interfere with spontaneity. On the other hand, most chemical contraceptives can be purchased without prescription in drugstores and family planning clinics. In clinics the materials are often distributed without charge.

Mechanical devices to block the sperm's progress through the vagina have long been used. A dome-shaped cap, the diaphragm, is designed to cover the cervix, which is the entrance to the uterus. Variation in the size and shape of female internal genitalia necessitates careful fitting and requires the services of a physician.

Diaphragm effectiveness depends upon a number of factors, including proper fitting, auxiliary use of a spermicide jelly or cream, proper insertion, and retention of the device over the cervix for at least six hours after the last ejaculation. Although a diaphragm is usually inserted manually, an inserter may be used.

A variation of the diaphragm, the cervical cap, is thicker, smaller, and less flexible. Popular in Europe, the cap requires less manipulation, is not so dependent on spermicide for effectiveness, and may be left in place for longer periods of time (up to a month for the new plastic one) than may the diaphragm. More difficult to insert, the cervical cap requires physician time both for fitting and instruction.

Usually made of synthetic rubber, the condom was originally developed in the sixteenth century by an Italian anatomist who suggested using a moistened linen sheath over the penis for protection against venereal disease during intercourse. It also served as an effective contraceptive. Two hundred years later parts of the intestines of sheep and cattle were used. Animal membrane condoms are still available today, although they cost about twice the price of rubberized condoms.

By the late nineteenth century vulcanized rubber had been employed in condom manufacture; rubber and other synthetics are still popular in condoms today. Legally, condoms are sold as prophylactics, for protection against venereal disease. They are readily available to anyone without prescription. In fact, they are commonly available in washroom dispensers. Although they were replaced by the pill as leader on the contraceptive popularity list, the accessibility of the condom and its low cost keep it in demand, particularly among single people.

The interruption of foreplay while the condom is put on and the elimination of direct penis-vagina contact, with subsequent reduction of tactile sensation, cause many couples to bypass the condom and risk pregnancy. Furthermore, the condom is often improperly used. Effectiveness is lost when the male starts coitus without it, waits too long before putting it on, leaves it off ''just once,'' continues coital thrust after ejaculation, which may force sperm back out the open end, fails to leave a pocket at the end, or fails to remove it properly. Sound instruction should be sought prior to using the condom. Used as directed, it is an effective contraceptive.

All contraceptive methods discussed so far are designed to prevent the sperm from ever reaching the ovum. Intrauterine devices employ a different principle. They prevent implantation of the fertilized ovum. It is not known exactly why a fertilized egg will not become implanted in the uterine wall. There are two rather commonly suggested reasons. One is that in the presence of an IUD the egg moves too rapidly along the fallopian tube and is not mature enough to become implanted. Others feel that the IUD simply prevents the fertilized egg from implanting in the wall.

Made from soft, cylindrically shaped plastic or nickel-chromium alloy, IUDs are made in various shapes and sizes. Many of the plastic devices can be inserted in a forced straight line, yet return to their original coil form upon release in the uterus.

Two basic types of IUDs are popular: the closed devices, such as the Birnberg bow and the Hall-Stone ring, and open devices, such as the Lippes loop, Margulies coil, the Dalkon Shield, and the Copper Seven. The Shield and Seven grew in popularity among younger girls, probably because of few side effects,

Condom

IUD—Intrauterine Device

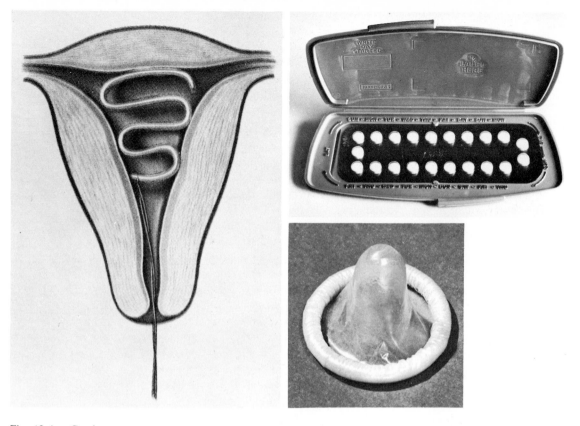

Fig. 12.4. Condom, intrauterine device, and pills. Regardless of which is used, fertility is usually restored with cessation of use of the device.

ease of insertion in childless women, low incidence of removal for medical reasons, potential long-term use, and high success rate. That was at first. Now the Dalkon Shield is under heavy suspicion as the cause of numerous and persistent problems and has fallen quickly from public favor.

The major side effects that limit the use of the IUD are involuntary expulsion, particularly among women who have had several children; perforation of the uterus; persistent bleeding or cramps; increased menstrual flow, especially during the first four months of use; loss of the retrieval string on the device inside the uterus; and low back pain. Most of these effects are short-term and far more prevalent in women who have never been pregnant.

Regardless of length of use, when the IUD is removed, fertility is usually restored. Rates of conception in women who have used the device and later had it extracted are within normal limits.

Pill

A brief review of the menstrual cycle will remind the reader that it is the FSH released by the pituitary gland that causes an ovarian follicle to mature. As the follicle matures, it secretes increasing amounts of estrogen; as the estrogen level increases, it suppresses further secretion of FSH. Ovulation then occurs, and progesterone levels increase. As the unfertilized egg disintegrates and as the corpus luteum cuts back its output, both the progesterone and estrogen levels diminish, and the pituitary gland responds with more FSH. The key to FSH production, then, appears to be the levels of estrogen and progesterone in the blood.

Oral contraceptives contain synthetic forms of estrogen and progesterone. Two major types are available: the combined pill (estrogen and progesterone taken together) and the sequential pill (estrogen followed by progesterone). Although the latter follows the natural body sequence more closely, the pregnancy rate is higher for the sequential pill than for the combination pill, although unwanted pregnancies are extremely low for both types. Sequential pills have lost popularity and are no longer being produced by many companies. The combination pill contains both estrogen and progesterone, with progesterone the major ingredient.

The major problem of administering the pill is that it must be taken daily for three weeks and then omitted for seven days while the female menstruates. Should the user forget to take the pill on two or more days, the contraceptive effect may be lost for the entire month.

Attempts have been made to simplify pill-taking by using either a placebo or an iron pill on the other seven days of the cycle. The user would then take a pill every day. More recently, a new mini pill has come into favor and is taken every day regardless of menstruation. It contains a low dose of progesterone only and is proving both popular and effective.

Medical concern about possible side effects of the pill has led doctors into a thorough study of thromboembolisms, cerebrovascular diseases, coronary-artery diseases, cancer, carbohydrate metabolism, hypertension, liver function, thyroid and adrenal function, headaches, emotional states, skin disorders, and subsequent reproductive function. The most significant findings are as follows:

1. Oral contraception use incurs an increased risk of thromboembolism. This risk is small and probably comparable to the risk of death in pregnancy occurring as a result of contraceptive failure with other methods.
2. Occlusion of cerebral or coronary arteries in the reproductive age group is rare, and a causal relationship to oral contraceptives has not been established.
3. There is not valid evidence that the oral contraceptives are carcinogenic. Conversely there is suggestive evidence that these agents exert a protective influence in regard to carcinoma of the endometrium and possibly breast.
4. Oral contraceptives lower glucose tolerance in initial months of use. These changes are only clinically significant in patients with latent diabetes; hence women with a family or clinical history predisposing to diabetes should have at least a postprandial blood sugar determination before using this method of contraception.
5. Hypertension may be produced by oral contraception in an occasional susceptible individual, but these changes are usually reversible. All patients employing these agents should have regular blood pressure determinations with discontinuance if significant hypertension is found.
6. No significant change in liver function has been found in women without an inherited or acquired defect in hepatic excretory function.
7. Ophthalmological abnormalities are no more frequent in users than nonusers.

8. Thyroid function is not altered although the results of some tests of thyroid function are changed by oral contraception. A similar conclusion is made in regard to adrenal function.

9. Etiologic relationships to subjective symptoms such as headaches, nervousness and depression are difficult to assess. Oral contraceptives apparently do initiate or aggravate migraine headaches in some patients and when this complaint or increased nervousness or depression is reported, oral contraceptives should be discontinued, at least temporarily, to allow the patient to act as her own control. Subsequent fertility is rarely altered by oral contraceptives with the occasional expectation of a patient previously showing evidence of gross ovarian deficiency.

Into the overall equation of side effects, and remote possibilities of significant ones, must be placed the positive value of totally reliable control of conception, and the prevention of certain dangers thereby.

Also some value must be assigned to the important embellishment provided in the exercise of one of nature's most rewarding privileges, by the removal of fear of pregnancy and the elimination of mechanical intervention and interruption.[2]

On the other hand, nausea, spotting, fluid retention, weight gain, vaginitis, and chronic depression are common complaints of women using the pill. Clearly, these are serious disadvantages and have major implications for the health of the user, and even for the health of the marriage itself. Some women simply cannot function at full capacity when they take the pill, and few men or women are willing to tolerate this for long.

Future Methods of Contraception

Contraceptive techniques are most successful when they satisfy the criteria of simplicity, safety, effectiveness, reversibility, and compatibility with normal sexual functioning. Any disturbance, potential or real, to the body image or life-style of the user is unacceptable, unless the disturbance is in a desirable direction. Some women, for example, use the pill as much for figure enhancement or rhythm regulation as for contraception; men, on the other hand, universally reject the male version of the pill because of its undesirable side effects— testicular shrinkage and testosterone reduction.

Current research is seeking new contraceptives that will be void of all undesirable side effects. The recent MIT announcement of a self-dissolving contraceptive capsule that is expected to work for a year or longer when implanted under a woman's skin is one example of such a search. Again, it places the burden on the female, and both partners should be responsible for contraception in any meaningful relationship.

Various drugs have been used in an effort to develop an effective postcoital method of birth control. Most research in this area has sought a drug that either accelerates the movement of the fertilized egg through the fallopian tube or interferes with ovum transplant. Some rather interesting compounds are presently being evaluated.[3]

Recent research has also focused on the development of hormonal drugs that would effectively lower the sperm count. It long has been felt that some method of fertility regulation in the male is necessary. Currently no male contraceptive measure is available that does not have undesirable side effects. One substance, *inhibin,* has been somewhat effective without detrimental side effects. It may become more widely used as a male oral contraceptive.[4]

Although male vasectomy gained rather sudden and intense popularity during the late sixties and early seventies, its incidence then declined somewhat. The advantages in terms of low cost, minimal risk, availability, and simplicity seem to fall short of the male's greater need—maintaining his ego. Undoubtedly, much of the early popularity was media-supported—vasectomy became a fad. The current decline is probably due to a leveling off of enthusiasm and a more realistic appraisal of the consequences of vasectomy. The incidence is still high and will probably remain so, but the age of the males undergoing the operation has risen to over thirty-five. Vasectomy appears to be more popular among university-educated males.

A rather simple operation, vasectomy involves the severing of the sperm ducts (vas deferens), thereby preventing the passage of sperm from the testes to the urethra. The operation affects neither the size nor the hormonal secretions of the testes. In theory, then, male sex function is unaffected by the operation. Sex drive should remain normal, or even increase, due to the new freedom from fear of impregnation. The man's ability to maintain erection, ejaculate, and enjoy intercourse should be just as before.

In fact, however, some psychological problems can occur, although they are usually caused by ignorance. The operation must be considered irreversible. Its finality seems to raise doubts among some men about their masculinity, particularly among those who equate masculinity with reproduction. A little education goes far in preventing this problem.

Vasectomy is a minor procedure, most often carried out in a physician's office or in a clinic. Side effects are few, and the patient generally resumes his daily functions the following day, if not sooner. All factors considered, it is a safe and sure method of contraception.

What happens to the sperm following vasectomy? How do the testes absorb the pressure of continuing sperm production? Spermatogenesis continues, but the trapped sperms become physically engulfed by the phagocytic leukocytes [see chapter 4] which accumulate in the epididymis. The rate of phagocytosis increases greatly, and pressure buildup is avoided. In fact in some men, autoimmunity develops to the point that even if surgical repair were possible the man's body would continue to inactivate his sperm.

Vasectomy is considered irreversible and is taken very seriously by physicians. Counseling of candidates generally precedes the operation, and the candidate is asked to sign a permission slip—one signifying that the operation has been requested by the patient and that its effect will be permanent. Although the operation doesn't guarantee sterility, the failure rate is extremely low, less even than with the pill.

Attempts to develop clips and on-off valves to block the flow of semen temporarily have been reported in the literature, especially in animal experimentation, but to date none has proven particularly effective in human subjects. The

Sterilization

Male
Sterilization:
Vasectomy

Fig. 12.5. Although the advantages of a vasectomy are many, the results must be considered as irreversible. A vasectomy should not be gone into hastily.

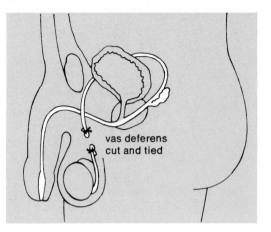

vas deferens cut and tied

problem of autoimmunity is a real one, and even when the vas deferens has been successfully reopened, fertility is only rarely restored. Even when fertility is restored, real fears persist that the sperm that do cause fertilization may be genetic mutants. Vasectomy should continue to be considered a permanent operation.

Female Sterilization: Laparoscopy and Culdoscopy

Female sterilization is achieved by removing or disrupting the function of the uterus, the fallopian tubes, and/or the ovaries. Surgical removal of the uterus, called hysterectomy, is a common operation, frequently performed for reasons other than sterilization, such as treatment of tumors and cancers or avoidance of future pregnancies that would endanger the mother's life. As a technique for sterilization alone, hysterectomy would seldom be the method of choice: the risk is too great. Tubal methods are preferable.

Removal of the ovaries (ovariectomy) and irradiation of the ovaries are both used to arrest imminently destructive diseases, such as cancer, but are far too drastic as sterilization procedures alone.

Fig. 12.6. The results of fallopian tube ligation by culdoscopy are shown in this diagram.

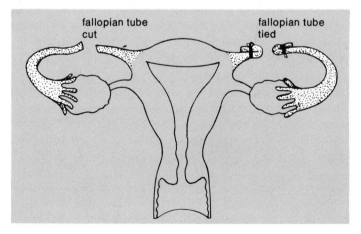

fallopian tube cut

fallopian tube tied

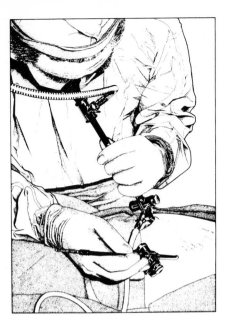

Fig. 12.7. Laparoscopy, one method of surgical sterilization for women, is used to sever the tubes and cauterize the ends. It also can be used for various other abdominal operations.

(From *Reproduction in mammals,* vol. 5, eds. C. R. Austin and R. V. Short, 1972, Cambridge University Press.)

When sterilization alone is desired, the method of choice is usually one designed to destroy the ovum-conducting function of the fallopian tubes. This action of severing the fallopian tubes and closing off the severed ends is called *tubal ligation.* Many techniques can be used, but the two most common ones are *laparoscopy* and *culdoscopy.*

Comparatively new, laparoscopy is performed with the aid of a laparoscope, a long tubelike device less than one-half inch in diameter that carries both a high intensity light beam and a magnifying lens system. By inserting it through a small incision into the lower abdominal cavity and sighting through it, the surgeon can readily identify the fallopian tubes. By means of another small incision, the surgeon uses a remote-control instrument with a surgical blade and electric cautery to cauterize a short segment of each tube. He then severs each tube at the center of the cauterized segment, and the tubes later become blocked with scar tissue. The entire laparoscopy requires less than thirty minutes, and the technique is being refined. A single-incision technique is being perfected.

A similar instrument, the culdoscope, can be used for tubal ligation via the vagina (the operation is entitled culdoscopy). The instrument is passed through an incision in the posterior fornix into the pelvic cavity, and the fallopian tubes are located and severed. Under local anesthetic the entire procedure takes only twenty minutes, and hospitalization is brief.

In still another technique under local anesthetic, a short incision is made in the vagina, and the uterus is pulled down until a fallopian tube is exposed. That tube is severed, using the Pomeroy technique; then the uterus is rotated until the other tube is exposed for severance. After this the uterus is returned to its normal position, and the vaginal incision is closed. Some doctors argue that this technique is too risky in terms of its contraceptive failure rate.

How can failure occur? Through recanalization, through the surgeon's failure to locate the proper tube, or through incomplete surgery. Regardless of circumstance and technique, however, failure rates are low and generally lower than the lowest rates recorded with oral contraceptives.

Like vasectomy, tubal ligation must be considered to be final. The operation is not reversible, but neither does it affect normal female physiological function. Ovum maturation and menstruation continue unchanged, and hormone function is normal. Released ova are absorbed into the body, and sexual drive, ability, and enjoyment should remain normal (in fact, records indicate an increase in all three areas, undoubtedly due to the relief from fear of pregnancy).

New techniques are being developed, including the use of tubal clips in place of cauterization or ligation as an approach to reversible female sterilization. Clips would greatly simplify the culdoscopic procedure.

Nonsurgical techniques have also been reported. Dr. Zipper (Santiago) has reported that injections of quinacrine through the cervix produce up to 92 percent sterilization effectiveness. Research continues.

Abortion

There are three different kinds of abortion. Early in many pregnancies the fetus is unintentionally expelled from the uterus. When this occurs, a *spontaneous abortion* results. This is normally referred to as a miscarriage.

Legal, intentional removal of the fetus by qualified personnel is referred to as *therapeutic abortion*. Historically most therapeutic abortions were performed to protect the health of the mother. In recent years, because of changes in legal regulations and the increasing feeling that a woman's personal right to bear or not to bear a child supersedes any rights of the fetus, therapeutic abortions are being performed for many other reasons.

A third kind of abortion is *criminal abortion*. These abortions are usually illegally performed by unqualified individuals. Many criminal abortions result in infection and death to the woman.

A last resort in family planning, and a practice that is frequently the result of either no family planning or ineffective family planning, is abortion. This is a widely practiced method of birth prevention in the world today. The right of a woman to obtain "abortion on demand" is a highly debated issue throughout North America. Many view abortion as immoral and as actual killing of human life (witness the right-to-life position). Others feel that there must be legal grounds for terminating a pregnancy when such a procedure is desired.

Various state laws regarding abortion have come into being since about 1967. The basic focus of these new abortion laws has been to liberalize older statutory regulations. Basically they would permit therapeutic abortion with certain medical restrictions.

The United States Supreme Court handed down a decision on abortion in 1973. This decision, which has been precedent-setting, legalized abortions during the first months of pregnancy. During the first trimester, the abortion must be recommended by a physician. The decision of the Supreme Court in effect held that under the U.S. Constitution a fetus is not considered to be a person. Therefore, the fetus has no legal right to life. The right of the woman to have an abortion was upheld. In the second trimester, the state may impose certain regulations related to maternal health. The effect of this decision was that antiabortion laws in numerous states were found to be invalid.

Many abortion problems have arisen since 1973. Those opposed to abortion of any kind have called for passage of a Constitutional amendment that would prohibit abortions. Some hospitals, particularly those with religious affiliations, have refused to permit abortions to be performed in their facilities. The question has been raised, Are they entitled to such refusal when they have received federal funds to construct their facilities? Another issue presently being discussed by Congress is whether Medicaid monies can be used to pay for abortions. Many politicians, as well as antiabortion supporters, feel such monies should not be so used. Such restrictions would, however, cause added burdens on the poor and disadvantaged.

The various issues surrounding abortion were raised in 1976 during the presidential campaign. This matter will continue to be controversial and often emotional for some time to come.

Before the End of the Third Month

Abortions performed during the first trimester are frequently done on an outpatient basis, or in a clinic, using a local anesthetic. In dilation and curettage, the physician expands the vaginal canal with a retractor, grasps the cervix with special forceps, and then passes a sound through the cervical canal and into the uterine cavity. Sound waves permit the experienced doctor to locate the exact position of the fetus and estimate its size.

The cervical canal is gradually dilated with the aid of muscle relaxants and appropriate instruments. Forceps are inserted into the uterus and used to remove the fetus; the uterus is then curetted (scraped). The entire procedure generally takes less than a half hour.

Imported from mainland China, the vacuum aspirator (see figure 12.8) has come into popular use in recent years. Usually performed under local anesthetic, the technique calls for application of a low suction force, with both duration and intensity carefully controlled. Under aseptic hospital or clinical conditions the operation is safe and fast (under fifteen minutes total); it reduces the risk of uterine perforation and blood loss involved in other techniques.

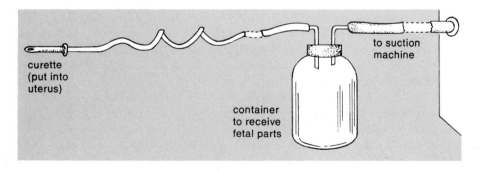

curette
(put into
uterus)

to suction
machine

container
to receive
fetal parts

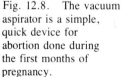

Fig. 12.8. The vacuum aspirator is a simple, quick device for abortion done during the first months of pregnancy.

After three months, abortion usually requires several days of hospitalization, and an abdominal hysterotomy is frequently the method of choice. Similar to a cesarean section, this operation involves making an incision in the lower abdomen, another incision in the uterus, and then removing the fetus and amniotic sac. Abdominal hysterotomy is the logical operation if late abortion is combined with tubal ligation.[5] This same operation can be done through the vaginal canal (vaginal hysterotomy) if the pregnancy is still less than sixteen weeks along. Vaginal hysterotomy has few advantages beyond that of not leaving a scar, and many disadvantages, not the least of which is lack of working space.

Intrauterine injections are useful for inducing abortion during the second trimester of pregnancy. The uterus can be approached through the vagina or, after sixteen weeks, through the abdominal wall. Full sterile precautions are essential, and a local anesthetic only is recommended. A two-way tap system is set up. From 50 to 200 ml. of amniotic fluid are drawn off and replaced by an equal volume of 20 percent saline or 50 percent glucose solution. The injection must be made very slowly and accurately. As further precaution, the antibiotic oxytetracycline may be added to the replacement fluid. Labor usually follows within a day or two, the products of conception are usually completely expelled, and curettage is seldom necessary.

Both abortifacient (abortion-causing) pastes and drugs are available, but overly dangerous at this time. Estrogens, quinine, and fluids that hasten contractions of the uterus have all proven unreliable and can produce physical defects in the fetus, such as displaced limbs and joints. Similarly the introduction of soap suds, alcohol, lye, lysol, potassium compounds, pine oil, soda pop, and hot water frequently result in severe tissue burns, shock, hemorrhage, and even death. As abortifacients, none is reliable.

The use of home techniques for abortion, like use of inserters (knitting needles, coat hangers, chopsticks), shock (falling down stairs, electric shock, a beating), and physical exertion (lifting heavy objects, running or swimming to exhaustion), may be damaging to the mother's health but will have little effect on the fetus. What effect they do have is neither predictable nor reliable.

In any case, abortion is not a method of choice for birth control. Safer, effective methods of contraception should be used.

Summary

We have examined family planning, primarily with a view to limiting the number of offspring. Although some current trends in family structure and function were discussed, the major focuses were fertility, contraception, sterilization, and abortion. New techniques were described, and some speculations about future means of contraception were aired.

It is important that we understand means of birth control for personal reasons. Yet, without birth control or some other method of adaptation, we also must begin to cope with the problem of an ever-increasing number of people in our world. Therefore, we shall examine next the issues of overpopulation and population control.

1. What factors may influence family size in the United States and Canada today?
2. Discuss some of the possible reasons for male infertility.
3. Why have we seen a gradual reduction in family size, particularly in North America, in recent years?
4. Why has the rhythm method proven to be one of the least effective in preventing conception?
5. If the condom is such a highly effective birth control method, why doesn't its failure rate indicate this effectiveness?
6. How do intrauterine devices differ from other mechanical birth control devices?
7. How does the pill prevent pregnancy? What are its possible side effects?
8. Describe the various forms of sterilization for the male and female. Explain the advantages and disadvantages of each.
9. If the IUD prevents the implantation of the fertilized egg in the wall of the uterus, is this not a form of abortion?
10. What is the legal status of abortion today in the United States?

Readings

Hubbard, W. *Family Planning Education*. St. Louis: C. V. Mosby Co., 1973.

McCary, J. L. *Human Sexuality*. 2d ed. New York: D. Van Nostrand, 1973.

Notes

1. William Masters and Virginia Johnson, "Intravaginal Environment: 1. A Lethal Factor," *Journal of Fertility and Sterility* 12 (1961): 560–80.
2. W. C. Andrews, "Oral Contraception: A Review of Reported Physiological Effects," *Obstetrical and Gynecological Survey* 16, no. 7 (1971): 477–99.
3. A. Kessler and C. C. Standley, "Fertility-Regulating Methods," *WHO Chronicle* 31 (May 1977): 190.
4. Ibid., p. 191.
5. J. Peel and M. Potts, *Textbook of Contraceptive Practice* (New York: Cambridge University Press, 1970).

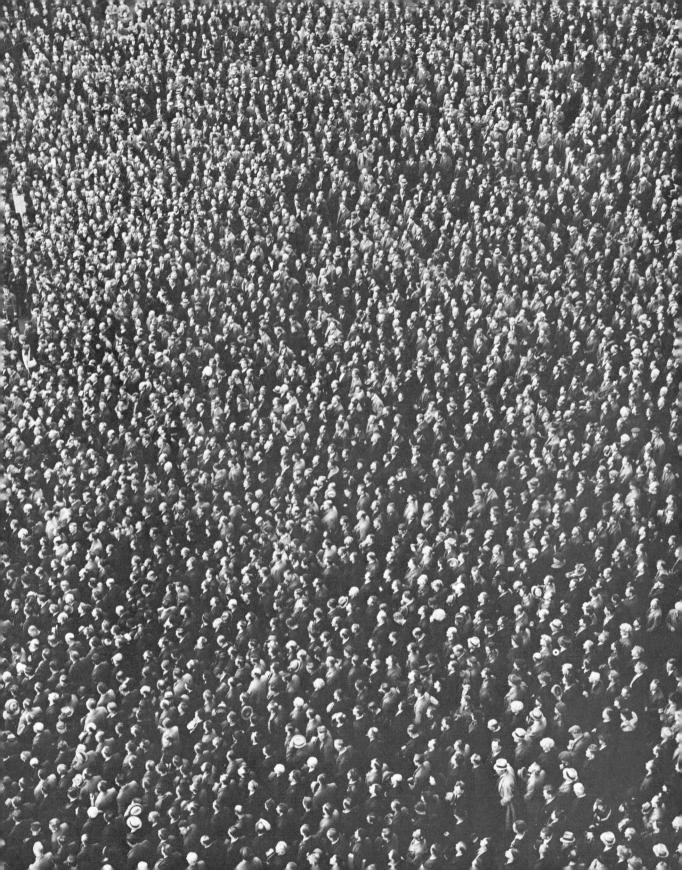

Population: Too Many People?

13

A serious problem to the well-being of the inhabitants of the world is increasing population. It is impossible to separate such concerns as malnutrition, problems of the environment, and many of the issues discussed in this book from the problems created by increased population. Simply stated, the presence of increasing numbers of individuals throughout the world will lead to more despoiling of nature, and hence to related health problems brought about by exposure to the various pollutants. In addition to environmental deterioration, the presence of more people in the world will result in greater problems of famine, malnourishment, sickness, and poor emotional adjustment.

Adaptation to greater numbers of people has no doubt been a part of the life experience of many who read this book. Certainly each of us has learned to adapt in some way to greater population. Some of those reading this chapter have waited in line for up to an hour for a four-minute ride at Disney World; others have spent two hours a day driving to and from work because they live in the suburbs. Our school classrooms have more than forty students crowded into rooms that should hold only twenty-five. Many other situations can be cited that are examples of the ways we have adapted to the present population level. What is of concern, and not at all clear, is an answer to the question: How many people can be sustained on the planet Earth without massive deterioration in the quality of life? What adaptations will you and your children need to make in the future as world population increases?

When it is realized that today there are more than 4 billion people alive and needing basic resources, one can begin to understand the problems of overpopulation and population control. An explanation of the growth rate of population throughout history will help to clarify the issue. There were only a quarter of a billion people in the world from the beginning of mankind until the discovery of the New World at the end of the fifteenth century. The doubling of the population to a half billion did not occur until the middle of the seventeenth century (approximately 1650). This doubling took more than 150 years. Interestingly, today there are more people in China (over 800 million people) and India (over 500 million) than populated the entire globe at the midpoint of the seventeenth century.

The next doubling time of the world's population was about two centuries. About 1850 the population of the world reached the 1 billion mark. The doubling period for the next billion was reduced to about 80 years as the 2 billion mark in world population was reached about 1930.

Table 13.1 Rate of Population Increase and Years Required to Double Present Population

	Rate of Population Increase (percent)	Years to Double at Present Rate
Canada	1.1	67
United States	.9	83
The World	2.1	32
Africa	2.7	26
East Asia	2.3	31
Europe	.7	95
Latin America	2.9	24
Near East	2.6	27
South Asia	2.8	25

Source: World Population Data, Agency for International Development, Washington, D.C.

At the present rate of world population growth—slightly over 2 percent—it becomes obvious that the number will double again in about thirty-two years. By the year 2000 there will likely be more than 7 billion people on our globe *unless* something happens to curtail population growth or unless worldwide calamity, either man-made or natural, occurs to bring death to millions of individuals.

The doubling rate is the amount of time it will take for the number of people in a given nation or locality to double if population growth continues at the current rate. At the end of the 1970s those nations where the most rapid growth is occurring, those that have the shortest periods of doubling time, are in the process of development. Latin American, African, and Asiatic nations will double in population between now and the year 2000.

In 1798 Thomas R. Malthus, an English clergyman and economist, wrote a book entitled *Essay on the Principle of Population, 1798.*[1] His basic thesis was that population increases more rapidly than resources. He suggested that unless there is an increase in deaths caused by war, disease, starvation, or some other means, overpopulation and its dire consequences result.

Malthus contended that food production could not keep up with the ability of the human race to reproduce. He stated that population when unchecked increases in a geometric ratio, while food production increases in an arithmetic ratio. Malthus pointed out that both food and sexual desire are necessary to the existence of mankind. Both are very clearly related to population increase.

The theories of Malthus have been a topic of debate in discussions about population growth since 1798. Many would suggest that technology has made his theories inconsequential. Food production has been increased, and further development will be able to keep pace with population growth. On the other hand, there is strong evidence that Malthus was correct. In a world where at the present time many are malnourished or starving and where geographic areas with rapidly doubling populations are already greatly overpopulated, the geometric rate of population increase postulated by Malthus is highly significant.

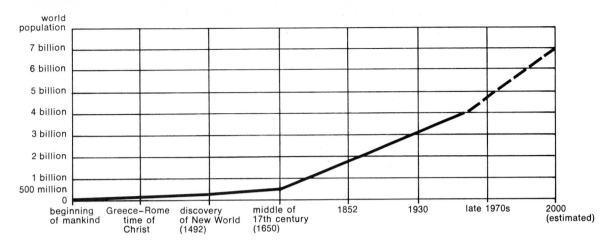

world
population

7 billion

6 billion

5 billion

4 billion

3 billion

2 billion

1 billion
500 million
0

| beginning of mankind | Greece–Rome time of Christ | discovery of New World (1492) | middle of 17th century (1650) | 1852 | 1930 | late 1970s | 2000 (estimated) |

Fig. 13.1. This graph represents the population growth pattern of the world since the beginning of mankind. The projection through the year 2000 is based on an assumed growth rate of slightly more than 2 percent.

As one travels across the open prairies of the western United States or the broad expanses of Alberta and Saskatchewan in Canada, it seems almost inconceivable that population growth should be of concern in our world. It is hard to imagine that in many parts of the world overpopulation is creating serious problems. How is it that many people are deeply concerned about the increase in population? Is it really possible that in some nations the growth in numbers of people is so rapid that the population will probably double in less than three decades? Without a building in sight and distances of fifty miles or more between small towns, it seems impossible to believe that uncontrolled population growth is a factor of prime importance in over two thirds of the nations of the world.

Present Increase of Population

The present annual increase in world population is approximately 70 million persons per year. That is the equivalent of adding *each year* three and a half times the number of people presently living in Canada or one third again the number of persons in the United States. To put it another way, the increase in human population *hourly* amounts to some 8,000 on a worldwide basis. The most rapid population increases are in the Third World nations. These are the developing countries, which in most cases are already greatly overpopulated, still troubled with famine and malnutrition, and lacking in vitally needed resources; disease is still a prime concern to almost everyone in these countries.

Population increase in the United States amounts to about 3 million persons per year. That is the equivalent of adding a city the size of Chicago *each year*. As one thinks of the resources needed to keep a city like Chicago operating, it can be seen to what extent increased population puts a stress on the natural resources and development.

The paradox of such astounding figures going through one's mind while traversing wide open spaces like those in the West is that so much of this astronomical growth is taking place in the urban areas of the world. With additional

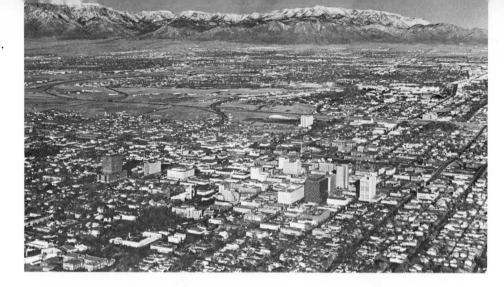

Fig. 13.2. Albuquerque, New Mexico, largest city in the state, has a metropolitan population of about 350,000. The business district and part of its residential areas are shown here.

population in areas already highly overcrowded, the numerous problems associated with large-city living are compounded. Three quarters of the United States population live in urban centers along the eastern coast and in the Great Lakes regions.

When an area—a region or a nation—is experiencing rapid population growth and is basically an agricultural entity, an interesting phenomenon often occurs. With increasing numbers of people, the amount of land that can be used for agriculture decreases. This means that many people, normally unskilled agricultural workers, cannot find employment. As a result, a migration to urban communities begins to take place. In the cities many of these people cannot find jobs; they have very poor housing, and crowded conditions, along with the many problems related to potential for disease, result.[2]

Many of the world's cities could be used as an example. Mexico City is such an urban area. Approximately a quarter of a million persons a year move to Mexico City. The population of this city has risen from 4.8 million people just a decade ago to 9.0 million today. Provision of basic services, such as water and sewage, is very difficult. Between 25 and 30 percent of these people cannot find work and live in very shabby, unhealthy environmental surroundings.

Table 13.2 Percentage of Total Population That Lives in Urban Areas

Canada	75%
United States	75%
The World	37%
Africa	14%
East Asia	29%
Europe	61%
Latin America	55%
Near East	39%
South Asia	18%

Source: World Population Data, Agency for International Development, Washington, D.C.

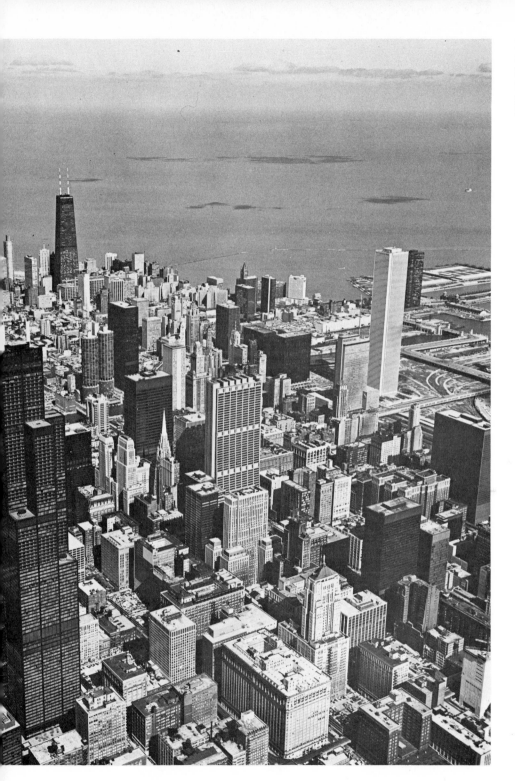

Fig. 13.3. Chicago's main business district, known as "the Loop," takes up only a small percentage of the city's 222.6 square miles.

Causes of Population Growth

There are numerous reasons for the increase in population throughout the world. Until the mid-1800s disease played a major role in maintaining a balance in the population level, that is, a balance between birth rates and death rates. Death rates were high because of numerous factors, such as exposure to many communicable diseases, high infant mortality, and famines. In the fourteenth century one fourth of the population of Europe died in an epidemic of bubonic plague. This happened in a period of about five years (1347–52).

With the development of the germ theory of disease and efforts to eradicate many communicable diseases, such as smallpox, malaria, yellow fever, cholera, and others, it came about that more people are living today who previously would have died from some disease condition.

In the days of high death rates due to disease it was not uncommon for a woman to bear many children to maintain the population—often as many as eight to ten. With the development of procedures to eliminate or at least reduce the incidences of dreaded disease, there more often than not was no accompanying reduction in births. Significant advances were also made in infant care. During the present century, much progress has been made in reducing infant mortality. Today the infant death rate is below 22 per 1,000 live births in Canada and approximately 17.6 in the United States. In several European nations, such as Sweden, Norway, Finland, Iceland, and England, the infant mortality rate ranges between 13 and 18 per 1,000. Recent statistics (1976) indicate that currently eight countries have less than a 13 per 1,000 infant mortality rate.

In many nations of the world, the infant mortality rate remains extremely high. In such African nations as Zambia, Tanzania, Senegal, and Liberia and the Asiatic countries of Cambodia, Indonesia, and Laos, the infant mortality rate is between 130 and 160 per 1,000 live births. These high rates must be lowered. Through improved programs of nutrition, disease control, and infant health care, one can hope that such extensive loss of infant life will be reduced. On the other hand, assuming that such does occur, what additional population pressures will this create? It is paradoxical to think that from a humanitarian viewpoint one should support and encourage improved health care to bring about a reduction in infant mortality, while realizing that when nations of the world that still have very high infant mortality rates approach the present levels of the United States, Canada, and most European nations, great population pressures will result.

Birth and Death Rates

The most commonly used measure for expressing the number of births in a given population group is the crude birth rate. Basically this statement of birth rate is an indication of the number of registered live births per 1,000 population. The statement of mortality that is most commonly used is the crude death rate, based on the number of deaths occurring during the year per 1,000 population.

Birth rates in the United States have dropped since the early 1960s from more than 23 to about 15 per 1,000.

Even though birth rates may be decreasing in some areas of the world, two potentially dangerous considerations are apparent. One is that there are a greater

Table 13.3 Birth Rates and Death Rates

	Birth Rate (per 1,000 Population)	Death Rate (per 1,000)
Canada	18	7
United States	18	9
The World	36	15
Africa	48	21
East Asia	41	18
Europe	17	10
Latin America	39	10
Near East	42	16
South Asia	44	16

Source: World Population Data, Agency for International Development, Washington, D.C.

number of women in the childbearing ages today. In 1968, when Paul R. Ehrlich wrote his now famous book on population, *The Population Bomb,* he stated that "roughly 40 percent of the population of the undeveloped world is made up of people *under fifteen years old.*"[3] This vast number of young people are those who today, in the late seventies, are of reproductive age. The majority of the population today in Latin America, for example, is below fifteen years of age.

Birth rates may have dropped, yet the number of births has not. When it is realized that such rates are expressions per 1,000 population, we see that the number of births continues to increase as overall population rises. This concept can be exemplified by taking two hypothetical communities with populations of 100,000 and 150,000 respectively.

Town A		Town B
100,000	Population	150,000
12.5	Birth rate	9.3
1,250	Actual births	1,400

As can be seen, Town B has the lower birth rate (9.3), so we might be tempted to conclude that population growth was less of a problem in that community, with a birth rate over one-third less than that of Town A. However, note which community contributed the most to the problem of population growth. This is what is happening on a worldwide basis. Birth rates may drop, but overall population continues to climb.

Throughout most of the nations of the world there continues to be an increase in the standard of living. As standards of living increase, as nutritional standards are improved, and as health resources and services continue to improve, longevity increases. This increase in length of life adds to the population problem.

Increases in the number of people lead to the need for more consumer products. This requires an increase in energy requirements and further use and depletion of natural resources. In the past the traditional notion has been that more

**Results
of Population
Increase**

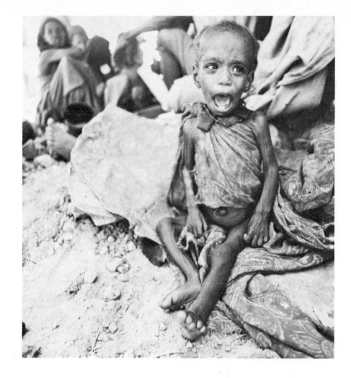

Fig. 13.4. Thousands of people have died and thousands more suffer from malnutrition and lack of water in Ethiopia and the Sahel region of Africa. This child is one of more than 1.5 million Ethiopians severely affected by a drought that swept the country in 1974.

people meant more business, greater prosperity, and a rise in standard of living. This idea is being widely questioned today by many people.

As has been emphasized since the latter part of 1973, the energy resources of our world are limited. If population continues to increase, there will be an accelerating growth in the resource demands of people. For example, in an average lifetime one American will consume or use 56 million gallons of water, buy 37,000 gallons of gasoline, and eat 5½ tons of wheat and another 5½ tons of meat.[4] It has been estimated that the average American will use thirty times more natural resources than the average person in India. If population growth is not curtailed in some manner, a number of conditions and situations might very well result. For example, as has been implied, further exhaustion of natural resources, such as coal, minerals, oil, and gas, will occur.

One cannot think seriously about the problems associated with population growth without facing the issues of mass starvation, hunger, and death. Many parts of the world are today experiencing difficulties in feeding the present population.

Efforts have been made to increase the food supply in the world. New strains of some crops that have been developed have helped. The work of Dr. Norman Borlaug in developing new strains of wheat in Mexico that greatly increased the yields per acre resulted in his receiving the Nobel Peace Prize in 1970. Dr. Borlaug was quoted as saying on this occasion, "We have only delayed the world food crisis for another thirty years. If the world population continues to increase at the same rate, we will destroy the species."[5] Resulting from the work

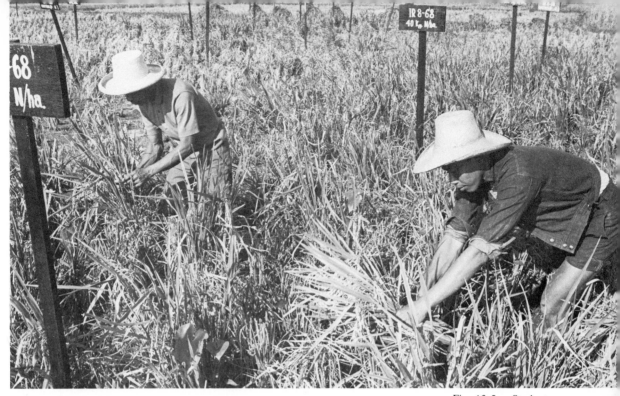

of Dr. Borlaug, there was a three times greater yield per acre than previously. Good soil fertilization is necessary for this to be effective.

Other similar technologic attempts have been taking place with such crops as rice, soybeans, and corn. A crop perfected in Canada involves a cross between wheat and rye. This newly developed species (called triticale) has a higher protein content than other cereals, is of value as a feed for livestock, has a better yield than either the normal rye or wheat, and can adapt to more extensive climate conditions.[6] Nevertheless, significant doubt has been expressed by many as to whether the starving and malnourished in the world can be properly fed. Possibly as many as one-half billion people are threatened by starvation.

Near the end of 1974 representatives of some 130 of the world's nations met in Rome at the United Nations World Food Conference. It was the purpose of this conference to focus attention on the problems of hunger in the world. Many speeches and discussions took place. However, one cannot be overly optimistic that any solidly fundamental programs for meeting the needs of hunger came from this meeting. Some speakers, such as the United States Secretary of State Henry Kissinger, spoke directly of the need to proclaim objectives such as ''Within a decade no child will go to bed hungry.'' Yet political conflict and international bickering seemed to result rather than the establishment of any direct programs of help. When one realizes that at least 10 million people will die each year during the 1980s from starvation, it seems paradoxical to think that some plan cannot be agreed upon. A decade would almost seem to be too long. The need is now!

Fig. 13.5. Students at the University of the Philippines count grains per stack of a fast-growing rice on an experimental farm. The United Nations sponsors many such programs to improve agricultural yields throughout the world.

Lifeboat Ethics

It has been suggested that the poorer developing nations should not be helped in their attempts to feed their multitudes of starving people.[7] This concept has been referred to as *lifeboat ethics*. In short, this notion says that each developed, rich country is a lifeboat. Worldwide survival will occur only if developed nations do not use their limited resources to feed the hungry masses. Only those "in the boat" will live, and the lifeboat is limited by size and resources. All others will be lost by starvation.

This theoretical ethic has its supporters as well as its opponents. The general concept of lifeboat ethics raises many difficult questions. Who shall determine who will survive or who will be lost? How can a person who truly treasures human life tell someone else they must "drown" in the morass of world population? Can you look on the world scene from your lifeboat of luxury and multiple resources and ethically permit little children and well-meaning people to "sink"?

It certainly is not a pretty picture. Also, one must seriously doubt that such a position is really the answer to worldwide hunger and famine. It is doubtful if any nation would sink into oblivion. As conditions became intolerable, revolt and rebellion would become more likely, leading to worldwide disruption in which the "haves" would most likely be the greatest losers.

Will increased population and a greater number of individuals crowded into smaller areas result in an increase in crime and in more aggressive human beings? There are many sociologists who suggest that this is the case. Some studies done with animals have indicated that those living in overcrowded conditions tend to be more aggressive. Other researchers found that rats living in crowded conditions became apathetic. It must be realized that these are animal studies, and that the adaptable nature of humans will no doubt make some adjustments to the increase in overcrowding as population increases. Nevertheless, we have seen an increase in crime, war, and other acts of aggression as people have become more crowded and as numbers have increased.

Possible Solutions

To resolve some of the problems related to population growth, it becomes obvious that efforts must be made to reduce the birth rate. This leads to the importance of establishing some kind of program of family planning. Education in the consequences of continued population growth might be helpful. As people come to realize the consequences of continued increases in numbers of people, it is hoped that they will better understand the need for family planning.

It seems important that efforts be made to determine how people can be motivated to *want* to have fewer children. This becomes a matter of attitude and of bringing about major changes in values for a large segment of our world's population. Many social mores come into play. For some it is a sign of virility or femininity to have a large number of children. For others it has been an economic necessity. This has particularly been the case in those cultures that are basically agrarian. Additional children are important in helping to farm the land.

Some of the governments of developing nations see the industrial nations' call for population limitation as a means of attempting to limit their countries'

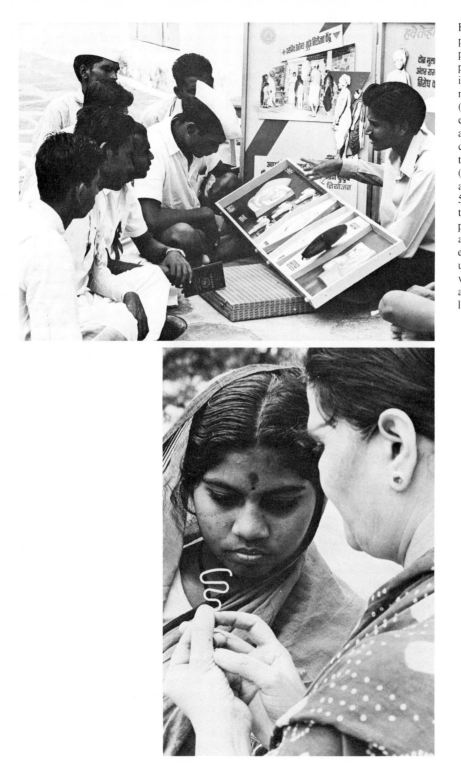

Fig. 13.6. Family planning and population control are part of economic policy in India. A class for men in family planning (left). A teacher explains the use of an intrauterine contraceptive device to a young mother (below). These people are part of a group of 56 couples selected by trade unions to take part in pilot population and family welfare education courses at a university near their villages. The men are all landless rural laborers.

economic development. This concept and the diversity of opinion among nations was highlighted in August 1974 at the United Nations World Population Conference. This meeting in Bucharest, Romania, was the first international conference involving the world's governments to discuss population problems. Several conflicting positions were presented at this conference. At least four general categories could be identified. There were those who said that:

1. Population problems are in reality problems of unequal distribution of world wealth. What is needed is a new economic order where inequities of world resources and wealth will be eliminated. Then fertility decline will be a natural result of true social development.
2. There is no need for population policies. Concern over population is in reality exploitation of the Third World nations, particularly by the capitalistic developed nations.
3. Some nations do in fact have population problems. The reason for these problems is lack of education, poor health, and poverty. As a result, socioeconomic development must be related to any population programs.
4. There are social and economic problems in the world. Population growth intensifies these problems. Therefore, population growth must be reduced to bring about better social and economic development. (The United States government supported this position.)

A number of the world's nations have refused to support officially the concept of family planning and population control. In those countries where support for population control programs is official policy, the objective for decreasing population growth is mainly to help meet plans for economic development. This was found to be true in more than half (thirty-three of sixty-three) of the countries supporting programs of family planning. The second most indicated reason for population control was based on grounds of health or of human rights.[8]

Religious values and beliefs have been obstacles to the reduction of births. While supporting the concept of responsible parenthood, the Roman Catholic church has historically opposed the use of contraception as a birth control measure. This has led to a serious dilemma for many people. On the one hand they recognize the need for some type of contraceptive action, while on the other hand they realize that the teachings of their faith prohibit such actions. A few Protestant groups oppose birth control and family planning activities; however, most of the Protestant denominations have given support to programs designed to limit population growth.

There is a need for making available information and the tools for contraception to the masses of people on a level that can be understood. This becomes no easy task, particularly in those developing countries of the world where the population growth rate is the highest. It is in these parts of the world that there is the greatest amount of ignorance and superstition regarding contraception. Many in these cultures see activities designed at limiting their population as attempts by others to obliterate their race or culture.

Numerous procedures for controlling birth have been discussed in the chapter dealing with contraceptive devices. Research continues on the development of

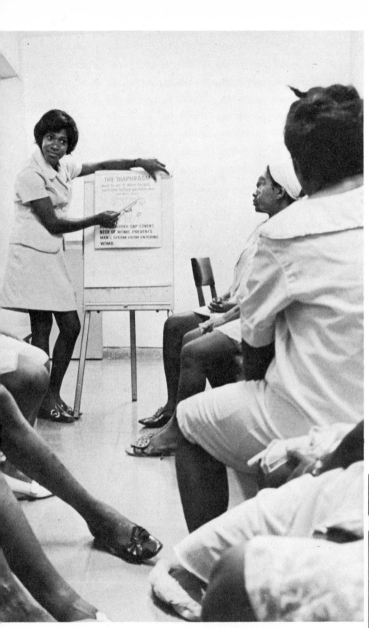

Fig. 13.8.   One purpose of the UN conference on human settlements in 1976 was to draw attention to the plight of people such as these in Bombay, India.

Fig. 13.7.   Population control is a major problem in many developing nations. Family planning sessions for new mothers are conducted in the crowded nation of Jamaica (above). Religious values and beliefs often block birth control policies. This Paraguayan family (right) is made up of sixteen members, soon to be seventeen.

newer, more effective, and more easily administered methods of birth control. However, these newer methods, when developed, will only be as effective as the ability of man to make them available and to educate the people who need them.

Another possibility for reducing the population in the United States has been the suggestion that tax incentives be used to help encourage limitation of population. At present there are greater tax incentives for those with larger families. The withdrawal of such tax incentives and the placing of a higher tax on those individuals with larger families might stimulate change. Of an economic nature would be the withdrawal of maternity benefits after a woman has given birth to a specific number of children. Obviously such economic sanctions might create other concerns and problems; yet limiting population may not be able to remain an individual, voluntary matter without some kinds of very dramatic incentives.

In 1969 the President of the United States, Richard M. Nixon, stated: "One of the most serious challenges to human destiny in the last third of this century will be the growth of the population." Following this the Commission on Population Growth and the American Future was formed, chaired by John D. Rockefeller III, to examine issues surrounding the matter of population and the American future. Many people had the opportunity to present data before the commission in public hearing. Numerous research projects were conducted, and the testimony of experts in many fields was evaluated by the commission. The final report of the commission was presented to the President and to the Congress in March 1972.

A number of recommendations were made. As would be expected, there was not unanimous agreement on all recommendations by all members of the commission. Several of the recommendations were also rejected by President Nixon. Specifically, he opposed the commission's recommendations regarding abortion.

It would be impossible to discuss the recommendations of the entire report. Some of the commission recommendations were:

1. There should be a Population Education Act that would assist school systems in establishing population education programs.
2. Sex education should be available to everyone. It should be presented in a reasonable manner through community organizations, the media, and the schools.
3. Adequate child-care services should be made available by both public and private agencies. These services should include health, nutritional, and educational components.
4. All legal restrictions on provision of contraceptive information, procedures, and supplies should be removed by all individual states. In addition, all states should be encouraged to pass legislation supporting such procedures.
5. Minors should be permitted to receive contraceptive information and services. These should be provided in settings sensitive to the needs and concerns of the young people.
6. Laws regarding abortion should be liberalized along the lines of the New York state statutes. Abortions should only be performed on request by duly licensed physicians in a proper medical setting.

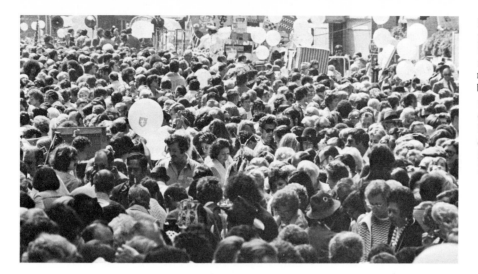

Fig. 13.9. The population explosion is the concern of all nations. There are more than four billion people unevenly distributed over the world's habitable areas. The crowd in the picture is at a bazaar in a New York City street.

7. A national policy should be identified that would reduce unwanted fertility, improve the outcome of pregnancy, and improve the health of children.
8. The nation must support and plan for a stabilized population. Population growth cannot continue indefinitely.[9]

Regardless of what action might result from the activities of this commission, at least the United States government has exemplified its concerns over population in the future by the formation of and the activities of the commission.

An organization formed in 1969, with Paul Ehrlich one of the principal founders, is known as Zero Population Growth (ZPG). It is the hope of this organization to encourage governmental action that would ultimately discourage childbearing. The concept of Zero Population Growth is that the number of births would not exceed deaths. If a replacement population of two children per family were to become universal, population would remain stable. Actually, if a replacement of two children per family became the norm, a reduction in population should occur. This is because of the fact that some children do not reach adulthood and some adults do not have children. For this reason it is felt that a replacement population of 2.1 children per woman should bring the population growth to a halt. Even if this level, 2.1 per family, could be achieved today, there would continue to be an increase in total numbers of people until about the year 2000. This would be the result of the fact that today, as we have noted earlier, a large number of young women are of childbearing age.

Zero Population Growth

Several private organizations and foundations have given extensive support to family planning programs and research throughout the world. The International Planned Parenthood Federation with its national and local associations has been very active in these concerns. Other private, nonprofit organizations providing

Private Organizations

research, training, and services in family planning activities are the Population Council, the Ford Foundation, the Rockefeller Foundation, and the Population Crisis Committee.

Summary

It might seem as though resolution of the problem of population control is beyond the scope of any one of us. After examining the potential for population increase and all of the ramifications associated with these concerns, one is left with a rather limp feeling of helplessness. No doubt, many reading this text can remember a time in their younger days when they were able to go out on the edge of town and hike through a woods, hunt rabbit or pheasant, or go for a family ride through areas where fields stretched for several miles. Today, for many, these areas contain suburban developments with houses, shopping centers, and *people*. One resolution to the population problem rests with *you*. You must examine your values, ethics, and beliefs regarding birth control in light of the data concerning population growth. Only then can you, the college student, take positive action to help curb the growth of population. Certainly population control is a personal health problem for each of us.

Review Questions

1. Although science and technology have made life easier, has the increase in population reduced the quality of life on earth?
2. What is Thomas Malthus' thesis of population growth? In light of our present situation, do you agree or disagree with it?
3. Should we as Americans share concern over the population problem that exists in other countries?
4. What factors have contributed to the rise in population growth?
5. How is it possible for birth rates to drop while overall population continues to increase?
6. Explain the close relationship that exists between population size and energy demands.
7. Do we as Americans have a responsibility to feed and share our food with the starving nations of the world?
8. What factors might be responsible for the fact that in overcrowded areas people tend to be more aggressive?
9. Since infant mortality is so high in underdeveloped countries, can we expect women to accept birth-control methods readily when we cannot assure them that those children already living will survive?
10. What is ZPG? What is your attitude toward it?
11. Do you support the concept of lifeboat ethics? Defend your answer.
12. What would your reaction be if the government began to regulate the number of children a family was allowed to have?

Books

Agency for International Development. *Population Program Assistance.*
Washington, D.C.: Office of Population, 1970.

Commoner, Barry. *The Closing Circle.* New York: Alfred A. Knopf, 1972.

Heer, David M. *Society and Population.* Englewood Cliffs, N.J.:
Prentice-Hall, 1968.

Phillips, John. *Environmental Health.* Dubuque: Wm. C. Brown Co., 1971.

Stockwell, Edward G. *Population and People.* Chicago: Quadrangle Books,
1968.

Articles

Barnett, Larry D. "Education and Religion as Factors Influencing Attitudes
Toward Population Growth in the United States." *Social Biology* 17
(1970): 26–36.

Hein, John. "World Population Growth and People's Well-being."
Conference Board Record, September 1973, pp. 7–10.

Hulett, H. R. "Optimum World Population." *Bioscience* 20 (1970): 160–61.

MacKenzie, V. Paul. "Evaluating Family Planning Programs in a Canadian
Context." *Canadian Journal of Public Health* 63 (1972): 228–36.

Ravenholt, R. T. "Facing Up to Population in 1974." *War on Hunger, A
Report from the Agency for International Development* 8 (1974): 4–7.

Wadia, Avabai B. "Population and Environment." *Journal of Family
Welfare* 19 (1973).

1. Thomas Robert Malthus, *Essay on the Principle of Population, 1798* (facsimile reprint with notes revised by James Bonar, New York: Macmillan Co., 1966).

2. Malcolm H. Merrill, "An Expanding Populace in a Contrasting World," *Journal of the American Medical Association* 197 (1966), pp. 114–19.

3. Paul R. Ehrlich, *The Population Bomb* (New York: Ballantine Books, 1968), p. 28.

4. *As We Live and Breathe: The Challenge of Our Environment* (Washington, D.C.: National Geographic Society, 1971), p. 205.

5. Ibid., p. 210.

6. Richard H. Wagner, *Environment and Man* (New York: W. W. Norton and Co., 1971), p. 437.

7. Garrett Hardin, "Lifeboat Ethics: The Case Against Helping the Poor," *Psychology Today* 8, no. 4 (September 1974): 38–43, 123–26.

8. *Population and Family Planning Programs: A Factbook* (New York: Population Council, 1947), p. 91.

9. Commission on Population Growth and the American Future, *Population and the American Future* (New York: Signet Books, 1972).

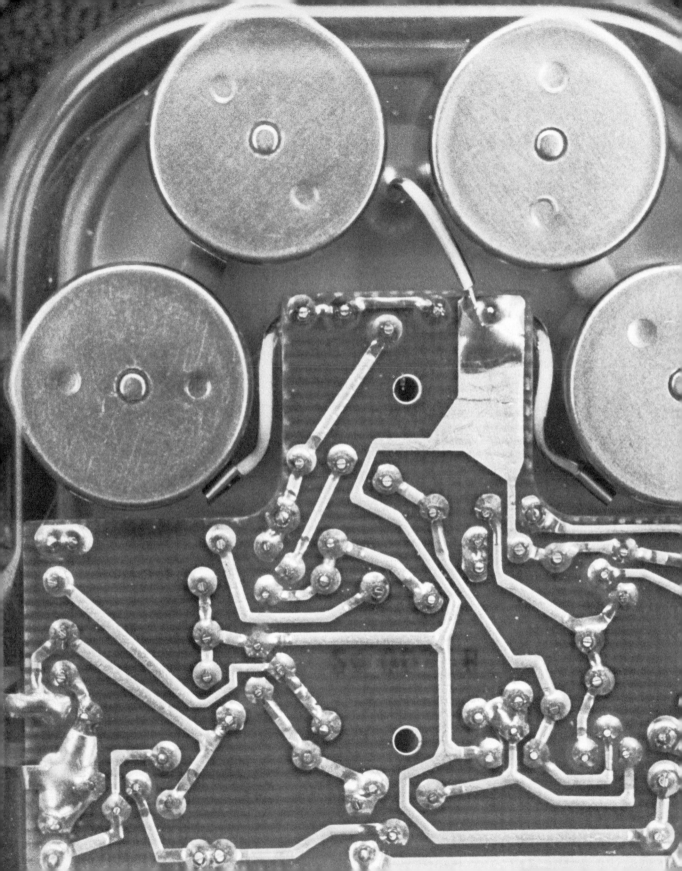

Cardiovascular Diseases: Preserving the Beat

14

Health-threatening aspects of life are now recognized as major contributing factors in the incidence of many noncommunicable diseases in North America. Increasingly, affluence, modern living conditions, ignorance, and irresponsibility are being identified as the culprits in auto accidents, alcoholism, obesity, most heart disease, and even infant mortality.[1]

Although few people have viewed life-style as a major health problem in the past, it is apparent that many of our daily habits and modes of living, such as our increased consumption of animal fats and sugar-rich foods, our decreased expenditure of muscle energy, our persistent reliance upon cigarettes, drugs, and alcoholic beverages, and our susceptibility to tension, have combined to assault young, middle-aged, and older Americans alike. The responses have been, and will probably continue to be, a series of maladaptations. These are manifested slowly yet progressively over a period of years as heart and blood vessel diseases, serious conditions of overweight, malignant tumors, emphysema and chronic bronchitis, and drug dependencies. Such noncommunicable diseases are typically *chronic,* that is, long lasting and often permanent. Moreover, they are difficult to prevent, frequently have no known single cause, and are difficult to control because a maximum of human adaptation is too often involved. For instance,

> protecting a man against smallpox by vaccination is quick, simple, and effective. Asking this same man to protect himself from heart disease by losing twenty-five pounds and jogging several miles a week is a complex request which demands a change in his entire style of living.[2]

And yet, it is through such *adaptive, risk-reducing activity* that many of our noncommunicable diseases can be prevented and controlled. Although

> the adoption of a risk reduction program does not guarantee that one will not develop the disease, it does increase his chances of adding productive years to his life and/or reduces disability and discomfort.[3]

The advantages of adaptation are universally recognized, but changing human behavior is a difficult task, even when the individual is confronted with the prospects of serious, disabling noncommunicable diseases.

Among the noncommunicable diseases are the heart and blood-vessel disorders known as cardiovascular diseases. In this chapter we will focus on these

In patients with slow or irregular heart action, a pacemaker may be implanted to supply electrical impulses at regular intervals, causing the heart to beat regularly.

diseases, the leading cause of death in America. The next chapter will identify other chronic noncommunicable diseases.

The umbrella term *cardiovascular diseases* includes specific disease entities, such as *atherosclerosis, hypertension, rheumatic heart disease,* and *congenital heart defects.* These in turn may result in *heart attack, stroke,* and *congestive heart failure.* Together the cardiovascular diseases afflict more than 29 million Americans and claim more than a million lives each year in the United States. This latter figure actually represents more deaths than for all other causes combined, nearly 53 percent.[4] In terms of lost wages, lost productivity, and expenses for medical care, the cardiovascular diseases cost more than $28 billion annually.

The Heart and Blood Vessels

Food and oxygen are supplied to the body's cells and waste materials are removed from them by means of a special fluid tissue called *blood*. Composed of living cells (oxygen-carrying red blood cells, phagocytic white blood cells, and clot-inducing platelets) plus various chemical substances in solution, the approximately six quarts of blood are circulated again and again throughout nearly 60,000 miles of a closed network of tubelike blood vessels, the *arteries, veins,* and tiny interconnecting *capillaries*.

Arteries are thick-walled blood vessels that carry blood away from the heart to various parts of the body; veins are thin-walled and convey blood from various body parts back to the heart.[5] To accomplish this movement of blood, a muscular four-chambered pump, the *heart,* beats almost 100,000 times each day.

In reality, the heart functions as a double pump. The two chambers on the right side—the upper *atrium* and the lower *ventricle*—receive oxygen-poor blood from the returning veins and pump the blood to the lungs. There, the blood's waste gas of carbon dioxide is exchanged for an optimal level of oxygen. The left heart pump receives the oxygen-rich blood from the lungs in its upper chamber, the atrium. Then after passing into the lower left ventricle, the blood is pumped out through the major artery, the *aorta,* to be distributed eventually to all body cells by smaller arteries and the capillaries. To prevent the blood from any backward flow, the heart is equipped with four sets of *valves*—one between each atrium and ventricle, and one at the outlet of each ventricle. "Proper function of these small flaps of tissue spells the difference between health and sickness or life and death."[6]

As blood courses through the arteries, capillaries, and veins, it exerts a force against the blood vessel walls. Termed *blood pressure,* this force is greatest in the arteries and their branches, much lower in the capillaries, and lowest in the veins. In normal usage, however, the term blood pressure usually refers to the pressure in the arteries that supply the body, collectively referred to as the systemic circulation. Various factors influence blood pressure, including the amount and rate of blood flow, the capacity of the blood vessel itself, the heart's output of blood, the contraction of the muscle fibers in the walls of the smallest arterial branches, the activity of the autonomic nervous system, and the production of hormones (norepinephrine and epinephrine) by the adrenal glands positioned atop the kidneys. These several mechanisms function adaptively in regulating

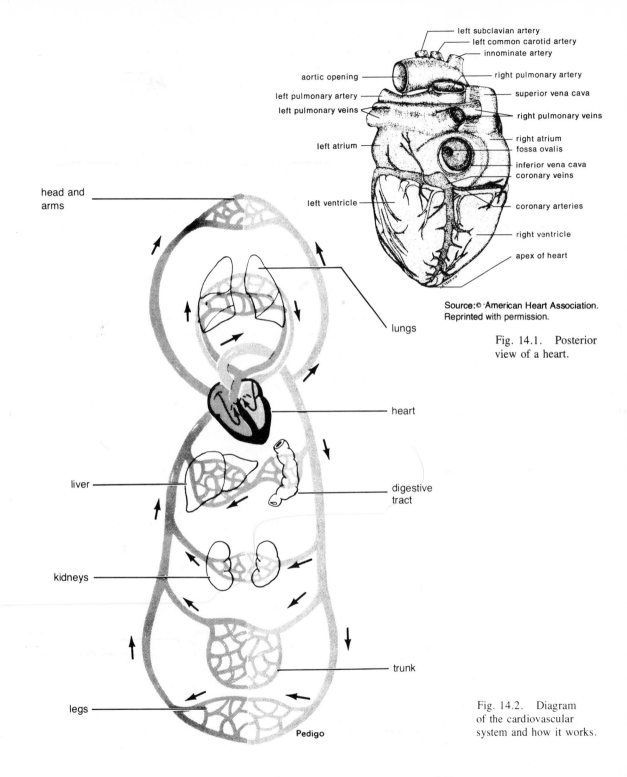

left subclavian artery
left common carotid artery
innominate artery
aortic opening
right pulmonary artery
left pulmonary artery
superior vena cava
left pulmonary veins
right pulmonary veins
left atrium
right atrium
fossa ovalis
inferior vena cava
coronary veins
left ventricle
coronary arteries
right ventricle
apex of heart

Source:© American Heart Association.
Reprinted with permission.

Fig. 14.1. Posterior view of a heart.

head and arms

lungs

heart

liver

digestive tract

kidneys

trunk

legs

Pedigo

Fig. 14.2. Diagram of the cardiovascular system and how it works.

heart action and systemic blood pressure to meet the changing circulatory needs of body organs and tissues.

Blood pressure is most often recorded with an instrument known as a *sphygmomanometer,* consisting of an inflatable cuff attached to a mercury meter. The blood pressure reading, expressed in millimeters of mercury, is a combination of two numbers:

> The higher of the two is the arterial pressure recorded during the heart's pumping stroke, or systole, and is called the systolic blood pressure. The lower number represents the arterial pressure prevailing while the heart relaxes and refills between beats and is called the diastolic pressure.[7]

In a relaxed, resting, young adult, the normal *systolic pressure* approximates 120 mm. of mercury, while the normal *diastolic pressure* is about 80. The blood pressure reading would be recorded as 120/80. However, other blood pressure readings somewhat below or above this average are also considered within the range of normalcy.

> For example, a blood pressure of 140/90 is within the normal range, whereas 150/95 is a little high. Systolic pressure tends to increase with age in healthy subjects. The rule of thumb—100 plus your age in years—provides a fairly good index of normal systolic pressure in adults.[8]

Unstable or persistently elevated blood pressure above a normal range is called high blood pressure or *hypertension.*

The precise and direct control of heart pumping action, and hence, the circulation of blood, is provided by a small mass of specialized cells, the *sino-atrial node* in the upper right chamber of the heart. This pacemaker node is controlled by brain stimuli and gives rise to electrical impulses that initiate contractions of the heart. "As the impulse charges through, the heart muscle contracts, and as it tightens, it compresses the blood-filled chambers to force blood out through the heart valves."[9]

For all the blood that passes through the chambers of the heart, none of it actually helps the living cells of this muscular pump. The heart is nourished, significantly, by the two *coronary arteries* arising from the aorta. These coronary arteries are primary targets of a degenerative process known as atherosclerosis.

Atherosclerosis
Underlying many tragic instances of *coronary artery disease, hypertension,* and *stroke* is a general pathological condition that causes the artery walls to become thick and hard and lose their elasticity. Known as *arteriosclerosis* or hardening of the arteries, it is responsible for nearly 84 percent of the deaths from cardiovascular diseases.[10] The most common form of arteriosclerosis is referred to specifically as *atherosclerosis,* a slow, progressive change in the inner layer of the artery wall. Characteristically, the smooth arterial lining becomes rough and thickened by soft fatty deposits called *plaques.* These plaques in turn are covered by a cap of fibrous scar tissue.

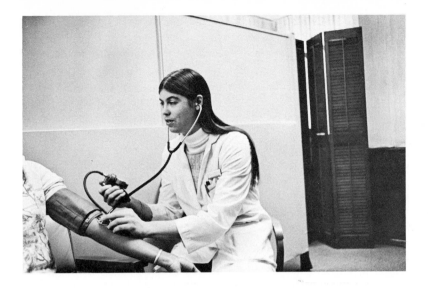

Fig. 14.3. A young doctor working in a health clinic of a large hospital takes a patient's blood pressure with a sphygmomanometer.

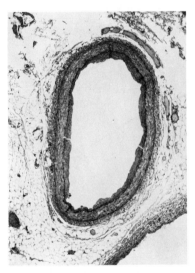

Fig. 14.4. The deterioration of a normal artery (left) is seen as *atherosclerosis* develops and begins to deposit fatty substances and to roughen the channel lining (center) until a clot forms (right) and plugs the artery. This deprives the heart muscle of vital blood and results in a heart attack.

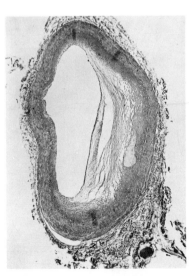

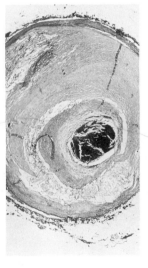

Cardiovascular Diseases: Preserving the Beat

Often beginning in childhood, the development of atherosclerosis "...may produce no symptoms for 20–40 years or longer. Even in advanced stages, it may be discovered only at post-mortem examination."[11] Although every artery is subject to the process of atherosclerosis, the most frequent and most severely affected targets are *the aorta, the coronary arteries that feed the heart, and the arteries that supply the brain and kidneys*. Unfortunately, nearly all adult American males and postmenopausal women are afflicted to some degree, indicating, perhaps, that this disease of blood vessels is the "disease of living."

Blood may infiltrate or hemorrhage into the plaque tissue, or an additional accumulation of blood fats may occur. Both of these actions may thereby contribute to growth of the plaque. More common, though, is the formation of blood clots on the plaque surface itself. (If a clot forms at the site of obstruction in an artery, the clot is called a *thrombus,* while a circulating clot that is carried to a smaller vessel before it blocks the arterial passageway is termed an *embolus.*) Eventually the innermost diameter of the artery is decreased in size, and the flow of blood through the arterial channel is slowed down or blocked altogether. As a consequence, the organ or tissue supplied by the diseased artery is deprived of oxygen and other life-sustaining substances and may die. The tissue area that is damaged or dies is termed an *infarct*.

Sometimes, though, cell death is avoided if *collateral circulation* develops. This is a remarkable form of blood flow in which

> neighboring arteries carry more blood than formerly to compensate for a narrowed vessel, and new arterial branches open up to help transport blood to where it is needed.[12]

Collateral circulation helps explain why many persons, even those with severe arteriosclerosis of the coronary arteries, do not suffer heart attacks and why some do not even experience the pain when the blood supply to the heart muscle is decreased. Recently scientists have used a newly developed mechanical pump, the counterpulsator, to speed the opening of the collateral vessel network in heart attack victims.

Coronary Heart Disease

When atherosclerosis occurs in the coronary arteries that supply the heart muscle (myocardium), the condition is described as *coronary heart disease* or CHD. Typically, there may be a narrowing of the artery reducing blood supply to the muscles, a saclike bulging (aneurysm) of the weakened arterial wall, or a rupture of the artery with loss of blood (hemorrhage) into the surrounding tissues.

With a decreased supply of blood flowing to the heart muscle, the result may be experienced as a pain located in the chest or arm. Such discomfort is termed *angina pectoris* and occurs intermittently with exercise, exposure to cold, and emotional stress, all of which temporarily increase the myocardium's demand for blood beyond the available supply. This pain usually subsides with rest or drug therapy. Nitroglycerin is often given to the individual to dilate the coronary arteries and thus relieve the pain.

If one of the large coronary arteries is blocked by a thrombus and heart muscle is suddenly deprived of its blood, the event is known as a *coronary occlusion*

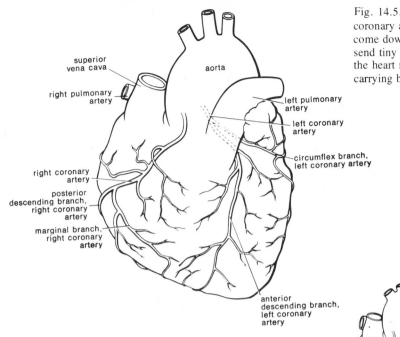

Fig. 14.5.   Coronary circulation. The main coronary arteries with their many branches come down over the top of the heart and send tiny branches down into all parts of the heart muscle to supply it with oxygen-carrying blood.

superior vena cava

aorta

right pulmonary artery

left pulmonary artery

left coronary artery

circumflex branch, left coronary artery

right coronary artery

posterior descending branch, right coronary artery

marginal branch, right coronary artery

anterior descending branch, left coronary artery

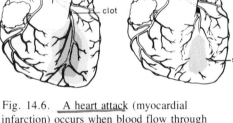

clot

scar

Fig. 14.6.   A heart attack (myocardial infarction) occurs when blood flow through the coronary arteries is obstructed, such as by formation of a clot. The clot (left) has blocked a main coronary branch, depriving the shadowed area of blood. The patient must remain quiet to speed the healing process at this early stage. Eight weeks or so later, (right) scar tissue has formed, and the patient may resume activities under a doctor's care.

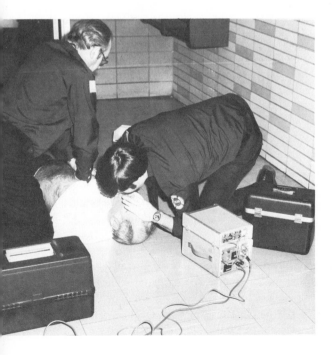

Fig. 14.7.   The men are members of the Fire Department's emergency intensive care unit, and have received the necessary training for emergency cardiopulmonary resuscitation.

(obstruction) or *coronary thrombosis*. The resulting damage or death of heart tissue is a *myocardial infarction* or *heart attack*. Another type of heart attack may occur when a fragment of the obstructing thrombus breaks off and continues to travel through a small artery until it (the clot fragment) becomes wedged in at a narrow point and thus forms a new blockage. Severe chest pain and pressure often occur prior to and during the heart attack. Like the symptoms of angina pectoris, the pain is usually strongest in the center of the chest and often radiates to shoulder, neck, jaw, and down the arms with a crushing, squeezing quality.

> Unlike anginal pain, however, it is not relieved by rest or the drugs generally used to treat angina, and it is usually much more intense and is frequently associated with other symptoms, particularly sweating and nausea.[13]

A person sustaining a suspected heart attack should be assisted in taking a comfortable position—usually halfway between lying down and sitting up. Do not attempt to lift or carry the individual. Keep the heart attack victim calm, loosen all tight clothing, and protect from overheating or chilling. Notify a physician or arrange for transportation of the victim to the nearest medical facility.

If extensive damage to heart muscle has occurred, the pumping performance of the heart may be so impaired that inadequate blood flows to various body organs. Kidney failure is a common complication along with accumulation of fluid in the body and congestion in the lungs. Abnormal heart rhythms also develop just after the myocardial infarction. The immediate mechanism of sudden death due to heart attack is thought to be total incoordination of heart contractions (ventricular fibrillation) with only feebly twitching ventricles or less frequently, cardiac standstill with motionless ventricles.[4]

Risk-Factors
in Coronary
Heart Disease

Findings from a long-term follow-up study of 5,209 Framingham, Massachusetts, adults (both men and women) begun in 1950 indicate that coronary heart disease occurs with increased frequency in association with certain constitutional and environmental characteristics. These characteristics have been termed risk-factors. The presence of one or more of these risk-factors in any individual will likely increase the possibility of atherosclerosis and its complications of coronary heart disease and stroke. Likewise, the modification or removal of one or more of these risk-factors will likely diminish the risk of such diseases.[15, 16, 17]

Age and Sex   Males are likely to develop more CHD earlier in life and in a more severe form than females. The relative immunity of females decreases with age, however. Despite this different incidence, CHD still constitutes the chief cause of death in both sexes.

Blood Lipids (Fats)   The risk of heart attack is proportional to the overall level of cholesterol, a fatlike substance, in the blood. A man with a blood cholesterol level of 250 mg. percent (250 mg. of cholesterol per 100 ml. of blood) or above has nearly three times the risk of CHD and stroke than does the man with a cholesterol reading below 194 mg. percent. Several other blood fats have also

What You Should Know About Heart Attack

An estimated 4,120,000 have coronary heart disease. 642,700 died of heart attack in 1975—350,000 before they reached the hospital. Many thousands of these might have been saved if the victims had heeded the signals.

Delay spells danger. When you suffer a heart attack, minutes—especially the first few minutes—count.

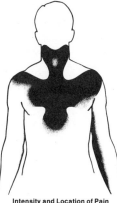

Intensity and Location of Pain

The signals of heart attack

- Uncomfortable pressure, fullness, squeezing or pain in center of chest lasting two minutes or more.

- Pain may spread to shoulders, neck or arms.

- Severe pain, dizziness, fainting, sweating, nausea or shortness of breath may also occur. Sharp, stabbing twinges of pain are usually not signals of a heart attack.

What You Should Know About Stroke

An estimated 1,840,000 persons are afflicted by stroke. Almost 200,000 suffered fatal strokes in 1975. Many fatal strokes can be prevented if high blood pressure, a leading cause of stroke, is diagnosed and controlled. Many major strokes are preceded by "little strokes" or warning signals experienced days, weeks, or months before the more severe event. Prompt medical or surgical attention to these symptoms may prevent a fatal or disabling stroke from occurring.

The warning signals of stroke

- Sudden, temporary weakness or numbness of the face, arm and leg on one side of the body.

- Temporary loss of speech, or trouble in speaking or understanding speech.

- Temporary dimness or loss of vision, particularly in one eye.

- Unexplained dizziness, unsteadiness or sudden falls.

Act immediately

Sometimes these symptoms subside, then return. When you experience one or more warning signs, call your doctor and describe these symptoms in detail. If he's not immediately available, get to a hospital emergency room at once. Be prepared to act. Instruct others to act if you cannot. Keep a list of numbers—doctor, hospital, ambulance or other emergency services and police—next to your telephone, and in a prominent place in your pocket, wallet, or purse.

Fig. 14.8. What you should know about heart attack and stroke. (Reprinted from *Heart Facts, 1978* with permission. © 1977, American Heart Association.)

Fig. 14.9. Hypertension prevalence by sex and race in U.S. adults age 20 and over, based on a 1975 estimate. Hypertension is often called the silent, mysterious killer, because it has no characteristic symptoms and in "90 percent of the cases the cause is unknown."

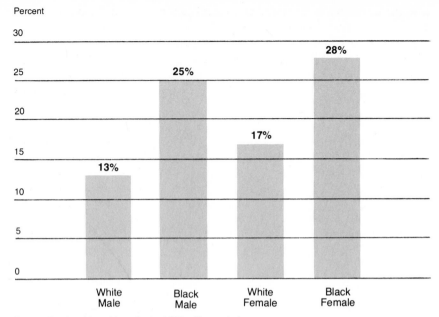

Source: Reprinted from *Heart Facts*, 1978, with permission.
© 1977, American Heart Association.

been incriminated in the development of atherosclerosis, although the exact blood fat responsible for plaque formation remains in doubt.

While the overall level of cholesterol remains a valid indicator for heart attack rate and stroke, medical research has revealed that one of the major fractions or subdivisions of cholesterol plays a protective role against coronary heart disease. This protective type of cholesterol, referred to as high-density lipoproteins (HDLs), decreases in the human body with age, as the damaging type of cholesterol—low-density lipoproteins (LDLs)—increases. However, with sustained and strenuous exercise, the level of beneficial HDLs can be maintained and developed.

Hypertension   The higher the blood pressure, the greater the risk of CHD in both males and females, especially when associated with blood fat abnormalities. The level of blood pressure, together with blood-fat values, apparently determines the general tendency to deposit plaques in the arterial walls.

Considered a disease process itself, *essential hypertension* is a persistently elevated blood pressure—a diastolic pressure in excess of 95 mm. of mercury—that cannot be attributed to any specific organic cause. More than 85 percent of all cases of hypertension fit into this category. The remainder constitute *secondary hypertension,* which is related to many possible factors: reduced arterial elasticity, kidney diseases or obstruction, excessive secretion of aldosterone (a hormone) that promotes retention of salt and water by the kidneys, emotional stress, and obesity (excessive deposition and storage of body fat). Sometimes tumors of the adrenal glands are thought to accelerate production of norepineph-

Chapter Fourteen

rine and epinephrine, hormones that raise blood pressure by stimulating heart action and constricting blood vessels.[18]

The higher and more sustained the blood pressure, the greater is the likelihood of damage to the blood vessels and the occurrence of CHD and stroke. In hypertension, the small peripheral arteries lose their elasticity and create resistance to normal blood flow. To overcome such resistance, the work load of the heart is increased. Unfortunately, with this added burden, the heart muscle often grows larger, weaker, and less efficient. Affecting an estimated twenty-three million adults in the United States, nearly half of whom are unaware of their problem, hypertension has no outstanding signs or symptoms. Although widely distributed in the general population, it is more prevalent among those twenty-five years of age or older, among males, and in the black population, with both males and females experiencing greater mortality rates than do their white counterparts.[19]

Antihypertensive drugs, and restriction of caloric intake and/or the exclusion of sodium from the diet have been successful in controlling high blood pressure if undertaken with the supervision of a physician.

Diabetes Mellitus and Impaired Carbohydrate Tolerance   Those persons with a tendency to diabetes mellitus (insulin deficiency, resulting in the body's inability to use carbohydrates, particularly sugar) have an increased risk of coronary heart disease. The exact relationship between diabetes mellitus and atherosclerosis remains unknown, although blood fat abnormalities usually appear several years before the onset of overt diabetic conditions.

Electrocardiogram (ECG) Abnormalities   Traits of atherosclerosis, especially critically narrowed coronary arteries, are often detected by electrocardiogram (ECG) examination prior to symptoms of the disease. The electrocardiograph is a device that measures the progress of the electrical impulse generated by the heart as the electric wave spreads throughout the heart chambers. The device produces a graphic representation (electrocardiogram) of the heart's electrical activity by means of a tracing recorded on graph paper. Diseased heart tissue gives rise to an electric pattern very different from that of healthy tissue.[20]

Diet   Evidence linking the occurrence of CHD with the quality of diet is presently lacking. Nevertheless, many scientists believe that relatively high blood cholesterol levels are related to high intake of animal fat and cholesterol in one's diet. It is probable that

> the excess of calories, which is derived largely from high in-take of saturated fat and refined carbohydrate, has contributed to the generally high blood lipid concentrations, impaired carbohydrate tolerance, and hypertension, and certainly to the obesity which may to some extent underlie them all.[21]

Because of the current interest in altering the amount and kind of fats consumed by the American population, the following definitions of fats are given:[22]

1. *Saturated fat*—a fat chemically constituted so that it is not capable of absorbing any more hydrogen. Usually solid fats of animal origin, saturated fats are

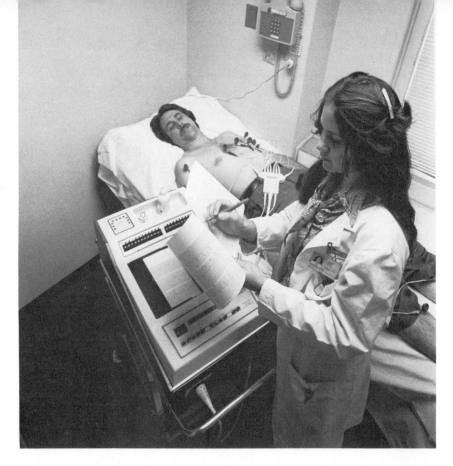

Fig. 14.10. An electrocardiogram is a graphic representation of the heart's electrical activity. The ECG pattern of a diseased heart is different from that of a healthy heart.

present in milk, eggs, butter, and meat. A diet high in saturated fat tends to increase the amount of cholesterol in the blood.

2. *Monounsaturated fat*—a fat chemically constituted so that it is capable of absorbing additional hydrogen but not as much as does a polyunsaturated fat. These fats, contained in olive oil, peanuts, chicken, turkey, and duck, have little effect on the amount of cholesterol in the blood.

3. *Polyunsaturated fat*—a fat chemically constituted so that it is capable of absorbing additional hydrogen. These fats are usually liquid oils of vegetable origin, such as corn oil, safflower oil, soybean oil, and sunflower oil, and herring oil and other fish oils. A diet with a high polyunsaturated fat content tends to lower the amount of cholesterol in the blood.

Physical Inactivity   The most sedentary (physically inactive) persons appear to have a significantly higher death rate due to CHD than individuals who exercise regularly. Among the many benefits of physical activity are a reduction of stress, possible protection against heart attacks, and the promotion of collateral circulation, which prepares the cardiovascular system to survive a coronary thrombosis or myocardial infarction should one occur. However, a program of activity for sedentary individuals should be initiated gradually. Persons over forty should undertake such a program only after a physician has determined the functional capacity of their cardiovascular system.

Obesity Formerly described in terms of desirable weight in relation to height and age, obesity is more properly defined qualitatively as "...an excess relative fat content."[23] Results of the Framingham study indicated that the risk of CHD—particularly angina pectoris and sudden death—was significantly increased in obese persons, and the risk increased with the degree of obesity. Such an increased risk is associated not only with excessive consumption of sugar-rich foods and animal fats—and hence elevated blood cholesterol levels, but also with the increased work load placed upon the heart, perhaps already damaged by atherosclerosis.

Cigarette Usage Inhaled cigarette smoke contributes to the incidence of heart attack as well as stroke. Males who smoked one pack of cigarettes or more per day had nearly twice the risk of sustaining a heart attack and three or more times the risk of a sudden death than did nonsmokers. However, no relationship was evident between CHD and either cigar or pipe smoking. While the duration of cigarette smoking was not significant in the study, the risk of heart disease increased with the number of cigarettes smoked per day. Framingham data further suggest that

> cigarette smoking has a relative immediate effect, triggering coronary attacks in susceptible persons rather than an influence which promotes atherosclerosis.[24]

A more complete analysis of cigarette use in relation to cardiovascular and other diseases is presented in the chapter on smoking.

Psychosocial Tensions Personal life situations inherent in cultural circumstances may also play a part in the origin of heart disease. Studies have revealed that social and geographic mobility, urbanization, emotional crises, and unusual fatigue serve to condition, aggravate, and even precipitate acute events of heart attack and stroke. This is especially true in individuals with preexisting severe atherosclerotic disease.[25] However, these findings were not derived from the Framingham data, and the actual involvement of the central nervous system in the development of CHD remains a controversial possibility.

In a prospective study on CHD among 3,524 subjects, researchers have identified a specific overt behavior pattern, designated pattern type A, that appears to be a significant risk-factor when found in combination with elevated blood pressure or elevated blood fats.[26] Additional studies by Friedman and Rosenman have clearly demonstrated that type A traits are closely linked with the origin of coronary artery disease and heart disease. They describe the type A behavior pattern as

> an action-emotion complex that can be observed in any person who is *aggressively* involved in a *chronic, incessant* struggle to achieve more and more in less and less time, and if required to do so, against the opposing efforts of other things or other persons.[27]

Type A behavior is neither a psychosis nor a neurosis, but a frequently praised and socially acceptable form of conflict. The coronary-prone type A person is characterized by excessive drive and aggressiveness and is subject to vocational deadlines and similar pressures. Afflicted with the so-called "hurry sickness," such an individual attempts to undertake too much or participate in too many activities in the amount of time allotted for such events. Thus the type A person is time-conscious—preoccupied with saving time or stretching time. The type A individual is also more likely to be restless, perfectionistic, impatient, self-centered, unobservant of the environment, and a rapid walker and eater.[28]

In contrast, the type B person, who is less coronary-prone, is characterized by the relative absence of type A behaviors. Type B individuals are generally more easygoing, less impatient, and less competitive. Additionally, they have no free-floating hostility, are less concerned with climbing the social ladder, and can relax without feeling guilty and can work without agitation or irritation.

| Reducing the Risks of Coronary Heart Disease | Multiple risk-factors in the same individual indicate high vulnerability to atherosclerosis, CHD, stroke, and peripheral artery disease. Because there is not much one can do about age, sex, and genetic factors influencing body chemistry, it does seem wise to correct certain of the risk-factors as early as possible, even during young adulthood. Such adaptive endeavors substantially reduce the chances of sustaining cardiovascular diseases and increase the potential for recovery should a coronary thrombosis occur. In fact, during the past twenty years, the death rate from cardiovascular diseases has dropped by nearly 25 percent among American men and women. In one recent year alone, the death rate for heart disease was lower by 5 percent and that for stroke by 9 percent over the previous one-year period.[29] Scientists generally credit such increasing freedom from heart attack and stroke to healthy changes in life-style, such as those listed below. |

1. Stop smoking cigarettes. If you cannot refrain from smoking, then cut down on the number smoked and try not to inhale the smoke.
2. Engage in some strenuous physical activity on a regular basis. A high amount of energy expended weekly in exercises that demand "bursts of energy output" appears to provide some protection against premature heart attacks. In addition, a high level of activity promotes collateral coronary circulation and helps "...prevent overweight problems with the attendant benefits of lower fat levels, lower blood pressure and reduced cardiac work load."[30]

   Activities such as jogging, walking, swimming, bicycling, backpacking, basketball, handball, and squash—those that cause sustained cardiovascular stress—are popular activities that promote fitness for the heart and blood vessels. Some research physiologists now believe that the protective effect resulting from physical activity alone seems to hold even when other risk factors are still present in an individual. Tennis, golf, bowling, baseball, and volleyball do not seem to provide sustained stress on the cardiovascular system and are significantly less beneficial.

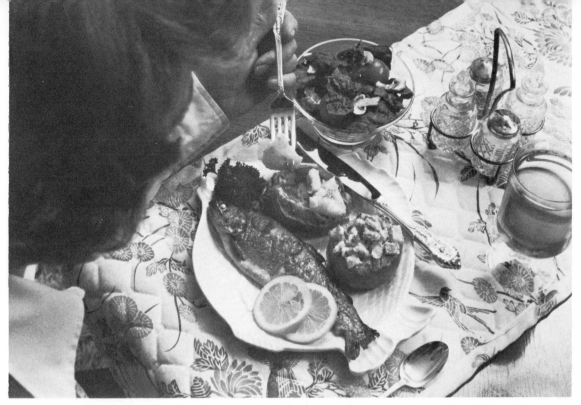

Fig. 14.11. This meal of fish, potato, tomato, spinach salad, and iced tea is well balanced and low in fats and calories—just the menu for a person who wants a healthy heart.

3. Adjust caloric intake to achieve and maintain optimal weight. However, one's diet should be nutritionally balanced in terms of the basic four food groups: *milk and dairy products,* two cups or the equivalent; *meats,* two or more servings; *fruits and vegetables,* four or more servings; and *breads and cereals,* four or more servings. (Number of servings represent daily adult recommendations.)

4. Substitute polyunsaturated fats for a portion of the saturated fats in the daily diet. Increase the use of poultry, fish, and lean cuts of red meat; low-fat dairy products, salad and cooking oils; soft margarines low in saturated fat; grains; fruits; vegetables; and legumes. Reduce consumption of fat cuts of meat, egg yolks, bacon, lard, suet, and butter.[31]

5. Get regular medical checkups to detect hypertension and early evidence of atherosclerosis. Then follow the instructions of your physician in relation to recommended therapies and other preventive activities.

6. Reduce stress through modifications in life-style, such as regularly planned, vigorous, physical exercise, which tends to relieve anxiety and tension. Consideration should also be given to setting more realistic life goals that can be attained, perhaps even a change of residence or occupation if your response to stress is health-damaging. Free yourself of "hurry sickness" by eliminating as many events and activities as possible that do not contribute to your social and economic well-being.[32] Counter feelings of hostility by developing a sense of humor and learning to laugh at yourself. Learning to control one's

Cardiovascular Diseases: Preserving the Beat   359

emotional reactions to daily events may also be useful in reducing stress. When someone advises you to "keep your cool," it may be good advice. Consult the chapter on mental health for more specific ways of coping with stress in your daily life.

Cerebrovascular Accidents (Stroke)

The blood vessels supplying the brain, the cerebral arteries, are sometimes ravaged with atherosclerosis and/or hypertension. When either condition exists, there is the possibility of a reduction of the cerebral circulation. Such an impeded blood supply to the brain is known as a cerebrovascular accident (CVA), stroke, or cerebral apoplexy. Cerebral thrombosis or embolism may contribute to the blockage of the arterial passageways. Sustained hypertension frequently results in the rupture of a blood vessel wall with hemorrhage into the surrounding tissues, thus interfering with normal blood supply to brain cells. The severity of a CVA is usually determined by the extent of cell damage (cerebral infarction) and the body's ability to repair or restore the blood supply to the injured area via collateral circulation.

Because different areas of the brain control various physical and mental functions, the symptoms of a CVA may include paralysis of a limb, loss of speech, loss of balance, visual disturbances, difficulty in swallowing, and disturbed mentation. Such effects may be slight or severe, temporary or permanent. Major CVAs kill about 200,000 persons each year in the United States—mostly among the elderly. But at least a quarter million individuals between twenty-five and sixty-four years of age are crippled physically or mentally by strokes annually.[33]

Risk-factors of CVA are similar to those of coronary heart disease, as are the risk-reduction activities. The recent decline in deaths due to stroke is the result of advances in the control of hypertension, detected by a physician and treated with appropriate drugs or modern blood vessel surgery. Through intensive and early rehabilitation procedures, many stroke victims have been restored to full or partial functioning.

Rheumatic Heart Disease

Formerly one of the most dreaded diseases of children and young adults, rheumatic heart disease has been largely prevented by antibiotic drug therapy. Heart damage sustained can often be repaired through surgical procedures. Nevertheless, more than 1.7 million children and adults are victims of this heart disease today.[34]

Typically, the individual is infected with disease-inciting streptococcal bacteria that produce a severe sore throat (strep throat) or scarlet fever (strep throat with a skin rash). Following recovery, an allergic reaction develops into a chronic inflammation of several body areas. This inflammatory condition, rheumatic fever, often attacks the joints, lungs, brain, and heart. If the heart is afflicted, the valves are damaged, scar tissue is formed and circulation of blood through the heart chambers is impaired. Only one to three of every 100 patients with strep infections develops rheumatic fever and ". . . only half of those who do will develop heart disease."[35]

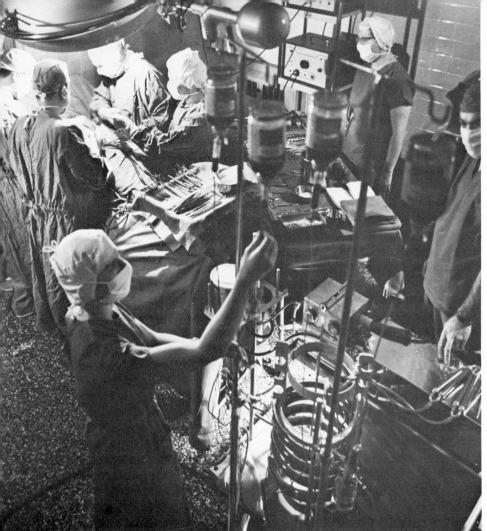

Fig. 14.12. Significant advances have been made recently in repairing congenital and acquired cardiovascular abnormalities. Surgery is often used as a treatment to repair and replace damaged portions of the heart and blood vessels. In some instances, surgical techniques have been useful in preventing the later development of more serious heart-blood vessel disorders.

Fig. 14.13. In cardiac catheterization, shown here, either the heart or its blood vessels may be studied by injecting a radiopaque dye directly into the heart chambers or into the coronary vessels. Then the function and circulation of the heart are studied with X rays.

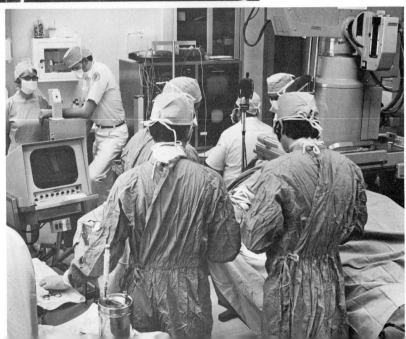

In the past, victims of rheumatic heart disease were treated as "cardiac cripples." Today, in many cases, severe restriction of physical activity is not considered desirable, and a return to normal functioning is encouraged. However, one
attack of rheumatic fever seems to predispose to another, so prolonged antibiotic
administration is continued on a daily basis to keep the strep bacteria under control. A recurrence of rheumatic heart disease can be stopped only by preventing
another strep infection.

Other
Cardiovascular
Diseases

Structural heart abnormalities due to faulty embryonic development and present
at birth are referred to as *congenital heart disease*. Both heredity and hazardous
environmental factors, such as viral infections and drug-induced trauma, have
been identified as possible causes. In general, the fetal heart or major blood
vessels near the heart fail to mature normally before birth. Due to advances in
surgical procedures, many such defects can be repaired, including holes in the
dividing walls between ventricles, narrowing of the aorta, prenatal channels that
continue to function after birth, and misplacement of the aorta. A common abnormality is manifest as a *blue baby*. The congenital defect permits returning
venous blood to leave the heart via the aorta without first being oxygenated in the
lungs. The low oxygen content of the blood accounts for the blueness of the skin,
a physiological condition known as *cyanosis*. Fortunately, this blue-baby condition can be surgically corrected today.

An arterial wall with weak spots due to heredity, injury, or disease sometimes
balloons out dangerously in the weakened area. This ballooning condition is
called an *arterial aneurysm* and poses a threat of rupture and hemorrhage if not
surgically treated. In addition to aneurysm, arteries near the periphery of the
body, that is, in the legs, can sustain arteriosclerosis. This results in impaired
circulation (arteriosclerosis obliterans) and in some rare instances leads to gan-
grene or tissue death, thus necessitating amputation.

A common blood-vessel disorder is a condition in which the veins become
dilated and tortuous. Known as *varicose veins*, they are prevalent in people who
stand for long periods of time. This uncomfortable condition is often accompanied by malfunctioning venous valves, which results in stagnation of blood
within the veins and swelling. Effective treatment usually includes the wearing
of elastic stockings or surgical removal of the affected superficial vessels.

A blood clot (thrombus) may obstruct the veins, giving rise to an inflammatory
condition referred to as *thrombophlebitis*, a frequent complication of pregnancy.
If a thrombus fragments in a vein, a circulating clot or embolus may be carried in
the blood to the lungs where blockage of a blood vessel occurs. Termed *pulmonary embolism*, this obstruction can result in physiological shock or death. Recognizing that both thrombophlebitis and pulmonary embolism can occur as undesirable side effects in women taking oral contraceptives, most physicians agree
that "...nine months of the use of oral contraceptives by a *normal* woman is
statistically less hazardous in respect to thrombophlebitis than normal pregnancy."[36] Of course, the use of oral contraceptives is not generally recommended for any patient with a history of heart or blood vessel disease, including
thrombophlebitis.

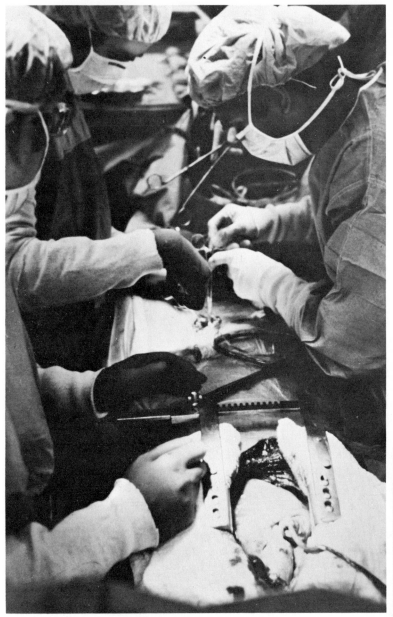

Fig. 14.14. Cardiovascular surgery is a complicated procedure. The chest is opened completely through the breastbone and held open with large metal retractors. The blood vessels for the heart and lungs are connected by tubes to a heart-lung machine, which temporarily takes over their functions. The heart looks white in this photo because it is not functioning.

Fig. 14.15. By taking over the functions of both heart and lungs, the heart-lung machine permits surgeons to operate on and inside the heart. As the machine pumps and oxygenates the blood, the relaxed heart can be opened to correct defects.

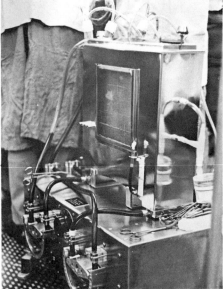

Cardiovascular Diseases: Preserving the Beat

Cardiovascular Treatment As Adaptation	Many persons seem unwilling or unable to implement a risk-reduction program in relation to cardiovascular disease. Indeed, the nature of such adaptive behavior might appear spartan or even austere to those who have tasted the life-style of affluence and luxury. Self-discipline and denial are somewhat foreign to a modern life of self-indulgence. And yet, physiologically, it is apparent that a life of scarcity and a life of activity are truly beneficial to the human organism. The chances for a disabling illness or a premature death can be reduced through preventive measures.

In 1978, Americans showed a lower mortality rate from heart disease and lower levels of cholesterol and fats in the blood. These improvements were attributed to the use of medication and healthful changes in life-style.

When risk reduction is not undertaken or proves ineffective, heart and blood vessel diseases sometimes occur. Now the adaptation is focused on the diseased organ or tissue, to restore reasonably normal function. Drug therapy has proven most successful in treating hypertension. High blood pressure is reduced through administration of mild sedatives or tranquilizers, diuretics, and drugs that suppress the activity of the sympathetic nervous system. Anticoagulant drugs delay clotting and thus reduce the chances of recurring strokes and heart attack. Digitalis, one of the oldest known drugs, is still used to increase the pumping function of the heart muscle. Antibiotics are most effective in combating heart infections.

Defective heart valves are replaced with artificial devices made of precious metals, Dacron, and plastic. Worn-out areas of the aorta and other blood vessels are repaired with Teflon. Irregular and inefficient heartbeats can be made smooth and even by the surgical implantation of an artificial pacemaker with long-lasting batteries or piezoelectric crystals that change mechanical energy to electricity. Ventricular assist devices, including the DeBakey left ventricular bypass pump, have a great potential for saving lives of heart attack victims.[37]

Various surgical techniques have been developed to correct many of the congenital heart defects and to remove localized arterial obstructions. However, none has proven as spectacular or as challenging to medical scientists as that of human heart transplantation. The operation involves the removal of a healthy heart from a dead donor and its rapid transplantation into a recipient with a diseased heart. Unless the blood-tissue type between donor and recipient is quite similar, the recipient may reject the transplanted heart whose tissues are chemically recognized as foreign invaders. In fact, certain white blood cells of the recipient produce antibodies that fight the donor's gift and eventually destroy the heart transplant. To reduce the rejection process, large doses of X rays or immunosuppressive drugs and antilymphocyte globulin are administered to the recipient.[38]

While human heart transplants have added months and even years of productive life to a limited number of heart disease victims, the future use of completely artificial hearts holds even greater promise for the population at large. Presently being researched is an implanted auxiliary pump or booster heart that can ease the work load of a patient's heart until it is able to resume its normal function.[39]

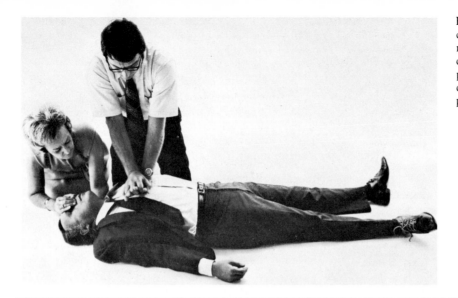

Fig. 14.16. Emergency cardiopulmonary resuscitation, as demonstrated in the photo, should only be done by a trained person.

If someone close to you experiences the warning signals of either heart attack or stroke, your immediate care and action may mean the difference between life and death. In every case, a physician should be called or the victim should be transported to the emergency room of the nearest hospital. So be familiar with the telephone numbers of the potential victim's doctor, an emergency ambulance service, or the local police. Other basic life support techniques vary according to the warning signs displayed by the victim.

In the event of a probable heart attack, in addition to summoning emergency care, you may try the following:

1. Administer to the conscious victim prescribed heart medication. Persons known to be subject to heart attack often carry with them the proper medication. When giving such medicine, be sure to read the label on the container first and then give the victim only the recommended dose.
2. Place the victim in a comfortable position, usually partially sitting up, especially if shortness of breath accompanies the heart attack.
3. Loosen tight-fitting clothing, such as ties and collars.
4. Stay with the victim and offer reassurance to calm fears and the sense of impending death that sometimes occurs.
5. Perform basic life support techniques of cardiopulmonary resuscitation (CPR) in certain instances. Such a procedure should be administered only by a trained individual and then only when the victim is not breathing and there is no heartbeat or pulse. As described by the American Heart Association:

CPR involves a combination of mouth-to-mouth breathing, or other ventilation techniques, and chest compression. This technique provides basic emergency life support until more advanced life support is available. More important, it keeps oxygenated blood flowing to the brain until appropriate medical treatment can restore normal heart action.[40]

Emergency Care As Adaptation

In the event of a probable stroke or cerebrovascular accident, in addition to summoning emergency care, you may try the following:

1. Place the victim in a reclining or semireclining position on a bed or sofa.
2. Avoid moving the individual any more than is absolutely necessary.
3. Remove any loose dental bridges or false teeth.
4. Elevate the conscious victim's head slightly. However, if breathing is difficult, be sure to turn the head to one side so as to allow fluids in the mouth to drain out. If the victim is unconscious, keep the person flat or turned on the side to allow secretions to drain from the mouth.

Your wise, appropriate, and immediate actions may help you preserve the pulse of life, the flow of blood, and the beat of the heart. What a wonderful way to show someone how much you care and how much you love!

Summary

Specific cardiovascular diseases, which kill more individuals than any other noncommunicable disease processes, have been described in this chapter. Emphasis was placed on coronary heart disease, with a description of known or suspected risk-factors together with risk-reducing activities. Various treatments for cardiovascular diseases as well as emergency care procedures were examined as adaptive countermeasures for victims of heart and blood vessel disorders. In the following chapter other noncommunicable diseases that plague Americans will be considered.

Review Questions

1. Why are present-day cardiovascular diseases harder to prevent and cure than the major communicable diseases of the past?
2. How does *adaptation* play a vital role in preventing disease today?
3. Explain the various parts of the heart. Follow the flow of blood from the heart throughout the body.
4. What is hypertension? How is it detected?
5. Differentiate between atherosclerosis and arteriosclerosis. Which specific areas do they affect?
6. Discuss the risk-factors associated with coronary heart disease. How can they be avoided?
7. Differentiate between saturated fats, mono- and polyunsaturated fats. Which one is potentially most harmful to the body?
8. What are the symptoms of cerebrovascular accidents (CVA)? Is their damage always permanent?
9. Why have we seen a large increase in cardiovascular diseases in the past fifty years?

Notes

1. Anne R. Somers, "The Nation's Health: Issues for the Future," *The Annals of the American Academy of Political and Social Science*, January 1972, p. 161.
2. Carter L. Marshall and David Pearson, *Dynamics of Health and Disease* (New York: Appleton-Century-Crofts, 1972), p. 129.
3. Wesley P. Cushman, *Reducing the Risk of Noncommunicable Diseases* (Dubuque, Iowa: Wm. C. Brown Co., 1970), p. viii.
4. American Heart Association, *Heart Facts, 1978* (Dallas, Texas: The Association, 1977), pp. 2–3.
5. U.S. Department of Health, Education, and Welfare, *A Handbook of Heart Terms* (Washington, D.C.: U.S. Government Printing Office, 1968), pp. 5, 63.
6. Brendan Phibbs, *The Human Heart* (St. Louis: C. V. Mosby Co., 1967), p. 5.
7. National Heart Institute, *Hypertension: High Blood Pressure* (Washington, D.C.: U.S. Government Printing Office, 1969), p. 4.
8. Ibid., p. 5.
9. American Heart Association, *1973 Heart Facts* (New York: The Association, 1973), p. 3.
10. National Heart and Lung Institute, *National Heart, Blood Vessel, Lung, and Blood Program*, vol. 1 (Washington, D.C.: U.S. Government Printing Office, 1973), p. 6.
11. National Heart and Lung Institute Task Force on Arteriosclerosis, *Arteriosclerosis*, vol. 1 (Washington, D.C.: U.S. Government Printing Office, 1971), p. 3.
12. National Heart and Lung Institute, *Hardening of the Arteries: Cause of Heart Attacks* (Washington, D.C.: U.S. Government Printing Office, 1975), p. 8.
13. Christiaan Barnard, *Heart Attack: You Don't Have to Die* (New York: Dell Publishing Co., 1973), p. 103.
14. National Heart and Lung Institute Task Force, *Arteriosclerosis*, p. 6.
15. William B. Kannel and Thomas R. Dawber, "Contributors to Coronary Risk Implications for Prevention and Public Health: The Framingham Study," *Heart and Lung*, November-December 1972, pp. 797–809.
16. Tavia Gordon and William B. Kannel, "Predisposition to Atherosclerosis in the Head, Heart, and Legs," *Journal of the American Medical Association* 221 (14 August 1972): 661–66.
17. National Heart and Lung Institute Task Force, *Arteriosclerosis*.
18. National Heart Institute, *Hypertension*, pp. 10–12.
19. American Heart Association, *1973 Heart Facts*, p. 4.
20. Phibbs, *The Human Heart*, pp. 158–59.
21. Kannel and Dawber, "Contributors to Coronary Risk," p. 802.
22. U.S. Department of HEW, *Handbook of Heart Terms*, pp. 54, 40, 49.
23. Jean Mayer, Introduction, "Obesity," *Postgraduate Medicine*, May 1972, p. 66.
24. Kannel and Dawber, *Contributors to Coronary Risk*, p. 804.
25. Inter-Society Commission for Heart Disease Resources, "Primary Prevention of the Atherosclerotic Diseases," *Circulation*, December 1970, p. A-71.
26. Ray H. Rosenman, Meyer Friedman et al., "Coronary Heart Disease in the Western Collaborative Group Study," *Journal of the American Medical Association* 195 (10 January 1966): 86–92.
27. Meyer Friedman and Ray H. Rosenman, *Type A Behavior and Your Heart* (Greenwich, Conn.: Fawcett Publications, Inc., 1974), p. 84.
28. Ibid., pp. 100–102.
29. National Center for Health Statistics, *Monthly Vital Statistics Report* 25 (11 February 1977): 2.
30. Cushman, *Reducing the Risk of Noncommunicable Diseases*, p. 5.
31. Inter-Society Commission for Heart Disease Resources, "Primary Prevention of the Atherosclerotic Diseases," p. A-87.
32. Friedman and Rosenman, *Type A Behavior and Your Heart*, p. 236.
33. National Heart and Lung Institute, National Heart Program, p. 6.
34. American Heart Association, *Heart Facts, 1978*, p. 10.
35. Phibbs, *The Human Heart*, p. 42.
36. J. Edwin Wood, "The Cardiovascular Effects of Oral Contraceptives," *Modern Concepts of Cardiovascular Disease*, August 1972, p. 39.
37. National Heart Institute, *Cardiovascular Surgery* (Washington, D.C.: U.S. Government Printing Office, 1968), p. 46.
38. William A. Nolen, *Spare Parts for the Human Body* (New York: Random House, 1971), pp. 61–62.
39. American Heart Association, *Heart Facts, 1978*, p. 14.
40. Ibid., p. 19.

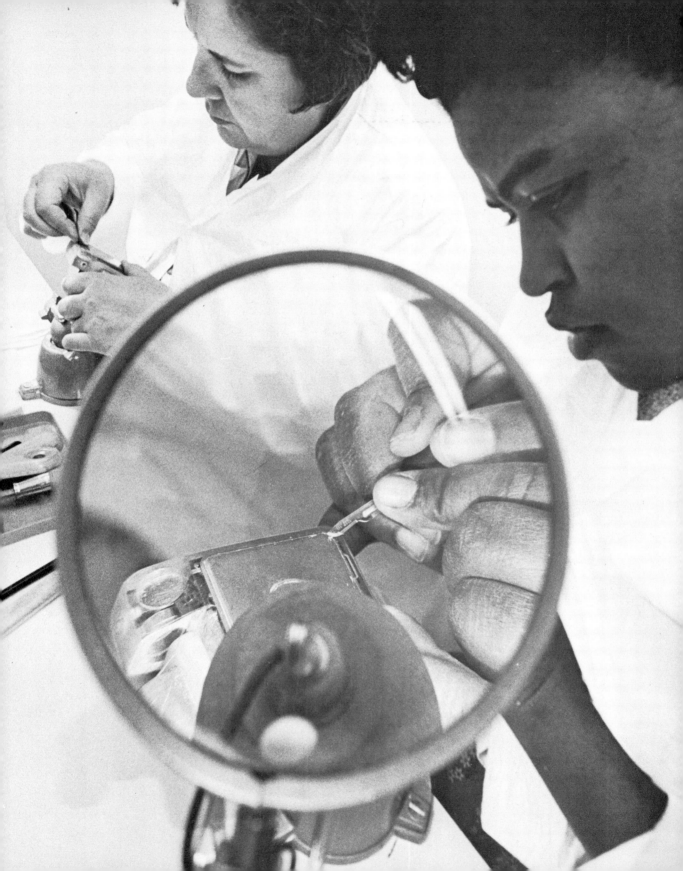

Modern Plagues: Cancer and Other Noncommunicable Diseases

15

In addition to the heart and blood vessel conditions discussed in the preceding chapter, there are many other noncommunicable diseases that have challenged the coping ability of millions of persons. These modern plagues can affect an individual in different ways, at varying phases in the human life cycle, and for diverse lengths of time.

No doubt the most feared of these diseases is cancer. So little is known by many people about this dreaded affliction, yet it ranks only behind the cardiovascular diseases as the major cause of death among Americans. However, public attitudes about cancer are changing. Now it is being talked about, dealt with, and in many cases conquered. Fortunately, early detection and improved treatment give promise of controlling, if not eliminating, many cancerous conditions that contribute significantly to disability and death.

Cancer

Throughout the human life cycle new cellular growth occurs, for example, in the increase in size during adolescence, in tissue repair and the formation of scar tissue following injury, and in the enlargement of a kidney after removal of its diseased partner. All these are generally favorable adaptations to some physical condition or the result of genetically controlled and regulated cellular reproduction. However, cells sometimes proliferate without control and produce a mass of new cells that serve no useful function. This abnormal, unwanted, nonfunctional new cell mass is called a *tumor* or *neoplasm*.[1]

What Is Cancer?

A tumor is described as *benign* if the new cell mass remains a localized, nonspreading, and usually nonlife-threatening growth. Such a growth is enclosed by a limiting fibrous membrane. Once removed by surgery, benign tumors do not recur.

Nomadic Anarchists   Unfortunately, some tumor cells have such a "lust for life" and exaggerated need for living space that they invade nearby tissues with clawlike protrusions and interfere with the function and nourishment of neighboring organs. A tumor with such behavioral characteristics is referred to as a *malignancy* (malignant tumor) or *cancer.* Sometimes the cells travel through the bloodstream and lymphatic system to establish distant colonies of secondary growths called *metastases.* This process of colonization is termed *metastasis* and is responsible for the reappearance of the growth after the original cell mass has

369

been removed surgically. Showing total disregard for the rights of other cells to function without disturbance, cancer cells are truly the nomadic anarchists of the human body.

Cellular Autonomy   Cancer cells grow rapidly in an uncontrolled manner. Their invasive qualities permit them to attack and destroy normal tissues and organs, often resulting in the death of the afflicted person. This display of semi-independent behavior is called cellular autonomy and is related to the cells' loss of growth control processes.

> Normal cells stick to one another and have a "home" of their own. A kidney cell stays in the kidney and a lung cell in the lung. Cancer cells may be said to belong nowhere, to have no proper residence, no "home."[2]

Anaplasia   When cancer cells are viewed under a microscope, they are identified by their loss of normal appearance, a characteristic known as anaplasia.

> The individual cells vary in size and shape, and the orderly orientation of normal cells is replaced by disorganization that may be so complete that no recognizable structures remain.[3]

Cellular Phases   Manifest by autonomy and anaplasia, cancer is now considered to be the result of changes in cellular metabolism (chemical processes) and cellular reproduction. Both of these functions are governed by the nucleic acids, DNA and RNA. Once genetic alterations have occurred, the changed cell may die; it may divide and evolve into a malignant tumor; or it may remain dormant unless some environmental stimulus causes it to start dividing.[4] While the precise mechanism for such changes in human cells remains a mystery, the cancerous process is usually distinguished by three *cellular phases*.[5]

- The *initiation* phase of genetic modification
- The *promotion* phase from dormancy to visibility
- The *progression* phase leading to the irreversible state of abnormality

These three stages of cancer cell development allow for the concept of reversibility in cellular changes and the commonly observed phenomenon of *regression,* the cessation of growth or disappearance of the neoplasm (tumor) with a decline of symptoms.

As we have seen, the cancerous mass of abnormal cells undergoes something of a progression. Beginning as a localized disease, the disordered cells divide and form the enlarged neoplasm. The majority of cancerous growths typically remain at the site of origin, that is, "in situ." Then after a variable time, some of the cancer cells penetrate adjoining tissues. The growth has become invasive. Even after this act of expansion, cancer cells often remain intact before metastasis occurs. But regional involvement ensues and eventually the advanced stage of cancer is reached wherein the nomadic anarchists spread to distant body parts. If cancer is not arrested or destroyed before advanced metastasis sets in, death often occurs.[6]

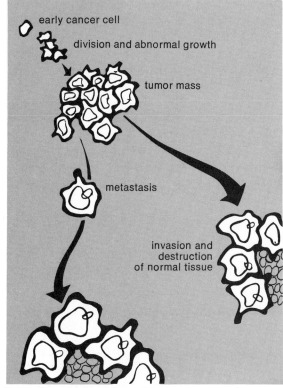

early cancer cell

division and abnormal growth

tumor mass

metastasis

invasion and
destruction
of normal tissue

Source: National Advisory Cancer Council

Fig. 15.1. Cancer cells
progress by division,
abnormal growth,
and destructive
invasiveness of nearby
normal tissue. At an
advanced stage, cancer
cells spread through
the blood or lymph to
other sites to form
new growths.

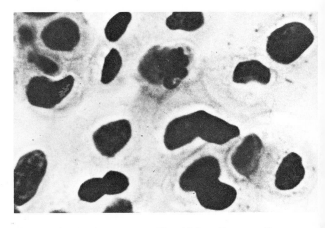

Fig. 15.2. Cancer cells
of the uterine cervix,
true nomadic
anarchists

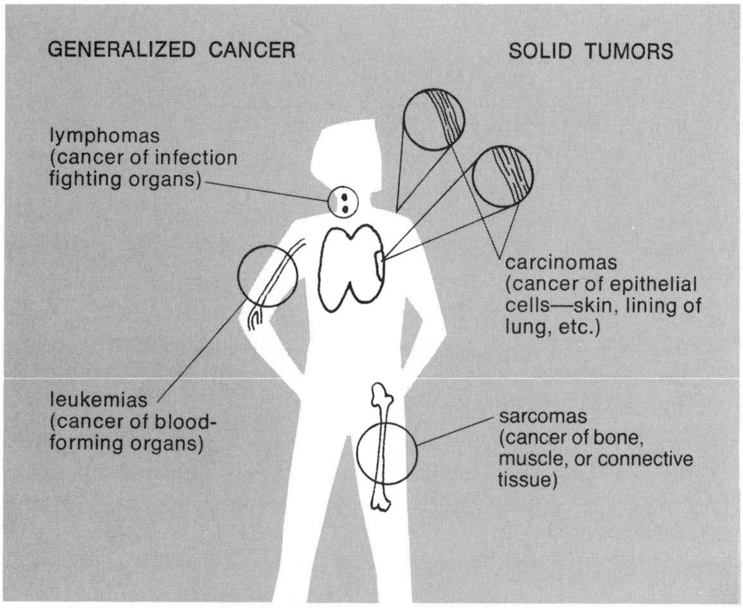

GENERALIZED CANCER   SOLID TUMORS

lymphomas
(cancer of infection
fighting organs)

carcinomas
(cancer of epithelial
cells—skin, lining of
lung, etc.)

leukemias
(cancer of blood-
forming organs)

sarcomas
(cancer of bone,
muscle, or connective
tissue)

Source: National Advisory Cancer Council

Fig. 15.3.
Types of cancers

Classifications   Cancer is an umbrella term that covers many specific disease entities. In general, both benign and malignant tumors are named after the tissue from which they arise. Consequently, there can be cancers of the epithelium or lining tissues; of fibrous, connective tissue; of fat; of bone and cartilage; of the muscles; of the blood vessels; of nerve tissue; and of lymph nodes. However, a traditional scientific classification of malignant neoplasms includes the following major types:[7,8]

Carcinoma Cancer of the skin or mouth or of the surface lining the cells of many body organs, including the lung, breast, and liver, and the secreting glands in the mucous membranes of the stomach, intestine, and uterus. This most common class of all malignant tumors metastasizes to other tissues and organs via the lymph system and the bloodstream.

Sarcoma Cancer of the connective tissues, such as muscle, bone, cartilage, and fat cells, with distant spread occurring through the bloodstream and metastases appearing in the lungs.

Lymphoma Cancer of the infection-fighting organs, the lymph nodes. Known as Hodgkin's disease, the malignancy often begins as a localized condition but may quickly become widespread.

Leukemia Cancer of the blood-forming organs in which there occurs a great and abnormal increase in the production of immature white blood cells.

Melanoma Skin tumor filled with dark pigment, sometimes jet black in color. Often beginning as a mole—a form of benign tumor—the growth undergoes a malignant change later in life and is noted by an increase in size, pigmentation, and itching.

Mortality   Generally considered the second leading cause of death in America, cancer kills
and Morbidity   more than 390,000 persons each year. Although cancer occurs more frequently among the aged, it can affect children as well as adults. Leukemia is actually the leading cause of death due to disease among persons between three and fourteen years of age. One estimate of cancer mortality and morbidity in the decade of the 1970s indicates that there were 3.5 million cancer deaths, 6.5 million new cancer cases, and 10 million persons under medical care for cancer.[9]

At the turn of the century, few cancer patients survived after diagnosis (identification of a disease) by a physician. Today, the survival rate is one in three, mainly due to early detection and diagnosis and to significantly more effective treatment methods. The American Cancer Society claims that of every six persons who develop cancer today, two will be saved and four will die. Moreover, one of the four who will die could have been saved if proper treatment had been received in time. Currently, nearly 2 million living Americans have been cured of cancer.

Trends in the occurrence of cancer and in cancer death rates since the 1950s show the following sex, age, and race differences.[10]

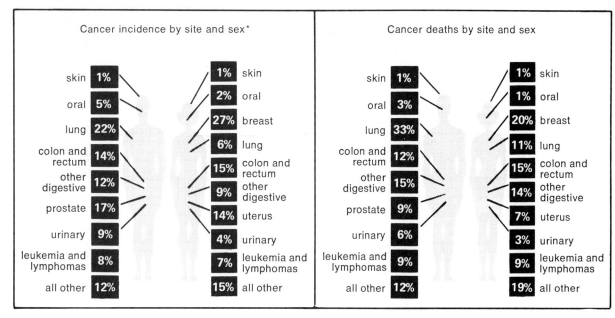

Cancer incidence by site and sex*

skin	1%
oral	5%
lung	22%
colon and rectum	14%
other digestive	12%
prostate	17%
urinary	9%
leukemia and lymphomas	8%
all other	12%

1%	skin
2%	oral
27%	breast
6%	lung
15%	colon and rectum
9%	other digestive
14%	uterus
4%	urinary
7%	leukemia and lymphomas
15%	all other

Cancer deaths by site and sex

skin	1%
oral	3%
lung	33%
colon and rectum	12%
other digestive	15%
prostate	9%
urinary	6%
leukemia and lymphomas	9%
all other	12%

1%	skin
1%	oral
20%	breast
11%	lung
15%	colon and rectum
14%	other digestive
7%	uterus
3%	urinary
9%	leukemia and lymphomas
19%	all other

*Excluding superficial skin cancer and carcinoma in situ of uterine cervix.

Fig. 15.4. Cancer morbidity and mortality in the United States. Reprinted from *1978 Cancer Facts & Figures* with permission. © 1977, American Cancer Society, Inc.

1. For women, a decrease has been noted in the occurrence of cancers of the uterus, including the cervix, and of the bladder and stomach. Incidence of breast and colon cancers remains unchanged, but lung cancer has steadily increased. Since 1950, the cancer death rate has actually declined by 5 percent for blacks and 10 percent for whites. This difference is due mainly to a sharp reduction in deaths caused by cancer of the uterine cervix, which is attributed to increased use of Pap tests and regular checkups. Cancer of the breast remains the leading site of cancer incidence and the leading cause of cancer death among females.

2. For men, there has been a much higher incidence of lung cancer, amounting to an increase of over 125 percent in twenty-five years. Slight increases occurred for cancers of the colon, prostate, pancreas, and bladder, while a decrease in stomach cancer has been noted. Since 1950, the cancer death rate per 100,000 population has increased by over 60 percent for blacks and by 20 percent for whites. The increased death rate is mainly the result of lung cancer.

3. For children, cancer is responsible for more deaths in the three- to fourteen-year-old group than any other disease. Each year, cancer will account for the deaths of about 2,500 children, about half of them from acute lymphocytic leukemia, a cancer of the blood-forming tissues.

4. The occurrence of cancer in blacks is considerably higher than it is in whites. This is especially true with regard to cancer of the lung, colon-rectum, prostate, and esophagus. Most of the differences in black and white cancer rates are related to environmental and social factors. Because blacks predominate

in the lower socioeconomic groups, many are exposed to industrial carcinogens. They also tend to have less education and therefore are less likely to know how they can help prevent cancer and detect it early.

Factors in Carcinogenesis Through scientific research and epidemiology (the study of the occurrence and distribution of diseases in human populations), it is now possible to identify various factors or agents that function in *carcinogenesis,* the production of cancer. The individual agents that cause cancer are termed *carcinogens.* Some of these agents may initiate chemical changes within the cell; others promote the cancerous process only after intracellular changes have begun; still others must act jointly with yet another agent to cause cancer. Environmental carcinogens may be chemical, physical, or biological in nature.

Chemical Carcinogens   Among the first agents causally associated with the incidence of cancer were chemical carcinogens. In 1775, Sir Percival Pott, a prominent English surgeon, attributed the high rate of cancer of the scrotum among chimney sweeps to their long exposure and contact with soot.[11]

Since that time, chemical components of tar, smoke, smog, air pollutants, and automobile exhaust fumes, especially hydrocarbon compounds, have been found to have carcinogenic properties. Recent research also has revealed that diethylstilbestrol (DES), a drug taken by nearly 2 million expectant mothers to avoid miscarriage (and also used as a morning-after birth control pill), appears to increase the risk of fatal cancers, especially of the breast. In addition, daughters of women who took DES often develop a rare form of vaginal and cervical cancer.

Nitrogen mustard, aminoazo dyes, vinyl chloride, phenols, and the deposits on smoke-preserved meat and fish also have cancer-producing activity. However, no chemical carcinogens have proven more deadly than those found in cigarette smoke, particularly benzo(a)pyrene and chrysene. These and other cancer-causing components retard the action of the bronchial cilia and then are deposited on the bronchial tube linings where they act as irritants and eventually produce cellular changes characteristic of early cancer.

The excessive use of alcohol has also been reported as increasing the chances of developing cancers of the esophagus, mouth, throat, larynx, and liver. For those who both smoke and drink heavily, the cancer risk is even greater. Scientists are also investigating the role of diets high in fats and cholesterol and low in dietary fiber in the occurrence of cancer of intestinal tract, especially the colon and rectum.

Physical Carcinogens, Radiation   Physical energy from the sun, X rays, radium, and nuclear weapons gives rise to cancers in both humans and animals. X rays, gamma rays, fast electrons, alpha particles, and ultraviolet rays all carry high amounts of energy. These radiations can change the chemical bonds within cells[12] and give rise to cells with altered genetic composition (mutations) and to abnormal and uncontrolled cell growth.

Incidence of skin cancer is related to the amount of sunshine in the area. It is highest among fair-skinned whites living in the southern and western parts of

Table 15.1   Reference Chart: Leading Cancer Sites, 1978*

Site	Estimated New Cases 1978	Estimated Deaths 1978	Warning Signal If you have one, see your doctor.	Safeguards	Comment
Breast	91,000	34,000	Lump or thickening in the breast	Regular checkup; monthly breast self-exam	The leading cause of cancer death in women
Colon and Rectum	102,000	52,000	Change in bowel habits; bleeding	Regular checkup, including proctoscopy, especially for those over 40	Considered a highly curable disease when digital and proctoscopic examinations are included in routine checkups
Lung	102,000	92,000	Persistent cough or lingering respiratory ailment	80 percent of lung cancer would be prevented if no one smoked cigarettes	The leading cause of cancer death among men and rising mortality among women
Oral (Including Pharynx)	24,000	8,000	Sore that does not heal or difficulty in swallowing	Regular checkup	Many more lives should be saved because the mouth is easily accessible to visual examination by physicians and dentists.
Skin	10,000**	6,000	Sore that does not heal or change in wart or mole	Regular checkup; avoidance of overexposure to sun	Skin cancer is readily detected by observation and diagnosed by simple biopsy.
Uterus	48,000***	11,000	Unusual bleeding or discharge	Regular checkup, including pelvic examination with pap test	Uterine cancer mortality has declined 65 percent during the last 40 years, with wider application of the pap test. Postmenopausal women with abnormal bleeding should be checked.
Kidney and Bladder	45,000	17,000	Urinary difficulty; bleeding, in which case consult doctor at once	Regular checkup with urinalysis	Protective measures to workers in high-risk industries are helping to eliminate one of the important causes of these cancers.
Larynx	9,000	3,000	Hoarseness or difficulty in swallowing	Regular checkup, including laryngoscopy	Readily curable if caught early
Prostate	57,000	21,000	Urinary difficulty	Regular checkup, including palpation	Occurs mainly in men over 60. The disease can be detected by palpation and urinalysis at regular checkup.
Stomach	23,000	15,000	Indigestion	Regular checkup	A 40 percent decline in mortality in 25 years for reasons yet unknown.
Leukemia	22,000	15,000	Leukemia is a cancer of blood-forming tissues and is characterized by the abnormal production of immature white blood cells. Acute leukemia strikes mainly children and is treated by drugs which have extended life from a few months to as much as ten years. Chronic leukemia strikes usually after age 25 and progresses less rapidly.		
Lymphomas	33,000	21,000	These cancers arise in the lymph system and include Hodgkin's disease and lymphosarcoma. Some patients with lymphatic cancers can lead normal lives for many years. Five-year survival rate for Hodgkin's disease increased from 25 percent to 54 percent in 20 years.		

*All figures are rounded to nearest 1,000.
**Estimated new cases of nonmelanoma skin cancer about 300,000.
***If carcinoma in situ is included, cases total over 88,000.
Incidence estimates are based on rates from N.C.I. Third National Cancer Survey.

Reprinted from *1978 Cancer Facts & Figures* with permission. © 1977, American Cancer Society, Inc.

America; lowest in the northern regions and among blacks, who are protected by skin pigmentation. ''Furthermore, skin cancer occurs more frequently among people who work outdoors, such as sailors and farmers, than among people who can guard themselves against exposure to the sun.''[13]

Before adequate protection was provided, individuals exposed to high doses of X rays were frequently afflicted with skin cancer and leukemia. During the 1920s, women who were employed to paint clock and watch dials with luminous radium paint later died of bone cancer because they had ingested the radioactive paint while pointing the brush tips with their lips. The survivors of the atomic bombing of Hiroshima and Nagasaki experienced increased incidences of leukemia (a tenfold increase) and cancer of the lung, breast, and thyroid.

Biological Carcinogens, Viruses The possible role of the virus, a cellular parasite, in carcinogenesis has stimulated scientific research for many years. While at least a dozen cancers among laboratory animals have been confirmed as viral in origin, it has proven difficult to establish the same virus-cancer link in humans. As yet, no virus has been discovered that causes cancer in human beings.

However, there is now evidence that the herpes group of viruses (one of which, herpes simplex, causes fever blisters of the mouth) is involved with some extremely malignant human cancers,[14] including Hodgkin's disease and leukemia. Adenoviruses that cause the common cold and upper respiratory infections have also been known to produce some tumors. While the exact method by which cancer is initiated remains obscure, it is thought that a virus disrupts the normal regulating mechanism of chromosomes and genes in a healthy cell.

> It may well be that a molecule of viral nucleic acid, without its protein overcoat, might so closely resemble a gene that it could slip into the cell's chromosomal lineup, displacing a normal gene, and make the cell reproduce abnormally.[15]

Having first demonstrated the presence of specific antibodies against the herpes simplex virus in the blood serum of advanced cancer patients, a prominent medical researcher contends that in addition to the viral factor in carcinogenesis, "...there must be at least one other contributing factor, and perhaps more, involved."[16] Such a statement affirms the general belief that no one factor is responsible for the development of cancer. A complex interaction of two or more factors or cocarcinogens is probably necessary. Perhaps the viral infection enhances chemical carcinogenesis, or maybe the virus remains latent until awakened by the effects of radiation or some other physical factor.

Based upon present knowledge, human cancer is not thought to be communicable, though it is possibly infectious in some forms.[17] Nevertheless, the detection of antibodies against the herpes virus in cancer patients holds out the promise that some forms of malignant neoplasms can be eliminated or reduced by the development of appropriate vaccines and by breaking the pathways of infection.

Inheritance In addition to chemicals, radiation, and possibly viruses, several other factors appear to play a role in carcinogenesis. While most forms of cancer and precancerous conditions do not show any evidence of being transmitted from parent to offspring, two exceptions have been noted:

> Retinoblastoma, a rare tumor of the eye, is inherited through a dominant gene; and intestinal polyposis, a benign condition which may become malignant, is definitely inheritable.[18]

The inheritance of a predisposition or susceptibility to certain cancers is probable, especially with reference to skin cancer and coloration of skin. However, the occurrence of breast cancer or leukemia in "familial aggregations," in which

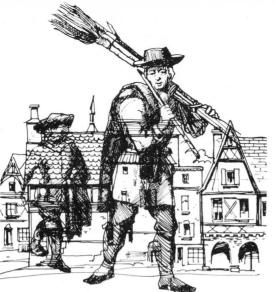

Fig. 15.5. The first environmental pollution victims to be reported were the chimney sweeps of 18th century London. Their high rate of scrotal cancer was related to their exposure to soot over a long period of time.

Source: National Advisory Cancer Council

several family members and succeeding generations develop the same type of disease, is likely the result of environmental influences as much as heredity.

Other Environmental Conditions　Other environmental conditions have often been associated with some cancers, although the exact cause or causes are not known. For instance, uterine cancer is more prevalent in females who have borne children than in females who have never given birth. The risk of breast cancer is higher in women than in men, but among females, the risk tends to be higher for those who have not borne children than for those who have. Cancer of the penis, possibly due to the irritating effect of accumulated smegma, is more frequent in uncircumcised males than in those who are circumcised. Pipe smokers experience an increased incidence of tongue and lip cancer related perhaps to the prolonged exposure to the heat and irritating pressure of the pipe stem. Occupational hazards have also been noted: asbestos workers experience increased incidences of lung and gastrointestinal cancer, dye workers exposed to certain chemical substances (aniline dyes) are likely to develop cancer of the bladder, and individuals working with or near radioactive materials run the risk of skin cancer.

Although psychological factors have not been linked traditionally with the incidence of cancer, widely circulated reports claim that personality plays a role in the development of the disease. As yet, there is no proof that a cause-and-effect relationship exists between cancer and despair, neglectful parents, loneliness, or the loss of loved ones.[19] Clearly, the primary causes of cancer are environmental carcinogens, not the patient's personality or character.

Until more is known about the causes of malignant neoplasms, the best weapons in the fight against cancer are (1) avoidance of known or possible carcinogens; (2) early detection and diagnosis; and (3) treatment under the supervision of

Countermeasures

Modern Plagues: Cancer and Other Diseases　　　377

medical personnel. If cancer is detected, diagnosed, and treated in its early stages before it spreads to other body parts, the chances for survival and cure are greatly enhanced. But the initial step in a program of risk-reduction must begin with the individual.

Avoidance of Known Carcinogens   Regularly inhaled cigarette smoke is one of the most harmful carcinogens known as a cause of otherwise preventable disease and death. In comparison with nonsmokers, regular cigarette smokers have a death rate for lung cancer alone that is nine times higher. The death rate is twenty times higher if the smoker consumes two or more packs per day. With the elimination of smoking, three out of four deaths from lung cancer would not likely occur. Cigarette smokers also tend to have a greater incidence of cancer of the lung, larynx, lip, oral cavity, esophagus, and bladder than do nonsmokers.[20] By not smoking, the chances of having a cancer-free respiratory system are greatly enhanced.

Cancer-causing chemicals have also been found in the air pollution of large urban centers. Sources of such carcinogens are industrial wastes, auto exhausts, and incinerator output that introduces high concentrations of polycyclic hydrocarbons into the atmosphere. Some of these compounds have proved to be lung carcinogens or cilia-toxic agents in the air passageways.

A reduction of air pollution is essential for maintaining the quality of life. To accomplish this goal, clean air standards have been set for both state and municipal areas to improve one of our most precious natural resources, the air we breathe. Solutions that require individual citizen support and cooperation may involve reliance upon mass public transportation rather than private automobile use, dispersal of population and/or industry, installation of control devices on all emissions into the atmosphere, and development and use of nonhydrocarbon energy sources. If air pollution cannot be reduced, the ultimate solution would be to escape from the hazardous environment—if a less hazardous one exists.

Skin cancer is the most common form of all cancers reported. Most of the 300,000 new cases reported annually in the United States can be cured if treated early. While many substances that produce skin cancer have been identified, their use in industry and medicine have been carefully regulated. The sun remains the most significant and leading cause of skin cancer. And yet, each year, millions of persons engage in deliberate, excessive tanning that not only increases the risk of skin cancer but also contributes to the aging appearance of the skin.[21] Fair-skinned persons are particularly susceptible because they lack sufficient skin pigmentation to protect their skin from ultraviolet radiation. Avoidance of excessive sun and the use of physician-recommended lotions or ointments to help shield the body from the sun are definitely advised.

Although the level of man-made radiation in the environment is cause for concern, the wise and prudent use of X ray in the detection, diagnosis, and treatment of diseases and injuries is justified. X-ray techniques have been refined so that unnecessary whole body irradiation can be prevented or minimized by medical and dental personnel. However, the indiscriminate use of X ray, as found in old shoe-fitting devices, is certainly to be discouraged.

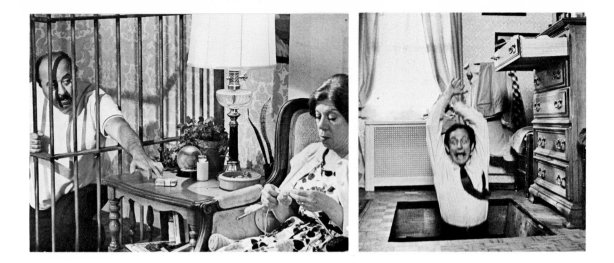

Detection and Diagnosis If warning signals develop, consult a physician. Signs and symptoms of cancer differ with the location of tumors. General symptoms, such as weight loss and weakness, may occur, but these are often dismissed because of their nonspecificity. In other instances, symptoms may not appear at all, or they may appear only after invasive cancer has taken its toll within the body. It is important to remember that *pain does not often occur in the early stages* of cancerous disease.

However, the body frequently speaks to a cancer victim in terms of early warning signals as defined by the American Cancer Society. While these signals do not conclusively prove the existence of cancer—they can be due to many other causes—the persistence or progression of one or more of them for two weeks is justification for seeking medical attention. Do not panic, but be sure to get to a doctor. If a warning signal develops, only a physician can distinguish between a false alarm and the real thing. Only a physician can help!

Fig. 15.6. Giving up the smoking habit is very difficult, and some people resort to elaborate means to quit, as shown humorously in these American Cancer Society TV spots.

The Warning Signals of Cancer Spell CAUTION

- Change in bowel or bladder habits
- A sore that does not heal
- Unusual bleeding or discharge
- Thickening or a lump in the breast or elsewhere
- Indigestion that persists or difficulty in swallowing
- Obvious change in a wart or mole
- Nagging cough or hoarseness

In reality, the seven danger signals are help signals. Listen to your body when it calls for help.

Take advantage of screening tests and medical examinations. At present there is no general test for cancer. There are, however, a number of special screening tests that can be used to detect early evidence of cancer on an organ-to-organ basis.

Fig. 15.7.

Breast self-examination

is vitally important
for women of child-bearing
age and women
after menopause.
A few minutes spent
each month can save
a life.

Looking

Stand in front of a mirror with the upper body unclothed. Look for changes in the shape and size of the breast and for dimpling of the skin or "pulling in" of the nipples. Be aware, too, of any discharge from the nipples or scaling of the skin of the nipples. Abnormality in the breast may be accentuated by a change in position of the body and arms.

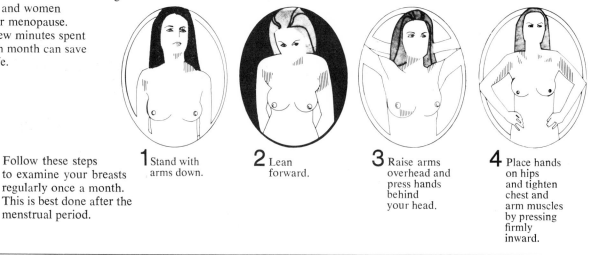

Follow these steps
to examine your breasts
regularly once a month.
This is best done after the
menstrual period.

1 Stand with arms down.

2 Lean forward.

3 Raise arms overhead and press hands behind your head.

4 Place hands on hips and tighten chest and arm muscles by pressing firmly inward.

Screening Tests

1. *Breast self-examination,* which can be easily accomplished without expense to determine the presence of lumps in the breast. Such a screening technique is recommended for women once each month after menstruation and should be continued after menopause.
2. *Chest X ray* to detect lung cancer.
3. *Papanicolaou (Pap) test* for early uterine and cervical cancer and precancerous conditions. Named for its originator, George Papanicolaou, the Pap test involves the microscopic examination of cells collected from a sample of vaginal fluid. If abnormal cells are detected, a biopsy is performed in which small pieces of uterine tissue are removed for further examination and diagnosis by a physician. The Pap test should be administered at least yearly to every woman twenty years of age or older and to younger women who have become sexually active.[22]
4. *Examination of the oral cavity* by a physician who utilizes a long-handled laryngeal mirror to detect cancer of the throat and mouth.
5. *Blood tests* for evidence of leukemia.
6. *Rectal examination,* involving digital insertion and exploration to discover cancer of the colon,

bladder, and prostate gland. Cancer of the prostate occurs most frequently in men over sixty.
7. *Use of proctosigmoidoscope* (a slim, lighted tube through which a physician can look directly inside the rectum and bowel) to detect cancer of the colon and rectum.
8. *Barium enema X-ray examination* for cancer of the large intestine.
9. *Mammography,* the X-ray examination of the breast to reveal lumps or lesions before they can be felt and before the possible cancer can spread to the lymph nodes. Presently the American Cancer Society and the National Cancer Institute recommend that routine mammograms be used only by women over fifty years of age and by those under fifty who are identified as having a high risk of getting breast cancer.
10. *Thermography* is the taking of a heat-sensitive photograph of the breast to detect tumors that cannot be felt. Developed from military and space technology, thermography operates on the principle that the human body broadcasts health signals through changes in temperature. "Thermograms can detect minute amounts of heat given off by a cancer or inflammation within the breast."[23]

Feeling

Lie flat on your back with a pillow or folded towel under your shoulders and feel each breast with the opposite hand in sequence. With the hand slightly cupped, feel for lumps or any change in the texture of the breast or skin; also, note any discharge from nipples. Avoid compressing the breast between the thumb and fingers as this may give the impression of a lump which is not actually there.

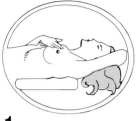

1 Place the left arm overhead. With the right hand, feel the inner half of the left breast from top to bottom and from nipple to breastbone.

2 Feel the outer half from bottom to top and from the nipple to the side of the chest.

3 Pay special attention to the area between the breast and armpit including the armpit itself.

4 Repeat this same process for the right breast using your left hand to feel.

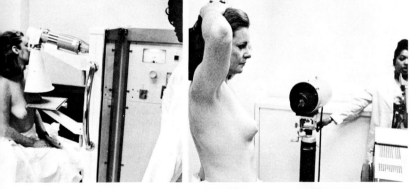

Fig. 15.8. In mammography, left, the breasts are placed alternately on a metal plate and X-rayed from the side and from above. For a thermogram, right, three positions of the breasts are X-rayed.

Fig. 15.9. Typical black-and-white thermogram, left. Lightest shades reflect warmest areas. Thermograms, middle and right, show abnormal pattern and temperature elevation in both breasts of patient with infiltrating carcinoma and lobular carcinoma in situ of the right breast. Arrows point to hot quadrant and dilated vein produced by this cancer.

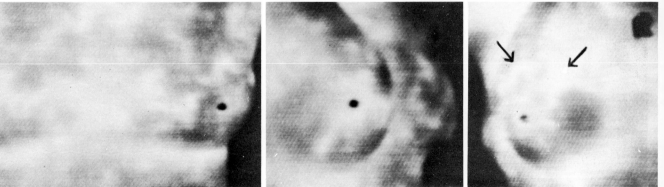

It is apparent that with the exception of the breast self-examination, these screening tests can be conducted only by medical personnel. The results can be interpreted only by a physician. As a consequence, regular comprehensive medical examinations assume added significance in the fight against cancer. Your physician will determine which screening techniques are appropriate. The need for such a medical examination, even with no symptoms, increases with age.

The earlier that cancer or precancerous conditions are detected and confirmed by diagnosis, the sooner treatment can begin. And earlier treatment increases the survival rate and the probable success of control and curative measures.

Treatment of Cancer Based upon a diagnosis, a physician must determine which treatment or therapy is best suited for the individual cancer patient. Consideration will be given to the type of malignancy, its extent and location, as well as to the age and general health of the person. Some therapies are more effective than others in curing the patient.

> The decision as to when a patient may be considered cured is one that must be made by the physician after examining the individual patient. For most forms of cancer, five years is the accepted time. However, some patients can be considered cured after one year; others after three years, while some have to be followed much longer than five years.[24]

Other treatment modalities prolong the life of the patient by producing a remission of the disease in which signs and symptoms are temporarily reduced. Frequently, combinations of therapeutic measures will be employed. Current cancer therapies include surgical removal of the tumor, radiation of diseased tissues, chemotherapy, and immunotherapy.

Surgical removal of localized benign tumors has been completely successful. However, malignant tumors, such as those of the breast, require the removal of not only the original cell mass but also, because of invasiveness, as much of the surrounding tissue as deemed necessary. To prevent distant metastases, surgeons may sometimes also remove regional lymph nodes in the armpit and musculature underlying the breast. This massive removal of tissue surrounding the original site of the malignancy is referred to as a "radical" mastectomy (surgical removal of the breast). The precise amount of adjoining and underlying tissue that should be removed in a mastectomy is still somewhat of a medical controversy, with some surgeons recommending much less tissue removal than is generally performed in a radical procedure. Unfortunately, the presence of distant cancer colonies often indicates that surgical treatment cannot produce a cure.

Radiation, already identified as a carcinogenic agent, has also proved to be a valuable tool in treating certain forms of cancer. Radiation has a *selective action* on cancer cells, that is, amounts of radiation that can be tolerated by normal, healthy cells have a destructive effect on more rapidly growing cells. Sources of radiation include low-voltage and super-voltage X-ray machines, radioactive cobalt machines for treating deep-seated tumors, radium elements introduced directly into tumors, and radioisotopes. Radioisotopes (radioactive elements that emit radiation) are often introduced in liquid form or embedded as solid needles, seeds, or wires in tissue.

Chemotherapy, the treatment of cancer by drugs, has been useful in controlling leukemia, lymphoma, and prostatic tumors.[25] Rather than producing cancer cures, drugs primarily function to slow the growth of malignancies, to relieve symptoms, and to extend the survival of the patient. Alkylating drugs apparently interfere with cancer cell division, and the antimetabolite drugs interrupt the chemical processes of cancer cells. One antimetabolite, methotrexate, has proven successful in effecting a very high cure rate in one rare form of uterine cancer known as choriocarcinoma. Hormones have also been useful in treating cancerous tissue normally under their influence, including the breast, uterus, and prostate. Chemotherapy has its limitations inasmuch as the relief produced is usually temporary and the undesirable side effects often predispose the patient to infection and hemorrhage.

Researchers have developed a concept that the sensitivity of cancers to drugs is related to the rate at which the tumor cells divide. Cancers with a large fraction of cells dividing at any one time, acute lymphocytic leukemia and Hodgkin's disease, are thought to be drug sensitive. Most of the highly active cancer drugs act on cells only during the division cycle. Cancers with few cells in the dividing state, lung, breast, and colon cancers, are thought to be drug insensitive. Researchers are trying to produce drugs that will act on slow-growing cancers.

Immunotherapy, although still a new and experimental treatment, may become a major weapon not only in curing cancer but also in its prevention. Immunotherapy is based upon the demonstrated fact that the human body possesses natural mechanisms for its own defense and protection. Such mechanisms reject foreign substances, proteins, and cells that endanger the body's self-integrity. The actual treatment "...uses a biochemical strategy designed to trick the body's own natural defenses into fighting cancer."[26] Experimentation is continuing to determine what agents or techniques are most useful in stimulating the body's rejection factors. The outcome may see the use of immunotherapy in conjunction with more established treatments or as a preventive vaccine.

Arthritis

A major cause of painful disability and incapacitation among the general population, but among the aged in particular, is arthritis, the inflammation of the body's joints. (A joint is the place in which bone ends meet or come together.) Although there are several arthritic diseases, including gout, ankylosing spondylitis, and systemic lupus erythematosus, the most common are osteoarthritis and rheumatoid arthritis. Both of these conditions produce painful and deformed joints.

Osteoarthritis

Osteoarthritis is a slow, progressive deterioration of the joints and will likely occur in all individuals if they live long enough. Sometimes called "wear and tear" arthritis, it is often noticed for the first time after an injury to the joint. Attempted joint movement, weight placed upon the joints, and inclement weather tend to aggravate the painful condition and the accompanying stiffness.

The joint is injured, with damage occurring to the smooth lining membrane (the synovium) and to the pads of tough, elastic cartilage that cover the bone ends. Three stages of the destructive process have been noted.[27] First, the cartilage cells become swollen and filled with abnormal amounts of fluid. Second, the cartilage begins to erode as it loses its dense homogeneous nature. Third, in response to strain produced at the outer margin of the bones, extra calcium is deposited and builds up slowly over several years as enlarged bony spurs. Eventually, these permanent alterations within the joint limit movement and make any motion somewhat painful. Occasionally, a small fragment of a bony spur will break off and work its way between contacting surfaces where the irritation results in severe pain.

No single cause of osteoarthritis has been noted, but age, trauma, heredity, abnormal use, diet, and impaired blood supply to the joint may be factors in the

Fig. 15.10. Understanding inflammation—a giant step in understanding arthritis.

The body's normal → protection system. Enemy agent (A) is contacted by defender blood cell (B) which gets "turned on" (C) and produces antibodies (D). Antibodies latch on to enemy agents (E), attract and join with complement (F). This triple complex is swallowed by eating cell (G) and brought in contact with lysosomes (H) which put their enzymes to work chewing up and digesting the complex (I and J).

The body attacks itself. → Section A. Confused defender cell attacks synovial lining cell of the joint. Section B. As complexes are gobbled in by eating cell, it becomes gorged. Powerful enzymes are vomited out and escape into surrounding joint fluid . . .where they seek and damage joint tissue.

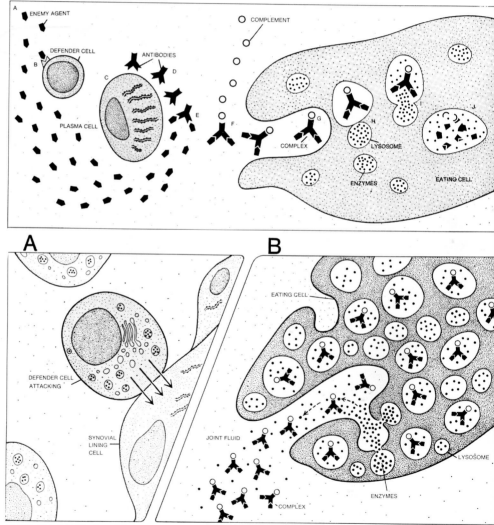

Source: The Arthritis Foundation

Chapter Fifteen

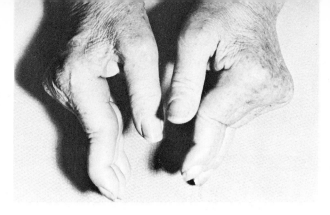

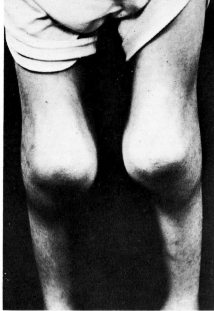

Fig. 15.11. Severe arthritic conditions often result in painful, deformed joints, as seen in these photos of knees and hands.

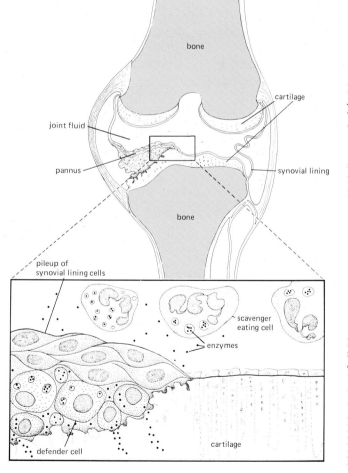

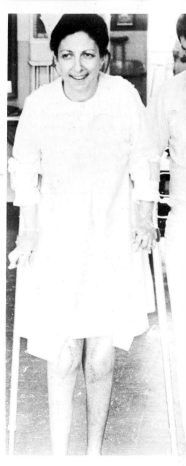

The joint inflamed. Cartilage, which protects bone ends in a joint, is eaten away and destroyed in the area of inflammation by a "rain" of enzymes from various sources, and by substances released from cells which multiply and pile up on it (pannus).

Fig. 15.12. An arthritis patient walking, after surgery, with the aid of a physical therapist. New surgical techniques, such as total knee replacement, provide relief from pain and allow previously disabled people to walk.

development of this disease. Serious disability is rare, as the condition frequently stabilizes at a plateau for several years. While the condition cannot be cured, the inflammation of the surrounding tissues and the discomfort can be reduced by aspirin and other drugs (including cortisone, muscle relaxants, and sedatives), local heat, rest with mild exercise, and weight reduction.[28]

Warning Signs of Arthritis
- Persistent pain and stiffness upon arising in the morning
- Pain, tenderness, or swelling in one or more of the body's joints
- Recurrence of these symptoms, especially when more than one joint is involved
- Noticeable pain and stiffness in the neck, knees, lower back, and other body joints
- Tingling sensation in the hands, fingertips, and feet

Rheumatoid Arthritis

Rheumatoid arthritis is considered an inflammatory joint disease of the whole body rather than a degenerative process as in osteoarthritis. The exact cause or causes have not been determined. It can occur at any age but often begins between the ages of twenty and thirty-five years. For unknown reasons, rheumatoid arthritis is three to four times more prevalent in women than in men. The onset of soreness and stiffness may be gradual or acute, with inflammatory attacks coming and going without apparent reasons. If treatment is not effective or if a remission does not occur, permanent joint deformities often result in disability.

The inflammation is first evident in the membranous synovium that normally generates the lubricating fluid of the joint. More and more fluid is secreted and more synovial cells are produced until the entire joint is swollen. With this increased synovial growth, a thick, sticky fibrous layer forms between the cartilage surfaces of each bone head.

> Now, if this inflammatory layer . . . persists any length of time, the cartilage with which it is in contact is destroyed. At the same time, the inflamed blood vessels in the ends of the bone are attacking the cartilage from beneath.[29]

The results are extensive destruction of the cartilage pads and the growing together of the two bone heads to form a stiff joint.

One theory explains the development of rheumatoid arthritis in terms of autoimmunity, that is, the normal defensive mechanisms of arthritic patients react against their own cells, resulting in additional joint damage. An antigen-antibody reaction apparently occurs in an adaptive response to some foreign substance. Unfortunately, the antibody in synovial tissue cannot distinguish between healthy cells of the body and the abnormal ones of enemy invaders. In addition to joint involvements, inflammation of muscles is commonly accompanied by soreness, general weakness, and fatigue.

Treatment of rheumatoid arthritis generally includes rest, an exercise program, posture rules, splints, walking aids, heat, corrective surgery, and a medication program. Several anti-inflammatory drugs have proved effective with various patients. Among those drugs commonly used are aspirin, indomethacin, ibuprofen, phenylbutazone, gold salts, and antimalarials.[30] Cortisone also suppresses pain and inflammation dramatically but may produce undesirable side effects.

Although rheumatoid arthritis is considered a chronic disease, many patients experience sporadic remissions and improve within several years after the first episode. Varying degrees of permanent disability occur, but only a small number of patients are totally incapacitated.[31]

The nature of arthritis is such that many people with this condition will look anywhere for relief and help. As a result this is one of the diseases in which the victim is most susceptible to misconceptions and quackery. Further discussion of this matter will follow as we discuss consumerism in the health-related products and services in a later chapter.

One of the natural defense mechanisms of the human body is the antigen-antibody reaction. When a foreign substance, such as a bacterium or a virus, invades the human organism, the host is stimulated to produce chemical antibodies that lock in on the invader and destroy it. The body is now sensitized to that antigen. A second exposure to that same invading antigen stimulates additional antibody formation. The resulting biochemical condition is thus described as *hypersensitivity* to the foreign invader.

Allergy

In addition to microorganisms, dust, dog dander, pollens, grasses, mold spores, and many other substances—collectively termed *allergens*—also may function as antigens and stimulate antibody production within the host. When next exposed to the same allergen, the antibodies trigger the secretion of a powerful defensive chemical, *histamine,* by specialized cells throughout the body. The histamine that is produced locally, as in the nose, causes dilation of blood vessels, increased secretion of mucus and other fluids, tissue swelling, sneezing, itching, and numerous other discomforting signs and symptoms. Thus an allergy or allergic reaction is a special sensitivity to some ordinarily harmless substance.[32] Although anyone can develop an allergy after repeated exposure to some offending allergen, it is thought that some individuals inherit the tendency or predisposition.[33]

Hay fever, which rarely results in fever, is an allergic reaction to tree and grass pollens, ragweed, hay, and many other wind-borne substances. The allergy usually involves the lining of the nose and results in prolonged and repeated sneezing; stuffy and watery nose; redness, swelling, and itching of the eyes; and itching of the nose, mouth, and throat. Breathing difficulties due to nasal obstruction are common at night.

Hay Fever

Usually a seasonal allergy, hay fever can be controlled by avoiding the allergen, use of air conditioning and air purification devices, and the administration of antihistamine drugs that counteract the effects of histamine produced by the allergen-antibody reaction. Skin tests to determine the offending allergens are followed by specific desensitizing injections that provide considerable relief to many individuals. Though hay fever is not dangerous and causes no permanent damage itself, it can cause great discomfort and lead to some troublesome complications, including bronchospasms.

Asthma   Many hay-fever sufferers develop a condition known as *asthma*. Described as chronic, reversible airway obstruction, this disease is manifest by attacks of breathing difficulty (shortness of breath) due to generalized narrowing of the small airways of the respiratory system.[34] There are many causative factors, apparently including allergens in the environment, cigarette smoking, and possible infection by microorganisms. The allergic reaction consists of bronchospasms, excessive secretion of mucus, and swelling of the air passageways.

Prevalent in both young and old, asthma is a remarkably common and particularly uncomfortable illness. It may last for years, even a lifetime. Treatment involves avoidance of known allergens, movement to a drier climate, and use of drugs that dilate the air passageways to the lungs and liquefy the mucous secretions. Cortisone treatment has proved very effective in controlling this disease. In some instances, oxygen must be given during an attack, although asthma is seldom a cause of death.

Chronic Obstructive Pulmonary Disease   The respiratory diseases of emphysema and bronchitis are increasing in prevalence and are described in detail in the chapter on smoking. Together they constitute a condition known as chronic obstructive pulmonary disease, commonly seen in persons who have smoked cigarettes excessively for many years. Each

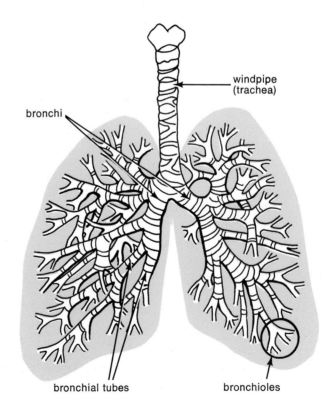

windpipe
(trachea)

bronchi

Fig. 15.13. Schematic diagram of the respiratory tree. The lungs are the site of emphysema and chronic bronchitis.

Source: National Center for Chronic Disease Control, United States Public Health Service

bronchial tubes   bronchioles

year, these crippling lung diseases claim the lives of more than 40,000 Americans. Nearly a quarter million new chronic lung disease cases are reported annually, and an estimated 15 million persons are now suffering from emphysema, chronic bronchitis, and other lung diseases.[35]

Emphysema is marked by a gradual destruction of the tiny air sacs (alveoli) of the lungs. The thin alveolar walls lose their elasticity and tear apart, resulting in large, nonfunctioning air spaces. Breathing becomes progressively more difficult as the patient attempts to squeeze trapped air out of the lungs. Exchange of oxygen for carbon dioxide is impaired, necessitating more rapid breathing. Eventually, the limp air spaces fill with used air and produce the barrel-chest effect so typical of this disease.

Emphysema

Treatment of emphysema is focused on relieving inflammation of the respiratory tract, slowing or stopping the progress of the disease, and the relief of symptoms. Drugs that tend to open up constricted air passages are often administered by inhalers or nebulizers. Expectorant drugs thin the sputum blocking the airways and make the mucus easier to raise and expel. Portable oxygen devices and intermittent positive-pressure breathing apparatus are employed to reduce severe breathing distress in victims. At present, little can be done to help those with advanced emphysema. However,

> training in breathing exercises helps victims make better use of their limited vital capacity, and enables them to resume activities formerly beyond their endurance. Similarly, general physical conditioning, with exercises tailored to the limitations of the patient, may help.[36]

Chronic bronchitis (inflammation of the bronchial tubes) is caused by prolonged irritation of the moist linings of the air passageways. With repeated insults by air pollutants (including cigarette smoke), chest colds, influenza, and allergens, the protective action of the cilia is suppressed, and the patient develops a chronic cough, excessive secretion of mucus or phlegm, and shortness of breath. Coughing, which is an attempt to force up the mucus secretions, becomes violent and wheezing occurs even with the slightest exertion.

Chronic Bronchitis

Common among males, urban dwellers, and heavy smokers, chronic bronchitis develops slowly and is often dismissed as "smoker's cough" or a "winter cold." Unfortunately, the coughing and spitting become more frequent and are usually more severe in the morning and at night and in cold, damp weather. Prolonged disability is probable without treatment, which is similar to that used in cases of emphysema. Rehabilitation depends on avoidance of irritants to the air passageways and the use of assistive breathing devices.

While most persons believe that lung disease affects only the elderly, it is quite common among children. According to the American Lung Association, thousands suffer from, and more than 29,000 children under five years of age die each year from, lung diseases such as the respiratory distress syndrome (hyaline membrane disease), the mysterious crib death or Sudden Infant Death Syndrome (SIDS), and pediatric asthma, a seriously disabling disease quite common among inner-city youth.

Pediatric
Lung Disease

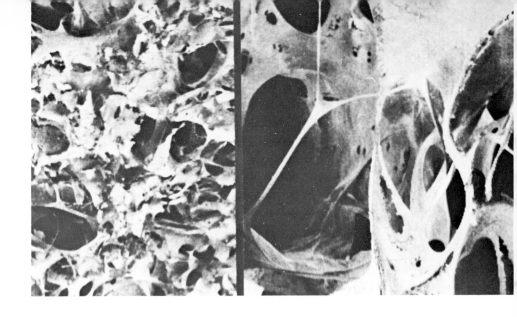

Fig. 15.14.
Photomicrograph of
a human lung magnified
150 times. Normal lung
tissue is on the left.
Lung with emphysema
showing large,
nonfunctioning, and
ruptured alveolar sacs
is on the right.

Diabetes

In a normal individual, the carbohydrate or starch foods that are eaten are converted to a common form of sugar, called *glucose,* by the action of various digestive enzymes. Distributed to the various cells of the body by the bloodstream, glucose, with the assistance of *insulin,* is either burned for immediate energy or stored for future use. Insulin, a natural hormone, is produced by specialized cells of the pancreas, a large glandular organ positioned behind the stomach. The function of insulin is "...to provide molecules of glucose in the bloodstream with a passageway through cell barriers which otherwise are essentially impervious to them."[37]

Although the exact mechanism of the action is unknown, insulin apparently interacts with certain molecules at the surface of the "hungry" cells and thus enhances the entry of glucose. Skeletal, diaphragm, and heart muscles must have insulin for efficient sugar transfer.

Diabetes mellitus is a disease in which the pancreas fails to produce sufficient insulin or makes insulin that cannot effectively perform its intended task. As a consequence, the blood-sugar level increases "...until some of the surplus is eliminated by the kidneys and passed off in the urine. Hence, sugar in the urine and too much sugar in the blood are signs of diabetes."[38] Detection of diabetes is frequently made by testing the urine for glucose. However, a medical diagnosis is made on the basis of the blood-sugar level. Common symptoms of diabetes include excessive thirst, frequent urination, constant hunger, loss of weight, tendency to tire easily, changes in vision, and slow healing of cuts and scratches.

Ordinarily, diabetes appears as the juvenile (youth-onset) type or the more common adult (maturity-onset) type. Abnormalities in the structure and function of blood vessels, particularly those in the retina of the eye and the kidneys, frequently occur as part of the diabetic picture in both types. Diabetes apparently

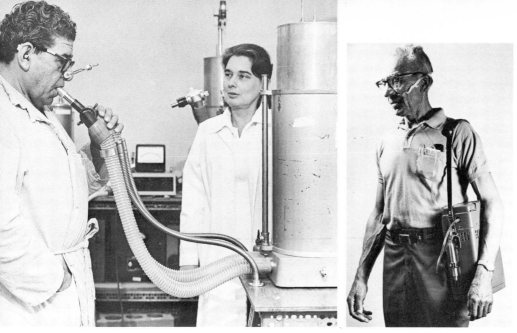

Fig. 15.15.   Emphysema patient undergoing a test
for pulmonary function. The vital capacity of the lungs
is tested by a machine called a spirometer.

contributes to other health problems, such as blindness, atherosclerosis, CHD,
and stroke. It also lessens the chance of a successful pregnancy and may significantly shorten one's life expectancy.

Although not all the possible causative factors have been discovered, diabetes is
often associated with:

Causative Factors

- A family history of the disease, suggesting that the chemical defect is an inherited condition
- Obesity (overweight) which precedes nearly 85 percent of the cases detected
- Advancing age, with a majority of diabetics discovering their abnormal insulin
  function at forty years of age or older.

Treatment usually controls but does not cure the diabetic. Proper dietary management is an important therapeutic tool for some individuals, especially those
whose diabetes appeared in middle age. The outlook for many diabetics remained bleak until the laboratory discovery of insulin by Frederick Banting and
Charles Best of Toronto, Canada, in 1921. Injections of insulin preparations now
available replace the deficient supply in the body and make it possible for diabetics
to utilize sugars and starches in their diets. Convenient orally administered compounds have been developed to lower blood-sugar levels by stimulating the pancreas to secrete insulin. Orally administered medication is not usually successful
for long-time diabetics.

Treatment

Occasionally, if diabetics do not carefully manage their food intake or fail to take their insulin, the available insulin decreases and a poisonous systemic condition, *acidosis,* gradually develops. This undesirable chemical condition results from the excessive use of diet and body fats as an energy source in lieu of carbohydrates. If not corrected in time, acidosis may lead to coma and then to death.

More common is the condition of *insulin reaction* that occurs in regulated or controlled diabetics. Insulin is present, but because of excessive exercise, failure to eat, or an overdose of insulin, the blood-sugar level is not in balance with the insulin level. Consequently, the diabetic experiences a sudden body reaction in response to excessive amounts of insulin. The individual will likely have moist skin and be very hungry, excited, and pale. The conscious person can be given a small amount of sugar, cola drink, or orange juice to restore blood sugar to an optimal level that will be in balance with the insulin present.

Epilepsy

The word epilepsy is derived from *epilēpsia,* the Greek term for seizure. Among the ancients, the "strange behavior" of seizing was attributed to evil spirits or the blessings of the gods. Today, epilepsy is more accurately viewed as a symptom of a brain disorder in which nerve cells of the brain (neurons) become overactive and irregularly release abnormal amounts of electrical energy.

Selected Noncommunicable Diseases: Description and Treatment

- Cataract—A cloudiness or opacity in the lens of the eye that interferes with vision. A cataract is *not* a film or membrane that grows over the eye, but the result of a change in the chemical composition of the lens. Surgery is the only method used in treating cataracts.

- Cerebral palsy—A term identifying a group of chronic, nonprogressive disorders of the brain that cause an impairment of motor function, including movement and coordination. Involuntary movements of the extremities are common, as are gross disturbances of articulation, speech, and chewing. Behavior disturbances and seizures can be controlled by drug therapy, although prolonged dependence and custodial care are the probable outcomes.

- Cirrhosis of the liver—The progressive, chronic destruction of liver tissue, accompanied by the formation of fibrous scar tissue. In time, the liver becomes smaller, hardened, and "hobnailed" in appearance and is impaired in its normal functioning. This form of chronic liver disease may be due to viral, toxic, or deficiency inflammatory conditions. Nutritional deficiency, frequently in combination with alcoholism, is a common causative factor. High protein diet, rest, and abstinence from alcoholic beverages are ef-

fective in reversing early cirrhosis. However, advanced cases often terminate in death within two years.

- Cystic fibrosis—An inherited disease and common cause of death in white children. The condition is rare among blacks. This genetic defect results in the thickening of the mucous secretions of the mucous glands of the body, particularly the pancreas, lungs, and liver. As a consequence, the ducts of the glands become clogged and deprive the body of important chemical regulators. Thickened mucus frequently obstructs the intestines, the bile duct of the liver, and the air passageways of the respiratory tree. Treatment consists of enzyme replacement, drugs that dilate the air passageways, mist tents, breathing exercises, and antibiotic inhalants.

- Dental caries—A progressive breakdown of tooth structure due to demineralization resulting in the production of cavities in tooth enamel. Bacteria in the mouth act on carbohydrates to form an acidlike substance that dissolves the enamel. Tooth integrity can be restored with a filling that seals off the cavity. Emphasis should focus on prevention via reduced sugar intake, tooth brushing, use of dental floss, and fluoridation of water.

This disturbance can suddenly spread to neighboring areas or jump to distant ones or even overwhelm the brain. When it spreads, a seizure results. The great majority of the neurons soon begin working in harmony again and the seizure is over.[39]

Although there are several types of seizures with many variations, the following are the more common forms.

Grand Mal or Major Seizure   The attack is often preceded by a shrill cry. Then as consciousness is lost, the person falls to the floor and experiences convulsive body movements, that is, the person thrashes about with jerking body motions. Excess salivation may occur as well as involuntary urination and defecation.

Petit Mal or Minor Seizure   In this seizure there are no convulsions. Loss of consciousness is so short that former activity is resumed within a few seconds. These seizures often go unnoticed and are commonly mistaken for daydreaming or the loss of one's place in reading.

Psychomotor Seizure   Such an attack involves both mental processes and muscular movements. The epileptic often enters a dreamy state of mental confusion,

---

- Glaucoma—A leading cause of blindness, due to increased pressure of the fluid within the eye. Initially, the increased pressure damages only those nerve fibers that permit side vision, but gradually it destroys nerves that permit front vision. Medication and surgery effectively check glaucoma.

- Goiter—Enlargement of the thyroid gland, which influences body growth, development of the brain, sexual maturity, and pregnancy. The most common form of goiter is due to iodine deficient diets. Goiter is endemic where soil is poor in iodine, such as the St. Lawrence River Valley and the Great Lakes region of North America. Thyroid enlargement is compensatory in nature, the result of production increase in order to perform necessary work load with inadequate supplies of raw material. Treatment involves administration of iodine or surgical removal of the gland, followed by thyroid hormone replacement.

- Huntington's disease (HD)—A progressive degeneration of brain cells manifested by fidgety nervousness, involuntary jerking or twisting, or spasms of facial, tongue, or limb muscles.[42] This hereditary neuromuscular disorder is often called Huntington's chorea and resembles multiple sclerosis, epilepsy, and schizophrenia. In general, symptoms usually occur between the ages of thirty-five and forty. At present there is no way to detect HD before symptoms occur; there is no known cause; and there is no treatment to halt its progression.

- Kidney disease—A general term covering such specific diseases as infections, kidney stones, uremia (urine in the blood) due to kidney failure, benign tumors, nephritis, and nephrosis. Sometimes called Bright's disease, nephritis is a nonbacterial inflammation of the blood vessels of the kidney, induced by a streptococcus infection of the upper respiratory tract.[43] Common symptoms are blood and albumin protein in the urine, elevated blood pressure, and swelling of the body. Treatment consists of bed rest, administration of fluids, and restriction of protein and salt in the diet. Nephrosis is a condition of the kidney that occurs when the tubes of the kidney malfunction, rather than the blood vessels as in nephritis.[44] Basic symptoms are swelling of body parts, especially the face, abdomen, ankles, and feet, and anemia. Treatment includes a high protein, low salt diet, and blood transfusions, often in combination with cortisone drug therapy.

- Multiple sclerosis (MS)—A disease of unknown causation characterized by widespread loss of the insulating myelin sheath that normally covers nerve fibers. Recent investigations suggest that MS is a

accompanied by quasi-purposeful actions, such as chewing, lip smacking, undressing, or searching the floor.

Jacksonian Seizure   This seizure begins with localized twitching on one side of the body and spreads progressively from the angle of the mouth, for instance, to the arm, hand, leg, and foot on the same side of the body. If the trembling crosses to the other side of the body, consciousness is lost and a grand mal seizure occurs.

Origins of Epilepsy   About half of the cases of epilepsy are of unknown origin. These are classified as *idiopathic epilepsy*. All others are labeled as *symptomatic* of some organic or toxic brain disease related to congenital abnormality, brain trauma, inflammation of the membranes covering the brain, drug and chemical poisoning, brain tumor, allergy, or arteriosclerosis. It is probable that heredity predisposes some individuals to convulsive tendencies.[40] However, it is also probable that some environmental stimulus, such as extreme nervous tension, bright flickering lights, or a sudden noise, must be operable before seizures occur.

Public Attitude Toward Epilepsy   The important thing about epilepsy is that with modern drug therapy and medical supervision, the vast majority of seizures can be measurably controlled, and

delayed reaction to a viral infection and may be related to prior exposure to pet dogs. Manifestations of visual disturbances, weakness, stiffness, speech difficulties, and involuntary movements are often followed by significant improvement or remission. No specific treatment is available, and although there are exceptions, average life expectancy is only twenty years after onset of symptoms.

- Muscular dystrophy—The progressive weakening and wasting of the muscles. Among children, the muscles first affected are those of the calves, resulting in difficulty in rising to a standing position. Often, after prolonged invalidism, the patient dies of an infection. The disease is probably an inherited disorder with no specific treatment available.

- Otitis media—Chronic middle-ear infection, the result of an upper respiratory infection that has been extended to the middle ear through the eustachian tube. Damage to the eardrum and bones of the middle ear and interference with sound transmission can be prevented with antibiotic treatment.

- Otosclerosis—Abnormal growth of spongy tissue that hinders the movement of the tiny bones of the middle ear and thus results in a conductive hearing loss. Although this disorder cannot be prevented, damage can be corrected surgically.

- Peptic ulcer—A small crater or erosion in the lining of the stomach, upper portion of the small intestine, or in the esophagus. Pain, relieved by the taking of foods and alkalis, is the major symptom of peptic ulcer. The lining tissue is somehow injured, dies, and then is "digested" by the acid gastric juice. Death may result from hemorrhage, obstruction of the organ, or perforation of an organ wall, resulting in inflammation of the abdominal cavity. Treatment includes drugs, diet therapy, and surgical intervention.

- Periodontal disease—A disorder affecting the structures surrounding and supporting the teeth. Hardened bacterial plaque or calculus causes the gums to recede, creating small pockets around the teeth that trap bacteria and food particles. Such entrapped substances inflame the gums, enlarge the pockets, infect and destroy the bones supporting the teeth. Teeth already loose in their sockets are easily lost.

- Refractive errors—Inability of the eye to focus images on the retina, which results in varying degrees of indistinct vision. Common refractive errors include hyperopia (farsightedness), myopia (nearsightedness), and inability to maintain entire visual field in focus (astigmatism).

- Silicosis—One of the oldest and most serious occupational hazards, commonly occurring in gold, coal,

epileptics can live as normal a life as possible. Medications vary and are prescribed according to the type of seizure pattern displayed and the patient's total health status. Many anticonvulsant drugs are now available, including Dilantin, phenobarbital, Mysoline, and Tridione. Sometimes these drugs are administered in combination so as to control the seizure activity while producing only minimal side effects, such as drowsiness.

Despite lengthy seizure-free periods, epilepsy remains a disease that cannot be cured. However, some individuals may gradually reduce their medications and never sustain another seizure.

First-aid procedures for epilepsy involve the removal of nearby objects that may injure the person during a seizure, loosening of clothing around the neck, keeping the individual down on the floor, maintaining an open airway, and turning the person's head to one side or having the individual lie on his or her stomach to prevent inhalation of vomitus into the lungs. Because the epileptic has experienced a great deal of movement during a grand mal seizure, it is advised that such a person be allowed to sleep or rest for a considerable time.[41]

The only major problem remaining is not the brain disorder, but the ignorance, fear, superstition, and general reaction of the public toward epileptics. As a consequence, epileptics are often more handicapped by the public's attitude of rejection and fear than by their own disability.

---

and tin mining industries and among stone and sandblasting workers and metal grinders. Silica dust particles are inhaled and irritate the alveolar sacs of the lungs. Fibrous tissue forms, which destroys the functional operation of the lungs.

• Strabismus—Imbalance of the muscles that control eye movements, leading to squinting, cross-eyes, or walleyes. Unless corrected by glasses, orthoptic muscle exercise, or surgery, the condition can result in double vision and suppression of vision in the "weaker," unused eye.

• Ulcerative colitis—Extensive ulceration and inflammation of the lining of the large intestine (the colon) and the rectum. Characteristically, the chronic condition worsens, then undergoes a remission. Symptoms include abdominal pain and diarrhea with mucus, pus, and blood in the fecal discharge. Although the patient is often hypersensitive to certain foods and of "high-strung temperament," no causative agent has been discovered. Treatment with bland diet, drugs, and surgery has been successful. Because of the possible psychogenic factor, psychotherapy is sometimes advocated.

Summary

Several common noncommunicable diseases have been discussed in this chapter. Cancer, probably the most feared, has been revealed as having many possible causes. Treatment for malignant tumors involves surgery, chemotherapy, and the use of radiation. The most positive adaptation to cancer is early diagnosis and treatment. Knowledge of the early warning signals will help to identify tumors and cancers when treatment may still be effective.

Other chronic diseases that plague humans are arthritic conditions, allergies, asthma, certain respiratory diseases, and epilepsy. Diabetes is of no small concern to many in our culture today. These noncommunicable diseases, which have been examined in this chapter, necessitate that all of us make numerous adaptations in our life-style.

Review Questions

1. Differentiate between a malignant and a benign tumor. Which one poses a real problem?
2. It has been said that cancer cells have "no home" and exhibit a behavior known as cellular autonomy. What does this mean?
3. What are the various scientific classifications of cancer? What part of the body does each one affect?
4. Why did survivors of Hiroshima and Nagasaki experience high rates of cancer and leukemia?
5. Since no cure for cancer has yet been found, what preventive measures can one take to reduce or eliminate carcinogenic factors?
6. List the seven warning signals of cancer.
7. Describe some of the various screening tests used to detect early evidence of cancer.
8. What preventive measures can one take to control hay fever?
9. Describe the more common forms of epileptic seizures.
10. Is there any common profile of those persons more likely to develop diabetes?
11. Explain how diabetes can be cured? If such is not possible, why not?
12. Distinguish between the terms osteoarthritis and rheumatoid arthritis.
13. What possible role does "autoimmunity" play in the development of rheumatoid arthritis?
14. What common preventive measures can be employed to reduce the occurrence of emphysema and chronic bronchitis?
15. What is physiologically occurring in the lungs when one has emphysema?

Readings

American Lung Association. *Introduction to Lung Diseases*. New York: The Association, 1973.

Brody, Jane E., and Holleb, Arthur I. *You Can Fight Cancer and Win*. New York: Quadrangle/The New York Times Book Company, Inc., 1977.

Jayson, Malcolm I. V., and Dixon, Allan St. J. *Understanding Arthritis and Rheumatism*. New York: Dell Publishing Co., Inc., 1974.

Sands, Harry, and Minters, Frances C. *The Epilepsy Fact Book*. Philadelphia: F. A. Davis Company, 1977.

Notes

1. William Boyd, *An Introduction to the Study of Disease*, 6th ed. rev. (Philadelphia: Lea & Febiger, 1971), p. 211.
2. Victor Richards, *Cancer: The Wayward Cell* (Berkeley: University of California Press, 1972), p. 69.
3. Michael B. Shimkin, *Science and Cancer*, rev. ed. (Washington, D.C.: U.S. Government Printing Office, 1969), p. 4.
4. National Advisory Cancer Council, *Progress against Cancer 1970* (Washington, D.C.: U.S. Government Printing Office, 1970), p. 20.

5. Richards, *Cancer: The Wayward Cell*, p. 95.

6. American Cancer Society. *1978 Cancer Facts & Figures* (New York: The Society, 1977), p. 4.

7. National Advisory Cancer Council, *Progress against Cancer 1970*, p. 80.

8. Boyd, *Introduction to the Study of Disease*, pp. 224–29.

9. American Cancer Society, *1978 Cancer Facts & Figures*, p. 3.

10. Ibid., p. 6.

11. Richards, *Cancer: The Wayward Cell*, p. 85.

12. Ibid., p. 103.

13. Shimkin, *Science and Cancer*, p. 60.

14. Keen A. Rafferty, Jr., "Herpes Virus and Cancer," *Scientific American*, October 1973, pp. 26, 32.

15. Boyd, *Introduction to the Study of Disease*, p. 215.

16. Albert Sabin, quoted by Don A. Schanche, "Countdown to a Significant Cancer Advance," *Today's Health*, July 1973, p. 48.

17. Shimkin, *Science and Cancer*, p. 79.

18. George E. Moore, *The Cancerous Diseases* (Belmont, Calif.: Wadsworth Publishing Co., 1970), p. 8.

19. Mary G. Marcus, "The Shaky Link Between Cancer and Character," *Psychology Today*, June 1976, pp. 52–54, 59, 85.

20. U.S. Department of Health, Education, and Welfare, *The Health Consequences of Smoking* (Washington, D.C.: U.S. Government Printing Office, 1973), pp. 74–77.

21. National Cancer Institute, *Cancer of the Skin* (Washington, D.C.: U.S. Government Printing Office, 1972), p. 5.

22. American Cancer Society, *1978 Cancer Facts & Figures*, p. 17.

23. "Meeting the Menace of Breast Cancer," *Cancer News*, Spring 1973, p. 7.

24. American Cancer Society, *1978 Cancer Facts & Figures*, p. 3.

25. Richards, *Cancer: The Wayward Cell*, pp. 213–15.

26. "Toward Cancer Control," *Time*, 19 March 1973, p. 64.

27. Darrell C. Crain, *The Arthritis Handbook: A Patient's Manual on Arthritis, Rheumatism, and Gout*, 2d rev. ed. (New York: Exposition Press, 1971), pp. 22–23.

28. Henrik L. Blum and George M. Keranen, *Control of Chronic Diseases in Man* (New York: American Public Health Association, 1966), p. 106.

29. Crain, *Arthritis Handbook*, p. 31.

30. The Arthritis Foundation, *Arthritis: The Basic Facts* (New York: The Foundation, 1976), pp. 9–11.

31. Blum and Keranen, *Control of Chronic Diseases in Man*, p. 111.

32. American Lung Association, *Hay Fever: The Facts* (New York: The Association, 1973).

33. Ibid.

34. National Heart and Lung Institute, *Respiratory Diseases*, Task Force Report on Problems, Research Approaches and Needs (Washington, D.C.: U.S. Government Printing Office, 1973), p. 64.

35. American Lung Association, *Lung Disease Changes Everything* (New York: The Association, 1976), pp. 11–12.

36. National Heart and Lung Institute, *Emphysema* (Washington, D.C.: U.S. Government Printing Office, 1973), p. 4.

37. *Diabetes Mellitus*, 7th ed. rev. (Indianapolis: Eli Lilly and Co., 1973), p. 23.

38. American Diabetes Association, *Fact Sheet on Diabetes* (New York: The Association, 1970), p. 3.

39. National Institute of Neurological Diseases and Stroke, *Epilepsy: Hope through Research* (Washington, D.C.: U.S. Government Printing Office, 1972), p. 9.

40. Walter Brain and John Walton, *Brain's Diseases of the Nervous System*, 7th ed. rev. (London: Oxford University Press, 1969), p. 922.

41. American National Red Cross, *Standard First Aid and Personal Safety* (Garden City, New York: Doubleday & Company, Inc., 1973), p. 176.

42. Abby Belson, "Little-Known Diseases," *Family Health/Today's Health*, May 1977, p. 44.

43. Gordon D. Oppenheimer and John G. Keuhnelian, "The Kidneys and the Urinary System," in *Symptoms: The Complete Home Medical Encyclopedia*, ed. Sigmund S. Miller (New York: Thomas Y. Crowell Company, 1976), p. 385.

44. Ibid., p. 388.

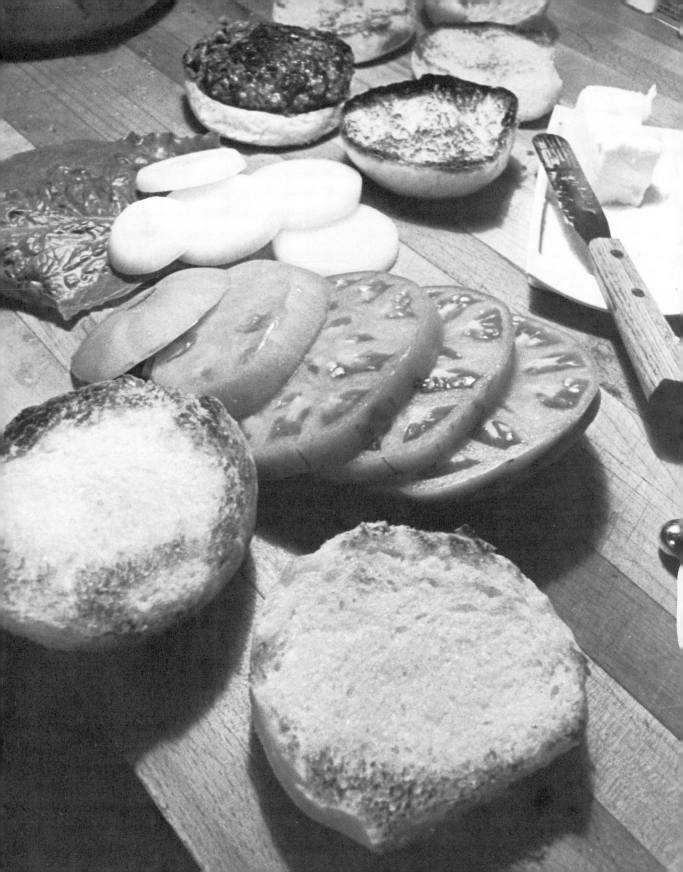

Eating: The Good and the Bad of It

16

Man doesn't live by energy alone—but he can't survive without it! Everything we do, from sleeping through running, breathing through dreaming, resting through working, uses energy. These various activities rely on oxidation to convert foodstuffs into little packages of dynamite, awaiting ignition. In this chapter and the next we shall examine the fascinating interaction between our basic need to eat and the sociocultural factors that influence our energy intake and output patterns, body types, and life-styles.

Food patterns reflect geography and climate, local flora and fauna, religion, superstitions and taboos, wars and invasions, victories and defeats, memories and expectations. In short, food is a looking glass revealing a thousand phases of personal, national, and international history. The food habits of a group are merely the product of its contemporary environment and historical development. Consequently, anyone who would change a food habit must first comprehend the deep meaning of that particular habit for a people.[1]

Dietary patterns frequently have little relationship to scientifically calculated nutritional principles. Few human groups habitually consume all the edible foodstuffs within their reach. Usually they arbitrarily categorize edibles as foods and nonfoods. Whereas grasshoppers and grubs are commonly eaten in many sections of Africa and Australia, they are only gourmet food to Americans. Conversely our staple commodities of hamburger and steak, although readily available in India, are forbidden to Hindus. Chinese students arriving for the first time in America may become ill at the sight of students drinking cow's milk at lunch—but on the other hand, few Americans would ever dream of joining Bantu friends in a gourd of warm cow's blood.[2]

Choice exists mainly in the midst of plenty; food taboos and restrictions are usually lessened in famine. Thus, where there is sufficient supply so that choices can be made, "there develops a set of food habits and foodways with their attendant taboos and prejudices."[3] Supply alone does not determine food patterns, however, and a host of sociocultural factors deserve consideration. Money is not the most important of them.

When unexpected financial gains occur suddenly within the lower classes, much of the money is spent on prestige items. An FAO study in Dakar revealed that when peasants' earnings increased due to profitable groundnut crops, the

Food around the World

What we eat is frequently decided more by chance than by choice.

Fig. 16.1. Fast food and drink businesses are very successful. They are compatible with a fast-paced life-style that often demands instant gratification of food desires.

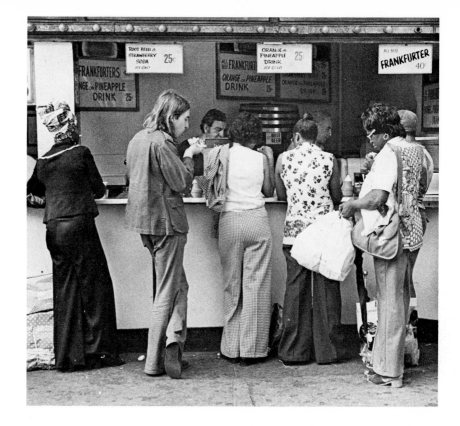

bonus was rarely spent on food. Rather it was used to increase social prestige through larger, more elaborate weddings, birth ceremonials, and funerals. During the Great Depression, New York's Italian community tended to spend money first on pasta, oil, cheese, and other foods of questionable nutritional value, but obvious cultural value; simultaneously, New York Puerto Ricans bought clothing and jewelry, often "forgetting" to allocate sufficient sums for food.[4] In the Gezira area of Sudan, where the average income from cotton tripled with irrigation, and again in the South Pacific, where the population's nutritional status actually deteriorated as copra prices and incomes rose, the *nouveaux riches* suddenly switched from local foods to refined wheat, flour, sugar, canned fish, and beef. A similar problem has been reported in Basutoland, where, now that women are working, the majority of their total incomes are given to home improvements. Also, weaning occurs much earlier now, and the supplementary diet of rich cereals has insufficient protein content for developing youngsters.[5]

Early
Feeding Habits

Early feeding patterns are critical in habit formations. Societies in which children are fed lovingly, and where food is a source of great pleasure, later become highly resistant to change. A major obstacle in relieving protein-calorie malnutrition is the innate resistance of cultures to the introduction of extra foods, and

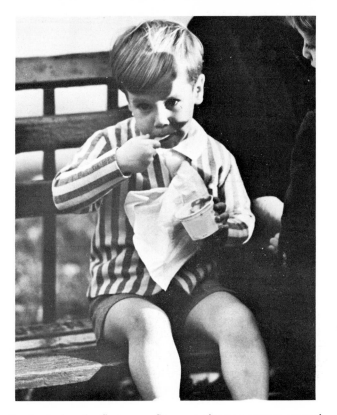

particularly protein foods, during the first year. Strong resistance centers around different types of foods: (1) foods generally avoided at all ages, such as milk in Thailand; (2) foods deemed unsuitable for infants and toddlers, like meat in Guatemala; (3) foods linked to physiological processes, permitted only after certain traditional ceremonies, such as puberty rites; (4) overvalued foods, such as plantain in Uganda or rice in Thailand; (5) disease-associated foods: mangoes are thought to produce jaundice in India. The style of living of the entire community is frequently a decisive factor in how the children are fed and how often.

Certain other cultural factors work against sound nutritional habits, and are a source of conflict when health-interested outsiders suggest changes. In Malaysia, for example, fish is among the best sources of animal protein, and yet is deemed unsuitable for young children because of its alleged capacity for producing intestinal worms. Similarly in Burma, the pregnant female's diet is severely restricted "to have a smaller baby and an easier delivery." The fetus in this case suffers a decrease in its supply of needed nutrients. More often than not, however, these cultural restrictions are harmless, as in Canada where a cultural taboo restricts the intake of protein-rich grasshoppers; the diet is already rich in meats anyway.

Cultural Factors

As a cult, vegetarianism has sprung up somewhat sporadically in the past few decades, and not always on religious grounds. The eighteenth-century scholar

Vegetarianism

Joseph Ritson contended that even the "sight of animal meat is unnatural and disgusting," that meat reminds the pensive individual of dead bodies along the roadway being feasted on by vultures and ravens. He argued that animal fat is not essential for the attainment of strength and size, that it endangers health, and that the very killing of animals leads eventually to human sacrifice and, ultimately, cannibalism.[6] In fact, a real danger may lurk among vegetarians—through ignorance they may not consume enough essential amino acids to fulfill dietary needs. (This does not necessarily follow, as we shall see later.) Also, in the case of infants and young children, animal products are an obvious source of both protein and calcium.

Religion   Religion has always played a prominent role in food patterns, especially in rituals and customs. The acts of giving or abstaining from food have been used as means of insuring the good will and protection of the All-Powerful on behalf of the individual and his people. Fortunately, many of the taboos characteristic of the world's five great religions do not have any direct effect upon young children, but inasmuch as they influence child-rearing patterns up to the age of six, they will be considered. One apt example of the influence of religion on food patterns might be the Hindus, who in early times sacrificed and ate animals as the main substance of their diet. Gradually, however, vegetarianism grew in popularity among the Hindus, encouraged largely by the principle of nonviolence, and stimulated indirectly by the growth of Buddhism and Jainism.

Other Cultural Factors   Other cultural factors are less obvious. In Morocco, people eat the liver of wild bear to gain the animal's strength and to prevent syphilis in children.

Striking differences in physique and relative state of health among geographical neighbors are often found to correlate with the amount of animal protein consumed. In northwest India, for example, where vegetarianism is less prevalent, a healthy, vigorous, well-developed populace has grown, but to the southeast, the vegetarian populace is poorly developed, disease-ridden, and apathetic. Granting the oversimplification of direct relationships, one might conclude that the flesh-eating northwesterners do consume a more nutritious diet.

Again, in Africa, the pastoral Masai of Kenya drink milk and blood, and eat animal flesh; they are a tall, vigorous, and relatively healthy tribe. Their Kikuyu neighbors, who thrive on millet, maize, sweet potatoes, and yams, are smaller, weaker, and less resistant to tropical diseases. It is said that the average Masai female is stronger than the average Kikuyu male.[7]

In 1972 Dr. Alexander Leaf, chief of medical services at Massachusetts General Hospital, visited three areas of the world where unusual longevity of a surprisingly large number of people was reported. Under the auspices of the National Geographic Society, he was able to examine the effects of geography, climate, and way of life on the life span of many of these regions' older inhabitants. In so doing, he also provided some interesting insights into the diet of these older people.[8] In the state of Hunza in Pakistan, he found that the diet was low, not only in calories, but also in animal protein. It consisted primarily of vegetables and grains.

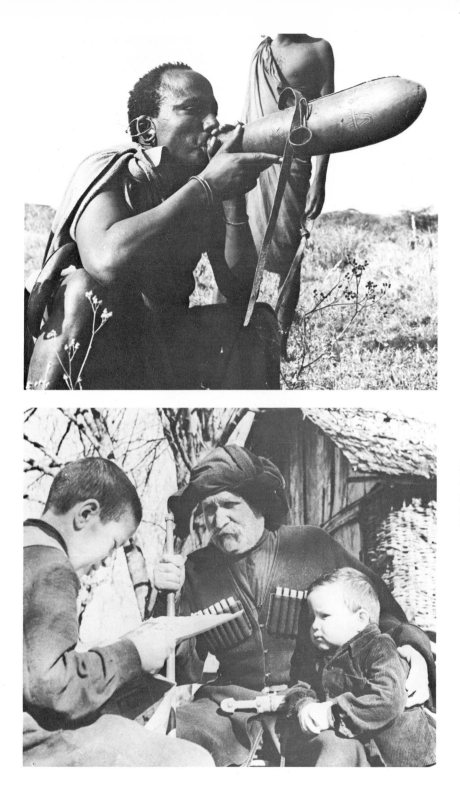

Fig. 16.3. The Masai drink a protein-rich mixture of cow's milk and cow's blood. The blood is obtained from the jugular vein and is caught in a gourd, which then serves as a glass.

Fig. 16.4. This 122-year-old man in Soviet Abkhazi, shown with two of his grandchildren, is a farmer, chairman of the village elders, and a member of a chorus composed of men of age 100 and older.

In the Caucasus Mountains of Russia, there are probably more centenarians than anywhere else in the world. Here, Dr. Leaf found the diet of the oldsters to be both varied and plentiful. Meat, dairy products, sweets, and an abundance of fresh vegetables were consumed. In addition, many of the oldsters he saw not only smoked but also drank.

In the village of Vilcambamba, high in the Andes Mountains of Ecuador, the diet was much more limited, essentially vegetarian. While undernutrition was apparent, the villagers subsisted on a low-protein and low-calorie diet. While there was no common dietary pattern for all three areas, the essential common thread was a vigorous, physically active existence.

Definition of Food

The way in which food is defined by one's culture may be illustrated further in the reactions of people who, having enjoyed a delicious meal of what they thought was fish, quickly alter their opinion upon discovering the dish was actually rattlesnake, or learn that the very palatable stew was really made of dog meat, muskrat, or some other objectively edible, but culturally rejected substance. Yet, even an American gourmet house will feature chocolate-covered ants, French-fried grasshoppers, preserved bumblebees, rattlesnake meat, and so forth, and the "cultured" will savor them.

Few if any societies treat the partaking of food as a purely casual, unregulated affair. The culture not only determines what and where one eats, but also with whom one eats, in what order, and even in what proportion. "Every society has its own etiquette pertaining to food and people who eat with their fingers or out of a common bowl may observe a very rigid code of manners."[9] Truly to understand the role of food in a society requires a knowledge of the society as a whole and the social ramifications of the total nutritional system.

Fig. 16.5. Culture helps determine not only what we eat, but also how we eat it.

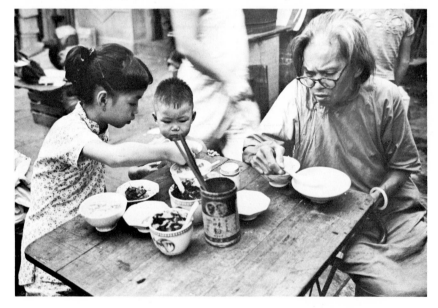

Carbohydrates, fats, proteins, vitamins, minerals, and water are the basic constituents of foods; all are essential, and merit attention. A discussion of each follows.

Most food is made through photosynthesis. Using energy from the sun, carbon dioxide from the air, and water from the soil, the leaves of green plants manufacture glucose, and from this the other sugars, starches, and cellulose of the plants. Carbohydrates account for close to 45 percent of our total caloric intake in North America. They are relatively inexpensive and may comprise more than 80 percent of the energy intake for poorer nations.

Carbohydrates
sugars & starches

The most common sugar in our diet today is *sucrose*, or white sugar; brown (unrefined) sugar is less common, but equally potent as a source of energy. Sucrose is composed of two simple sugars, or monosaccharides: *fructose*, found in fruits, and *glucose* (or dextrose), found in honey, candy, maple syrup, and very fresh young vegetables.

Glucose is by far the most important monosaccharide. As "blood sugar," it is absorbed from the intestine and stored in the liver and muscles as glycogen. In addition, the tiny but important amount of sugar in our blood is glucose. Our primary source of energy, glucose provides fuel for all body cells and is essentially the sole form of energy available to the brain.

Sucrose foods generally contain little more than calories, whereas starches, found in cereals, bread, and potatoes, are far more complex nutritionally. Regardless of structure, however, all carbohydrates must be broken down to monosaccharides in digestion.

Some of the water and carbon dioxide is synthesized into complex acids, or fatty acids, which are the chief constituents of fats, the second major energy source in North American diets. They comprise about 40 percent of our caloric intake. The body is able to synthesize all of the fatty acids it uses except the unsaturated fatty acid called linoleic acid, which must be provided from our diet. This is called the *essential* fatty acid. This polyunsaturated fat, plus others we are able to manufacture, is critical to the maintenance or reduction of cholesterol levels, and retards the deposition of cholesterol in the arteries.

Fats

Proteins contain nitrogen, whereas fats and carbohydrates do not. Essential to virtually every body structure, only proteins can provide the essential materials for tissue maintenance, growth, and repair. Proteins comprise about 15 percent of the American diet.

Proteins

Programmed by DNA, thousands of the twenty-two nitrogen-bearing acids, or amino acids, are arranged in a variety of patterns to form body proteins. Of the twenty-two, eight cannot be synthesized by the human body, but are essential to life (the *essential* amino acids). They must be imported to the body via food intake. From them the body can build the remaining fourteen. Complete proteins are generally more readily available from meat sources than from plant sources, as the animals have already manufactured the essential amino acids for us.

In producing energy, the body oxidizes carbohydrates and fats first. When there is a deficiency of carbohydrates and fats, proteins must be used, and growth is impeded. An adequate supply of carbohydrates and fats frees the proteins from energy production, and permits them to work in their area of greatest competence, body-building.

Vitamins

The lowest forms of life synthesize, or make within themselves, most of their nutrient requirements, and require few ready-made raw materials from their environment. Higher forms, like man, depend almost entirely on other organisms to supply many vital constituents of the diet. This is particularly true of vitamins.

Vitamins are either water-soluble (B complex, C) or fat-soluble (A,D,E,K).

Although vitamin E deficiency causes some sterility in lower animals, its relationship to sexual functioning in humans is a myth. It has been amply demonstrated that people subsisting on low vitamin E levels, as in many underdeveloped nations, do *not* have problems associated with low birth rates. The only therapeutic use of vitamin E in humans established by a well-controlled clinical trial is the treatment of hemolytic anemia in premature babies. Some physicians prescribe it as a precautionary measure in a few rare diseases involving fat-absorption impairment, but otherwise its value as a dietary supplement for common ailments is doubtful.[10]

One should not take vitamin pills to make up for deficiencies in the diet. Overdoses of vitamins can be harmful. Excessive vitamin D is toxic, for example, and may result in vomiting and dysentery. Similarly, an overdose of vitamin A may create joint pain, loss of appetite, loss of hair, dryness of skin, and irritability. Nor is vitamin C a cure for the common cold; at best, it is simply an expensive psychological aid.

Most foods are susceptible to nutritional loss both in storage and preparation. In general, they should be cooked briefly, and in as little liquid as possible. Further, whenever convenient, the cooking liquids should also be consumed, as they frequently hold vitamins B_1, B_2, and C and a variety of minerals. The accompanying table has been developed to summarize the role of various vitamins in nutrition.

Minerals

The soil gains its minerals from disintegrating rocks. Plants pick them up from the soil, and pass them on to us directly in vegetables, fruits, and grains, or indirectly through meat and dairy products. Nine principal minerals are present in humans: calcium, chlorine, iodine, iron, phosphorus, potassium, sodium, sulfur, and magnesium. Other trace elements are found in minute amounts: cobalt, copper, chromium, manganese, molybdenum, fluorine, selenium, zinc.

Since minerals are absorbed, used, and excreted by the body, they must be replaced continuously.

Water

Water is a required medium for all of the body's chemical reactions. It transports enzymes into the digestive tract, and provides the conveyor-belt lubrication for circulation, digestion, and excretion. With over 50 percent of total body weight accounted for by water, no one can survive for long without it.

How Were Vitamins Named?

Vitamins were first called *accessory factors* by Hopkins, who demonstrated in 1906 that normal foods contain, in addition to the nutrients then recognized—carbohydrates, proteins, fats, minerals, and water—minute traces of other substances essential to health. The curative effects of diet on scurvy, rickets, beriberi, night blindness, and other disorders had been observed from time to time for centuries and speculated upon. In 1911 Funk, who believed that the antiberiberi factor he isolated from rice polishings was an amine, proposed changing the group name to *vitamines* to emphasize the fact that the factors are essential to life and not merely accessory to other nutrients. It was Funk who formulated the vitamin hypothesis of deficiency disease. Classification by solubility was suggested in 1915 by Osborne and Mendel, as well as McCollum and Davis. Thus the *fat-soluble A,* which cured nutritional eye disease, was differentiated from the *water-soluble B,* which prevented beriberi in pigeons. An antiscorbutic substance was not taken into account. These workers rejected the term *vitamine,* having found that the fat-soluble A lacks an amine group. In 1920 Drummond proposed a compromise terminology, using *vitamin* without the final *e* as the generic term, labeling the antixerophthalmic factor *vitamin A* and the antiberiberi factor *vitamin B,* and adding a third factor, the antiscorbutic principle *vitamin C. . . .*

Confusion Worse Confounded

Successive letters of the alphabet were assigned to new vitamins as they were characterized and isolated, and some letters were assigned out of order; vitamin K, for example, refers to the Scandinavian word *Koagulation* and vitamin H to the German *Haut* (skin). It became evident that the original vitamin B was not a single vitamin but a group of vitamins, and subscripts were added for identification of separate factors as they were isolated. The nomenclature was confused when subscripts were used also for the fat-soluble vitamins, but for a different purpose. The subscripts here, instead of differentiating separate factors, merely label closely related chemical compounds having identical or nearly identical physiological actions. Further confusion was introduced when some vitamins were named as growth factors for test organisms. Many concentrates thought to be new vitamins and so named were afterward proved to duplicate prior vitamins. The recent trend has been toward chemical names; vitamin B_1 has become thiamine, vitamin B_2 riboflavin, and so on. Vitamin C, however, took a new name based on its antiscorbutic function—ascorbic acid.

It has been argued that vitamins that undergo transformation in the body should be called *provitamins,* but since a vitamin is by definition a dietary factor this could only introduce more confusion. Other terms, probably more confusing than useful, that have been proposed for the purpose of relating vitamins to their various properties include *nutramine, advitant, exogenous hormone, food hormone, ergin, ergon, catalin, biocatalyst* (as a comprehensive name for a vitamin, a hormone, or an enzyme), *vitazyme* (a vitamin-containing enzyme), *nutrilite* (a vitamin for any kind of organism, and not higher animals only), and *vitamer* (a specific form, or isomer, of a vitamin).

Like vitamin research, vitamin nomenclature is still in the developmental stage and will undoubtedly undergo many more modifications in the future. The present alphabetical confusion may someday give way to a rational and self-consistent nomenclature.[11]

Cellulose from vegetables contributes bulk to digested foodstuffs, increasing the mobility of ingested material and stimulating secretions from the intestinal walls. This indigestible roughage serves the useful purpose of maintaining consistency and bulk in feces.

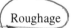 Roughage

Even at total rest the body requires some energy to maintain its circulation, temperature, and other biological functions. Such energy is usually measured in calories, which in turn are used as a gauge for estimating food values.* Foods vary greatly in their caloric content, depending upon their composition. A pound

Measuring
Nutrition

---

*One calorie is the amount of heat required to raise the temperature of a gram of water 1 degree Centigrade (1.8 degrees Fahrenheit). Nutritionists generally refer to kilocalories, which are larger units (1000 calories). They are the amount of heat required to raise 1 kilogram of water 1 degree Centigrade. These larger calories are what are usually called "calories."

of fat contains more than twice as many calories as a pound of either proteins or carbohydrates. For example, there are four calories each in a gram of proteins or carbohydrates, while there are nine calories in a gram of fat.

Adequate Diet

What diet is adequate for the average person? It depends upon many factors, including age, health, size, sex, climate, occupation, and activity patterns. Generally speaking, caloric requirements diminish with age; women, except during pregnancy, require fewer calories than men; and caloric needs decrease in warm weather. But quantity is only one factor. The way foods are prepared and the conditions under which they are eaten also affect the utilization of calories. Fried foods usually contain far more fat than broiled foods. Rates of digestion vary with tension, disease, and other factors. Some people may process food so quickly that they actually gain very little from it, and hence eat like horses, yet resemble wisps. Basal metabolic rate may have something to do with that.

Basal metabolic rate (BMR) is the minimum amount of energy a given person can use, in a resting, postabsorptive state, ideally measured while the person is sleeping peacefully in the early hours of the morning. It is measured by comparing the oxygen of the air expired with that inspired. Since all energy requires oxidation, the amount of oxygen used by a person during a period of time is an effective measure of energy output.

Not all calories taken in are given directly to energy output. Some are expended by our bodies in processing food. In any case, this loss is minimal, and often overlooked. The technical name for it is Specific Dynamic Action of food, or SDA. As a subject of controversy, it is unresolved, but probably accounts for well under 10 percent of caloric output. It is mentioned here only to advise the reader of its existence, as it should be added into the energy-output column. In the determination of the total energy expenditure of our bodies, BMR, SDA, and activity provide a measure of one's Total Metabolic Rate (TMR), as depicted in figure 16.6.

Fig. 16.6.
Determination of Total
Metabolic Rate (TMR)

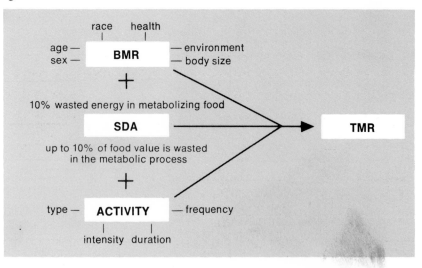

Chapter Sixteen

Table 16.1 Nutrients: Functions and Sources

Key Nutrients	Important Functions	Important Sources
Protein	Builds and repairs all tissues Helps build blood and form antibodies to fight infection Supplies energy	Meat, fish, poultry, eggs Milk and all kinds of cheese Dried beans and peas Peanut butter, nuts Bread and cereals
Fat	Supplies large amount of energy in a small amount of food Helps keep infant's skin healthy by supplying essential fatty acids Carries vitamins A, D, E and K	Butter and cream Salad oils and dressings Cooking and table fats Fat in meat
Carbohydrate (Sugars and Starch)	Supplies energy	Bread and cereals Potatoes, lima beans, corn Dried beans and peas Dried fruits, sweetened fruits; smaller amounts in fresh fruits Sugar, sirup, jelly, jam, honey
Minerals Calcium	Helps build bones and teeth Helps blood clot Helps muscles and nerves to work Helps regulate the use of other minerals in the body	Milk, ice cream Cheese, but less in cottage cheese, Sardines, other whole canned fish Turnip and mustard greens Collards, kale, broccoli
Iron	Combines with protein to make hemoglobin, the red substance in the blood that carries oxygen to the cells	Liver, other meat and eggs Dried beans and peas Green leafy vegetables Prunes, raisins, dried apricots Enriched or whole grain bread and cereals
Iodine	A constituent of thyroxine, a hormone that controls metabolic rate	Seafoods, iodized salt
Vitamins Vitamin A	Helps keep skin clear and smooth Helps keep mucous membranes firm and resistant to infection Helps prevent night blindness and promote healthy eyes Helps control bone growth	Liver, eggs Dark green and deep yellow vegetables Deep yellow fruits, such as peaches or cantaloupe Butter, whole milk, fortified skim milk, cream Cheddar-type cheese, ice cream
Thiamin or Vitamin B₁	Helps promote normal appetite and digestion Helps keep nervous system healthy and prevent irritability Helps body release energy from food	Meat, fish, poultry—pork supplies about 3 times as much as other meats, eggs Enriched or whole grain bread and cereals Dried beans and peas Potatoes, broccoli, collards
Riboflavin	Helps cells use oxygen Helps keep eyes, skin, tongue and lips healthy Helps prevent scaly, greasy skin around mouth and nose	Milk All kinds of cheese, ice cream Enriched or whole grain bread and cereals Meat, especially liver Fish, poultry, eggs
Niacin or Its Equivalent	Helps keep nervous system healthy Helps keep skin, mouth, tongue, digestive tract in healthy condition Helps cells use other nutrients	Peanut butter Meat, fish, poultry Milk (high in tryptophan) Enriched or whole grain bread and cereals
Ascorbic Acid or Vitamin C	Helps make cementing materials that hold body cells together Helps make walls of blood vessels firm Helps in healing wounds and broken bones Helps resist infection	Citrus fruits—orange, grapefruit, lemon, lime Strawberries and cantaloupe Tomatoes Green peppers, broccoli Raw or lightly cooked greens, cabbage White potatoes
Vitamin D, The Sunshine Vitamin	Helps absorb calcium from the digestive tract and build calcium and phosphorus into bones.	Vitamin D milk Fish liver oils Sunshine on skin (not a food)

The basal metabolic rate (BMR), expressed on a per-pound-body-weight basis, increases from birth to about two years of age, and thereafter gradually decreases until death. In general, we stop growing during our late teens, and as a consequence, the body's basic energy needs are reduced. Unfortunately, many of us simultaneously experience a decrease in activity, particularly when organized sport gives way to organized business, and social life moves from the outdoors to the indoors. As a consequence, too many people typically experience a gradual increase in body weight in their adult years. This unfortunately leads to many health problems.

What Is
Good Eating?

Basically, we require the essential nutrients in sufficient quantity to maintain health, growth, vigor, and emergency storage. There are two approaches to determining what is a satisfactory diet.

A simplified approach utilizes a chart such as that shown in figure 16.7. By judicious selection of foods from all four food groups, one can be reasonably sure that one's diet is adequate.

The more complicated approaches utilize Recommended Dietary Allowances (table 16.2). One must determine the nutritive value of all foods eaten. This requires detailed food composition tables, and necessitates some rather lengthy calculations. An individual serious about evaluating his diet should evaluate the quality of his daily food intake by employing the recommended dietary allowance tables and a food composition guide. (The latter table is found in most nutrition textbooks.) Many people are surprised to learn that the quality of their food is far lower than what they expected it to be.

Fad diets abound today. In fact, there are so many—old and new—that keeping up with all of their claims would be truly time-consuming. Whatever their claims, the regimes are usually followed by dieters with exaggerated zeal for short periods of time.

Some diets are based on excessive claims for a specific food, others purport to solve a special problem, and still others maintain that they can restore or contribute to good health. The fact is such exaggerations are false. Fad diets do none of these things. The best diet is a well-balanced one based on sound principles of good nutrition.

Why then do fad diets continue to be so popular? There are several reasons. Many people have little knowledge about nutrition and have little basis for accepting or rejecting superclaims for special foods or diets. They can easily be exploited as a result of their ignorance.

We live in a quick-fix, technological society and have come to expect remedies for most problems. It often seems that no matter what the problem, it will be solved if we are just patient enough to wait for scientific minds and sophisticated machines to give us the answers. Fad diets as quick cures or sure solutions fit right into this frame of modern expectations.

For many of those who are suffering from a long-term or incurable illness, a diet that promises a cure can be irresistible. By following a regime that offers them help, they can maintain hope. Likewise, those who are dissatisfied with the

A GUIDE TO GOOD EATING

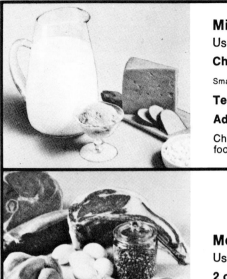

Milk Group

Use daily:

Children—3 or more glasses milk

Smaller glasses for some children under 8

Teenagers—4 or more glasses

Adults—2 or more glasses

Cheese, ice cream, and other milk-made foods can supply part of the milk

Meat Group

Use daily:

2 or more servings

Meats, fish, poultry, eggs, or cheese—with dry beans, peas, nuts as alternates

Vegetables and Fruits

Use daily:

4 or more servings

Include dark green or yellow vegetables; citrus fruit or tomatoes

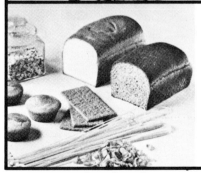

Breads and Cereals

Use daily:

4 or more servings

Enriched or whole grain
Added milk improves nutritional values

Source: National Dairy Council

Fig. 16.7. These foods form the foundation for a good diet. However, young children, teenagers, and women need more iron than do men. Liver, eggs, meat, legumes, dried fruit, dark green leafy vegetables, enriched or whole grain breads and cereals are good iron sources. Include vitamin D for infants and children, pregnant and lactating women, and adults who get little sunshine. Milk and fish liver oils are good sources of vitamin D.

This is the foundation for a good diet.
Use more of these and other foods as needed for growth, for activity, and for desirable weight.

Eating: The Good and the Bad of It   411

Table 16.2 Recommended Daily Dietary Allowances,[1] Revised 1973

	Years		Weight		Height		Energy	Protein	Fat-Soluble Vitamins		Vitamin D	Vitamin E Activity[5]
									Vitamin A Activity			
	from	up to	(kg)	(lbs)	(cm)	(in)	(kcal)[2]	(g)	(RE)[3]	(IU)	(IU)	(IU)
Infants	0.0	0.5	6	14	60	24	kg × 117	kg × 2.2	420[4]	1400	400	4
	0.5	1.0	9	20	71	28	kg × 108	kg × 2.0	400	2000	400	5
Children	1	3	13	28	86	34	1300	23	400	2000	400	7
	4	6	20	44	110	44	1800	30	500	2500	400	9
	7	10	30	66	135	54	2400	36	700	3300	400	10
Males	11	14	44	97	158	63	2800	44	1000	5000	400	12
	15	18	61	134	172	69	3000	54	1000	5000	400	15
	19	22	67	147	172	69	3000	52	1000	5000	400	15
	23	50	70	154	172	69	2700	56	1000	5000		15
	51+		70	154	172	69	2400	56	1000	5000		15
Females	11	14	44	97	155	62	2400	44	800	4000	400	10
	15	18	54	119	162	65	2100	48	800	4000	400	11
	19	22	58	128	162	65	2100	46	800	4000	400	12
	23	50	58	128	162	65	2000	46	800	4000		12
	51+		58	128	162	65	1800	46	800	4000		12
Pregnant							+300	+30	1000	5000	400	15
Lactating							+500	+20	1200	6000	400	15

Source: Food and Nutrition Board, National Academy of Sciences-National Research Council

[1]The allowances are intended to provide for individual variations among most normal persons as they live in the United States under usual environment stresses. Diets should be based on a variety of common foods in order to provide other nutrients for which human requirements have been less well defined. See text for more-detailed discussion of allowances and of nutrients not tabulated.
[2]Kilojuoles (KJ) = 4.2 × kcal
[3]Retinol equivalents
[4]Assumed to be all as retinol in milk during the first six months of life. All subsequent intakes are assumed to be one-half as retinol and one-half as B-carotene when calculated from international units. As retinol equivalents, three-fourths are as retinol and one-fourth as B-carotene.

high cost of medical care, with the difficulty in promptly securing an appointment with a physician, or with the lack of communication between busy doctors and their patients may find the accessible fad diet attractive.

Capitalizing on our personal desires also may make food fads more appealing. Desires to lose weight, to find an aphrodisiac, to have a clear complexion, or even to transcend the consciousness of ordinary humans have all been appealed to by various fad diets.

Weight-loss diets have been consistently popular. It is understandable how regimes that promise quick weight loss have such widespread appeal. Low-carbohydrate programs have been among the most popular. Such diets generally claim to be high protein but should be called high fat and protein. Carbohydrates, which supply energy, are discouraged in these diets because supposedly they are rapidly converted to body fat in overweight persons. Fat and protein are said to be utilized in metabolic processes rather than stored, and hence these become the substance of the weight loss diet. In reality the initial weight reduction is due to loss of body water. Continued weight loss does occur on low-carbohydrate diets, but the loss is due to reduced caloric intake and not to any special properties of

Water-Soluble Vitamins							Minerals					
Ascor-bic Acid	Folacin[6]	Niacin[7]	Ribo-flavin	Thiamin	Vitamin B$_6$	Vitamin B$_{12}$	Calcium	Phos-phorus	Iodine	Iron	Mag-nesium	Zinc
(mg)	(ug)	(mg)	(mg)	(mg)	(mg)	(ug)	(mg)	(mg)	(ug)	(mg)	(mg)	(mg)
35	50	5	0.4	0.3	0.3	0.3	360	240	35	10	60	3
35	50	8	0.6	0.5	0.4	0.3	540	400	45	15	70	5
40	100	9	0.8	0.7	0.6	1.0	800	800	60	15	150	10
40	200	12	1.1	0.9	0.9	1.5	800	800	80	10	200	10
40	300	16	1.2	1.2	1.2	2.0	800	800	110	10	250	10
45	400	18	1.5	1.4	1.6	3.0	1200	1200	130	18	350	15
45	400	20	1.8	1.5	1.8	3.0	1200	1200	150	18	400	15
45	400	20	1.8	1.5	2.0	3.0	800	800	140	10	350	15
45	400	18	1.6	1.4	2.0	3.0	800	800	130	10	350	15
45	400	16	1.5	1.2	2.0	3.0	800	800	110	10	350	15
45	400	16	1.3	1.2	1.6	3.0	1200	1200	115	18	300	15
45	400	14	1.4	1.1	2.0	3.0	1200	1200	115	18	300	15
45	400	14	1.4	1.1	2.0	3.0	800	800	100	18	300	15
45	400	13	1.2	1.0	2.0	3.0	800	800	100	18	300	15
45	400	12	1.1	1.0	2.0	3.0	800	800	80	10	300	15
60	800	+2	+0.3	+0.3	2.5	4.0	1200	1200	125	18+	450	20
60	600	+4	+0.5	+0.3	2.5	4.0	1200	1200	150	18	450	25

[5]Total vitamin E activity, estimated to be 80 percent as a-tocopherol and 20 percent other tocopherols. See text for variation in allowances.

[6]The folacin allowances refer to dietary sources as determined by *Lactobacillus casei* assay. Pure forms of folacin may be effective in doses less than one-fourth of the RDA.

[7]Although allowances are expressed as niacin, it is recognized that on the average 1 mg of niacin is derived from each 60 mg of dietary tryptophan.

[8]This increased requirement cannot be met by ordinary diets; therefore, the use of supplemental iron is recommended.

the diet. There is no evidence of any greater loss on this diet than on a well-balanced diet, if the total number of calories is the same.

Dr. Stillman's Quick Weight Loss Diet and Dr. Atkins' Super Energy Diet are both low-carbohydrate plans. People on these regimes often complain of fatigue and lassitude. Increased blood cholesterol levels, acceleration of atherosclerosis, and increased risk of heart attack are among their hazards.

High-fiber diets are a recent addition to our repertoire of food fads. Fiber is important in the diet. High-fiber foods include vegetables, fruits, and whole grains. Inclusion of these foods allows for regular bowel movements and has also been associated with lower levels of intestinal cancer. More research is being carried out in this area.

These foods do give a full feeling and may encourage one to push away from the dinner table sooner. But to claim that high-fiber diets push foods through the gastrointestinal tract faster, minimizing the absorption of calorie-containing foods, is ridiculous.

Vegetarian diets can range from healthy, sensible eating to dangerous fanaticism. They exclude meat, poultry, and fish. A pure or vegan vegetarian excludes

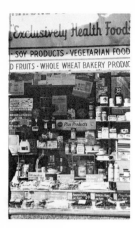

all animal products, while an ovo-lacto-vegetarian may eat eggs and dairy products as well as vegetables and a lacto-vegetarian will add dairy products only.

These diets can be nutritionally adequate if the variety of permissible foods is wide enough to guarantee a proper mixing of vegetable proteins. A vitamin B_{12} deficiency is a serious hazard for a vegan vegetarian. This vitamin is found only in foods of animal origin. So, for ovo-lacto-vegetarians and lacto-vegetarians there is less threat of B_{12} deficiency.

The Zen-macrobiotic diet is one that progresses through several stages, first excluding meat and eventually every other food except brown rice and tea. It was invented by George Ohsawa, and it is claimed that it will provide spiritual enlightenment and freedom from disease for its followers. It has absolutely nothing to do with Zen Buddhism.

Strict followers of this diet are rare, which is fortunate, since it is one of the most dangerous diets. Vitamin deficiencies, mineral deficiencies, loss of kidney function due to restricted fluid intake, starvation, and death have been reported in macrobiotic dieters.

Massive doses of vitamins have also been advertised as important today in the maintenance of health and the prevention of disease. The claims for vitamin E have gone even further, holding that it prevents sterility, miscarriages, and muscular weakness, among other things. The American Dietetic Association recognizes the scientific evidence that these claims are unfounded and that massive doses of vitamins should be discouraged. A well-balanced diet is the most sensible and safest way to guarantee an optimum vitamin intake. Vitamin poisoning and kidney-stone formation are among the many side effects associated with vitamin self-therapy.

Summary

We have taken a cross-cultural look at eating patterns around the world, emphasizing North America. The essential food elements have been examined. We have also discussed some of the more hazardous pop diets of the twentieth century. Such considerations will require you to make dietary adjustments and decisions about your food intake throughout your life. Your knowledge of foods, tempered by your various personal attitudes, will influence how you eat. And as you eat, so will you grow, usually in spots where you wish you would not.

Review Questions

1. Describe how food patterns reflect much more than nutritional principles and income.
2. How do cultural factors sometimes work against the establishment of sound nutritional habits?
3. Discuss how religion plays a prominent role in food patterns.
4. List the four basic food groups and give examples of each.

5. Why is vegetarianism potentially hazardous to one's health?

6. What are the functions of vitamins A, B, C, and D? From what foods can they be obtained?

7. What factors determine the caloric requirements of an individual?

8. Discuss a few fad diets that are popular today. Are there health hazards involved?

Readings

FAO Third World Health Survey. *Freedom From Hunger.* Basic Study No. 11. Rome, 1963.

Gambrell, W.; Haggerty, J.; and *Life* Editors. *Food and Nutrition.* New York: Time-Life, 1967.

Harper, A. "Recommended Dietary Allowances: Are They What We Think They Are," *Journal of the American Dietetic Association* 64 (1974): 151–57.

Mayer, J. *Overweight: Causes, Cost, and Control.* Englewood Cliffs, N.J.: Prentice-Hall, 1968.

Robson, J.; Larkin, F.; Sandretto, A.; and Tadayyon, B. *Malnutrition: Its Causation and Control.* New York: Gordon & Breach, 1972.

Notes

1. J. May, *The Ecology of Malnutrition in the Far and the Near East* (New York: Hafner Publishing Co., 1961), pp. 3–7.

2. I. C. Brown, *Understanding Other Cultures* (Englewood Cliffs, N.J.: Prentice-Hall, 1973), pp. 22–24.

3. M. Lowenberg et al., *Food and Man* (New York: John Wiley & Sons, 1968), p. 11.

4. A. Burgess and R. Dean, *Malnutrition and Food Habits* (New York: Macmillan Co., 1962), p. 26.

5. Ibid., p. 28.

6. F. Simoons, *Eat Not This Flesh* (Madison: University of Wisconsin Press, 1961), p. 11.

7. Ibid., p. 8.

8. "Search for the Oldest People," *National Geographic Magazine,* January 1973, pp. 93–119; "Observations of a Peripatetic Gerontologist," *Nutrition Today,* September-October 1973, pp. 4–12.

9. Brown, *Understanding Other Cultures,* p. 15.

10. "Vitamin E: What Is Behind All Those Claims for It," *Consumer Reports,* January 1973, pp. 60–66.

11. Upjohn Company, *Vitamin Manual,* SCOPE Monograph, 1965, p. 2.

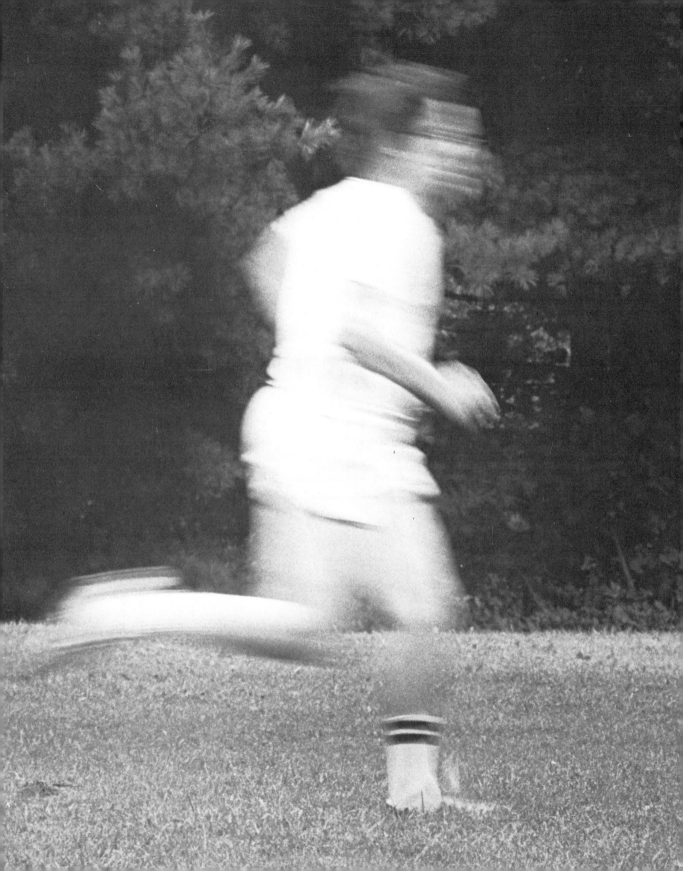

Fitness: Better Appearance and Ability to Function Optimally

17

Walk along the nearest beach or spend a day at a family amusement park and notice the shape of our citizens. They come in great variety. Many of their sizes and shapes are not those of persons one would think of as being fit. Individual shapes often are unattractive and no doubt less than totally fit, physiologically speaking.

The most obvious indication of poor fitness is overweight. However, there are many other indications. A person might not be able to pick up a fifty-pound bag of grass seed without discomfort or possibly mow the lawn without feeling fatigued. An eight-year-old child asks Daddy to toss a ball around after supper. Tragically, Daddy might find himself out of breath after running a couple of pass patterns. These and thousands of similar occurrences can be noted daily and are signs that most adults in our society today lack physical fitness.

While the most obvious outward sign of lack of fitness is probably overweight, closer physiological examination would no doubt reveal decreased optimal functioning of many of the physiological activities of the body. There may well be a buildup of cholesterol and triglycerides in the blood vessels, causing reduced effectiveness of the circulatory system. The oxygen capacity of the lungs may be reduced as the result of smoking, environmental pollutants, or lack of exercise. These and many other deficiencies, though not immediately apparent, have a detrimental effect on a person's ability to function at an optimal level.

The need to exercise regularly as an adult may be brought on by many factors, but basically Americans are a sedentary people. Mechanization has relieved us of many physical labors, tremendously reducing our energy output. For example, today we use riding mowers, expending much less energy to mow the lawn than if we pushed a hand mower. Many houses have automatic garage-door openers. Instead of stepping out of the car, walking to the door, and raising it, the driver simply pushes a button and the door automatically goes up; the driver expends little energy. For many Americans, their recreation and relaxation involves sitting in an armchair watching television or riding a motorized cart around the golf course. The motorized boat or snowmobile, though exciting to ride and fun to use, consumes very little physical energy. These and numerous other labor-saving devices have reduced individual energy output for most Americans.

Anyone who has traveled to other parts of the world must be amazed at how active adults in other cultures are in carrying out various normal functions of life. In Holland hundreds of people bicycle to work, to the store, and to school each day. Lifting and carrying loads of various sizes for long distances is commonplace in many countries of the world. Recreation for the Scandinavian involves many vigorous outdoor sports—hiking, skiing, orienteering—all of which necessitate the use of much physical energy.

Total Fitness

The concept of total fitness includes the several interrelated dimensions of health—social and emotional as well as physical. The fitness pattern might be likened to a wheel. Each component—social, emotional, and physical—is a different part of the wheel. As long as each part is functioning effectively, we can say that a person is healthy or fit. However, when one part of the wheel is damaged, the effectiveness of the entire tire is reduced. So it is with the individual whose total fitness is reduced by poor functioning along one dimension.

The measures of physical fitness include agility, body composition, balance, coordination, endurance, flexibility, power, reaction time, speed, and strength. Four of these dimensions are closely related to health and well being and will be examined in this chapter: muscular strength, muscular endurance, flexibility, and cardiovascular endurance. Also related to these components of physical fitness is weight control.

Definition

Physical fitness may be defined as the ability to perform the normally expected functions of life and have energy left over to meet emergency situations that might arise. A high level of physical fitness gives the individual the physical capacity to live a quality life. Fatigue and lack of strength should not limit one's daily activities as is so often the case. Maintenance of a reasonable level of physical fitness must be considered a type of preventive medicine. Fitness cannot be achieved overnight by taking a pill or some other medicine. It involves hard work, time, personal discipline, commitment, and a positive attitude.

Establishing a program of physical fitness is individual and personal in nature. The needs and aspirations of each person's program will vary. For this reason, one planning a program of physical fitness will need to identify his or her specific needs. This, then, will establish the specific goals to be achieved. The goal may be losing weight, improving respiratory functioning, lowering pulse rate, achieving greater flexibility, or eliminating body fat on the hips and thighs. A person may have one or many objectives in establishing a physical fitness program.

You can use several measures to identify your physical fitness needs. Before you begin to participate in any active physical fitness program you should have a thorough medical examination. One major purpose of the physical examination is to determine if there are any conditions present that would be aggravated by physical exercise.

Medical Examination

The medical examination should include at least the making of a complete health history. Height, weight, pulse, and blood pressure should be measured. Other basic exams should include a blood sugar test, urinalysis, a chest X ray, and an electrocardiogram (ECG). It is also useful to have tests of blood cholesterol and pulmonary functioning. Take no shortcuts in an effort to reduce the cost of the

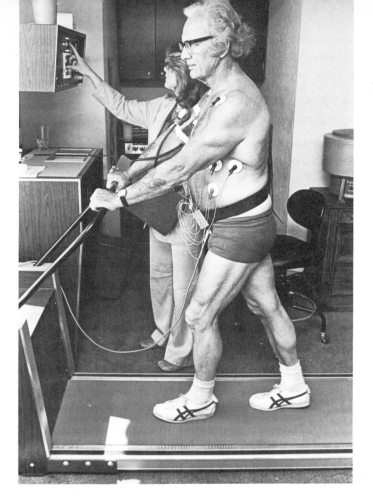

Fig. 17.1. A person's capacity for strenuous exercise may be measured by ECG while the subject walks on a treadmill. The device is gradually speeded up to test the reaction of a person's heart to physical stress.

examination. It is vitally important that your physical status be known before you start any regular exercise program.

Other important physical indicators are helpful in ascertaining one's physical status, which usually are not included in a medical examination unless requested. If an expert in physiology and exercise is available, certain physiological functions related to fitness should be measured. The exercise physiologist can help ascertain individual maximum oxygen consumption, the functioning level of the cardiovascular system, body fat composition and density, and take other useful measures of physical fitness.

Identification of physical fitness needs may simply be listing one's personal needs observed in the course of day-to-day living. One young man, who had previously been active in college track, discovered three years after graduation that he became short of breath when shoveling the driveway after a heavy spring snowfall. He realized something was wrong, began a fitness program of jogging, and today is in good condition. When one can no longer perform functions that one previously could, it may be time to make note of a personal fitness need.

Other
Physical Indicators

Muscular Strength   One component of fitness that many people are interested in improving is *muscular strength*. Muscles function by contracting and extending. When one wishes to lift an object from the floor, the muscles of the upper arm (biceps) contract, and force is exerted. The same muscle extends as the object is lowered to the ground.

The amount of force exerted in a single contraction is known as the strength of that muscle. Muscular strength is important for performing the many functions of daily living. In particular the large muscle groups of the arms, legs, back, trunk, and abdominal region are used in everyday activities. Muscular strength can be measured by instruments called tensiometers and dynamometers. These instruments record the amount of force in a single, maximum movement pattern. Any muscle of the body will become stronger with use. Whenever a muscle is not used, the muscle fibers weaken and eventually atrophy.

The average adult usually does not perform any activity on a regular basis that strengthens the muscles. Many college students are involved in sports activities, which help develop the muscles. However, once out of school, a person's activity level is usually greatly reduced. Though one's muscles usually retain enough strength to carry out common activities, when a person is called on to lift or move a heavier object than one is normally accustomed to moving, the muscle strength may not be there.

People often strain and injure themselves trying to lift or move objects that are too heavy for them. A pulled back muscle or other such injury can incapacitate a person for weeks. It is important that a person develop an exercise program that will help strengthen the large muscle groups so that one can perform with ease the various tasks that might occur each day. Once a reasonable degree of fitness is achieved, it is also vital to continue exercises that will maintain muscular strength.

Most men will show some interest in developing their muscular strength. However, women often are not interested because they think such activity will develop unattractive, bulging muscles, not at all in keeping with the traditional feminine image. This has been shown to be untrue. Regular strength exercises lead to better muscle tone and improved total fitness. Women have no need to worry that exercise will result in an unsightly, masculine appearance. Two different types of exercise may be used to develop muscular strength: *isometric exercises* and *isotonic exercises*.

Isometric Exercises   Isometric exercises build strength in muscle groups. This can be accomplished with a minimum amount of equipment and in a rather short time. However, even though they do help build strength, isometric exercises contribute very little to the development of other muscular fitness components such as flexibility and endurance. They also have little effect on cardiopulmonary fitness. Furthermore, many people consider isometric exercises boring.

The principle underlying isometric exercises is that muscles may be strengthened by contraction against some resistance with little or no movement of the body part involved. For example, as you sit at a desk that is fastened to the

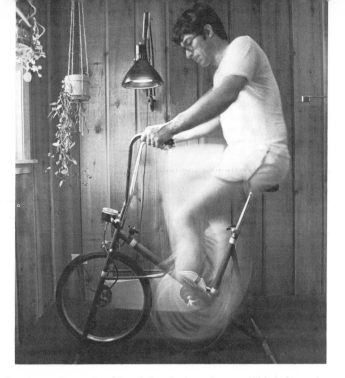

Fig. 17.2. Regular strength exercises lead to better muscle tone and improved total fitness. Prolonged cycling can have beneficial cardiovascular effects, too.

floor, place your hands on the underside of the desk and exert lifting force for several seconds (usually five to ten seconds). Doing this several times a day will strengthen the biceps.

In designing an isometric exercise program identify the muscle group to be exercised, then find or design a device against which force may be exerted with some resistance. However, keep in mind that people who have diagnosed heart disease, who are obese, who are prone to strokes, or who faint easily should not perform isometrics.

Isotonic Exercises

Isotonic exercises are more popular than isometrics, particularly among college students. These exercises involve movement similar to the many daily movements of an individual and involve contraction of muscle groups with movement of the body parts involved. The increase in strength occurs as a result of *overload,* which is achieved by either adding weight or increasing the number of times the exercise is performed. To develop further muscular strength, one should use increased resistance, more weight, and fewer repetitions. To improve muscular endurance, the weight should be kept constant or reduced and the number of repetitions increased.

In an effective isotonic program, exercises must be performed against resistance. Weight training is most commonly used. A specific set of muscles is selected to be exercised, an appropriate weight level is identified, and a certain number of repetitions are chosen, say sets of six to ten. Usually two to four sets of repetitions are considered satisfactory. As this measure is performed comfortably, sets of repetitions are added or weight is added depending on the objective of the activity program.

In the absence of weights, timed calisthenics are useful. For example, pushups contribute to strength development of the triceps and chest muscles. Chinups strengthen the back and biceps. Curlups (properly executed situps) are useful for abdominal strength development. Other calisthenics strengthen specific muscle groups when performed regularly and in a proper manner.

Muscular Endurance

Muscular endurance is the ability to contract the muscles repeatedly. After continual repetition of contraction of a given muscle or muscle group, fatigue will set in. The body part will no longer contract on demand. Endurance is important in a general sense, related as it is to cardiovascular functioning and respiratory capacity.

Flexibility

The place where two or more bones come together is known as a *joint*. All of a person's movements involve motion at a joint. The range of motion at a joint is referred to as *flexibility*. The more flexible an individual, the greater one's ability to perform a variety of body functions.

A number of factors can limit flexibility at a joint. Injury to tissue around a joint will often reduce flexibility; this often happens with athletic injuries. The knee is often injured by football, basketball, or hockey players; the elbow commonly is affected in the case of a baseball pitcher. Many diseases, such as arthritic conditions and infectious diseases, inhibit joint flexibility.

When there is lack of exercise, joint flexibility is reduced. The muscles become weak; ligaments and connective tissues shorten. The result is a decrease in flexibility. Sedentary living patterns contribute to decreased flexibility.

To improve flexibility, it is necessary to stretch the specific joint. Slow, sustained stretching exercises cause the muscles to relax and lengthen. One should not use quick, bouncing exercises to develop flexibility. Select a given set of muscles for development and begin by steadily and slowly stretching them. Examples of flexibility exercises are touching the toes, which stretches the hamstring muscle, sitting and curling the back with the head between the knees, and trunk-twisting movements. There are many other movement patterns that contribute to improved flexibility.

Cardiovascular Fitness

Though not the only component of physical fitness, cardiovascular fitness may be the most important. An efficient cardiovascular system (heart, blood vessels, lungs) not only is important for good health, but also may determine how long a person will live. Heart disease is the leading cause of death among adults over forty. Regular exercise helps reduce the risk of coronary heart problems.

The cardiovascular system supplies the cells of the body with oxygen and removes the waste products. This physiological process requires proper functioning of the heart, the blood vessels, and the lungs. Many maladaptations can interfere with the efficiency of this system, including hypertension, arteriosclerosis, atherosclerosis, emphysema, and various other heart and lung diseases.

The ability of the heart, lungs, and blood vessels to function efficiently is known as *cardiovascular endurance*. Exercise has been shown to improve cardiovascular endurance. Most medical personnel agree that regular exercise will produce the following physiological results:

1. A stronger, more efficient heart muscle
2. A slower heartbeat, which means that the heart does not work as hard to handle the same amount of blood—a more efficient use of energy
3. Fewer triglycerides and less cholesterol (fatty substances) in the blood. Triglycerides have been associated with clotting of the blood, and some medical experts consider them more important in causing atherosclerosis than cholesterol. However, both substances are factors in atherosclerosis.
4. Greater oxygen intake capacity, which means that oxygen consumption is lower for a given task and one does not have to breathe as rapidly or as deeply to perform it
5. Development of collateral circulation through the formation of new blood vessels or the enlargement of small capillaries around diseased or damaged vessels, which maintains the flow of blood to a given organ. (Collateral circulation is of particular value in maintaining coronary circulation.)
6. A reduction of high blood pressure

There are two different types of exercises that relate to the cardiovascular system: *anaerobic* and *aerobic*.

Anaerobic Exercises

Anaerobic exercises are physical activities that do not require the use of great quantities of oxygen over long periods of time. Such exercises are of short duration and do not depend on the body's cardiovascular efficiency. For example, running at full speed for a short distance is anaerobic exercise. When the activity demands too much oxygen, an oxygen debt results, and the individual stops exercising. Oxygen recovery occurs after the exercise is halted. There is little cardiovascular fitness value in anaerobic exercises. They are useful to individuals who want to develop a high level of fitness for activities involving short bursts of speed or strength.

Fig. 17.3. Swimming is one of the best activities for developing and maintaining cardiovascular endurance.

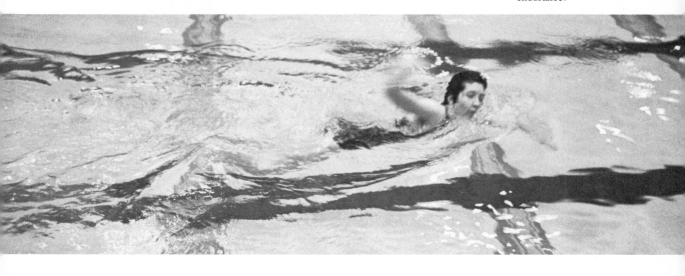

| Aerobic Exercises | Aerobic exercises require immediate and constant use of oxygen. These exercises last long enough to have beneficial physiological effects on the cardiorespiratory system. Activities that help improve cardiovascular fitness include jogging, cycling, walking, swimming, racket sports, and others. |

Aerobic training has been popularized by Dr. Kenneth H. Cooper.[1] Cooper studied extensively the effects of exercise on the human body. Two of his many findings should be noted. If a particular activity is to have a training effect, it must require a sustained heart rate of about 150 beats per minute, or 180 beats minus the subject's age. The training effect will begin about five minutes after the sustained heart rate is reached and will continue as long as the exercise is performed. Second, Cooper noted that a training effect can occur even if a heart rate of 150 beats per minute is not reached. In this case, there must be increased oxygen consumption for a longer period of time than five minutes.

Cooper originally designed a point system based on the amount of oxygen consumed in particular activities. In 1970 Cooper expanded his program.[2] He identified a number of different aerobic exercises, determined their point values, and noted activity differences in various age categories for both men and women. Cooper suggests that a person should earn thirty points a week and that these points should be earned over the whole week, not compiled in one or two activity periods.

Before starting Cooper's program of cardiovascular fitness activities, individuals determine their own level of fitness. They walk, run, or jog for twelve

Table 17.1 Fitness Categories for Men and Women Based on Running Times for 1.5 Miles*

1.5-Mile Test—Men

Fitness Category	Under 30	30-39	40-49	50+
I. Very Poor	16:30+	17:30+	18:30+	19:00+
II. Poor	16:30-14:31	17:30-15:31	18:30-16:31	19:00-17:01
III. Fair	14:30-12:01	15:30-13:01	16:30-14:01	17:00-14:31
IV. Good	12:00-10:16	13:00-11:01	14:00-11:31	14:30-12:01
V. Excellent	<10:16	<11:01	<11:31	<12:01

1.5-Mile Test—Women

Fitness Category	Under 30	30-39	40-49	50+
I. Very Poor	17:30+	18:30+	19:30+	20:30+
II. Poor	17:30-15:31	18:30-16:31	19:30-17:31	20:30-18:31
III. Fair	15:30-13:01	16:30-14:01	17:30-15:01	18:30-16:31
IV. Good	13:00-11:16	14:00-12:01	15:00-12:31	16:30-13:31
V. Excellent	<11:16	<12:01	<12:31	<13:31

*Times given in minutes and seconds
Source: Reprinted in P.E. Allsen, J. M. Harrison, and B. Vance, *Fitness for Life: An Individualized Approach* (Dubuque, Ia.: Wm. C. Brown, 1976), p. 10. Adapted from Kenneth H. Cooper, M. D., *The New Aerobics*, p. 31. Copyright © 1970 by Kenneth H. Cooper. Reprinted by permission of the publisher, M. Evans & Company, Inc., New York, New York.

Chapter Seventeen

minutes. The distance traveled in this time determines one's specific fitness category: I—very poor; II—poor; III—fair; IV—good; V—excellent. Once the fitness category is determined, individuals design their own activity programs based on activities in which they wish to participate.

Though Cooper's aerobics program has become the most widely known and used for development of cardiovascular fitness, there are other programs.[3] Also, individuals who understand some of the concepts underlying cardiovascular fitness can design their own programs.

Exercise activity choices will differ from one person to another. Some people cannot play basketball, tennis, or handball well. Others may not be able to swim. For some people, social relationships are so important that jogging by themselves is unthinkable. Regardless of the activities chosen, they should be activities that the person enjoys. In addition, one should carry out aerobic exercises on a regular basis. This will make for a more consistent activity pattern. Allsen, Harrison, and Vance maintain that "a person should receive training stimuli no less than forty-eight hours apart in order to maintain cardiovascular endurance."[4]

Weight control has become almost an obsession in contemporary America. Newspapers, movies, magazines, billboards, radio, television, and other media continuously stress the theme that an ever-increasing proportion of our citizens are overweight. Obesity has become a moral vice, leanness a virtue. | **Weight Control**

To understand the intricate mechanism of weight control, it is necessary to examine the relationship between caloric intake and expenditure and the role of physical fitness. Different theories of weight loss produce various reduction schemes. This chapter offers some "exchange" plans for the maintenance of an energy intake-output balance.

Weight control is really a simple problem. It demands that one maintain a balance between energy intake and energy output. Since both can be calculated fairly accurately and without elaborate equipment, the conscientious individual should have no problem maintaining an acceptable weight. | **The Scales of Conscience**

Caloric intake is the sum nutritional value of all foods and liquids taken into the body; *caloric output* includes Basal Metabolic Rate (BMR), Specific Dynamic Action (SDA), and activity. Food intake is easily measured and can be regulated by consulting charts on caloric intake. Determining and regulating energy output, on the other hand, is slightly more complex. | Caloric Intake

Basal metabolic rate is relatively stable for a given individual, although it does vary according to age, sex, state of health, climate, and physical condition (well-conditioned people tend to have a higher BMR than fat people). To a large degree, BMR is genetically determined. Although it can be modified by drugs or even physical activity, it is relatively constant over time, and therefore quite predictable. | Energy Output

The really perplexing thing about BMR is its relationship to weight control. Some people simply have high BMRs and seem to be able to eat anything without gaining weight. Others gain weight almost by looking at food. BMR is important—in sedentary people it can account for 50 to 70 percent of their total caloric requirements.

On the basis of previous tests, BMR may be estimated from height and weight figures. For persons of average body build only, an estimate based on body weight—1 kilocalorie per kilogram of body weight per hour—gives a value that corresponds well with those obtained on actual tests. It does not work as well for either lean or fat people, however; an estimate of fat-free weight must be used for them.

Basal metabolism can be calibrated directly by measuring the precise amount of heat given off by the body in a respiration chamber. Assuming the individual is in a postabsorptive, resting state, the heat produced represents the minimum energy need of the individual. A simpler method involves indirect calorimetry, in which the oxygen consumption is measured to determine basal metabolism. By comparing the exhaled air with that inhaled and noting the amount of oxygen consumed, one can estimate the energy expenditure during the time of the sampling. All energy expenditure requires oxygen—so the measure is quite accurate. A protein-bound iodine (PBI) test on a blood sample is the measure most commonly used today.

Fig. 17.4. Basal metabolic rate in females and males

As mentioned in chapter 16, the Specific Dynamic Action (of food) factor is a constant and varies little, if at all, over time. Nor can we do very much to change it. Activity, however, is a different story.

CALORIES PER HOUR PER SQUARE METER

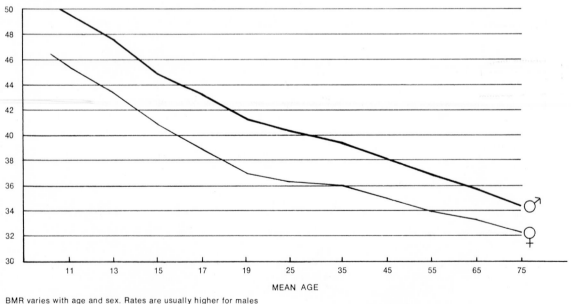

BMR varies with age and sex. Rates are usually higher for males and decline proportionately with age for both sexes.

Source: L. L. Langley, *Physiology of Man*, Toronto: Van Nostrand Reinhold Company, 1971, p. 576.

Table 17.2 Energy Equivalents of Food Calories Expressed in Minutes of Activity

Food	Calories	Walking	Riding bicycle	Swimming	Running	Reclining
Apple, large	101	19	12	9	5	78
Bacon, 2 strips	96	18	12	9	5	74
Banana, small	88	17	11	8	4	68
Beans, green, 1 c	27	5	3	2	1	21
Beer, 1 glass	114	22	14	10	6	88
Bread and butter	78	15	10	7	4	60
Cake, 1/12, 2-layer	356	68	43	32	18	274
Carbonated beverage, 1 glass	106	20	13	9	5	82
Carrot, raw	42	8	5	4	2	32
Cereal, dry, ½ c, with milk and sugar	200	38	24	18	10	154
Cheese, cottage, 1 tbsp	27	5	3	2	1	21
Cheese, Cheddar, 1 oz	111	21	14	10	6	85
Chicken, fried, ½ breast	232	45	28	21	12	178
Chicken, "TV" dinner	542	104	66	48	28	417
Cookie, plain, 148/lb	15	3	2	1	1	12
Cookie, chocolate chip	51	10	6	5	3	39
Doughnut	151	29	18	13	8	116
Egg, fried	110	21	13	10	6	85
Egg, boiled	77	15	9	7	4	59
French dressing, 1 tbsp	59	11	7	5	3	45
Halibut steak, ¼ lb	205	39	25	18	11	158
Ham, 2 slices	167	32	20	15	9	128
Ice cream, ⅙ qt	193	37	24	17	10	148
Ice cream soda	255	49	31	23	13	196
Ice milk, ⅙ qt	144	28	18	13	7	111
Gelatin, with cream	117	23	14	10	6	90
Malted milk shake	502	97	61	45	26	386
Mayonnaise, 1 tbsp	92	18	11	8	5	71
Milk, 1 glass	166	32	20	15	9	128
Milk, skim, 1 glass	81	16	10	7	4	62
Milk shake	421	81	51	38	22	324
Orange, medium	68	13	8	6	4	52
Orange juice, 1 glass	120	23	15	11	6	92
Pancake with sirup	124	24	15	11	6	95
Peach, medium	46	9	6	4	2	35
Peas, green, ½ c	56	11	7	5	3	43
Pie, apple, ⅙	377	73	46	34	19	290
Pie, raisin, ⅙	437	84	53	39	23	336
Pizza, cheese, ⅛	180	35	22	16	9	138
Pork chop, loin	314	60	38	28	16	242
Potato chips, 1 serving	108	21	13	10	6	83
Sandwiches						
Club	590	113	72	53	30	454
Hamburger	350	67	43	31	18	269
Roast beef with gravy	430	83	52	38	22	331
Tuna fish salad	278	53	34	25	14	214
Sherbet, ⅙ qt	177	34	22	16	9	136
Shrimp, French fried	180	35	22	16	9	138
Spaghetti, 1 serving	396	76	48	35	20	305
Steak, T-bone	235	45	29	21	12	181
Strawberry shortcake	400	77	49	36	21	308

Reprinted by permission from 'Food Energy Equivalents of Various Activities' by Frank Konishi.
J. Am. Dietet. A. 46:186, 1965. Copyright The American Dietetic Association.

Fitness: Better Appearance and Optimal Functioning

The critical characteristic for any weight change program is the caloric balance, and that balance results primarily from the constant interplay between food (intake) and activity (output). Diet *and* exercise—not diet *or* exercise—seems to be the most logical model in a long-range weight control scheme. Most people understand diet as a factor; indeed, calorie charts are common. But few people truly comprehend exercise and the real significance of duration, intensity, and frequency of activity for weight change.

Whereas the average man burns around 2,000 to 2,500 calories per day, and the average woman around 1,600 to 2,000, few really alter their dietary patterns over time. Since BMR itself tends to decrease about 3 percent annually after the person reaches twenty-four or twenty-five, if all other factors remain stable, individuals should expect to add a little body weight each year. Couple this diminishing BMR with reduced activity and heavier eating and drinking patterns, and the result is obvious: beginning obesity.

Obesity

What is obesity? Medically it is "a condition of the body characterized by overaccumulation of fat under the skin and around certain of the internal organs."[5] In this text we use the term to describe a body condition in which fat content is 20 percent above normal. The term "overweight," then, represents that portion of the weight scale that lies between normality and obesity.

How is normal weight determined? Tables of desirable weights have been made available by numerous sources for years. Usually such tables take age, body type, and height into account, and they are relatively accurate for the population at large. But individuals vary, and many people hedge on their body types in the direction of the more favorable category. This gives them a false sense of security.

The major problem is not weight itself, anyway; it is fat. Weight is a measure of the entire body, including muscle. The calculation of *fat-free weight* is the only really important measurement. It can be estimated with calipers or pinching, or measured by means of buoyancy tests, injection techniques, X rays, and other sophisticated methods, some of which are both expensive and hazardous.

Since about 50 percent of the body fat is stored beneath the skin, an estimate of the fat content can be obtained by measuring a double skinfold. The double layer of skin is approximately 1 millimeter in thickness. Thus the double thickness minus 1 millimeter is a good indication of the quantity of fat stored at the particular location in question. Calipers, applying constant pressure, can be used for the triceps skinfold, the subscapular skinfold, the hip skinfold, and the biceps skinfold, and the measurements totaled. Comparing that total to the table in figure 17.5 provides a reasonable estimate for fat content.

Body density is another factor. Whereas bones, fat, and air tend to be buoyant, muscle sinks. The total immersion body weight of an individual, therefore, provides an indication of body density. As an operational method, it demonstrates the inaccuracy of using height-weight tables alone to estimate fat content. Men or women of equal age and height can weigh vastly different amounts. In fact, the leaner person may even be heavier. The key is *muscle*. Muscle weighs far more

	Height (with shoes on) 1-inch heels Feet Inches	Small frame	Medium frame	Large frame	
	5 2	112–120	118–129	126–141	Fig. 17.5. Desirable weights for men and women of ages 25 and over
	5 3	115–123	121–133	129–144	
	5 4	118–126	124–136	132–148	
	5 5	121–129	127–139	135–152	
	5 6	124–133	130–143	138–156	
	5 7	128–137	134–147	142–161	
Men	5 8	132–141	138–152	147–166	
of ages 25	5 9	136–145	142–156	151–170	
and over	5 10	140–150	146–160	155–174	
	5 11	144–154	150–165	159–179	
Weight in pounds	6 0	148–158	154–170	164–184	
according to frame	6 1	152–162	158–175	168–189	
(in indoor clothing)	6 2	156–167	162–180	173–194	
	6 3	160–171	167–185	178–199	
	6 4	164–175	172–190	182–204	
	2-inch heels				
	4 10	92– 98	96–107	104–119	
	4 11	94–101	98–110	106–122	
	5 0	96–104	101–113	109–125	
	5 1	99–107	104–116	112–128	
	5 2	102–110	107–119	115–131	
	5 3	105–113	110–122	118–134	
Women	5 4	108–116	113–126	121–138	
of ages 25	5 5	111–119	116–130	125–142	
and over	5 6	114–123	120–135	129–146	
	5 7	118–127	124–139	133–150	
	5 8	122–131	128–143	137–154	
	5 9	126–135	132–147	141–158	
	5 10	130–140	136–151	145–163	
	5 11	134–144	140–155	149–168	
	6 0	138–148	144–159	153–173	

For girls between 18 and 25, subtract 1 pound for each year under 25.

Courtesy, Metropolitan Life Insurance Company.

than fat, and a true mesomorph may be categorized as obese by height-weight tables when he or she actually has little fat. This is one major problem with the tables, and further testimony to the need for measurement of fat-free weight.

In fact, some people may weigh the same at fifty as they did at twenty-five, yet be obese at fifty whereas they were ''lean'' at twenty-five. A well-tuned body is taut and dense; years of inactivity permit muscles to atrophy and fat to increase. Should these developments happen to parallel each other, it is possible for an individual to become obese despite maintaining a constant weight. That's one reason why ''I haven't gained a pound in forty years'' really isn't that meaningful a statement.

For research purposes fat may be measured through isotope dilution techniques, which depend on differential fat solubility, or total body densiometry (based on Archimedes' principle) in which the land and water weight of the individual are compared. Obviously, such methods require sophisticated apparatus and are of little use to the lay public. Calipers to measure fat are frequently used in schools, in YM-YWCAs, and fitness clubs, and height-weight tables are common for virtually everyone. Interpretation is the problem—not estimation itself. The major principles are that overweight does not necessarily imply overfat, and weight alone is not a good predictor of fitness.

What Is Fat? Body fat is formed from excess calorie intake, regardless of source (carbohydrate, fat, or protein). It is stored as a liquid oil (triglyceride) in special cells (adipose tissues). About 50 percent of the total body fat is stored immediately under the skin (subcutaneous); the rest surrounds the body organs, and is often deep inside.

> An important point that has recently emerged is that the number of fat cells in the body is determined early in life, and an excessive number are created by overeating in infancy. Later, these fat cells can be empty or full, depending on the state of nutrition. The implication is that the person who was overfed as a baby can more easily convert energy to stored fat and find somewhere to put it.[6]

In other words, one can almost program obesity from birth. After puberty, we either fill or do not fill the fat cells, but before puberty we have some control over how many fat cells we will later have.

When fat is burned in the body, additional oxygen must be supplied by the cells to combine with all the carbon and hydrogen atoms, thus producing more heat. For this reason, a gram of fat gives the body approximately 9 calories of energy, whereas carbohydrates or proteins yield only 4 calories per gram. So, although fat will keep you warm, once accumulated, it is very difficult to get rid of.

Fat has many advantages: it cushions the bones and organs, contours the body, insulates, and provides emergency energy and mass, which can be beneficial in activities requiring momentum. Males tend to have less fat than females; young people usually have less than older people.

Unfortunately, fat also has many disadvantages. Besides the obvious problems of awkwardness and possible social embarrassment occasioned by it, fat is closely linked medically to shortened life span and an increase in both morbidity and mortality. Cardiovascular disorders, diabetes, liver and kidney diseases, accidents, and a wide variety of other health problems are all linked with fat. The greater the obesity, the greater the risk.

Obesity is also a complicating factor in atherosclerosis. Cholesterol is closely linked with high caloric intake but, more important, with circulation per se. Whereas it is a fact that serum cholesterol levels are high in many well-trained athletes, deposition within the arterial walls tends to be minimal and the buildup of fatty deposits slow. As fat buildup increases, however, activity tends to decline; as activity declines, deposition rates increase. As blood flow declines and cholesterol increases, hypertension, coronary occlusion, and peripheral constriction all become more possible, and the risk of early death or invalidism increases with every cubic centimeter of body fat. Roughly speaking, life expectation decreases 1 percent below the normal for every pound of fat above normal.[7]

How Prevalent Is Obesity? In a large-scale nutrition survey undertaken in Canada from 1970 to 1972, the investigators concluded,

Table 17.3 Prediction of Percent Total Fat in College Students from Subcutaneous Fat Thickness Measurements

Female: 6 site total (in mm)	% Body fat	Classification	% Body fat	Male: 6 site total (in mm)
28.4-46.5 mm	8%	Very Thin	3%	0-3.0 mm
55.6-73.7 mm	8-12%	Thin	4.0-6.0%	4.0-24.0 mm
82.8-100.9 mm	14-18%	Desirable	6.5-8.5%	30.0-50.0 mm
109.9-128.0 mm	20-24%	Average	9.0-11.5%	55.0-80.0 mm
137.1-155.2 mm	26-30%	Plump	12.0-14.5%	85.0-112 mm
164.2-182.3 mm	32-36%	Fat	15.0-17.0%	118-138 mm
191.4+ mm	38% +	Obese	17.5-20.0%	143-170 mm

Double skinfold measurements must be taken at 6 sites as follows:
females: tricep, subscapular, suprailiac, umbilical, front thigh, rear thigh
males: chest, tricep, subscapular, suprailiac, umbilical, front thigh

Data derived from M. S. Yuhasz, *Physical Fitness Appraisal Laboratory Manual*, London, Ontario, The University of Western Ontario, revised 1974, with permission of the author.

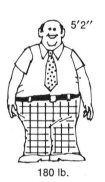
5'2"
180 lb.

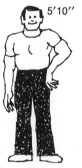
5'10"
180 lb.

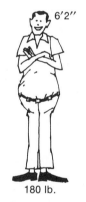
6'2"
180 lb.

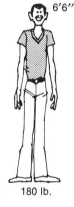
6'6"
180 lb.

Fig. 17.6. Weight alone can be misleading.

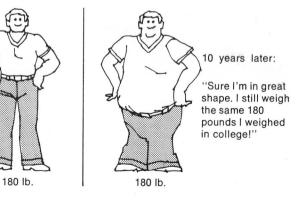

Fig. 17.7. Weight does not equal mass.

180 lb.

10 years later:

"Sure I'm in great shape. I still weigh the same 180 pounds I weighed in college!"

180 lb.

Fitness: Better Appearance and Optimal Functioning

The problem of overweight plagues very large proportions of adults in Canada. The initial analyses of the data show that calories alone do not account for the overweight problem. Those who are overweight and those who are not do not differ greatly in the number of calories they consume. The main cause is likely to be a sedentary life, and therefore both factors, caloric intake and physical activity, need to be considered. Over the past few decades, Canadians have reduced their physical activity to minimal levels because of changes in life-style and the misuse of advances in technology. The impact of such changes on metabolism and the consequences to health are indeed complex and remain only partly understood. Since the level of physical activity and the amounts and types of foods consumed are matters of personal choice, overweight may be viewed as a self-inflicted health problem.[8]

About one in every four women and one in five men are seriously overweight. The prevalence rises sharply with age, being relatively uncommon in primary school children (1.3 percent), low in pubescence (5 percent), and moderate in late adolescence (15 percent). By middle age close to 50 percent of the American population is obese.[9]

The Society of Actuaries' "Build and Blood Pressure Study" provides a long-term follow-up of five million insured persons.[10] When compared with the low-risk group, the mortality of men aged fifteen to sixty-nine who were 20 percent or more overweight was found to be 50 percent greater; that of men 10 percent overweight (i.e., greater than the normal range for age and body build) was 30 percent greater. The effect on women was slightly less, but highly significant.

Other insurance data on American policyholders indicate that 50 percent of American men aged thirty to thirty-nine are at least 10 percent overweight. Twenty-five percent are at least 20 percent overweight. The greatest prevalence is in the fifty to fifty-nine group, where 60 percent are at least 10 percent overweight and a third at least 20 percent. The figures for women are slightly lower up to age forty, equal throughout the next decade, and greater at fifty and above. Figures for children are sparse, although the link between generations is well known. In homes where neither parent is obese, approximately 7 percent of the children are obese; when one parent is obese, the number of obese children increases to about 40 percent; and when both parents are obese, 80 percent.

Contrary to popular notion, obesity is more common in the working class than in the middle or upper classes of society.[11] Nearly twice as many middle-class people have reported trying to lose weight as lower-class people. The reasons are subject to conjecture; they range from the theory that eating and drinking are really all the working classes have for entertainment, to the oversimplified ego-embellishment idea. Body consciousness may be more acute among the wealthy. Certainly the opportunities for middle- and upper-class people to visit beaches, participate in organized fitness endeavors (clubs), and pursue their recreational interests on a more formal basis are greater. And in that light, body image may assume an important place. Regardless of explanation, fat is less visible among the wealthy.

One must question the link between heredity and environment in producing obesity. The evidence is sparse. Studies in Boston and London suggest that gene-

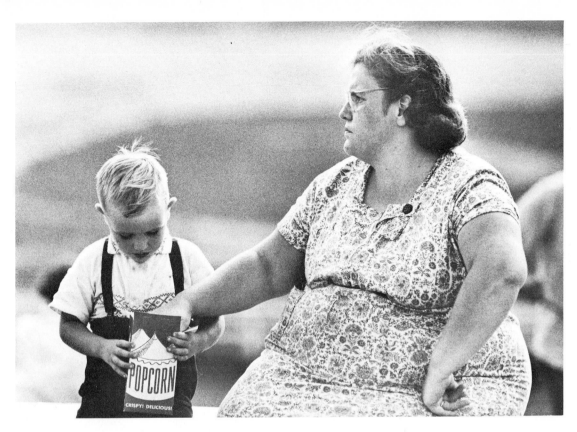

Fig. 17.8. Eating habits begun in childhood are partially responsible for weight problems in adult years.

Excess* for Principal Diseases Among Persons About 20 Percent or More Overweight		
	Men	Women
Heart disease	43%	51%
Cerebral hemorrhage	53%	29%
Malignant neoplasms	16%	13%
Diabetes	133%	83%
Digestive system diseases (gallstones, cirrhosis, etc.)	68%	39%
*Compared with mortality of Standard risks (Mortality ratio of Standard risks = 100%)		

Courtesy, Metropolitan Life Insurance Company.

Fig. 17.9. Overweight shortens life. Excess mortality due chiefly to heart and circulatory diseases.

tics is the dominant factor. The weight of children adopted in infancy shows little association with that of the adopting parents. Similarly, identical twins separated at birth and raised in different environments still tend to maintain similar weights. Body type probably accounts for much of this.

Fitness: Better Appearance and Optimal Functioning

Identical twins, Ada and Ida, were separated at three and lived very different lives—Ada in cities, Ida on farms. Ida had goiter, married at thirty-four, and led a quiet married life; Ada had no goiter, married at seventeen, and lived a stormy life until her divorce at twenty-seven. They lived different lives, and apart, yet at age fifty-nine Ada weighed 208 pounds, Ida 221.

"When environment is not greatly different, genetic factors are paramount. Even when extremes in environment occur, genetic traits, if powerful enough, will override them as in the cases of Ada and Ida."[12]

What Regulates Weight

There appear to be two weight-regulating systems—remote and immediate. The remote system is concerned with weight regulation over weeks, months, and years; the short-term one is related to more immediate factors, such as hunger, eating patterns, and the quantity/quality content of each meal. Oddly enough, the immediate factors (the time, content, and quality of any particular meal) bear little relationship to the actual energy used that day, or even on the previous day. The maintenance of a stable body weight in fact depends on the energy intake/energy output (Ei/Eo) balance over periods of at least a week. Daily weight fluctuations are usually caused by differences in liquid (water) retention levels.

The key to long-term weight control probably lies in the *hypothalamus*, that tiny section of the brain lying just above the pituitary. Within the hypothalamus lie the so-called feeding and satiety areas, and beside these, the feeding center. Scientists feel that under normal conditions the feeding center is under the control of the satiety center. Eating, however, is influenced by far more than simple hunger. Habit and environment are probably more important and play a critical role in weight. Some people, for example, eat frequently but only in small amounts; others save up for the big supper. In fact, small meals taken frequently are far less likely to cause obesity than the same amount of food taken in one large meal.

Why Do We Eat?

Why do we eat? A sensation of gastric activity, which can sometimes feel quite uncomfortable and may even be heard as a rumble, sometimes occurs. In fact, this is the empty stomach contracting vigorously, literally calling for food. This contraction is frequently felt a few hours after a very heavy meal, and hence is not always indicative of any real need for food. Many people who usually eat small meals rarely experience such gastric distress, even if they fast.

Blood-sugar levels are also important in "hunger," although the relationship is complex. Hunger clearly does increase following any reduction in blood-sugar levels, but this occurs in the recovery phase when the level is already on its way back to normal.

Finally, the relationship between climate, body temperature, and the heat regulation mechanism within the body is interesting. We tend to eat less in warm weather and more in the winter. Energy intake is obviously linked with body temperature regulation.

So far we have looked at what makes us eat, but little has been said about what tells us to stop eating, beyond the obvious factor of physical space.

Certainly the physical aspects of eating are important. Subjects fed intragastrically (directly through the stomach) do not report feeling as satisfied or full after their meals as subjects eating the same amount of food naturally. Obviously, tasting, chewing, and swallowing foods have some influence on satiety.

The physical swelling of the stomach undoubtedly adds to any feeling of fullness, and blood-sugar levels may also be important. The increasing sugar level appears to act on the satiety center and causes it to inhibit the feeding center. As the sugar level recedes, the feeding center again takes over.

Skin temperature rises slightly as food is digested and may influence the satiety center. Eventually it returns to normal, following digestion. Such interplay between the satiety and feeding centers appears to be an adaptation mechanism for the maintenance of consistent body weight.

While the evidence is incomplete, indications are that genetic traits in man largely influence the potential for overeating (or undereating) and obesity. (In contemporary America we have ideal conditions for realization of genetic potentialities, or for the phenotype to be an expression of the genotype.) But while genes enhance the potential for obesity, actual overeating and underexercising still must take place before obesity develops. In part, an acceptance of the genetic influence should provide us with a positive basis for preventive treatment. If it is recognized that children with one obese parent are likely candidates for obesity and that children with two obese parents are even more likely prospects, there is an opportunity to develop early eating and activity patterns that will help minimize this condition.

A variety of factors influences eating patterns. Host, agent, and environment interact in both the input and the output phases of energy utilization.

Mayer grouped obesities into two major categories: "regulatory" and "metabolic." [13] In the former the central mechanism regulating food intake is impaired; in the latter there is an inborn or acquired error in the metabolism of the tissues themselves. In the first case, habitual overeating can lead to secondary metabolic abnormalities; in the second, peripheral metabolic dysfunction may interfere with the regulating centers in the brain. As is already apparent, the physiological factors are complex and beyond the scope of this text. Activity, on the other hand, is crucial in weight control. The facts overwhelmingly demonstrate that exercise is the great variable in energy expenditure, and exercise does not necessarily increase one's food intake.

Like eating, physical activity is cumulative, a fact too frequently ignored by those who claim it is of little value. Whereas an average-size man may only burn 300 calories in an hour of volleyball (3,500 calories = 1 pound), if he repeats that activity three times a week throughout the year, the calorie equivalent will be $300 \times 3 \times 52 = 46,800$ calories, or over 13 pounds. Remember, pounds do not come and go by the day but by the week, the month, and the year. In any weight-control program, the long-term calorie balance is far more critical than the immediate or short-term balance. Even a week of stringent dieting will have little effect on long-term weight control. Following a week of crash dieting, Big

Bertha bounced into the classroom and announced in her most audible tone, "I've just lost ten pounds." From the back of the room came the response, "Turn around, I think I've found it!" People are loath to accept extravagant claims by the advocates of them.

Interestingly, if excess body weight impedes mobility, the energy cost of any specific exercise may actually be higher for an overweight person (swimming is a likely exception here, since fat increases buoyancy and may actually reduce the work load for a given individual). An increase in calorie intake above the balance level may create little weight change in an active person, because the energy lost in moving the extra poundage will be greater. It has been demonstrated that about 99 percent of the energy expended in playing tennis is involved in moving the body about the court; only about 1 percent is used for hitting the ball. Provided the activity level is stable, therefore, long-term weight gain will be minimal. For sedentary individuals, on the other hand, the opposite is probably true—the more they eat, the less they move, and the more weight they gain.

Does appetite increase with exercise? Within limits, yes. Moderate exercise, and even strenuous exercise up to but not surpassing the exhaustion level, appears to stimulate appetite proportionately. On the way up this is of little consequence, as balance is maintained; on the way down it is of grave consequence, as people are reluctant to cut back on eating in the face of diminishing activity. Herein lies a problem.

Mayer unequivocally cites inactivity as the single most important factor explaining the frequency of creeping overweight in North American society. "Our bodies' regulation of food intake was just not designed for the highly mechanized sedentary conditions of modern life."[14] In short, many people do not expend even the minimum energy required to keep their food-regulating mechanisms functioning properly.

So I'm Obese—Help Me!

Weight gains and losses vary directly with caloric balance, i.e., energy intake/energy output (Ei/Eo); body weight remains constant only when these two components are in balance over time. If intake rises or expenditure declines, weight gain follows, and vice versa. The balance is delicate, and the effects long-term—weight is easier to put on than to take off.

The critical step in any reducing program is reversing the caloric balance, i.e., creating a situation in which $Eo > Ei$. To do this, one must have a medical check-up and establish a personal total caloric balance chart. The use of a table for intake estimates and a table for output and a table of desirable weights (see table 17.2) may be of some assistance.

The next question is, how fast do you want to lose the weight? Be careful here. Ideally we should develop a weight-reducing scheme that establishes new lifelong patterns, so the weight will stay lost. Crash diets can work, but usually don't in the long run. In fact, many see them as simply a "rhythm method of girth control." Similarly Metrecal, Ayds, Regimen, and other gimmicks may help in the short run, but like chewing (Fletcherism) they soon get boring and begin to wear on you. Over time their value diminishes.

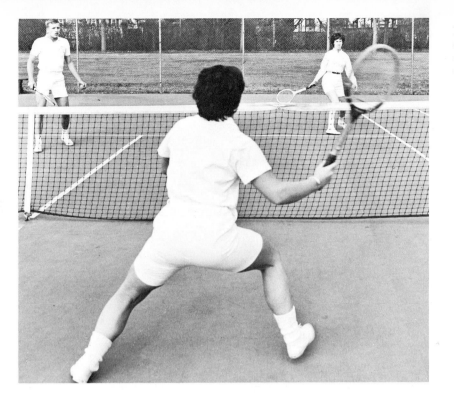

The key to successful weight reduction is reversing the calorie balance over long periods of time. If one's weight is stable, a little exercise, coupled with refined eating patterns, can go a long way. Simply cutting back 150 calories per day (two buttered slices of bread), and walking to and from work (one mile in fifteen minutes) could result in a net difference of 225 calories per day, or $\frac{365 \times 225}{3,500} =$ 23+ pounds per year, all other factors remaining the same. These figures also represent a long-term pattern. True, BMR may continue to decline each year, and our new figure will provide us with greater efficiency in movement (and therefore reduced caloric expenditure per activity)—but the new image we create may encourage us to increase our activity still more. Oddly enough, more slim people participate in fitness programs than do fat people. A geometric progression is possible in which body image improves, activity level increases, interest perks up, and an ever-increasing number of activities are engaged in; the more we do, it seems, the less tired we are. Weight loss and figure refinement bring positive reinforcement, and positive reinforcement enhances drive.

Role of Increased Physical Activity

Diet
Ei down   Eo up
        +   = net difference of 225 cal./day or 2 lb./month
(−150)   (+75)

Fitness: Better Appearance and Optimal Functioning

If Mayer and others are correct, overeating may in fact be far less of a problem than underactivity. In a study of girls at a Massachusetts camp, for example, obese girls ate less than those of normal weight, but they also moved less. Oddly enough, their activity charts showed equal participation, but further probing revealed a critical variable: intensity. The fat girls swam, played volleyball, basketball, and even tennis, but they hardly ever moved. When a special camera was placed in one corner of the court and set to take three-second "shorts" every three minutes, the girls could be individually assessed. In 65 percent of the tennis sequences, 80 percent of the volleyball films, and even more of the swimming clips, the overweight girls were essentially motionless. Even more serious was the fact that the overweight girls were quite unaware of their inactivity.

In a situation where a constant attempt was made to render exercising pleasant, the girls professed great enthusiasm for sports and were, as a matter of fact, more vocal in their praise of exercise than the nonobese girls. Participation in sports thus appeared to present the obese girls with a conflict of which they were not aware. While they knew they were less active than their thinner peers, they failed to recognize their disinclination for active exercise, or else simply enjoyed the exercise periods as occasions for social contact, not for their intrinsic worth.

Fig. 17.11. Bicycling and jogging are good ways to expend excess calories and help tone the body. They are activities that can be done at all ages throughout one's life, but with care and with a doctor's knowledge.

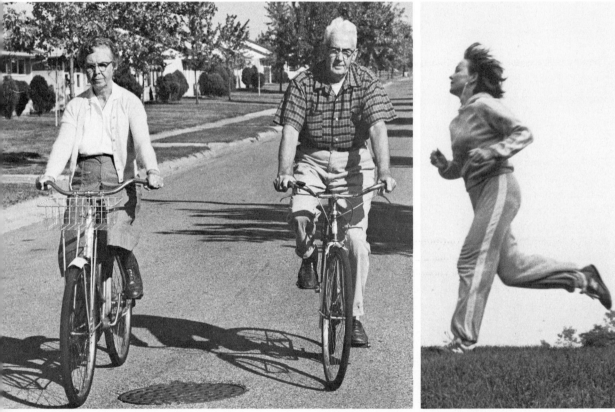

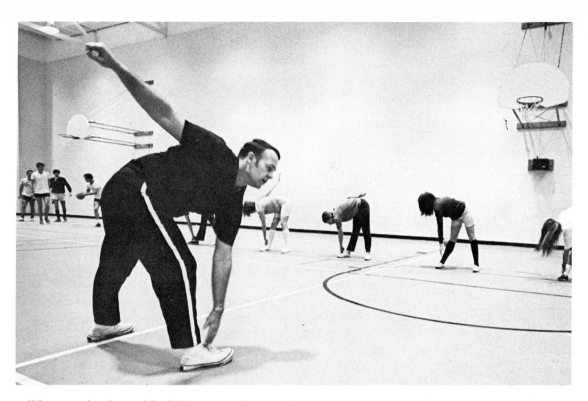

Whenever the obese girls did become active, weight reduction was achieved. Further, obese youngsters forced into activity inadvertently showed stable eating patterns, thereby creating a negative caloric balance.[15]

The camp-girl example might well serve as a model for middle-aged fitness club adherents, who go to the club daily but engage in little more than passive exercise, massage, and sauna, and wonder why their weight remains the same. Exercise must be active to be beneficial.

The question of just how to go about exercising can be of tremendous significance to someone interested in losing fat and increasing vitality. In fact, it may be such a perplexing problem that the individual will do nothing but think about it. Physical activity should be meaningful and fun. It should also be an activity that can be performed on a continued basis. The actual form it should take can be more easily determined if one has a particular goal in mind, such as improvement in cardiorespiratory function (heart, lungs, and circulatory system) or simply expenditure of calories to lose body fat.

Fig. 17.12. It is better to use simple progressive exercises than mechanical equipment.

Summary

The sedentary life-style of most Americans is a major contributor to their poor physical condition. Four dimensions of physical fitness are usually considered most directly related to health: muscular strength, muscular endurance, flexibility, and cardiovascular endurance.

Before undertaking any program of physical fitness improvement, one should have a complete medical examination. Several other tests and measures also can be used to ascertain the physical status of the individual in preparation for designing a specific activity program.

Individuals desiring to improve their level of physical fitness need to identify certain objectives. Then they should select specific activities, exercises, and movement patterns that will be most effective in meeting the identified needs.

Long-term maintenance of an ideal body weight is a result of a balance between energy intake (the foods we eat and drink) and energy expenditure. For most people, this should not be an unrealistic goal. However, the ideal is the exception rather than the rule in most advanced nations in the world. Our physical activity may be so little that our weight-regulating mechanisms cannot function properly, or we may be ignoring subtle internal signals that tell us we have eaten enough. Whatever the reason, weight control is an essential component of a happy, healthy life. The equation *energy intake − energy expenditure = change in body fat* is the key to achievement and maintenance of ideal weight. For those who are overweight or obese, the only sensible answer is a prolonged period of negative calorie balance arrived at, ideally, by a reduction in food intake and an increase in energy expenditure. The difficulty is that few people realize that obesity is a condition requiring years of diligent abuse. Too often we demand quick results, and failing this, we resign ourselves to the inevitable. The knowledge and practice of simple life-style modifications could easily result in a happier, healthier population.

Review Questions

1. What is your definition of physical fitness?
2. Explain the difference between muscular strength and muscular endurance.
3. What should be included in a medical examination that precedes the initiation of an exercise program?
4. How do isometric exercises differ from isotonic exercises?
5. What is flexibility as it applies to physical fitness?
6. Give several examples of anaerobic exercise.
7. Why is aerobic exercise of more importance and value than anaerobic exercise for cardiovascular fitness?
8. Does dieting necessarily mean losing weight? Explain.
9. What is the BMR? What factors influence it?
10. Explain how exercise plays an important role in weight control. Is dieting alone enough?
11. Differentiate between obesity and overweight.
12. How can overeating in infancy possibly affect one's weight in adulthood?
13. Discuss the advantages and disadvantages of fat.

14. How is obesity linked to heart disease?

15. What variables would you change to gain or lose weight?

16. What is the difference between hunger and appetite?

17. What would you describe as the most important causes of obesity in North America?

Readings

Allsen, Philip E.; Joyce M. Harrison, and Barbara Vance, *Fitness for Life: An Individualized Approach,* Dubuque, Iowa: Wm. C. Brown, 1976, 153 pp.

Cooper, Kenneth H., *Aerobics,* New York: M. Evans and Company, 1968, 253 pp.

Cooper, Kenneth H., *The New Aerobics,* New York: M. Evans and Company, 1970, 191 pp.

Corbin, Charles B.; Linus J. Dowell, Ruth Lindsey, and Homer Tolson, *Concepts in Physical Education,* Dubuque, Iowa: Wm. C. Brown, 1974.

Konishi, F. ''Food Energy Equivalents of Various Activities.'' *Journal of the American Dietetic Association* 46 (1965).

Notes

1. K. H. Cooper, *Aerobics* (New York: M. Evans & Co., Inc., 1968).

2. K. H. Cooper, *The New Aerobics* (New York: M. Evans & Co., Inc., 1970).

3. P. E. Allsen, J. M. Harrison, and B. Vance, *Fitness for Life: An Individualized Approach* (Dubuque, Ia.: Wm. C. Brown, 1976); C. B. Corbin, L. J. Dowell, R. Lindsey, and H. Tolson, *Concepts in Physical Education* (Dubuque, Ia.: Wm. C. Brown, 1974).

4. *Fitness for Life,* p. 36.

5. W. Thompson, *Black's Medical Dictionary* (New York: Harper & Row Publishers, 1974).

6. M. Yaffé, ''Inside Every Fat Man,'' *New Society,* June 1973, p. 675.

7. Ibid., p. 674.

8. Nutrition Canada National Survey, 1973, p. 112.

9. J. Mayer, *Overweight: Causes, Cost, and Control* (Englewood Cliffs, N.J.: Prentice-Hall, 1968), p. 27.

10. Society of Actuaries, *Causes of Excess Mortality Among Overweight Men and Women (Aged 15–69),* 1955, p. 675.

11. T. Silverstone, ''Obesity and Social Class,'' 8th European Conference on Psychosomatic Research, 1970, as quoted in Yaffé, ''Inside Every Fat Man,'' p. 675.

12. Mayer, *Overweight: Causes, Cost, and Control,* p. 54.

13. Ibid., p. 60.

14. Ibid., p. 82.

15. Ibid., p. 127.

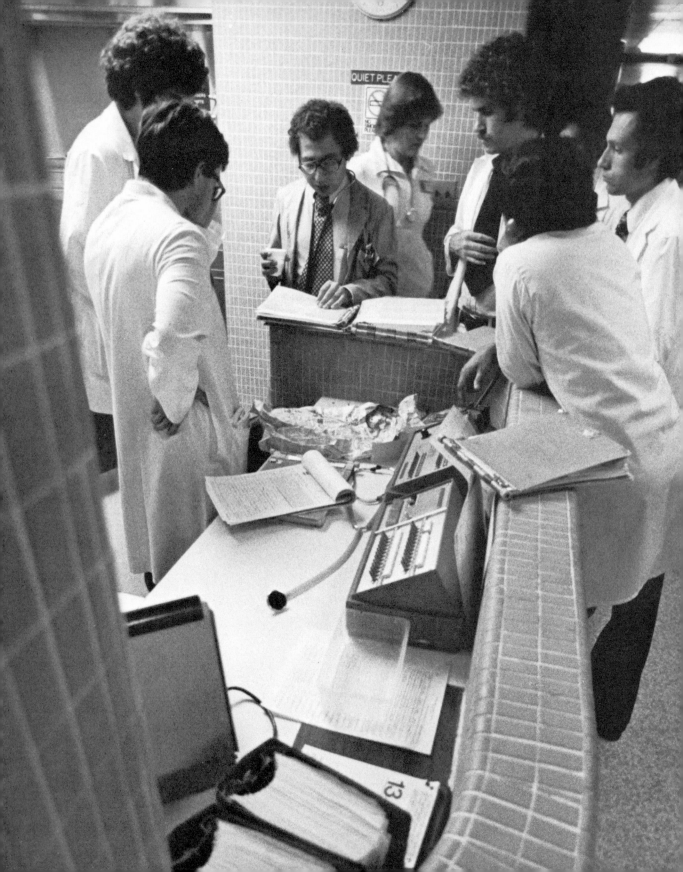

Consumerism: Selection of Health Providers

18

All too often people see themselves as health consumers only when faced with a physician's fee for service, a hospital bill, or the cash register tape in a pharmacy. Yet each one of us is confronted daily with myriad consumer choices that influence our health and welfare. For example, how do we respond to television commercials that encourage self-medication and suggest that overindulgence is permissible? Do we often believe advertising that tells us a certain food or drug can assure a prolonged life, and therefore we purchase the product? What criteria do we apply in our search for a new or different medical adviser? Do we faithfully follow the directions on the label of the container when taking medicines? Do we examine the nutritional information on packages of food products to assure a well-balanced diet? What safety features do we consider when we purchase a toy for our children or an automobile for ourselves? On what basis do we judge printed stories on losing weight, improving mental health, satisfying our sexual partners, and curing or preventing numerous illnesses? Indeed, consumers are at the crossroads of decision making when they enter the "marketplace of health."

As the cost of health care soars, the need for consumers to be informed and discriminating increases. However, the "marketplace of health" is not only more expensive than formerly; it is also more complicated and faster changing today. New health professions are emerging, new health services and facilities are available, new health products are multiplying, and new health claims must be analyzed for their validity or falsity. Hopefully, the consumer will adapt to the conditions of the marketplace by:

1. identifying and evaluating sources of medical assistance,
2. developing and implementing a personal program for procuring health information and services,
3. replacing fears and superstitions with scientific facts and objectivity in health-related matters, and
4. avoiding fraudulent health practices and worthless devices.

Such adaptive behaviors will require a good deal of private action and public support to make sure that health care and protection dollars are well spent. To accomplish this worthy endeavor, we devote this and the two chapters that follow to the promotion of your success in the marketplace of health.

The growing force of consumers may be expressed in other ways. In seeking some influence over the organization and function of the health care system, the "ultimate buyer" is beginning to win the opportunity to budget for and prepay all inclusive costs of health care, including services rendered outside the hospital. This retrieval of bargaining power, now diluted by intermediate health insurance agencies, may result in a major restructuring of the health delivery system.[1] This is further discussed in chapter 20.

Consumer protection is yet another example of the potential for adaptation in response to the current pitfalls of the health marketplace.

Consumer protection depends on carefully designed controls. The controls must be created by government, and government must be instructed by its one true paymaster—not the lobbyist, not the campaign donor, not the political boss, but the *citizen*.[2]

The opportunity for consumer action in the area of health is truly awesome. If people are willing to act wisely and responsibly on both an individual and cooperative basis, consumerism will likely be one of the noblest endeavors of the present generation. In the final analysis, our ability to utilize health products, services, and information wisely will affect the quality of our health. And it is this quality of health that we wish to consume in the pursuit of life's goals.

Health Care and Services

Much of the recent emphasis on consumer health education is the result of citizen frustration with past and present health care delivery systems. When citing reasons for their dissatisfaction, critics identify rapidly rising hospital charges, poor geographical distribution of physicians and medical facilities, overspecialization of practitioners, lack of accountability, performance of unnecessary surgical procedures, doctor error, exploitation of government health programs, the decline of the doctor-patient relationship, and the lingering belief that good health care is a privilege rather than a right.[3, 4, 5] In comparison with other nations of the world, America ranks relatively low on life expectancy and infant mortality—commonly accepted indexes of health—which has led still other citizens to despair.

Perhaps the most severe criticism of our health care programs is that most individuals receive only crisis care, which amounts to supplying sickness services rather than maintaining health.[6] There is no reward for physicians or insurance companies in keeping patients out of the hospital. This may not be the fault of the medical profession alone. More likely, this situation is the product of our long-term fixation on *rehabilitating sick people* rather than concentrating on *keeping healthy people well*. Health maintenance, or preventive medicine, is being adopted ever so slowly by both health professionals and the general public. These problems will be discussed more fully in the chapter on the health care system.

Providers

Whether health care is primarily disease preventive or rehabilitative in scope, such service is usually offered to the consumer under the direction or general supervision of *autonomous health professionals*, such as physicians, dentists, optometrists, and podiatrists. A more detailed account of these professional health care providers is presented later in this chapter. Working in support of the

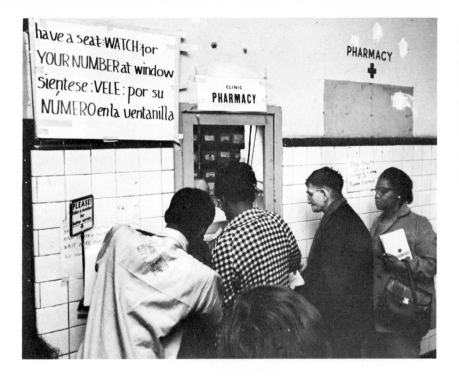

Fig. 18.1. A neighborhood clinic or hospital health clinic often has a pharmacy in the facility. Drug prices vary, depending on place purchased and whether the prescription calls for generic or brand names. The customer must decide how to get the most for his money.

independent practitioners are increasing numbers of *allied health professionals,* including registered and practical nurses, nurse-midwives, dental hygienists, dietitians, medical technologists, certified laboratory assistants, respiratory therapists, pharmacists, medical social workers, physical therapists, and X-ray technologists, to name a few.

Actual procedures of diagnosis and treatment are generally accomplished in the *private office* of a health professional, in a tax-supported *public clinic,* or in a *medical facility* or *hospital* that provides a full range of patient services. If patients require prolonged observation or nursing care, extensive use of laboratory and X-ray services in diagnosis and treatment, and rehabilitation services, they are admitted as *inpatients* and occupy hospital beds. Otherwise, patients receive various medical, dental, or auxiliary services on an *outpatient* basis and are not lodged in the medical facility.

Resources

Due in part to the difficulty of obtaining medical care from private practitioners, more and more individuals in an adaptive response are swarming to the emergency treatment departments of community hospitals for services formerly rendered by the family doctor. Consumers of these emergency services should be aware that they are likely to be billed both by the attending physician and by the hospital for use of its facilities.

Hospitals, medical centers which offer specialized diagnostic, treatment, and rehabilitation services primarily for inpatients, differ considerably from one another. Most are short-term community medical centers that provide comprehensive services for many health problems; others focus on specific areas of tuberculosis, psychiatric disorders, long-term care, and children's health problems.[7] A few deal with drug dependency or leprosy exclusively.

Hospitals also differ in terms of their ownership and management. Accordingly, medical facilities are classified as follows:

- *Voluntary*—Nongovernmental, nonprofit organizations for use by the general public. These hospitals are usually governed by a board of trustees from the local community and operated by a religious group, a philanthropic organization, or a community corporation.
- *Proprietary*—Privately owned hospitals established as profit-making organizations in the provision of general or specialized medical care to the public.
- *Governmental*—Tax-supported hospitals operated by federal, state, county, or city health agencies. These may be comprehensive in nature, such as the federal military and Veterans Administration hospitals, or specialized medical facilities, as represented by state mental institutions.

Certain health services formerly provided only in a hospital or physician's office are becoming available in new medical facilities. Such facilities are neighborhood health clinics, comprehensive mental health centers, mobile coronary care units, short-term surgery centers, and emergency treatment stations.

Increasingly, patients enter those hospitals that are near their homes, that have vacancies, and where their physicians have staff privileges. However, if any element of personal choice remains, the consumer will want to consider the *accreditation status* of the medical facility. In the United States, hospitals are periodically inspected to determine compliance with certain minimal standards of health care. Review of medical practices, cleanliness, records, laboratory operations, and other procedures is conducted by the Joint Commission on Accreditation of Hospitals (JCAH). The accreditation process is voluntary and may result in denial of approval, one year's provisional approval, or full two-year approval.

Other major health care resources are *nursing homes*. These facilities have grown in significant numbers recently to accommodate long-term patients with chronic disorders not requiring hospitalization. However, not all so-called nursing homes provide comprehensive nursing services. Some offer only personal care or institutionalization, while others make available varying types of nursing services ranging from catheterization to application of dressings and bandages. *Extended care facilities* offer more medical and nursing service than normally found in a nursing home and are approved for Medicare patients.[8]

Health Care Providers

Most often, through personal experience, individuals learn that the maintenance of health status cannot be achieved without qualified medical assistance. At some time during your life, then, you will most likely be confronted with choosing a physician to render some type of professional health service either for yourself or a member of your family. As a consumer, you will have several questions to answer in procuring the desired assistance.

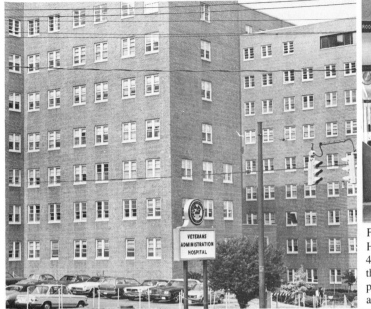

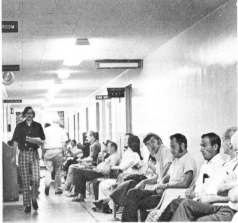

Fig. 18.2. The Veterans Administration Hospital, Syracuse, New York, a 438-bed general hospital affiliated with the State University of New York, and patients' waiting room for admitting area and one of the ambulatory-care clinics.

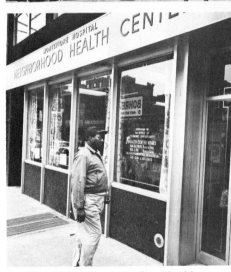

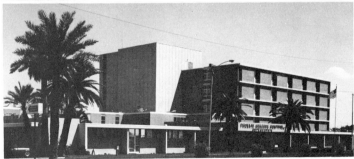

Fig. 18.3. A neighborhood health center (above) helps provide medical services for people who do not have their own family doctors.

Fig. 18.4. Carefully check out a nursing home (above right) before using its services to be sure its patients receive good care.

Fig. 18.5. This small community hospital (right) offers many of the same services as larger hospitals.

1. What type of physician is needed for a particular health problem?
2. Is there any way to evaluate physicians before they are consulted?
3. How does one go about choosing a medical adviser from a variety of physicians?
4. Just when should a physician be called?
5. What can be done if you are not satisfied with a physician's services or a medical bill?
6. What can other health specialists do in promoting health status, and what are the philosophical bases of their systems of healing?

Perhaps you can think of more questions. However, the ones posed above are those most frequently asked, especially by persons who are unfamiliar with the local community.

Medical Doctor

Responsibility for providing health services and safeguarding human life is centered in the physician, an independent health professional trained and licensed by the state: (1) to diagnose disease (i.e., to differentiate one disease from another), and (2) to prescribe and render treatment or therapy for disease conditions.

Commonly referred to as doctors, most physicians practicing today hold a Doctor of Medicine (M.D.) degree, indicating that they generally use medicines in their professional endeavors. Other diagnostic and therapeutic methods utilized in certain instances include operative surgery, X ray, psychotherapy, diet therapy, massage, exercise, and the physical agents of heat, cold, light, water, and electricity. Medical doctors subscribe to the "germ theory" of disease and the importance of preventive medicine, curative medicine, and rehabilitation procedures. This system of treating disease is referred to as *allopathy* because the agents (medicines) used in treating disease produce effects different from those of the disease treated. (*Allo-* means "other" or "different.")

The education and training of a modern medical doctor is a long and challenging process. After three or four years of undergraduate premedical study in a college or university, the student enters a medical school for four years—or the equivalent—of intensive professional training. The medical curriculum concentrates on the basic medical sciences of anatomy and physiology, biochemistry, pharmacology, psychiatry, internal medicine, diagnostic techniques, radiology, and surgery. In addition to this academic preparation, the medical student is familiarized with the actual practice of medicine in clinical situations in a teaching hospital.

Following graduation and the awarding of the M.D. degree, the physician enters a one-year apprentice training period, or internship at a hospital. As an intern, the physician may rotate through various clinical services or concentrate in a single area, such as pediatrics, surgery, or medicine.

Upon completion of the internship, the physician qualifies for state licensure. A passing score entitles the individual to function as a general practitioner of the medical sciences. However, many prefer to take advanced training in one of the specialty branches of medicine, which requires two to five years of additional

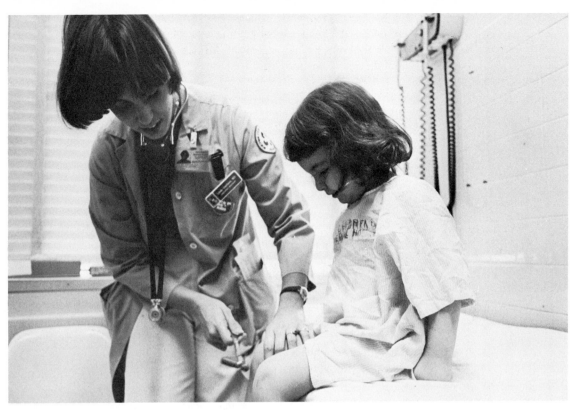

Fig. 18.6. Many physicians are attracted to pediatrics as a field of specialization.

preparation and experience as a resident in a hospital. At the conclusion of this residency program, a physician may submit to both written and oral examinations to qualify as a diplomate or board-certified specialist.

Listed below are some current medical specialists with short descriptions of their respective areas of specialization.[9, 10]

Allergist   Allergy involves diagnosis and treatment of unusual sensitivity of the body to a large variety of substances.

Anesthesiologist   Anesthesiology is the administration of chemical anesthetics (pain-killers) to cause insensibility to pain.

Dermatologist   Dermatology concerns the diagnosis and treatment of skin diseases.

Family practitioner   Family practice is the provision of medical care by a medical doctor who assumes comprehensive and continuing responsibility for the patient and the patient's family regardless of age.

Gynecologist   Gynecology deals with diseases of female reproductive organs.

Internist   Internal medicine deals with the nonsurgical treatment of diseases, especially those affecting internal organs, such as the heart, liver, lungs, and pancreas.

Laryngologist   Laryngology concerns diseases of the throat.

Nephrologist Nephrology deals primarily with kidney disorders.

Neurologist Neurology involves diseases and disorders of the nervous system.

Obstetrician Obstetrics concerns medical care of the woman during pregnancy, childbirth, and the period just after birth.

Oncologist Oncology deals with the treatment of irregular growths, such as tumors and cancers.

Ophthalmologist Ophthalmology concerns the treatment of diseases and injuries of the eyes.

Otologist Otology deals with diseases of the ear.

Pathologist Pathology concerns the nature, cause, and development of diseases and structural and functional changes they cause in the body.

Pediatrician Pediatrics concerns medical care for children from birth through adolescence, including aid in mental and physical growth and development.

Physiatrist Physical medicine and rehabilitation offer physiotherapy for physical, mental, and occupational rehabilitation of patients.

Proctologist Proctology deals primarily with diseases of the rectum and colon, the lowermost part of the intestinal tract.

Psychiatrist Psychiatry is concerned with mental disorders.

Radiologist Radiology concerns the use of X rays and other forms of radiant energy to treat diseases of the body.

Surgeon Surgery deals with the diagnosis and treatment of diseases, injuries, and deformities by manual or operative procedures.

Urologist Urology deals with diseases of the urinary tract.

Osteopath In contrast to the medical doctor, the osteopathic physician holds a Doctor of Osteopathy (D.O.) degree. The underlying philosophy of this method of healing originated with Andrew Still in 1892. It differs considerably from accepted medical science. Osteopathy focuses on

> . . . the biological mechanisms by which the musculoskeletal system, through the nervous and circulatory systems, interacts with all body organs and systems in both health and disease.
>   The emphasis is appropriate since osteopathic research and practice have demonstrated that disorders of the musculoskeletal system, in some degree, almost invariably are present when illness occurs.[11]

Any impairment of nerve function, caused by a pinching of the nerves as they leave the spinal column, results in a disturbance of the musculoskeletal system and thus places a stress on the body. Manipulative therapy is an attempt to restore the "structural integrity" of the skeletal system, which in turn will allow proper nerve transmission and blood circulation to diseased body parts. One of the important osteopathic principles is that the living body has an inherent capacity to resist many diseases and to a large extent to repair itself.

However, since its beginning, osteopathy has gradually modified many tenets of its original philosophy. Because of its emphasis on the relationship between body structure and organic functioning, osteopathic medicine contends that it offers something more than allopathic or orthodox medicine, not something else.

Accordingly, the American Osteopathic Association views osteopathic medicine as ''... today's most comprehensive and complete approach to man's health problems.''[12]

Osteopathic medicine now embraces all the scientific methods of treating diseases and injury, including use of drugs, operative surgery, radiation, physical therapy, and other physical means, in addition to manipulation. This alignment of osteopathy with orthodox medical practices has been achieved through a significant improvement in professional training in osteopathic colleges and hospitals. Like medical doctors, some osteopathic physicians specialize in certain fields, such as pediatrics, surgery, radiology, and physical medicine.

Osteopaths are now licensed to practice medicine and surgery in all states after passing the same examination given to medical doctors. Until recently, though, osteopaths were not permitted to care for patients at community hospitals. This restriction led to the establishment of osteopathic hospitals in certain parts of the United States. However, an ever-increasing number of accredited ''medical'' hospitals now grant staff privileges, internships, and residency programs to osteopathic physicians.

Because of the shortage of general practitioners, many individuals have turned to medical specialists for basic health care services. Due to their training, those most frequently consulted are the internist, the family practice specialist, and for children, the pediatrician. Perhaps the location or the shortage of physicians will limit your selection of a medical adviser. However, if the opportunity for free choice presents itself, the following suggestions may prove helpful in the selection process.[13] You will find that it is wise to investigate before you invest, even when procuring health care.

Selection of a Physician

1. The yellow page listing of the telephone directory will indicate the local medical doctors and osteopaths by name and professional address. Such a listing, though, does not indicate competency and may not be complete.
2. A telephone call to the local medical society or osteopathic association will generally reveal a list of several recommended physicians who are licensed and qualified to meet specific health problems.
3. Most public libraries will have a copy of the *American Medical Directory*, which presents a brief biographical and educational sketch of physicians who are members of the American Medical Association. From this information some ideas about age, experience, and training can be formed. It should be noted that some qualified medical doctors are not listed because they are not members of the American Medical Association.
4. *The Directory of Medical Specialists*, available at some public libraries, will list those physicians who are diplomates or board-certified medical specialists recognized by the proper American specialty board.
5. If membership in one of the national professional organizations, i.e., the American College of Physicians or the American College of Surgeons, can be determined, this would tend to indicate some degree of competence.

6. Ask the local hospitals for a listing of staff physicians together with their rank or level of privileges. Consulting and active staff privileges usually indicate that physicians are experienced, while associate rank is a general indication of less experience. Full or major surgical privileges are indicative of more experience than intermediate and minor surgical privileges. Competency, however, is not always a function of experience. The reputation of a hospital most often reflects the competence and expertise of its staff physicians. "Good hospitals" as a rule have "good staff physicians."

7. The accreditation status of a hospital, determined by an on-site inspection by the Joint Commission on Accreditation of Hospitals, is another indicator of the quality of medical care rendered by the hospital's professional medical staff. Hospitals with full accreditation on a continuing basis typically attract quality physicians, who in turn help the hospital maintain a favorable rating.

After a physician has been selected, do not wait until some major health problem arises before making the first appointment. Such delay could be frustrating because in some areas there is a critical shortage of medical advisers, and physicians are no longer accepting new patients on a minute's notice. Authorities agree that the first professional contact with a physician should be for a routine medical examination or a get-acquainted session. This will help establish a basis for a continuing physician-patient relationship and will provide an opportunity for both parties to evaluate each other. Before any service is performed, ask the office nurse or receptionist about the current charges for office visits and routine procedures. If any questions remain, bring them up with the physician.

Fig. 18.7. Don't wait until you are seriously ill before you visit the physician of your choice for the first time.

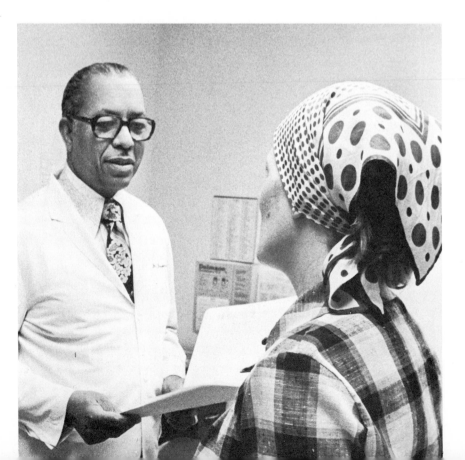

Now that you have some idea about costs, what can you expect for your money? A thorough medical examination generally consists of an extensive medical history of your past health status; a comprehensive head-to-toe physical inspection; diagnostic procedures appropriate to age, sex, and prior illnesses; arrangements for laboratory analysis of body fluids; X rays—usually of the chest, if indicated; an electrocardiogram; and the scheduling of a follow-up consultation. This first physical may be expensive from the consumer's point of view, but it is money well spent in determining health status.

Question the physician about the possibility of medical consultation or referral to other health specialists if needed. Also, your visit to the doctor's office will enable you to judge the manner and courtesy of both physician and staff, the efficiency of office management and scheduling of patients, the willingness of the physician to display a real interest in you, the patient, and the extent of explanations pertaining to diagnostic and treatment procedures. If you do not receive what you believe to be honest answers to your questions or are not favorably impressed with the professional conduct of either physician or staff, then you are ready to implement your selection process again.

Many persons are not prepared to act as smart patients and to participate as active and creative members of their own health care team. They see their physicians, bathed in "medical mystique," as providers of health services, but they do not recognize their own opportunities or responsibilities as intelligent consumer-patients.

To use physicians wisely and to your own advantage as a health consumer, you should ask plenty of questions, take notes when your physician gives you advice and directions, and seek out additional information about your own body, your symptoms, and specific disease processes. Belsky and Gross[14] also recommend that patients offer continuous feedback to their doctors by open expression of concerns, feelings, ideas, and even suggestions regarding health status and treatment alternatives. They suggest that smart patients will do the following:[15]

1. Tell the doctor when they do not understand the doctor's directions.
2. Write down specific directions and follow the recommended therapy.
3. Request that instructions be repeated if not completely understood.
4. Ask about alternative choices in treatment and the relative advantages and disadvantages of each.
5. Develop a degree of assertiveness in communicating with physicians.
6. Rehearse what they intend to say to their physicians.
7. Ask what prescribed medications are supposed to do and what side effects can be expected.
8. Inquire whether specific medicines can be taken with other drugs, foods, and drinks, especially alcoholic beverages.
9. Report any adverse side effects of medications and any changes in body functions to their physicians immediately.
10. Leave a physician when the doctor-patient relationship breaks down and becomes antitherapeutic, that is, when the patient is unhappy with care or

Using Your Physician Wisely

treatment, the patient loses confidence in the doctor's abilities, or personality conflicts give rise to antagonism or other forms of "mental cruelty."

Understanding the importance of treatment and the specific instructions of your physician, the limitations of modern medical practice and surgery, and the actual risks associated with any particular treatment will help you avoid some undesirable consequences in the health marketplace. As consumers, we often expect both physicians and hospitals to be fail-safe systems in rendering health care. Unfortunately, they are not! All too often, though, we as patients fail to follow the directions of our physicians; we tend to increase the dose of our prescribed medicine without medical advice, and we sometimes stop taking medication before the drugs have had time to work completely in controlling or curing a disease.

The Rights of Patients[16]

Each patient has a right to

- considerate, respectful, and compassionate care.
- continuing professional competence, including time, availability, and accessibility of a physician.
- knowledge of the physician giving care and his/her relationship to other health care providers and institutions.
- full information in understandable language about the nature and risks of, and alternatives to, treatment.
- question the physician, make suggestions, and even refuse treatment.
- privacy and confidentiality regarding medical care.
- reasonable response to requests for services.
- knowledge of and refusal to participate in human experimentation.
- explanation of bills and professional fees.
- education about one's illness and health status.
- compliance with one's request to have medical records transferred to a doctor of his/her choice.

Reducing the Costs of Health Care

Unplanned illness can cause considerable family disruption, loss of income, abandonment of career or educational plans, the sacrifice of home payments, and a permanent lowering of living standards. Yet physician and hospital bills—even minor ones—are rarely budgeted for as are the more ordinary expenses of living: food, clothing, shelter, energy, major appliances, and automobiles. Nevertheless, consumers often expect the best of medical care at the least possible expense whenever the need arises. Sick or injured consumers quickly learn that the bill for illness and health care includes not only physician and hospital charges, but just as frequently, expenses associated with drugs and medicines, medical supplies, convalescent care, immunization, periodic health examinations, screening procedures, dental care, nursing home services, and loss of income due to absence from the job.

Traditionally, many individuals have had the financial capacity to meet both minor and even major medical expenses of short duration either from savings or current income. However, with advances in medical science, the increased technology of treatment, and the higher value consumers now attach to health care, millions of Americans, even those not considered poor, are finding that "adequate medical care is becoming evermore elusive and evermore expensive."[17] Illness due either to disease or trauma precipitates a financial catastrophe for the average consumer. Various types of insurance to guard against such catastrophes are discussed in chapter 20, which deals with the health care system.

There are several steps you can take to keep your health care costs to a minimum.[18]

1. Have a family or personal physician to provide comprehensive and continuous health care and a program of health maintenance.
2. Try to have as many diagnostic tests as possible performed on an outpatient basis before you are hospitalized. Many health insurance plans now cover such prehospitalization procedures.
3. For truly minor surgical procedures, investigate with your family physician the possibility of utilizing short-term surgical centers rather than general hospitals.
4. Avoid relying on the emergency room facilities of a general hospital as a medical supermarket for nonemergency cases. Although convenient, emergency room medical care is much more expensive than that provided by your family or personal physician in a private office or clinic.
5. Do not utilize the hospital for the purpose of getting a rest or taking a vacation. In general, hospitals are noisy, unfamiliar places where time schedules are set for the convenience of the staff and physicians rather than for the patients.
6. Do not plead with your physician to admit you to the hospital over a weekend unless absolutely necessary. Hospitals typically gear down over weekends unless there is a real emergency.
7. Refrain from pressuring your doctor to let you stay in the hospital longer than necessary after treatment and recovery. Each extra day comes at a premium price of more than $100.
8. When surgery is recommended, insist on an independent consultation from another surgical specialist. Many surgical procedures performed today have been found to be unnecessary, especially hysterectomies and tonsillectomies.

The best way to reduce health care costs is to stay healthy. In particular, avoid those behaviors that tend to induce or predispose to illness, such as smoking, poor eating habits, alcohol abuse, inadequate sleep, and lack of moderate exercise.

There are some common tip-offs or signs of poor health care that wise consumers should consider before continuing a therapeutic relationship with any health care provider. Chisari, Nakamura, and Thorup offer several clues to the inadequate or unconcerned physician.[19] These include failure to spend adequate time with a patient; failure to perform an adequate medical history prior to diagnosis and

Detecting Inadequate Medical Care

treatment; performance of an inadequate physical exam; and refusal to answer questions to your satisfaction.

Additionally the inadequate physician is characterized as one who does not explain adequately the reasons for performing specialized tests or taking associated risks, who fails to educate patients about their particular illness, who neglects to caution patients about both common and serious side effects of prescribed medications, and who rarely refers patients to another doctor for consultation and is offended when asked for a second medical opinion, especially before surgery.

You should also be concerned about the quality of health care if your doctor prescribes three or more different medicines for you to take each day (except for a very serious condition), or if every visit to the physician involves an injection. Vickery and Fries further recommend that you as a consumer become suspicious

> . . . when any service costing a significant amount of money is promoted enthusiastically even though you were not aware of the need. If your questions go unanswered or if the physician fails to perform any physical examination at all, it's time to worry.[20]

However, patients should be cautious in applying their newly assumed rights as assertive health consumers. Physicians are also human and are constantly faced with treating diseases for which there are no cures. As a counterpoint, then, to the assertions of the health consumer, physicians suggest that patients not take trivial problems to their doctors or cause an erosion of medical ethics " . . . by requests for slightly misleading insurance claims, exaggerated disability statements, and repeated prescriptions for pain medication."[21] As in any relationship, each party has certain responsibilities, including the consumer in this case!

Challenging Medical Bills

Whether physicians' services are paid for directly by the patient or indirectly through insurance premiums, the consumer "foots" the bill. Therefore it is important that patients have some information to help them decide if they are getting a bargain, a fair deal, or a fleecing for their health care dollars.[22]

Although most people surround the physician with a mystique that would ordinarily prevent direct questioning of the health service charges, the best approach is to talk over the matter of fees and payment plans with the doctor before treatment is begun. Even though physicians set their own fees, they have to be somewhat comparable with those of colleagues. Therefore, it might be wise to contact several local physicians to determine their fees for service and then compare the average charge with that of your physician.

If the physician refuses to discuss fees or claims that the fees are fair in spite of your objection, insist on an itemized bill that indicates the portion to be paid by the insurance carrier and the part to be paid by the patient. Then submit the bill together with an *unsigned* claim form to your insurance carrier and protest what you think is unfair. Be as specific as you can in your descriptive statements. The insurance company will contact you about the matter and tell you if the bill is in line with other doctors' charges.

The ultimate appeal mechanism, short of legal action, is a "peer review" or grievance committee of the local medical society. Although this service is often inaccessible to complaining patients, your insurance company can protest more successfully those physicians' fees that are not usual, customary, or reasonable.

When to Seek
Emergency Care

Although you may schedule yearly physical examinations, there are likely to be times when you feel it is necessary to have medical attention immediately. Whether such an occasion occurs on a weekend or before, during, or after regular office hours of your physician, some criteria should be applied to differentiate major alarm signals from minor ills. It is evident that every time you become sick or experience some abnormality of body function, you cannot and should not call a doctor. But the task of distinguishing between imminent threats to health and relatively harmless symptoms can be a frustrating experience.

When is a delay in treatment justified? What usually demands immediate treatment? Whether to phone or postpone is the consumer's dilemma. The guidelines that follow may be useful in assuring you the best of health care when likely to be needed and the wise expenditure of your resources, to say nothing of your physician's time and efforts.[23]

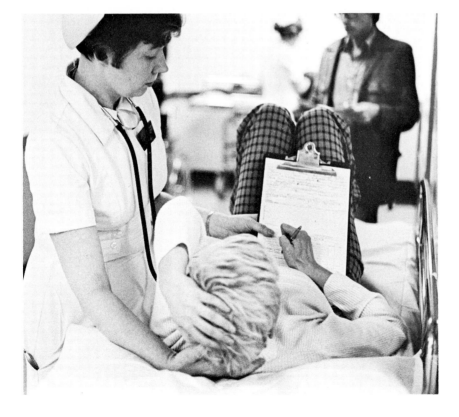

Fig. 18.8. Hospital emergency facilities should be used in an emergency only. Too many Americans use them when they should be using a family doctor.

Older children and *adults* do *NOT* generally require immediate medical care when these conditions are present:

1. Minor, self-limiting colds.
2. Mild rash unaccompanied by other symptoms.
3. Low fever, under 102° F or 39° C, unaccompanied by other symptoms.
4. Single episodes of diarrhea or vomiting unaccompanied by abdominal pains.

Young children are *NOT* likely to require immediate medical attention in these circumstances:

1. Single mild symptoms—one minor ache, one episode of vomiting without other symptoms, one loose stool, one sniffle, a few coughs.
2. A rash unaccompanied by other signs or symptoms.
3. Apparent constipation with no other symptoms.

Older children and *adults* generally *DO* need immediate medical care in these instances:

1. Serious accidents or injuries, such as animal bites, puncture wounds, wounds with great loss of blood, actual or suspected fractures, severe burns, actual or suspected poisoning.
2. Falls with possible head or spinal injury, followed by bleeding from the mouth, nose, or ears, headache, vomiting, visual disturbances, paralysis or convulsions, unusual behavior or drowsiness.
3. Sudden, severe abdominal pain or cramps, continuing or intermittent.
4. Noticeable increase or decrease in pulse rate.
5. Difficulty in breathing.
6. Loss of consciousness, however brief.
7. A mild fever that suddenly shoots up.

8. Headache that does not respond to ordinary or prescribed pain relievers.
9. An itch that becomes unbearable.
10. Unexplained discharge of blood or any other substance from any body opening.
11. Any sign of internal bleeding, including faintness, dizziness, weak or rapid pulse, shallow or irregular breathing, clammy skin.
12. Sudden neurological symptoms, such as impairment of vision or hearing, mental confusion, amnesia, numbness, or paralysis.
13. Any adverse reaction to a prescribed drug.
14. Fever above 102° F or 39° C, even when it is the only sign of illness.
15. Continuous diarrhea or vomiting.

Young children DO require immediate medical care for ALL THE SAME REASONS AS ADULTS, but special attention should also be given to these *major alarm signals:*

1. Failure to be aroused early from sleep, especially after head trauma.
2. Severe pain that persists anywhere in the body, but particularly in the abdomen, with or without trauma to the abdominal area.
3. Any earache that persists.
4. Fever over 103° F (39.5° C) orally or 104° F (40° C) rectally or, in an infant, over 100.5° F (38° C)—or any fever accompanied by stiffness of the neck.
5. Any combination of two or more of these symptoms: fever, rash, bad cough, stiff neck, swollen glands, markedly decreased appetite, acting miserably sick.
6. Diarrhea without let up or projectile vomiting.

Limited Health Practitioners	Various health care providers with limitations of practice exist throughout America today. Although they are licensed in most states to perform certain services, none is considered as a qualified medical adviser for the *entire range* of human diseases and disorders or preventive medical procedures.
Dentist	The *dentist** is concerned with the teeth, oral cavity, and associated parts, and the diagnosis and treatment of their diseases with medicines, surgical procedures, and radiation. The Doctor of Dental Surgery (D.D.S.) or the equivalent Doctor of Medical Dentistry (D.M.D.) is also trained to restore defective and missing teeth and other structures of the oral cavity. Fields of specialization are (1) dental

*Definitions marked with an asterisk have been derived from Indiana Health Careers, Inc., *Opportunities Unlimited* (Indianapolis: Indiana Health Careers, Inc., n.d.).

public health; (2) endodontics, the treatment of interior tooth tissues; (3) oral pathology, the diagnosis of diseased tissues of the oral cavity; (4) oral surgery; (5) orthodontics, dental development, and proper alignment of teeth; (6) pedodontics, or children's dental problems; (7) periodontics, the treatment of supporting tooth structures, i.e., the gums and bones; and (8) prosthodontics, the replacement of missing teeth with artificial dentures.

The *podiatrist** (formerly known as a chiropodist) diagnoses, prevents, and treats foot disorders through foot surgery, use of drugs, physical therapy, fitting of corrective devices, and prescription of proper shoes.

Podiatrist

The *optometrist** examines eyes for conservation and improvement of vision, prescribes lenses (including contacts) for correction of visual problems, and conducts visual training.

Optometrist

The *psychologist** studies the nonmedical science of human behavior for the purpose of diagnosing, treating, and preventing mental illness. Specialties include clinical, industrial, and school psychology, private counseling, and research.

Psychologist

The following practitioners base their services on systems of healing that are not founded in orthodox medical sciences.

The *chiropractor* functions within a nonmedical and nonsurgical form of therapy founded by Daniel Palmer in 1895. According to chiropractic theory, conditions of health are determined by the ''structural integrity'' of the small, movable bones of the spinal column, the vertebrae. Disease is the result of spinal subluxations, i.e., improper alignment or derangement of the vertebrae. These derangements within the spine and pelvis cause a disturbance of the nervous system that ''is often a primary or contributing causative, provocative and extending factor in the pathological process of many common and at times seemingly intractable human ailments.''[24]

Chiropractor

Through spinal manipulation or adjustment, the chiropractor returns the vertebrae to their proper position, thus restoring nerve transmission and normal functioning of body parts. Chiropractors typically use X ray (spinography) to detect subluxations. Some also employ clinical nutrition, physical therapy, psychological counseling, hygiene, and sanitation in the prevention and treatment of disease.

Chiropractic, which basically denies the ''germ theory'' of disease and the efficacy of medicines and surgery, has been branded as false and unscientific by the medical profession. Consequently, chiropractors are not allowed to practice in any hospital accredited by the Joint Commission on Accreditation of Hospitals.[25] Orthodox medicine contends that diseases having different causes require different treatments.

By contrast, chiropractic theory states that most or all illnesses come from a single source. The chiropractor may therefore believe that his task is not to identify the affliction but to roll the patient over and adjust the spinal subluxations that he rarely fails to discover.[26]

Although chiropractors can relieve some maladjustments of the spinal column and body joints, they should not be thought of as medical specialists or as family physicians.

Homeopath   The *homeopath* employs a method of treating disease by drugs, given in small doses, which produce in a healthy person symptoms similar to those of the disease. Therefore, the concept of "like cures like" is the foundation of this system of healing. In contrast, orthodox medicine uses agents that produce effects different from those of the disease treated.

Naprapath   The *naprapath* subscribes to a system of therapeutics based on the theory that many diseases are caused by connective tissue and ligament disorders. Primary treatments of manipulation and massage relieve muscular and ligamentous tension and thereby increase body resistance to disease. Diet therapy and other hygienic measures are also employed.

Naturopath   The *naturopath* embraces a system of healing that uses therapies of sunlight, manipulation, exercise, water, air, organic foods, nutrition supplements, and naturally occurring drugs in the promotion or restoration of normal body processes. Maintenance of an internal balance based on mechanical, mental, and physiological principles of life is the major precept of naturopathy. Only natural forms of treatment are used.[27]

Acupuncture   Recently, a form of alternative medicine has emerged on the health care scene. The ancient art of acupuncture, as practiced in the Orient for thousands of years, has generated considerable interest among physicians and dentists in America.

According to traditional Chinese definition, acupuncture is a procedure of treating certain diseases and alleviating pain by the insertion of extremely fine needles into the human body at specific points called loci.[28] After initial insertion, which causes only a slight feeling of soreness and swelling, the stainless steel or copper needles are twisted constantly by manual twirling or by electrical stimulation for varying lengths of time.

At present, intensive investigations are being undertaken by Western medical scientists to learn more about the therapeutic use of acupuncture. Its use has been investigated in treating nerve deafness, reducing the pain of withdrawal from heroin, and relieving chronic pain associated with neuralgia, muscular spasms, migraine headaches, osteoarthritis, and low back pain.

One experimental innovation of acupuncture practice that has been adopted by some modern medical specialists is the production of surgical anesthesia. The advantages of acupuncture anesthesia are obvious: the patients remain fully conscious during surgery; the death risk associated with general anesthetics is eliminated; the dangers of blood clotting and nausea after surgery are reduced; and the patients walk away from the operating table rather than having to be carted off to a recovery room. Clinical and research studies in the United States indicate that acupuncture anesthesia will likely have significant application in root canal work in dentistry, skin grafts, tumor biopsies, hernia repairs, tonsillectomies, appendectomies, abortions, and childbirth.[29]

Precisely how acupuncture works as a therapy for disease is not known. Its use in inducing anesthesia is also shrouded in mystery. In traditional Chinese medicine, it is thought that the body's internal organs are connected to points or loci on the skin by way of hypothetical channels or meridians that course throughout the body close to the skin surface. Stimulation of points or loci along a channel or meridian supposedly affects the internal organ attached to that channel.[30] In acupuncture, the stimulation is provided by the insertion of needles to a predetermined depth in a patient's skin. This action allegedly restores a balance in the flow of vital energy throughout the channels and various body organs.

Western medical researchers generally dismiss this unscientific explanation for the apparent functions of acupuncture. The efficacy of acupuncture, they contend, is probably based on the inserted needles' interference with the transmission of pain signals from the body to the brain. Other theories are based on hypnotherapy, needle hypnosis, and autosuggestion.[31]

Although acupuncture holds some promise as an anesthetic or—more precisely—an analgesic for certain surgical procedures and for the treatment of some acute and chronic painful conditions, this ancient form of alternative medicine has its limitations and is no panacea.[32] Perhaps the greatest immediate danger associated with acupuncture is "quackupuncture," with its costs and its health-threatening consequences, including infection, puncture of body cavities, mental trauma, and disfigurement.

Soon after several Western physicians returned from mainland China in the early 1970s with favorable impressions of the restored ancient medical art, acupuncture clinics and practitioners sprang up throughout the United States. False claims of cures for nerve deafness, sciatica, and asthma were made by therapists with dubious or nonexistent credentials.[33] To guard against the conversion of acupuncture into a new form of health quackery, medical authorities generally advise that this technique be considered an experimental procedure that should be performed only by a licensed physician or dentist trained in modern Western medicine.

Summary

When consumers enter the marketplace of health, they are at the crossroads of decision making. Health status will be affected by the ability of the consumer to utilize health products, services, and information wisely. Resources for health care include private health practitioners, public clinics, hospitals, nursing homes, extended care facilities, and public health departments. An evaluation of various health care providers reveals the training and philosophy behind those who call themselves doctors—the doctor of medicine, the osteopath, the dentist, podiatrist, optometrist, psychologist, chiropractor, homeopath, naprapath, naturopath, and practitioner of acupuncture. Each has a service to provide, but only as we learn how scientifically based that service is will we be able to make logical and rational decisions about health care throughout our life cycles.

Review Questions

1. What new health services, facilities, and professions have emerged in the last fifteen years? How does the consumer judge their reliability?
2. Discuss the citizen's role in assuring consumer protection.
3. Should good health care be considered a privilege or a right?
4. How does the concept of sickness or crisis service differ from that of preventive health care service?
5. Should our health care services be concerned with curative medicine or preventive medicine? What has the trend been?
6. Discuss the major functions of local health departments, nursing homes, voluntary agencies, health care clinics, and hospitals.
7. How has the doctor's role expanded in the past twenty years? Is the trend toward specialization?
8. What is the difference between an M.D. (Doctor of Medicine) and a D.O. (Doctor of Osteopathy)?
9. What factors should one consider before selecting a physician?
10. Describe the chiropractic theory. Does it differ greatly from osteopathy?
11. What is the allopathic theory of disease?
12. What is acupuncture? Explain its value as an anesthetic.

Readings

"Chiropractors: Healers or Quacks? Part 1: The 80-Year War with Science," *Consumer Reports* 40 (September 1975): 542–47.

"Chiropractors: Healers or Quacks? Part 2: How Chiropractors Can Help—or Harm," *Consumer Reports* 40 (October 1975): 606–10.

Editors of Consumer Reports. *The Medicine Show*. Rev. ed. Mount Vernon, N.Y.: Consumers Union of United States, Inc., 1976.

Klein, Aaron E. *Medical Tests & You*. New York: Grosset & Dunlap, 1977.

Tuck, Miriam L., and Grodner, Arlene B. *Consumer Health*. Dubuque: Wm. C. Brown Company Publishers, 1972.

Notes

1. William L. Kissick and Samuel P. Martin, "Issues of the Future in Health," *Annals of the American Academy of Political and Social Science* 399 (1972): 152–53.
2. John W. Gardner, quoted in James C. Conniff, "How You Can Make Big Business Care About the Little Man," *Today's Health* (December 1971): 18.
3. Aubrey C. McTaggart, *The Health Care Dilemma* (Boston: Holbrook Press, 1971), pp. 3–13.

4. Aubrey C. McTaggart and Lorna M. McTaggart, *The Health Care Dilemma,* 2d ed. (Boston: Holbrook Press, Inc., 1976), pp. 3–8.

5. Abigail Trafford Brett, "America's Doctors: A Profession in Trouble," *U.S. News & World Report* 83 (17 October 1977): 50–52, 55–58.

6. Marvin M. Kristein, Charles B. Arnold, and Ernst L. Wynder, "Health Economics and Preventive Care," *Science* 195 (4 February 1977): 457–62.

7. "The Nation's Hospitals: A Statistical Profile," *Hospitals* 45 (1971): 447–58.

8. Carter L. Marshall and David Pearson, *Dynamics of Health and Disease* (New York: Appleton-Century-Crofts, 1972), pp. 353, 356–57.

9. American Board of Medical Specialties, *Directory of Medical Specialists,* 17th ed. (Chicago: Marquis Who's Who, Inc., 1975).

10. U.S. Department of Health, Education, and Welfare, *Facts About Medical and Dental Practitioners* (Washington, D.C.: U.S. Government Printing Office, 1976).

11. American Osteopathic Association, *Osteopathic Medicine* (Chicago: The Association, n.d.).

12. American Osteopathic Association, *Fact Sheet* (Chicago: The Association, October, 1976), p. 2.

13. McTaggart and McTaggart, *Health Care Dilemma,* pp. 24–30.

14. Marvin S. Belsky and Leonard Gross, *How To Choose and Use Your Doctor* (New York: Arbor House, 1975), p. 102.

15. Ibid., pp. 154, 165–67.

16. Modified from the 1972 American Hospital Association Patient's "Bill of Rights."

17. Citizens Board of Inquiry into Health Services for Americans, *Heal Your Self,* 2d ed., rev. (Washington, D.C.: The American Public Health Association, 1972), p. 26.

18. Blue Cross Association and National Association of Blue Shield Plans, *How You Can Save Health Care $$$$* (Cincinnati: Hospital Care Corporation, 1976).

19. Francis V. Chisari, Robert M. Nakamura, and Lorena Thorup, *The Consumer's Guide to Health Care* (Boston: Little, Brown & Company, 1976), pp. 36–39.

20. Donald M. Vickery and James F. Fries, *Take Care of Yourself: A Consumer's Guide to Medical Care,* special ed. (Reading, Mass.: Addison-Wesley Publishing Co., Inc., 1977), p. 23.

21. Ibid., p. 24.

22. "Is Your Doctor Charging Too Much for His Services?" *Dayton Daily News,* 23 September 1973, p. 7-E.

23. Dodi Schultz, "When You Should (and Shouldn't) Call the Doctor," *Today's Health* (August 1972): 21–23, 50–61.

24. National College of Chiropractic, *Fact Sheet on Chiropractic* (Lombard, Ill.: The College, n.d.).

25. American Medical Association, *Did You Know That . . . ?* (Chicago: The Association, 1965).

26. Ralph Lee Smith, *At Your Own Risk: The Case Against Chiropractic* (New York: Pocket Books, 1969), p. 25.

27. McTaggart and McTaggart, *Health Care Dilemma,* pp. 98–100.

28. Joseph B. Davis and Lillian Yin, "Acupuncture: Past and Present," *FDA Consumer* 7 (1973): 1.

29. Peter Gwynne, "Acupuncture Update," *Today's Health* (January 1974): 19.

30. Victor W. Sidel and Ruth Sidel, "The Delivery of Medical Care in China," *Scientific American* (April 1974): 25.

31. Davis and Yin, "Acupuncture: Past and Present," p. 7.

32. Walter Tkach, "I Have Seen Acupuncture Work," *Today's Health* (July 1972): 56.

33. Samuel Rosen, "Beware of the 'Quackupuncturist' Who Operates for Profit," *Today's Health* (August 1974): 6; Harold Carron, Burton S. Epstein, and Bernard Grand, "Complications of Acupuncture," *Journal of the American Medical Association* 228 (1974): 1552–54.

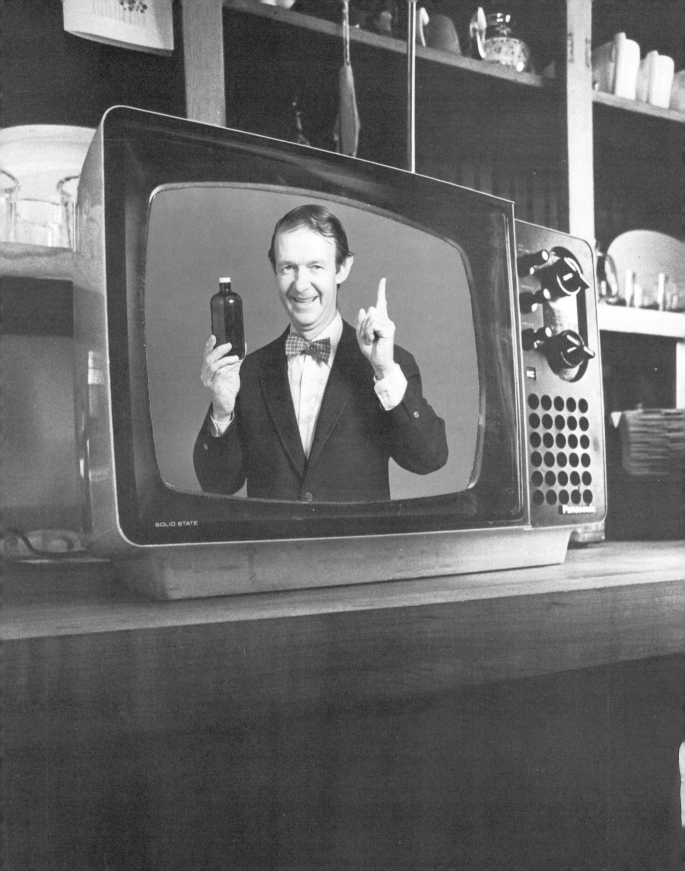

Consumerism: Products and Purchases of Concern

19

In the marketplace of health, the consumer is often faced with numerous alternative products. Certain knowledge must be possessed to help the individual make sound, rational choices and to avoid deceit and fraud. The danger lies in the multitude of useless or even dangerous substances, processes, and medicines that a person might come to rely upon. We will examine some of these health products and services and ascertain their use, uselessness, or hazards for the consumer.

Today many people are convinced that some miracle drug is available for nearly every human ailment. Such an expectation is reflected in the current demand for medications. In addition to the vast quantities of illegally marketed drugs, billions of doses of prescribed drugs and those purchased for self-treatment are used each year. Unfortunately, this fascination with drugs, especially those taken by mouth, carries certain penalties—adverse drug reactions, drug dependency, and hundreds of millions of dollars spent on ineffective or unneeded medications. Problems of drug usage are compounded by advertising that subtly and continuously encourages the general public to excessive and even irrational use of drugs.[1] Thus, of all the health care products, drugs pose one of the greatest potential hazards to the consumer's health and pocketbook.

Drugs can be wonderful substances. They aid in the diagnosis of illness; they can also be used to relieve symptoms of disease, including pain and fever. Some drugs are used to kill or inactivate disease-causing microorganisms; others—vaccines and toxoids—are employed to prevent disease. Drugs can depress or speed up body functions, as well as suppress them entirely, as seen in the effect of oral contraceptives on ovulation. While some diseases can be cured by drugs, others, including epilepsy and diabetes, can only be controlled by drugs. Drugs can also do harm to the body and impair health. Depending upon their use, drugs can act as poisons and intoxicants, alter the effect of other medications, and cause some very undesirable and unanticipated side effects.

According to law, drugs are classified as either *over-the-counter* (OTC) *drugs* or *prescription drugs*. Whereas OTC drugs can be procured without a physician's prescription and used safely if directions are followed, prescription drugs can be obtained only by the direction of a physician. Moreover, prescription drugs are to be used under a physician's supervision to assure safety and effectiveness of the

Drugs

Drug Classifications

465

medication. Each prescription is individualized for a patient in terms of dose and frequency of use according to the nature of the illness and the patient's age, weight, sex, general health status, and allergic reaction.

Over-the-Counter (OTC) Drugs   Many human ailments are only temporarily distressing and produce no permanent changes in the body. Used with care and discrimination, over-the-counter drugs can provide a degree of relief from these minor discomforts, experienced as headache, indigestion, constipation, mild aches and pain, and skin irritation. OTC drugs serve yet another function in overall health care. They permit physicians to concentrate their efforts on more serious problems of prevention, treatment, and rehabilitation. Without the wise and responsible use of OTC drugs and the application of home remedies, such as rest, sleep, hot water bottles, and ice-caps, physicians would be so overwhelmed with patients complaining of minor illnesses that their practices would be severely limited.

However, in the utilization of OTC drugs, the labels should be noted carefully and recommended doses should be observed. The same applies to prescribed drugs. Federal law requires OTC drug labels to list the following:[2]

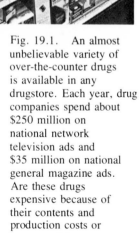

Fig. 19.1.   An almost unbelievable variety of over-the-counter drugs is available in any drugstore. Each year, drug companies spend about $250 million on national network television ads and $35 million on national general magazine ads. Are these drugs expensive because of their contents and production costs or because of the money spent on advertising?

1. Name or statement of identity of the product
2. Symptoms that the product will relieve
3. Net quantity of contents
4. Active ingredients
5. Name and place of business of the manufacturer, distributor, or packer
6. Directions—the amount of each dose, how frequently it can be taken, and how to take the medicine, for example, by mouth, with water, and so on
7. Warnings—total dose that should be taken in a day, limit on the length of treatment, statement of possible side effects, and circumstances under which a doctor's supervision is required while the medicine is being taken
8. Drug interaction and other precautions, including warnings about use if symptoms persist and about keeping medicines out of the reach of children

The abbreviations *N.F.* and *U.S.P.* may appear on some OTC drug labels. These symbols stand for the *National Formulary* and the *United States Pharmacopeia,* reference books containing official standards for identity, strength, and purity of various drugs.

> Whenever a drug label has these letters on it, it means that the drug was made according to official standards, and you can buy and use it with confidence. This provides the consumer with additional assurance that OTC drugs are of the highest quality.[3]

Prescription Drugs   These drugs require even more faithful adherence to the directions on the label. For the best possible results of prescribed medication, the consumer needs to know how often and when to take the drug, how much should be taken in one dose, and any special instructions regarding drug use. Therefore, prescription drug labels carry:

1. patient's name,
2. prescribing physician's name,
3. name, address, and phone number of the pharmacy,
4. pharmacy-designated prescription number,
5. specific directions for use, including size of dose and frequency of administration,
6. any special instructions for use,
7. name of the drug, only if requested by the prescribing physician.

Unlike the labels on OTC drugs, the labels on prescription medicines do not usually indicate what the drug will do for you, what possible side effects it may have, or any special precautions you should take. This information must come from the prescribing physician. However, the label of a prescribed drug will indicate the number of times the medication can be refilled. Under the provisions of the Controlled Substances Act of the United States, those drugs that have a significant potential for producing psychological or physical dependence are restricted according to the following schedule:[4]

Prescriptions for narcotics (opiates, morphine, methadone, and Demerol), certain short-acting barbiturates, and specific amphetamines may not be refilled. In order to obtain more drugs, the patient must return to a physician to obtain another written prescription.

Written or oral prescriptions for certain depressants (Doriden, Placidyl, Noludar, and long-acting phenobarbital) and minor tranquilizers (Equanil, Miltown, and Valium) may be refilled up to five times and any time within six months from the date of the initial filling, if the patient is so authorized by the physician.

Over-the-Counter narcotic preparations, such as antitussives (cough medicine) and antidiarrheals which contain codeine require no prescription, but the patient must be at least 18 years of age, must offer some form of identification, and must have his or her name entered in a special log maintained by a pharmacist.

Some prescription drugs may produce side effects. If any abnormal behavior or sensation develops, discontinue drug use until you can consult with your doctor. It is always wise to question your physician about possible side effects before taking a drug, especially if you plan to drive an automobile or operate machinery. Some medications cause drowsiness and thereby pose a safety hazard. Unless your physician indicates otherwise, the consumption of alcoholic beverages should be avoided when taking prescribed sleeping pills or tranquilizers. The combination of central nervous system depressants can be fatal.

Recently, consumer interest has developed into a skirmish involving drug purchasers, prescribing physicians, pharmacists, and pharmaceutical companies. The controversy surrounds the naming of drugs and the possible differences in quality between various brand names of medication.

Drugs have a chemical name based on chemical structure, a shorter generic name used by physicians and pharmacists, and a brand or trademark name used on the competitive market by the manufacturer.[5] According to drug companies'

Generic vs. Brand
Names

Fig. 19.2. Pharmacists prepare medicine, using the ingredients prescribed by the doctor.

"Is a brand name a guarantee that a drug will be good, while a generic name is an indication that the drug will be bad? In our experience it is not. On the basis of the data accrued to date, we cannot conclude there is a significant difference in quality between the generic and brand name product tested." (From the *FDA Consumer*, March 1973, Food and Drug Administration.)

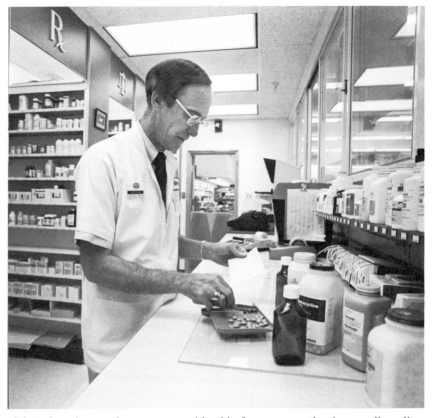

claims, brand-name drugs vary considerably from one another in overall quality, reliability, and predictability of effects. Some physicians and pharmacists contend, however, that generic drugs are in no way inferior to the same drugs sold under brand names. The consumer will probably find that if a physician prescribes medication by its generic name, the drug bill will likely be lower. For instance, one investigation revealed that while brand-name Tetracycline (a frequently prescribed antibiotic drug) sold for $58.50 per 1000 capsules, the generic tetracycline was priced at $8.40 for the same amount.[6] A large retail chain of drugstores recently surveyed its pharmacies' stocks and compared the cost of generic and brand-name drugs. On an average the generic drugs cost 57 percent less.[7] Such a difference can translate into significant savings, especially if you must take a drug over a long period of time.

Dangers of Self-Medication

Although the use of drugs can be very beneficial, self-medication carries some very real hazards. The adaptations sought through drug use—the relief of symptoms—sometimes result in maladaptations. Self-medication involves the use of drugs, prescription or over-the-counter,

> for the self-treatment of symptoms, without having a medical diagnosis of what those symptoms mean or how they are caused, and without medical advice about the drug being taken, its dosage, and its possible dangers.[10]

Some Facts about Medicines[8]

When you don't feel well, you shouldn't always reach for some medicine. Sometimes ads or commercials for OTC medicines may persuade you to take medicines, although you will do as well to let time and your body do the healing.

- Many prescription and OTC medicines relieve symptoms without actually curing illness. For example, cold remedies may make you feel more comfortable by reducing sniffles and sneezes, but the cold will last as long as it would with no medicine at all. If symptoms such as pain, fever, or headache persist, see a doctor.

- All medicines affect body functions. OTC medicines generally affect you less than prescription drugs because they are less powerful.

- A medicine that is safe and effective for most people may cause problems for others who have unpleasant or allergic reactions to it. For example, some persons get a skin rash if they take aspirin.

- Certain medicines cannot safely be taken together. Some prescription drugs for infections, for example, cannot be taken with certain OTC drugs for acid indigestion.

- Many medications lose or increase their strength as time goes by. Therefore, the large economy size may not be economical if it stands unused for a long time. However, if the doctor prescribes a drug you must take regularly and you can save money by buying a large quantity, ask your doctor or pharmacist how long it will keep.

- Many OTC medicines contain exactly the same ingredients and differ from each other only in brand name. This is particularly true of aspirin compounds and pain relievers, cold medicines, antacid preparations, acne remedies, and antiperspirants.[9] By checking ingredients, you can avoid buying identical medicines, thereby saving money and guarding against an overdose.

- Pills, gadgets, and wishful thinking seldom help you lose weight. Instead, eat fewer calories and exercise regularly. Your doctor can help you plan a program for losing weight.

- Most people do not need vitamin pills. A varied diet provides the vitamins and minerals most people need. If your doctor does recommend vitamins, take only the suggested amount—no more. Large doses of certain vitamins can have a toxic effect.

The dangers of self-treatment with drugs should be familiar to all those who occasionally act as their own physicians. Some of the common potential hazards follow:

1. The production of unintended, undesirable, and harmful side effects
2. The possibility of harmful and even fatal overdoses, as in aspirin poisoning, barbiturate intoxication, and excessive drug usage that can damage body organs
3. The treatment of the wrong disorder because of similar symptoms that arise from various disease conditions
4. The use of several medicines at the same time, which can alter the effects of one or all of the drugs
5. The repression of symptoms, thus effectively masking the progress of a minor ailment into a major disorder
6. The delay in treatment by a physician until the disease can no longer be controlled or cured
7. The unexpected and sometimes adverse reactions—or no effect at all—that can accompany use of old drugs that have changed in chemical composition or effectiveness
8. The unneeded prolongation of drug use, as is evident in the persistent reliance upon laxatives to produce "regularity."

Thus, the consumer who engages in self-medication has several concrete reasons for caution and concern. Indeed, the phrase ''let the buyer beware'' is most appropriate for drug users.

Before any drug is purchased, do yourself a favor and read the label to make sure the medication is appropriate for your health problem or symptoms. It is also good policy to reread the label before each dose to avoid taking the wrong medicine and to make sure that you follow directions. You are flirting with danger if you use someone else's prescribed drugs, so resist the temptation to borrow medications from friends and relatives.

Whether you are taking prescription or OTC drugs, consult your physician if symptoms persist. Furthermore, do not expect miracles from OTC drugs. Like prescribed medications, they do have limitations and may have varying effects in drug users due to individual differences. Be mindful, too, that advertising may exaggerate the need for a particular drug and thereby create a health problem for you that does not really exist.

Ask your physician to prescribe drugs by their generic names when possible, if you are interested in saving money. Also make sure that you get a written prescription that can be filled at a pharmacy of your choice. Since prices vary for the same drug at different pharmacies, some comparative shopping may result in considerable savings. Coded prescriptions and those directed to certain pharmacies only are possible violations of professional ethics.

Above all else, the main consumer responsibility is to follow the directions on the label. Altering dosage, failure to take medications at the specified time and in the appropriate manner, and disregarding warnings about availability to curious children may produce tragic results.

Advertising
Health Products
and Services

As a consumer, you eventually realize that many medications, products, and services are in fierce competition for your health dollars. Some items will be promoted through advertising, often described as ''the voice of free choice.'' Pain relievers, cold remedies, cough suppressants, vitamin pills, antacids, enriched and high-fiber cereals, laxatives, skin fresheners, diet aids, health club memberships, and low-calorie food and drink products are commonly presented so as to persuade you to seek out and buy the product or service. As one authority states, much of the advertising takes a predictable form.

> Virtually all promoters of health products proceed in the same pattern—inducing alarm so that they can offer reassurance, and then promising benefit with every bottle, jar, and tube.[11]

To create an illusion of superiority for a health product that is quite similar to other brands of the same product, a commercial or ad will use puffery, a common advertising technique. Legally, *puffery* is defined as

> advertising or other sales representations which praise the item to be sold with subjective opinions, superlatives, or exaggerations, vaguely and generally, stating no specific facts.[12]

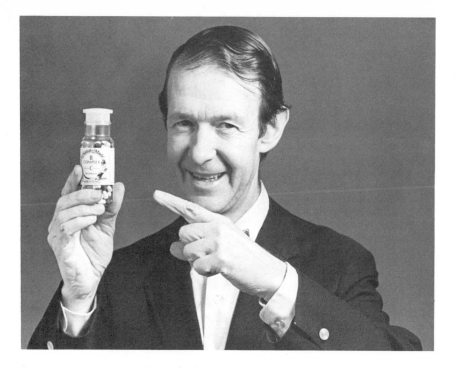

In other words, puffery is a means of puffing up a product to be greater than it actually is and exaggerating its effectiveness and benefits. Such technique is often used in promoting *parity products*—nearly identical items with numerous brand or trade names. As Schrank notes,

> in parity claims, "better" means "best" but "best" only means "equal to." If all the brands are identical, they must all be equally good, the legal minds have decided. So "best" means that the product is as good as the other superior products in its category.[13]

Consequently, be suspicious of advertising that proclaims that a product is "the greatest," "the best," and "the most frequently used." Be alert for ambiguous statements in commercials, such as those that assert that a product "works miracles," is "hospital tested," or is "government supported." Beware of claims that appear to be substantial on first notice but do not hold up under close analysis, such as "helps control dandruff," "fights bad breath," and "quality has not changed."

To give the impression of superiority, commercials will frequently use one or more of the following techniques or propaganda appeals.[14]

- Bandwagon appeal—everyone is doing it, so join the crowd by purchasing Brand X.
- Snob appeal—buy one of our products and be among the privileged few; go first class and get the very best.
- Glittering generality—make this your very last headache with the product to end all headaches.

- Testimony appeal—well-known persons extol the wonders of antacids, laxatives, fruit juices, and cereals.
- Brand loyalty appeal—accept no substitutes; pay just a little more to get the brand you have come to rely on.
- False image appeal—some desirable quality, such as improved love life, sex appeal, marital bliss, or occupational success, will result from use of a product.
- Reward appeal—purchase of a product will produce free merchandise offers and bonus stamps or coupons, and in combination with the false image appeal, will deliver personal security in the form of regained smiling ability or a slimmer waistline.
- Progress appeal—new features, formulations, ingredients, and sometimes packaging make an old product much better than before, according to the ads and commercials.
- Humor appeal—amusing slogans, jingles, or illustrations can capture the hearts and purse strings of many consumers.
- Just plain folks appeal—no gimmicks here, by golly, just simple, wholesome, good old natural ingredients for the common person.
- Scientific evidence appeal—the use of statistics, surveys, endorsements by doctors or professional health organizations, and laboratory tests to claim product superiority.
- Nonverbal appeal—pictures, gestures, and romantic or athletic activities are employed to entice the consumer to use a product and instantly be like and act like the persons in the ad or commercial.
- Underdog appeal—your support of the product is solicited so that Brand X can eventually achieve nationwide acceptance. Won't you please help in this worthy cause?

Remember, much of health advertising wants you to become a believer in and then a purchaser of a specific product. Be on guard! The advertising attack has been waged for many years, and you are the target. You are not immune to the subtle deception of the printed, verbal, or visual sales pitch.

Quackery

Perhaps the cruelest pitfall of the medical marketplace is the phenomenon of health quackery, the practice of deceit or fraud with regard to medical skills, health products, and devices. Quackery includes the "health practitioner" or quack who falsely represents ability and experience in the diagnosis and treatment of disease; the deceitfully promoted drug or nutritional supplement (the quack product); and the machine or appliance (a quack device) for diagnosis or treatment, which works only to exploit the victim's ignorance and bank account.

Basically, quackery is misinformation about health, whether or not it is intended to deceive. Much quackery comes from persons whose intentions may be honest though misguided. In everyday life experiences, quackery takes many forms: the promoter of unproven remedies for cancer; the fast buck schemer who sells health miracles by mail order; the phony nutritionist who relates all illnesses

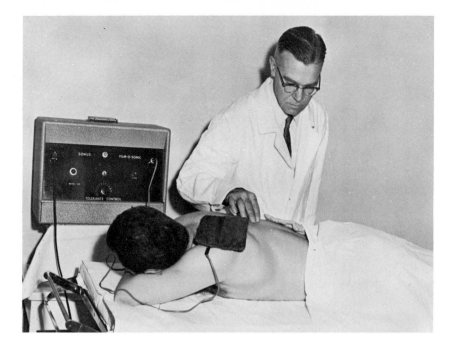

Fig. 19.4. A modern version of the chanting witchdoctor, the Sonus Film-O-Sonic used a playback tape mechanism that translated music into electric impulses through moistened pads on the patient's body. "Smoke Gets In Your Eyes" was the cure for cancer; for arteriosclerosis, "Holiday For Strings." About 500 machines at $500 each were sold to practitioners who used them to diagnose and treat serious diseases. The manufacturer went out of business after action by the Food and Drug Administration.

to faulty diet and promotes megavitamin therapy for all diseases; the door-to-door sales representative who pretends to be a health expert; the author of a book on folk remedies for heart disease and arthritis; the promoter of a rejuvenation program to restore sexual vitality; the advertiser who touts a special product to assure good health; and the modern version of the ancient medicine man who promises a reduction of excess weight through the use of a vibrator or the elimination of "cellulite" fat with its accumulation of toxic substances.

With the growing mistrust of scientific medicine and the upsurge of alternative forms of therapy supported by the medical freedom of choice movement, one observer believes that we are now entering the golden age of quackery.[15]

Identification of Quacks

The total cost of this business of half-truths, false claims, and phony treatments—all wrapped in pseudoscientific language and administered with tender loving care—has been estimated to exceed two billion dollars a year. The real tragedy, though, is not economic. Quackery offers false hope; it masks signs and symptoms of progressing disease; it delays proper diagnosis and treatment and encourages dangerous self-medication. While some quack preparations and devices are worthless and ineffective, others constitute a direct, major threat to health and life because they are used without diagnosis and supervision.

Although there is no foolproof way of recognizing a quack, the following clues have been suggested to help the nonmedical person identify a bogus practitioner.[16] The quack

1. uses a special machine or secret formula that is claimed to cure disease,
2. guarantees or implies that treatment will produce a quick or easy cure,

3. advertises or uses case histories and testimonials from patients to impress the public,
4. refuses to accept tried and proven methods of medical research and treatment,
5. clamors constantly for medical investigation and recognition by orthodox health practitioners,
6. claims that persecution by the medical profession is an attempt to suppress competition and innovation,
7. declares that traditional therapies of surgery, drugs, and X rays cause more harm than good,
8. employs high-sounding titles easily confused with qualified, scientific professionals and organizations.

Another common quack practice is worth noting. Much quackery is ''monistic,'' that is, it is based on the proposition that diseases are so alike that all or many can be attributed to a single cause, or diagnosed by one method, or treated by a single technique or medicine. The ancient Greeks had a word for this kind of oversimplification—''panacea,'' meaning cure-all. The use of a panacea invariably constitutes quackery.

The Vulnerable Consumer

In this age of proven medical techniques, fraudulent health practices and quackery should be regarded as aspects of a bygone era—the unscientific past. And yet these persist even today. Certainly the profit motive is behind the unscrupulous quack who thrives in a free enterprise economy. But the viability of the charlatan depends upon the gullible consumer. Many observers believe that quackery would cease if it were not for the cooperation of the consumer. In a certain sense, society indulges the quack who stands ever ready to ''help'' the vulnerable individual adapt to numerous human conditions and unmet needs. Reasons for consumer susceptibility are complex.

We are truly conditioned by significant advances in modern health care to expect medical miracles. Indeed, the accomplishments of medical science give us the impression that any human ailment can be controlled, if not conquered. Great expectations of the public thus form a solid foundation for the persistence of quackery. Now, add a large measure of ignorance, confusion, and false belief about health and disease; a liberal dose of uncontrolled and unremitting pain that often accompanies some disorders; some basic human fears of death and incapacitation and longings for survival and strength, and the ground floor of quackery is complete. The insulation for this cultural receptivity to fraud is provided by our predisposition to the practice of self-medication—aided and abetted by advertising—especially by those who view legitimate forms of medical care as too expensive. A primitive desire for the supernatural, manifest in the resurgence of the occult and the magical powers of spiritualism, fuels the structure of false devices and cures.[17, 18]

Not to be overlooked are the findings of a recent national study which concluded that millions of Americans make decisions on personal health problems, believing that ''anything is worth a try.''[19] Because there are individual differences in response to treatment—a well-known fact—many persons find it easy to believe that there is a chance that almost anything, no matter how outlandish, may be beneficial in their case. They do not realize the enormity of the odds against the success of a treatment that has not been scientifically proven and accepted. Faith in quackery is thus strengthened by the coincidences that constantly occur in which people feel better or get well for reasons other than the treatment they received.

Perhaps the all-embracing roof of quackery-proneness is fashioned by our personality structure.[20] Many people reflect a belligerent anti-intellectualism in their decision-making, while others display a deep-seated resentment against authority as reflected in orthodox medical practice. Of course, some people are easily frustrated and fall prey to the offer of get-well-quick schemes. Then too, there are the emotionally immature who carry over into adult life the magical thinking and fantasy common to childhood. These are the poor souls who perceive themselves as basically impotent and therefore vulnerable to the exaggerated power and influence of others. And how many of us are willing to bypass a bargain or still cling to the idea that we can really get something for nothing? Yes, there is also the lamentation of the hopeless, ''I have nothing to lose, but everything to gain.'' All these psychological factors play a role in the consumer's response to the lures of quacks.

Fakes and swindles in the health field come in every size and shape imaginable, and then a million more. Appeals are directed at every age group from the teenager with acne to the senior citizen with low back pain. Underweight weaklings and the overweight alike are targets of quacks. New scientific discoveries, such as radiation and nuclear energy, or resurrected concoctions of the ancients serve as the vehicles for quackery.

Forms of Quackery

Listed below are some of the recent fake treatments and health products identified by reputable organizations.[21, 22]

1. Air purifiers advertised to treat viral and bacterial diseases
2. Alcoholism treatments to cure the liquor habit
3. Anemia preparations to remedy fatigued blood
4. Baldness cures to feed hair roots or the scalp
5. Bust developers based on the principles of negative pressure and the stimulating whirlpool bath effect
6. Cold and cough medicines guaranteed to cure rather than to relieve symptoms
7. Colitis treatments utilizing laxatives to assure daily bowel movements
8. Cosmetic treatments that give a new complexion by chemical face peels
9. Dental plates and eyeglasses by mail order
10. Diabetes cures promoted by health food salespersons and diet books
11. Diets that indicate that calories do not really count in the process of weight control
12. Electrical and mechanical devices with which a person supposedly can diagnose or treat many different diseases merely by turning dials or applying electrical contacts to the body
13. Health books sold as a substitute for medical care obtained from a physician
14. Hemorrhoid ointments that are claimed to cure dilated veins without surgery

15. Impotency cures and health exercises to restore sexual vitality
16. Kidney medicines sold as OTC drugs to cure bladder trouble and kidney disorders
17. Pyorrhea cures for self-treatment of sore and bleeding gums
18. Reducing products that promise get-slim-quick results without control of food intake
19. Royal jelly contained in drugs and cosmetics for purposes of rejuvenation
20. Trusses sold as rupture remedies and cures
21. Ulcer cures, containing antacid ingredients good only for relief of pain
22. Wrinkle removers as contained in creams, lotions, masks, or plasters

But the best—or worst—of quackery is usually reserved for victims of arthritis, cancer, and food faddism.

Arthritis and Quackery   Arthritis presents the two absolute prerequisites for successful quackery: an incurable disease and a sufficient number of sufferers. Arthritis is characterized by pain and swelling of the joints and by sporadic remissions of symptoms. Exploiters of pain make hundreds of millions of dollars each year with numerous quack products and devices, and they conveniently attribute remissions to the curative properties of their phony remedies. Copper bracelets and electric heels have become best-sellers. Alfalfa tea, mineral water, condensed seawater, cod-liver oil and orange juice, honey and vinegar, and immune milk—from which all foreign substances have been removed—all have been popularized as arthritis treatments and have been proven worthless.[23]

Fig. 19.5. Suffering arthritis victims are the market for hundreds of quack products, ranging from wonder gloves and copper bracelets to massagers and secret tonics and food supplements. According to the Arthritis Foundation, for every dollar spent by legitimate research organizations seeking the cause and cure of arthritis, twenty dollars are wasted on quack products.

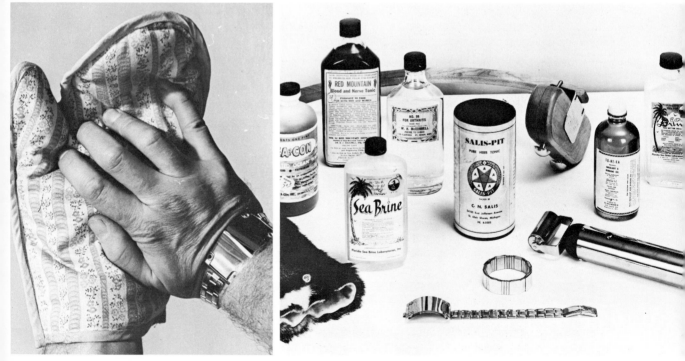

While aspirin is an excellent drug for temporary relief for some arthritics, certain manufacturers add small amounts of other materials, of little or no benefit, and market these "super aspirin" at many times the actual cost of production. More serious are the potent cortisone or synthetic steroid drugs sold in Mexico as wonder cures for arthritis. Unsupervised use can result in immediate improvement, but this is often followed by dangerous side effects, such as infection, cataracts, adrenal shock, thinning of the bones, compression fractures, and ulcers of the stomach.[24]

Useless gadgets and devices also abound in arthritis quackery. Stiff joints are bathed in "blue light"; patients pay to sit in "uranium tunnels" or wear radioactive gloves; crippled persons submit to colonic irrigations and Swedish massage—all to no avail.

Cancerous Diseases and Quackery   Cancerous diseases, marked by uncontrolled cell growth, also present a fertile field for quacks. Frustrated, confused, desperate patients often forego the proven methods of treating cancer—surgery, X ray, and chemotherapy—and seek out individuals who promise quick cures, wonder drugs, or secret therapies. Frequently, patients without cancer are convinced of its existence and then begin a series of expensive treatments to cure their nondisease. Although not all advocates of untested methods of cancer control are quacks, new drugs and remedies are not to be trusted until they have been thoroughly investigated and found to be safe and effective.

Cancer quackery has involved special diets, machines, drugs, and biological compounds from cancer tissue and animals. All have been proved ineffective and even harmful in some instances of cancer treatment.[25] One quack treatment, the "grape cure," consisted of a diet of grapes, unsweetened grape juice, fruits, raw vegetables, nuts, honey, and milk products. Grapes were also used as poultices for skin cancer, and the juice was sometimes used as a gargle or for enemas. Quack instruments, equipped with flashing lights, dials, noises, and electrical current, have also figured prominently in bogus cancer therapy.[26]

However, the most publicized unproven cancer cures have been drugs and biochemical preparations. The *Hoxsey Cancer Clinic* offered a concoction of herbs and a common laxative for treatment of internal cancer. Represented as chemotherapy, the treatment supposedly restored the original chemical balance of the body that would prove unfavorable for the survival of cancer cells. *Krebiozen,* another worthless cancer remedy, was obtained from horses' blood. Upon analysis by Food and Drug Administration chemists, Krebiozen was found to contain creatine, a normal constituent of animal tissue found in the human body. Eventually the drug was banned from interstate commerce.

Perhaps the most sensational unproven cancer cure of the modern era has been Laetrile, a substance derived from crushed apricot kernels. Promoted first as a drug, Laetrile was alleged to release cyanide within the human body and to kill off cancerous cells without damaging normal cells. More recently, Laetrile has been promoted as an astounding new vitamin, vitamin B-17 or amygdalin. According to one theory, sufficient daily intake of B-17 acts to prevent cancer, a disease thought to be caused by a specific vitamin deficiency.[27]

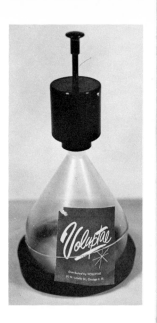

Fig. 19.6. Voluptae was one of scores of gadgets marketed with claims that it enlarged the female breasts. Operating on the principle of a vacuum pump, such devices are dangerous to women with incipient breast cancer, as well as being ineffective and fraudulent.

Fig. 19.7. Use of the Relaxacisor, a package of equipment to induce muscle contractions by mild electric shocks, "promised" effortless reducing. More than 400,000 were sold at prices from $100 to $400 each. Food and Drug Administration studies showed that the device was capable of aggravating such serious conditions as epilepsy, hernia, ulcers, varicose veins, heart disease, and could cause miscarriage.

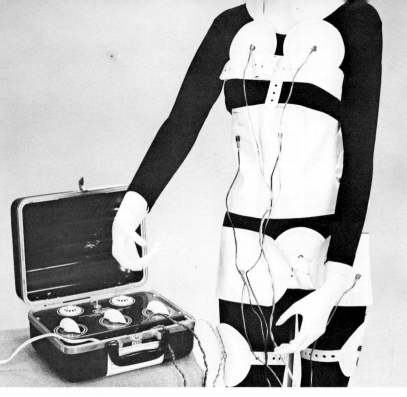

Despite the fact that extensive animal tests of Laetrile by the National Cancer Institute and the Sloan-Kettering Memorial Cancer Center have found the substance to be ineffective, the battle to legitimize Laetrile continues unabated. (The National Cancer Institute recently undertook the first government-sponsored human tests of this controversial substance.) What is behind the movement to legalize Laetrile?

A basic argument advanced by many Laetrile advocates is that patients have a right to choose the therapy they are to have. "Freedom of choice" has become the rallying cry of many Laetrile supporters. Much like the hucksters of old who promoted their patent medicines with patriotic pictures, Laetrile supporters have made the drug a symbol of alleged government suppression.[28]

Perhaps the real issue in the Laetrile promotion is one of consumer protection. Since the early 1900s, federal and state drug laws have been enacted to protect consumers from unproven, unsafe, and ineffective remedies. As Consumers Union notes:

Such laws are now being jeopardized by the pro-Laetrile forces and by the state legislatures that bow to their demands. In our opinion, approval of Laetrile as an anticancer drug would devastate the carefully structured consumer-protection drug laws enacted in modern times and would open the door to the legitimization of quackery.[29]

How much freedom do you think a person should have in choosing unproven remedies over conventional therapy? How much protection do we need from government? Perhaps the ultimate question is "How much protection do we need from ourselves?"

Food Faddism and Quackery For many years the value of dieting has been recognized by the lay public. Our fascination with slimness and the lessened need for physical activity in an affluent and sedentary society have helped to focus attention on weight control via food intake. In addition to this widespread general interest, the medical profession has acknowledged the effectiveness of special food additives and supplements in the treatment of certain diseases. Such developments have spawned the nutrition quacks with their food fads, crash diets, exotic vitamin preparations, concentrated minerals, super tonics, weight-reduction pills, spot-reducers, massaging devices, and the fast-multiplying health food stores where unlicensed individuals on occasion offer advice and recommend products in the casual practice of medicine.

Nutrition quackery has given rise to the so-called health foods that are claimed to have special health-giving properties. Actually, these foods have the same nutritional qualities that other food products have, but they usually are sold at exorbitant prices. Nevertheless, these products have been so widely promoted that millions of persons have turned to them for self-treatment of various disorders and nutritional deficiencies. One unhappy result of this preoccupation with nutrition is that many individuals who use "health foods" do not consume a nutritionally balanced diet. The food faddist often concentrates on a limited number of food elements and thereby excludes others to the point of deficiency.[30]

The common claims or myths of food quackery are presented here together with scientific facts by nutritional experts.[31]

1. *Claim:* You are what you eat.
   Fact: In one sense, yes. But you are also what heredity and environment have contributed.
2. *Claim:* Our soil has lost its vitamins and minerals, thus our food crops have little nutritional value.
   Fact: Plant nutrients are added to the soil in fertilizers, and food crops produced contain the expected nutritional value.
3. *Claim:* Chemical fertilizers are poisoning our soil.
   Fact: Modern fertilizers are needed to produce enough food for our population. There is no scientific evidence to indicate that the soil is being poisoned.
4. *Claim:* Natural, organic fertilizers not only are safer than chemical fertilizers, but also produce healthier crops.
   Fact: Organic and chemical fertilizers produce crops of equal quality and are equally safe. However, chemical fertilizers are easier to use than are organic fertilizers because organic ones cannot be absorbed as such by plants. They must be broken down by bacteria in the soil until they finally become the same chemical elements—potassium, phosphorus, and nitrogen—that are supplied directly and more quickly by modern fertilizers.
5. *Claim:* Modern processing removes most vitamins and minerals from foods.
   Fact: While any type of processing, including simple cooking, reduces to

some extent the nutrient content or quality of foods, modern processing methods are designed to keep such losses as low as possible. For some foods, nutrients are restored by enrichment after processing.

6. *Claim:* If you have an ache or pain or are just feeling tired, you are probably suffering from a vitamin deficiency.

   Fact: Most people feel tired or suffer aches and pains at one time or another. These are symptoms that may be caused by overwork, emotional stress, disease, or lack of sleep, as well as by poor nutrition. If such symptoms persist, you should see your physician.

7. *Claim:* You have to eat special foods if you want to lose weight.

   Fact: Successful weight control depends primarily on self-control of one's total food intake, while maintaining a reasonable level of physical activity. Your physician should prescribe any special diet you may need.

8. *Claim:* Vitamins from natural sources are much better than synthetic vitamins.

   Fact: Vitamins are specific chemical compounds. The human body can use them equally well whether they are synthesized by a chemist or provided by nature.

9. *Claim:* Everyone should take vitamins, just to be sure.

   Fact: Most healthy individuals whose diet regularly includes even modest amounts of meat and eggs, milk products, fruits and vegetables, any bread and other cereal products need not resort to dietary supplements. Some persons under a doctor's care or in an institution need dietary supplements because of special conditions that restrict their ability to eat a well-balanced diet. Modest supplementation with certain vitamins is also generally recommended during infancy, pregnancy, and while breast-feeding. But generally, if you eat a well-balanced diet, you do not need vitamin supplements.

Consumer Protection

To avoid the hazards of health quackery, the consumer must take some actions to assure that quality health care is provided for the investment of health care dollars. If the consumer is able to detect quack practices and products, evasive action can be taken. Therefore the wise person will become familiar with the characteristics of fraudulent and deceitful practitioners.

But just as significant in consumer protection is the discriminating choice of professional health personnel for medical care. Becoming informed about various healing arts, medical specialties, the limitations of scientific health care as well as of self-medication can also serve as a bulwark against exploitation. Learning authoritative sources of health information can also protect the consumer. Suggested sources include the family physician, the local or state medical society, the several voluntary health agencies, such as the American Cancer Society and the Arthritis Foundation, the local or state health department, and the federal food and drug law enforcement agencies.

The consumer should also develop criteria for the evaluation of health information. Consideration should be given to the motive behind the message or advertisement, the source of information, the qualifications of the author or speaker, the currency of the information presented, and the parallel between the content of the message and known scientific facts. For instance, no matter how hard you try you just can't melt away body fat, unless you undergo rapid incineration. This step-by-step analysis as applied to health information, advertising, and even to the sale of health products and devices will go a long way to counter the blind faith of many individuals.

Consumers have powerful allies in the war against fraud in the health marketplace. First, there are several private organizations that provide reliable information, engage in scientific research, and undertake antiquackery programs. Second, federal, state, and—in some instances—local governmental agencies play the role of official watchdog and can offer legal protection to consumers.

Professional Health Organizations   The American Medical Association, the American Dental Association, and their state and local affiliates set standards of education and professional conduct. Frequently they engage in public and school health-education programs to combat quackery.

Research Organizations   Consumers Union of United States, Inc., and Consumers Research, Inc., are nonprofit research associations. They offer subscribers information and counsel on consumer goods and services that are tested and rated on estimated overall quality.

Better Business Bureaus   These bureaus and their equivalents serve as voluntary self-regulating organizations to promote responsible sales and promotional activities of business members. They also provide the public with information on the reputation and reliability of business concerns and services.

Private Organizations with Consumer Interests

The Food and Drug Administration   A federal agency within the United States Department of Health, Education and Welfare is charged with the responsibility of protecting consumers against contaminants in food and against falsely represented, worthless, and dangerous drugs, medical devices, and cosmetics. New drugs must be proven safe and effective by the manufacturer before public sale is permitted.

Governmental Organizations with Consumer Interests

The Federal Trade Commission   This federal regulatory agency concerned with interstate commerce safeguards consumers by stopping false or deceptive claims made in advertising over-the-counter drugs, foods, cosmetics, and devices in newspapers and magazines and on radio and television. Frequently advertised health frauds that come under the jurisdiction of the Federal Trade Commission involve hearing aids, contact lenses, dental plates, hair restorers, and bust developers. However, this organization cannot act legally until fraud is detected.

The United States Postal Service   This service seeks to protect the public from medical quackery conducted through the mails. A special section of the service devotes full time to health frauds, including worthless medicines and devices, promotions of baldness cures and bust developers, and voodoo and other cult quackery. Formerly, proof of fraudulent intent was required before the Postal Service could prosecute. Presently, though, only proof of misrepresentation in advertising through the mails is required for conviction.

So if you, the consumer, suspect quackery, consult your local physician or report the incident to one of the appropriate agencies described above—or their regional, state, or local counterparts. Police officials will also be interested in fraudulent practices. Your action will be a great public service and may lead to the detection of a violation of law, to the seizure of products that break the law, and to the punishment of lawbreakers.

Summary

In this chapter we considered the classification of drugs as either over-the-counter or prescription drugs. Knowledge of the action and limitations of these health products and their judicious use can assist consumers in protecting not only their pocketbook but their health status too.

Dangers of self-medication were enumerated to alert consumers to potential dangers of this all too common health practice. The area of health quackery was also examined in some detail, and several criteria were offered in the identification of quack practitioners. Reasons for consumer susceptibility to health frauds were discussed along with resources that provide some consumer protection in the marketplace of health.

Why do so many individuals become involved with fraudulent health products and services? Do they not value health, or is it out of ignorance that they so act? It seems that if ever one must learn to adapt in a society where one can be easily misled, it is in the area of selection and use of health products and in the purchasing of health services.

Review Questions

1. What are the primary functions of over-the-counter drugs?
2. What information must be on the labels of all over-the-counter drugs?
3. What information should be present on the labels of prescription drugs?
4. What is meant by a drug carrying a generic name or a drug with a brand name? Which do you prefer to use?
5. Describe the potential hazards of self-medication.
6. What is quackery? What clues might aid a person in identifying a quack?
7. Describe some false treatments used for arthritis and for cancer.
8. Have you ever purchased items from a health food store? If so, discuss their benefits to you.
9. What organizations are available to help the consumer? What are their specific functions?
10. Identify several common propaganda appeals frequently used in health-related ads and commercials.

Editors of Consumer Reports. *The Medicine Show*. Rev. ed. Mount Vernon, N.Y.: Consumers Union of United States, Inc., 1976 (updated).

Schaller, Warren E., and Carroll, Charles R. *Health, Quackery & the Consumer*. Philadelphia: W. B. Saunders Company, 1976.

Notes

1. Food and Drug Administration, *First Facts about Drugs* (Washington, D.C.: U.S. Government Printing Office, 1972), p. 1.
2. Food and Drug Administration, *We Want You to Know About Labels on Medicines* (Washington, D.C.: U.S. Government Printing Office, 1976).
3. Food and Drug Administration, *We Want You to Know About Medicines Without Prescriptions* (Washington, D.C.: U.S. Government Printing Office, 1974).
4. William W. Vodra, "The Controlled Substances Act," *Drug Enforcement* 2, no. 2 (Spring 1975): 4.
5. Aubrey C. McTaggart and Lorna M. McTaggart, *The Health Care Dilemma*, 2d ed. (Boston: Holbrook Press, Inc., 1976), pp. 207–8.
6. *Drug Topics Red Book 1975*, as cited by Joe Graedon in *The People's Pharmacy* (New York: Avon Books, 1976), p. 291.
7. Revco Discount Drug Centers, *Generic Drugs Can Save You Money* (Twinsburg, Ohio: Revco D.S., Inc., 1977).
8. Modified from "A Primer on Medicines," reprinted from *FDA Consumer*, December 1973–January 1974.
9. Editors of Consumer Reports, *The Medicine Show*, (Mount Vernon, N.Y.: Consumers Union, 1976).
10. W. W. Bauer, ed., *Today's Health Guide* (Chicago: American Medical Association, 1965), p. 451.
11. Editors of Consumer Reports, *The Medicine Show*, p. 10.
12. Ivan L. Preston, *The Great American Blow-Up: Puffery in Advertising and Selling* (Madison, Wisconsin: The University of Wisconsin Press, 1975), p. 17.
13. Jeffrey Schrank, *Deception Detection* (Boston: Beacon Press, 1975), p. 4.
14. Warren E. Schaller and Charles R. Carroll, *Health, Quackery & the Consumer* (Philadelphia: W. B. Saunders Company, 1976), pp. 35–37.
15. Philip R. Alper, "The Golden Age of Quackery," *Medical Economics*, 19 September 1977, pp. 156–65.
16. American Medical Association, *Health Quackery* (Chicago: The Association, 1966), p. 3.
17. Jan Ehrenwald, "The Occult," *Today's Education*, September 1971, pp. 28–30.
18. "The Occult: A Substitute Faith," *Time*, 19 June 1972, pp. 62–68.
19. Food and Drug Administration, "Study of Health Practices and Opinions," *HEW News*, 9 October 1972.
20. James Harvey Young, *The Medical Messiahs* (Princeton: Princeton University Press, 1967), pp. 427–31.
21. Food and Drug Administration, *Your Money and Your Life* (Washington, D.C.: U.S. Government Printing Office, 1965).
22. American Medical Association, *Facts on Quacks: What You Should Know about Health Quackery* (Chicago: The Association, 1967).
23. Darrell C. Crain, *The Arthritis Handbook: A Patient's Manual on Arthritis, Rheumatism, and Gout*, 2d rev. ed. (New York: Exposition Press, 1971), pp. 138–40.
24. Terri Schultz, with Bard Lindeman, "The Pain Exploiters," *Today's Health*, October 1973, p. 30.
25. Victor Richards, *Cancer: The Wayward Cell* (Berkeley: University of California Press, 1972), p. 271.
26. National Cancer Institute, *Danger: The Cancer Quacks* (Washington, D.C.: U.S. Government Printing Office, 1969), p. 7.
27. Michael L. Culbert, *Freedom from Cancer* (Seal Beach, Calif.: '76 Press, in cooperation with The Committee for Freedom of Choice in Cancer Therapy, Inc., 1974, 1976), p. 136.
28. Food and Drug Administration, "Laetrile: The Making of a Myth," reprint from *FDA Consumer*, December 1976–January 1977, p. 4.
29. "Laetrile: The Political Success of a Scientific Failure," *Consumer Reports* 42, no. 8 (August 1977): 447.
30. Kenneth L. Jones, Louis W. Shainberg, and Curtis O. Byer, *Consumer Health* (San Francisco: Canfield Press, 1971), p. 55.
31. Food and Drug Administration, "Nutrition: Sense & Nonsense," reprinted from *FDA Consumer*, September 1972.

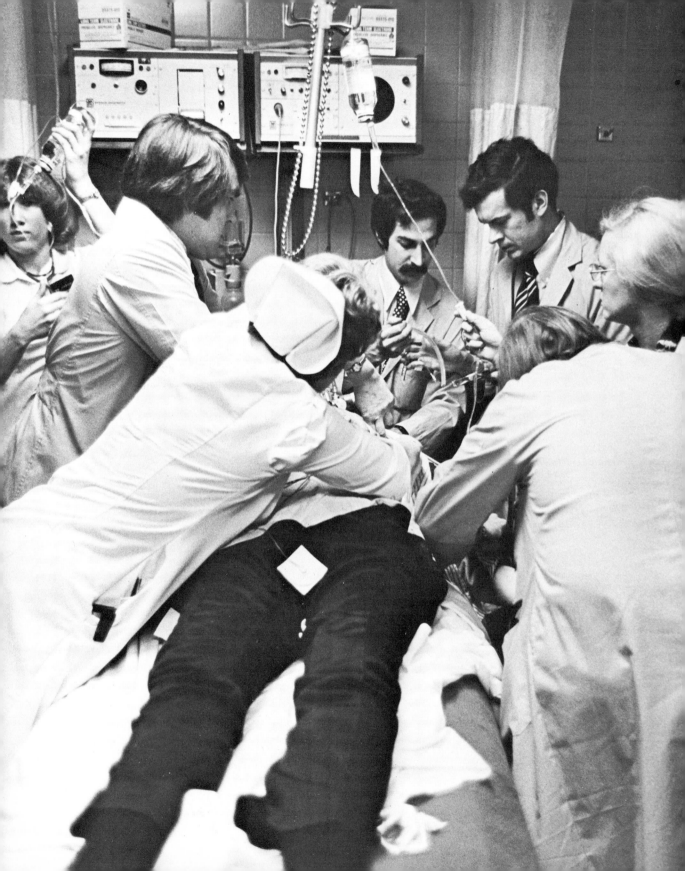

The Health Care System: Expensive and Fragmented

20

The consumer of health services is faced with a number of concerns and issues as he or she enters the health care system. Many individuals have little knowledge and awareness of this health system. For most people involvement with it is confined to visiting a physician or dentist when the need is present. The hospital is available, but most people hope they will not have to enter it. Beyond this, little is known by most citizens about the health care system in the United States.

It is becoming more evident in the United States that the health care system is not meeting the needs of the people as it should. Conflict, indecision, and differences of opinion exist as to just what the health care system should be like. There is little doubt, however, that some major changes and improvements are needed.

The cost of receiving needed health care has risen dramatically in the past decade. Hospital costs, physicians' fees, pharmaceutical expenses, and other economic considerations have made it difficult for many to obtain health care except in the most serious situations. Maintaining even an average level of health by receiving preventive health care is out of the question for most Americans for economic reasons, among others.

A person does not have to be living in poverty to realize that the cost of health care is a serious concern to many in our society. The greatest expenditures of health money is for hospital care. These expenditures have risen at double-digit rates annually for the past decade.[1] The cost of hospitalization may run from $100 to more than $150 a day. Between 8 and 9 percent of the gross national product is spent annually on health care in the United States. This amounts to approximately $140 billion in a recent year.

A question that is directly related to the problem of health care delivery in America is whether the availability of health care is a right or a privilege. The health delivery structure that has predominated throughout the history of America is based on the "fee-for-service" concept. Simply explained, this concept holds that when an individual receives health care by a physician, in a hospital, or at some other health facility, he is obliged to pay for the services rendered. This certainly would seem a reasonable premise realizing the free enterprise nature of the American economic system.

However, an ugly head is raised when one tries to ascertain how the individual who cannot afford the cost of needed health care services is to be provided for. Is

Problems of the Health Care System

Too many people receive medical care only in an emergency.

485

it correct and humane to suggest that this individual will not receive the needed health care *unless* he can pay for it? An increasing number of people in the United States, including your authors, would like to suggest that availability of health care is a *right* not to be denied specific individuals.

Related to the concerns about health care are several specific problems. One is that of health manpower. In many geographical areas, particularly rural and inner city regions, physicians and other health professionals are often unavailable. Whether there is a real shortage of health personnel (physicians, nurses, dentists, and others) is open to question and debate. Certainly the distribution of health manpower does present problems. The need today is to encourage physicians to enter primary-care, general, family-centered practice. Approximately three out of every four physicians in the United States are involved in some medical specialty, which does not help to further the concept of preventive health care and creates serious difficulties for many families in smaller communities in meeting primary health care needs. Numerous are the small communities through rural America that have no physician available.

Another problem associated with the health care delivery system is its fragmentation. Little effort at coordinated planning within the community has taken place, and competition rather than cooperation has been the keynote. As a result, wasted space and facilities may be developed with little thought to the real need for such services. The fragmentation of the health care system can be exemplified by the case of the woman who visited her family physician with a personal health problem. She was referred to a specialist, a gynecologist. After extensive tests and evaluation of her condition, she was referred to a urologist, then to a neurologist. Since they could find no problem, several other referrals took place, and finally corrective surgery was performed. However, months of discomfort passed with little effort at informing the woman what was being done. Of particular concern to her was the increasingly high professional rates charged by each specialist with seemingly no positive release of information. One, who had not seen her for half a year after indicating from his specialty point of view that she had no problem, visited her room for two minutes while she was being prepared for surgery, and in turn sent a rather large bill for "consultation." All he did was greet the lady, pass a few pleasantries with her husband, and depart. There is little doubt that such actions and the fragmentation of health care frighten many away from the health care delivery system as it exists in our communities today unless a medical emergency situation is present.

Related to the economic problems of health care is the matter of health insurance. Numerous insurance programs exist for the purpose of helping to cover the costs of health care.

In spite of the fact that 80 percent of Americans have some health insurance, much of this is inadequate coverage or "fragmented" policies. Through the past three decades in the United States there have been various efforts to provide a program of national health insurance coverage. Such a program has been available in Canada and in most European countries for a number of years. Many reasons could be offered as to why a federal plan has never been developed in the United States.

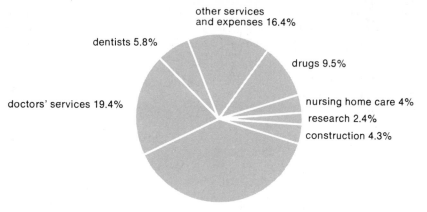

other services and expenses 16.4%

dentists 5.8%

drugs 9.5%

doctors' services 19.4%

nursing home care 4%

research 2.4%

construction 4.3%

hospital care 38.2%

Fig. 20.1. The approximate figures shown in this circle graph show how much of your dollar is spent for the various medical services.

Source: U.S. Social Security Administration, *Research and Statistics* Note (Note No. 3), 1974.

In the mid-1960s, with the passage of Medicare and Medicaid, the United States federal government for the first time became involved in a program of health insurance, but only for a selected segment of the American population. There would seem to be little doubt that the United States government will bring about some kind of national health insurance program in the future. The administration of President Carter is presently and openly committed to the establishment of a national health program. The scope, coverage, and types of coverage will no doubt depend on many political and economic variables.

Increasing emphasis has been given by those concerned about health care to preventive health activities. For a great number of citizens the only time they visit a physician is when they are ill. To give attention and care to measures designed to protect against poor health is of little consequence to them. It is paradoxical that the average American will take his automobile to the garage for periodic preventive checkups, yet so few give equal thought to their personal health maintenance.

In terms of manpower, the health care field is the third largest industry in the United States. Some 5 percent of the nation's labor force is involved in it in some way. This labor force is made up of almost 5 million persons. The average growth in the health care industry has averaged 4.8 percent per annum. This is a growth rate three times faster than that in the total employment field.

Problems exist in the health manpower area today. If you have ever been in need of a physician and been unable to find one, you have some idea of one of the problems. There is a significant lack of primary-care physicians. Less than a fourth of the nation's physicians are in primary care or general practice. Most, nearly three out of every four doctors, are specialists, such as surgeons, internists, neurologists, anesthesiologists, gynecologists, etc.

Health Manpower

The shortage of primary-care physicians is particularly acute in rural communities and in the central urban areas. Distribution and availability of physicians in rural localities is a problem in most of the nations of the world. There is no active physician providing medical care in 133 counties of the United States. Almost a half million persons live in these counties.[3]

Many suggestions have been made as to how the need for greater primary-care services could be met. One United States federal program started in 1971, known as the National Health Service Corps, was designed to make health personnel of the Public Health Service available in areas where current personnel are inadequate to meet the needs of the residents. The local community makes a request through either the state or the local health department for the specific personnel needed. The Health Service Corps personnel are then assigned for a definite period of time and salaried by the federal government. Those citizens receiving health care from the personnel employed in this program pay a service charge; this money is returned to the federal government. One long-range objective of this program is that the health personnel will remain in the community in private practice after the government obligation has been fulfilled. It is hoped that in this way the health manpower needs in rural and depressed urban areas can be resolved.

Another approach that has been used to attempt to get physicians into rural communities is for a community to contract with a student while still in medical school. The community will help to pay the student's schooling expenses during the last couple of years of training. In turn, the student will intern and practice in that community upon graduation from medical school.

Fig. 20.2. The lack of doctors, especially in general practice, is a serious concern. Many towns and rural areas have no medical personnel living there. In 1972 there were 371,434 physicians in the United States and Puerto Rico, or 1 physician for every 575 people.

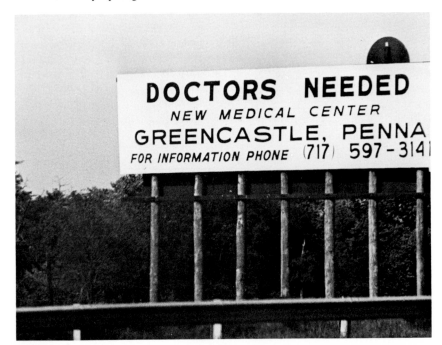

The use of paraprofessionals should help to meet the need for increased manpower in primary care. There is increasing use of the physician's assistant, a paraprofessional who functions at the direction of and under the supervision of a physician. The physician's assistant should be able to perform many primary-care procedures previously done only by the physician.

At least two questions must be answered before the physician's assistant can become accepted on a broad base, however. The first consideration is to clarify just exactly how the physician's assistant will fit into the present medical care team. What are the activities and responsibilities in which this individual will be permitted to become involved? It will be very important that physicians delegate appropriate responsibilities to the physician's assistant. This will be a difficult task for many physicians to accept.

Second, one must wonder how well the physician's assistant will be accepted by the patient. We have become so accustomed to having a physician care for our needs that it will necessitate some changes in attitude by the public to accept the physician's assistant.

Another development expanding paraprofessional manpower programs in recent years has been the use of nurse practitioners. Nurses with training beyond that which has been traditional are trained and then used to do certain kinds of diagnostic procedures. In addition, prescribing home medications and taking medical histories are often a part of the work activities of the nurse practitioner. Most of the existing nurse practitioner programs are in the pediatric field.[4]

Allied health personnel now constitute a majority of all persons working in the health care profession. Included in the allied health professions are nurses, various health technologists and technicians, therapists, dietitians, and nutritionists. Technical advances in the health care field have led to the establishment of many new and different health occupations. Technologists, such as inhalation therapists and circulation technologists, are trained to operate diagnostic and monitoring equipment and to perform needed rehabilitative services.

There are over one hundred occupational titles in the health field. However, the following sixteen allied health occupations represent approximately 90 percent of the total personnel employed in the allied occupations.[5]

1. Dental assistants
2. Dental hygienists
3. Dental laboratory technicians
4. Dietitians, nutritionists, and dietetic technicians
5. Health and hospital librarians
6. Health and medical record technicians, assistants, and aides
7. Medical laboratory technologists
8. Medical laboratory technicians and assistants
9. Nursing aides
10. Occupational and physical therapists
11. Practical nurses
12. Radiology (technologists, technicians, and assistants)
13. Registered nurses

14. Technologists and technicians
15. Therapy assistants and technicians
16. Other therapists

Expansion of knowledge and technology will continue to result in new and different occupational specialties in the health care field. All of these various health occupations play some role in the overall program of providing for better personal health for everyone. We should know and understand the role in health care of all professional and allied health personnel.

Private
Health Insurance

More than three quarters of the American population has some kind of hospitalization insurance and coverage for physician in-hospital visits. Less than half of all Americans have any prepaid private health insurance, however. Most insurance coverage is subject to deductible and coinsurance payments. The full cost of health care services is almost never met by third-party health insurance programs. As many as 20 percent of Americans under age 65 have no private health insurance coverage. Most of these are the disadvantaged, the poor, the unemployed, the nonwhite, and those with some kind of physical disability. Even though three out of every four Americans have some coverage, only 42 percent of the expenditures for personal health care were met by private health insurance in a recent year.[6]

Table 20.1 Personal Health Care—Third Party Payments and Private Consumer Expenditures: 1950 to 1972[1]

Item	1950	1955	1960	1965	1970	1971	1972
Personal health care expenditures[2]	10,885	15,708	23,680	34,821	62,322	68,785	76,466
Third party payments							
Total	3,752	6,576	10,690	16,768	38,525	43,848	49,260
Percent of total health care	34.5	41.9	45.1	48.2	61.8	63.7	64.4
Private health insurance	992	2,536	4,996	8,729	15,744	17,713	19,492
Percent of total health care	9.1	16.1	21.1	25.1	25.3	25.8	25.5
Government[3]	2,440	3,608	5,157	7,342	21,853	25,136	28,687
Percent of total health care	22.4	23.0	21.8	21.1	35.1	36.5	37.5
Philanthropy and others	320	432	537	697	928	999	1,081
Percent of total health care	3.0	2.8	2.3	2.0	1.5	1.5	1.4
Private consumer expenditures							
Total[4]	8,125	11,668	17,986	26,778	39,540	42,650	46,697
Percent met by private health insurance	12.2	21.7	27.8	32.6	39.8	41.5	41.7
Hospital care	1,832	2,997	5,119	8,135	13,123	14,049	15,623
Percent met by private health insurance	37.1	56.0	64.7	71.2	76.3	80.3	78.2
Physicians' services	[5]2,597	[4]3,433	5,309	8,181	11,045	12,270	13,434
Percent met by private health insurance	12.0	25.0	30.0	32.8	44.4	44.3	45.3

[1] In millions of dollars, except percent. Prior to 1960, excludes Alaska and Hawaii. Third party payments include private health insurance benefit payments, government expenditures (including those for health insurance for the aged), and philanthropy and the expenditures of employers to maintain industrial in-plant health facilities.
[2] All expenditures for health services and supplies except expenses for prepayment and administration, government public health activities, and expenditures of private voluntary agencies for fund raising activities.
[3] Beginning 1970, includes benefit payments under the health insurance for the aged program.
[4] Includes other expenditures not shown separately. Excludes expenses for prepayment.
[5] Includes small amounts for other types of professional services.

Source: U.S. Social Security Administration, *Research and Statistics Note* (Note No. 3), 1974, and unpublished data.

If one does have insurance coverage, it is important to know how extensive and what kind of coverage it is. Many different kinds of insurance programs are available, each with varying degrees of coverage. There are five basic different forms of health insurance coverage:

1. Hospital expense insurance
2. Surgical coverage
3. Medical insurance or physicians' expenses
4. Major medical insurance
5. Disability or loss-of-income coverage

Hospital expense insurance provides daily board and room benefits that cover room accommodations, food service, nursing care, and such procedures as laboratory tests and X rays. Maternity benefits are usually available and are paid in the form of a single or lump sum payment. In most cases limits of coverage are stated in the policy.

Surgical coverage provides for most kinds of operative procedures, with each policy listing the maximum benefits for each surgical procedure. Obviously, there is a wide range of benefits, predicated upon the seriousness and difficulty of the operation. Brain and heart surgery are the most expensive operative procedures.

The surgical benefits of a health insurance policy are usually identified for each individual occurrence, as shown in table 20.2. The figures in the left-hand column are the schedule of surgical expense coverage, and those in the right-hand column are the schedule of anesthesia expense.

Every person should examine the schedule of surgical benefit coverage on his or her health insurance policy. It is important to know if this coverage will be adequate for hospital costs in the community where one resides. If not, it is important to consider what steps should be taken to insure oneself more completely against the costs involved in surgery.

Insurance designed to cover the costs of visits to a physician for services not involving surgery is known as medical insurance. As with hospital insurance, there are usually limits and certain deductible sums that must be considered in determining how much of the total cost the policy covers.

Major medical insurance is designed to cover the costs of the catastrophic expense of an illness or accident. The overall maximum benefits are high, as high as $25,000 or more. Two cost-sharing features of this kind of insurance are the deductible clause and the coinsurance clause. The purpose of the deductible clause is to eliminate the small claim. A major medical policy may have a $200 amount deductible clause. This means that the insured person pays the first $200 of cost. Coinsurance indicates a sharing between the insurance company and the individual. The policy might indicate that after the insured has paid the deductible, he is to pay a certain percent, say 20 percent, while the company will pay the remainder—80 percent—up to the indicated maximum coverage.

Many major medical insurance plans prove to be inadequate for the long-range catastrophic illness because of the limits on maximum benefits. Also, too many people fail to carry any type of comprehensive major medical insurance.

Table 20.2 Surgical Benefits of a Health Insurance Policy (Excerpt)

Fractures	Surgery	Anesthesia
Musculoskeletal System		
Humerus: simple	100.00	*
compound or open operation	200.00	35.00
Radius, head or shaft: simple	75.00	*
compound or open operation	150.00	30.00
Radius and Ulna, distal ends, Colles': simple	75.00	*
compound or open operation	150.00	30.00
Radius and Ulna, shafts: simple	100.00	25.00
compound or open operation	150.00	30.00
Phalanx: simple	25.00	*
compound or open operation	50.00	20.00
Femur: simple	250.00	30.00
compound or open operation	350.00	50.00
Tibia, shaft: simple	100.00	20.00
compound or open operation	150.00	30.00
Tibia and Fibula, shaft: simple	125.00	30.00
compound or open operation	200.00	40.00
Respiratory System		
Septectomy: submucous resection	150.00	30.00
Maxillary sinusotomy, simple; antrum window		
operation	50.00	*
Maxillary sinusotomy, radical	150.00	30.00
Ethmoidectomy, intranasal	100.00	*
Bronchoscopy:		
diagnostic, with or without biopsy	75.00	10.00
with removal of foreign body	125.00	20.00
Total Pneumonectomy	450.00	75.00
Lobectomy, total or subtotal	450.00	75.00

Disability or loss-of-income coverage is designed to replace one's lost earning power. It provides a source of income while one is unable to work due to an injury or illness. Usually a specified benefit amount is indicated. In most instances this benefit will range between one third and two thirds of the person's normal income.

In considering disability insurance, it is important to know the definition of disability in the contract. Disability may be different for a laborer, such as a plumber, an electrician, or a carpenter, than it would be for an executive, a lawyer, or a teacher. Total disability might mean different things in different policies. Sometimes it means the inability to perform the duties of one's particular occupation. At other times it means the inability to perform duties of any occupation for which the person is suited by education, training, or experience. In some contracts it means the inability to engage in any occupation.

As one analyzes the health insurance coverage available to him, it is important to know how much of and what kind of coverage one has. What members of the family are covered? Another consideration that often goes unnoticed is how the benefits available in the policy compare with the level of health care costs in the local community. The coinsurance variables of deductibles and percentage of coinsurance must be understood. All too often failure to be familiar with these cost-sharing features of the policy results in serious misunderstandings when it comes time to pay the bills.

Some kind of comprehensive federal health insurance program will eventually be passed by the United States Congress. The extent of coverage, the coinsurance variables, the cost, and the effect on the health care system will depend upon the results of political maneuvering and compromise.

National Health Insurance in the United States

In recent years numerous proposals for some kind of national health insurance have been introduced into the United States Congress. The American Medical Association, the Health Insurance Association of America, the American Hospital Association, and the AFL-CIO have all sponsored some kind of national health insurance legislation. None of these proposals has ever gone beyond the committee level in either house of Congress.

It would be impossible to analyze every national health insurance proposal that has been submitted in recent years. Some programs, like the one sponsored by Senator Edward Kennedy, would establish a federally financed and administered health insurance program for everyone. Compulsory coverage of all persons would be required. A comprehensive range of services would be available with no financial limits, no deductibles, or no cost-sharing by the individual. Financing of this program would be by payroll taxes and general revenue monies. Built into this proposal are incentives for reorganizing the delivery of health services. No use would be made of individual, private carriers (health insurance companies).

A much less radical proposal is one that would encourage continuation of private health insurance policies as they are presently designed. This program would set minimum standards to be met by all private policies. A system of federal tax incentives would be designed to encourage the purchasing of private health insurance.

A number of basic questions must be considered in developing an effective national health insurance program. What is the proper role of the federal government in financing and administering health insurance? Financing the program is of paramount concern. The nature and the scope of benefits to be insured are varied and need clarifying. Another issue is the role of the private health insurance industry in a national program. These are just a few of the issues that must be resolved before a truly effective program can be designed that will receive the approval of both Congress and the people.

Regardless of what program the United States finally adopts, some provision for universal coverage without distinction as to income or premium contribution must be a part of it. A mechanism for consumer participation in the program planning must be included, along with an equitable means of financing. Some provision must be made to make the best use of resources and to discourage health care price inflation.

Fig. 20.3. Since the Medicare program was established in 1965, the average hospital charge per admission covered by the program has doubled. This woman is over 65, ill, has no private insurance, and lives on social security. Without Medicare, how would she pay the average hospital expense of $100 to over $150 a day?

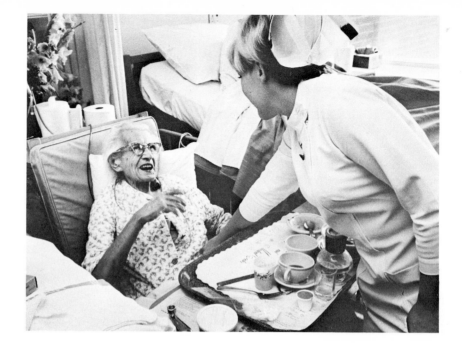

Many people today seem to be looking to national health insurance as a panacea for all our health cost problems. In actuality, they may well be greatly disappointed.

In 1965 the United States government established the Medicare and Medicaid programs of federally financed health insurance. This was the first time that the government provided a program to help pay for health services for a portion of the American public.

Table 20.3 Medicare Costs, 1978

Coverage	Time	You Pay	Medicare Pays
Hospital insurance	1st 60 days	1st $124	All covered costs
Extended care in nursing facility	1st 20 days 21st through 100th day	$15.00/day	All covered services Rest of covered services
Medical insurance	In each calendar year	All covered costs,	80% of remainder
Home health care	12 months after discharge from hospital or nursing facility	except for $31 per day	For 100 visits

Medicare provides hospital expense (Part A) and medical insurance coverage (Part B) for those senior citizens who are entitled to Social Security benefits.

Under the mandatory phase of Medicare (Part A), hospitalization expenses are covered. In addition, other related health services, such as nursing-home care, limited outpatient care, and home nurse visitations, are available on a deductible-sum basis (table 20.3).

The medical insurance coverage (Part B) is optional. An individual may elect to enroll voluntarily in this phase of Medicare. The enrollee pays a monthly premium that is deducted from the Social Security check. This monthly premium ($6.70 per month in 1975) is matched by the federal government. Physician's and surgeon's services, many diagnostic tests, rental of certain types of medical equipment, and other services are provided under Part B.

Medicaid is a program of medical insurance designed for those who are on public assistance (welfare) and for those who may not be on public assistance but are identified as being medically needy.

Medicaid is a federal-state program of medical assistance for the needy. This program provides such basic health services as inpatient hospital services, outpatient hospital services, physician's services, nursing-home services, and diagnostic tests. A number of other services may be provided, varying from one state to another. The federal government pays a certain percentage of the cost to the individual states, who must provide the remainder of the expenses. These services are available for persons on welfare and public assistance—the aged, blind, disabled, and members of families with dependent children.

Canada and the nations of western Europe have developed national programs of hospital insurance and medical care insurance, while the United States still has fragmented health care insurance coverage.

In Canada a national program of hospital insurance coverage was implemented in 1958. This program of prepaid hospital care and treatment covers more than 99 percent of the citizens of Canada. In 1968 Canada implemented a program of medical care insurance, and coverage throughout Canada today is almost 100 percent.

Under the health care plan, some residents of Canada pay a small premium, while citizens in several provinces pay no premiums at all. In the latter instance, coverage is paid for out of general or provincial revenue.

In Great Britain a program of universal health care has been in existence since 1948. Any British resident is eligible for health care under the provisions of the National Health Service. Basically, this health service is free, except for some cost-sharing features of the program. The National Health Service is funded principally by the government. Payroll deductions and cost-sharing provide the remainder of funds to support this national health program.

Hospitals, as part of the National Health Service, are governmental institutions. They are basically supported by general revenue. Medical specialists are usually salaried hospital employees.

The various Scandinavian countries for many years have had national programs of health insurance. All residents of Sweden are required to belong to that country's program, which is funded principally through taxation. Cost-sharing and payroll deductions provide some support for this program. Medical benefits are available to all residents of Sweden. Hospital care is provided free of charge.

All western European nations have some type of national health insurance program. Some are more decentralized than others; however, one would find that most of the population is covered in each country. Citizens would be eligible to receive medical and hospital care free or at a minimal cost. The economic status of an individual does not prohibit that person from obtaining health care when it is needed. Also, a major illness does not ruin an individual economically in those countries that have some national health insurance plan.

Preventive Health Care

When do *you* go to see a doctor? If you are like most individuals, you only go to see a physician if you are ill, have some health concern, or if for some reason it is necessary to have a medical examination. The concept of going on a regular periodic basis for preventive health care purposes is foreign to a majority of individuals, particularly college-age people. If we are well, we rarely give serious thought to our health or to prevention of health problems.

It is paradoxical that people are willing to spend time and money to take preventive measures to protect their personal belongings, such as their cars and their homes, while the quality of life for so many could be improved greatly if the same degree of effort and concern were applied to their health. Simply stated, our North American culture is just not oriented to the concept of preventive health care. It has been pointed out by one study committee that "in actual practice today, there is not much preventive care beyond immunizations, prenatal care, well-baby clinics, and some screening programs. The nation does not even have a tradition that emphasizes periodic checkups."[7] In recent years there has been increasing interest in the concept of preventive health care and concern expressed about the effect of our style of living upon our healthful well-being.

The causes of sickness and death are intimately related to human biology, environment, the availability of health care, and life-style. It becomes apparent that attention to these elements is necessary for the improvement of the health status of people. In supporting this concept, called the "health field concept," at a meeting of the Pan American Health Organization in 1973, Marc Lalonde, the Minister of Health and Welfare of Canada, pointed out that the leading causes of early death in Canada are: (1) heart disease, (2) accidents, and (3) lung cancer. The same could be said of the United States. Death in each of these three categories cannot be eliminated, but certainly attention to human biology, environment, and life-style will help to reduce the number of such incidences. Mr. Lalonde expressed the opinion that the health care system "is relatively helpless to reduce the number of early deaths compared to what we can do ourselves."[8] He pointed out that most attention and resources have been devoted to the health care system in the past. Greater attention must be placed on other factors, particularly life-style.

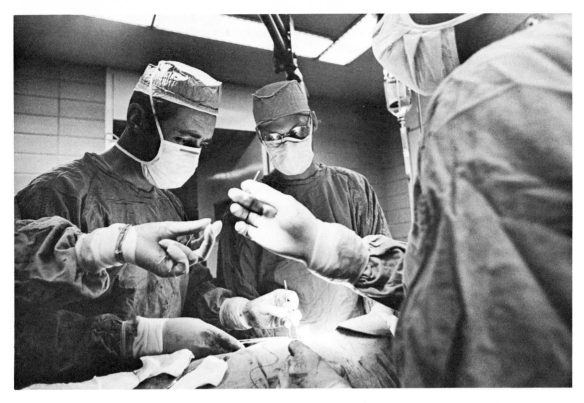

Human biology involves those matters resulting from basic biology that affect one's health—the organic makeup of the individual. What is necessary is basic research and application of the findings of biology to the betterment of the health of mankind.

Environment encompasses those conditions outside the human body that affect health. Concerns about air and water pollution, noise pollution, exposure to radiation and pesticides, plus other elements in the environment, are discussed in chapter 22. Certainly the individual has some control over these factors; however, the major impetus must come from corporate community action on behalf of everyone.

Life-style involves those decisions made by an individual that have some effect on health. The individual has some choice in the determination of these personal habits and decisions that are made. Traditional life-style in most of Canada and the United States has not been particularly conducive to a high quality of health. Lack of activity, use of tobacco, overeating, and excessive intake of alcoholic beverages by many are examples of the common life-style of a majority of people. This life-style relates to such health problems as heart attacks, lung cancer, and diabetes.

A person's life-style is affected by one's value system. What an individual values is directly related to his or her behavioral patterns. As a population begins to value the importance of improving and maintaining health, it does not seem so

Fig. 20.4. Less surgery would be required if more people followed a program of preventive maintenance rather than waiting until they are ill, in some cases seriously ill, before seeing a doctor.

strange to see adult men and women jogging, cycling, ice skating, and skiing. Increased activity by many in our society in the 1970s is an encouraging indication of the concern by many regarding life-style and improved health.

Health
Maintenance
Organizations

In an appearance before a Senate committee in 1971, where he was speaking on behalf of the idea of establishing prepaid group programs of health care, HEW Secretary Elliott Richardson stated that the concept of such programs, which he termed *health maintenance organizations,* was to "shift the medical care industry from its preoccupation with acute care in hospital settings . . .to the application of preventive measures."[9]

The basic idea involved in a health maintenance organization (HMO) is to bring together into a single health organization a comprehensive health care delivery system. This would include hospital facilities, clinics, and necessary medical and technologic manpower. A group of enrollees who are willing to pay a fixed fee for a specific period of time must be identified. Then the comprehensive health services of the HMO are available to all enrollees regardless of the frequency or extent of services needed.

In December 1973, President Richard Nixon signed a bill designed to encourage the establishment of health maintenance organizations. One major emphasis of this act was that it should make available preventive health services to a broad spectrum of individuals. In essence, what should occur is that people will have available facilities and services for providing preventive health maintenance in lieu of at some future time incurring the high costs that accompany a major sickness.

The idea of prepaid group health plans is not new. It is estimated that there are some 300 such programs in operation throughout the United States today. Such programs as the Kaiser-Permanente Medical Program have been operational for years. While individual group practice prepayment plans differ in some features, they generally share the following principles of operation:

1. Regular monthly flat-rate premiums that constitute a prepayment for the cost of health care on a per-person basis rather than on a "fee-for-service" basis
2. Predictability of expenses, which permits budgeting for health care— preventive, diagnostic, therapeutic, and rehabilitative
3. Provision of comprehensive health care with an emphasis on health maintenance and prevention of disease
4. Physicians' group practice of medicine as a cooperative team effort rather than as a competitive endeavor
5. Availability of services on a twenty-four-hour-a-day basis with most services under one roof in a clinic or hospital
6. Provision of services without the necessity of filling out claim forms

Several limitations do exist; some consumers object to various implementation procedures, and certain elements of organized medicine remain opposed. Nevertheless, group practice prepayment plans have emerged as a significant vehicle for providing high-quality, comprehensive health services at a reasonable cost. Experience has proved that members of prepaid group practice plans actually have a lower rate of hospital utilization than do subscribers of "fee-for-service" plans.

Not until 1970 were prepaid group plans referred to as health maintenance organizations. The objective of the 1973 legislation was to encourage the establishment of such programs throughout the United States so that they might eventually be available to anyone who desired to become an enrollee. By the late 1970s, however, the interest of consumers in HMOs was minimal. Government data showed that only about 4 percent of Americans are served by health maintenance organizations.

Summary

Needed health care should be within the reach of each person in our society. A number of obstacles seem to hinder the possibility of obtaining health care for many, however. Excessive and increasing cost, lack of availability of needed health resources, and other problems often stand in the way of proper care.

Health insurance has been developed historically to help meet some of the financial hardships created by health problems. In the United States such insurance programs have not been completely effective for all citizens. The United States cannot copy some other nation's model, but we would do well to use one as a focal point for developing a health insurance program that would help American citizens to cope better with the health care system.

You will no doubt be called upon in the years ahead to make your voice heard regarding what shape the health care system of your nation will take. What approaches can be established that will help make the availability of health care a goal that all citizens, regardless of status in life, can attain? This is the challenge that awaits each of us in the years ahead.

Review Questions

1. Discuss whether the provision of health care is a right or a privilege.
2. Do you agree with the current notion that there is an inadequate number of health care personnel in the United States today? If you do not agree, wherein do you believe the problem lies?
3. What is a primary-care physician? When in need of a medical service, at which point do you enter the health care system (physician, specialist, clinic, hospital, emergency room, etc.)?
4. Think of possible solutions to the problem of health manpower shortages in rural communities. How can these communities attract physicians and other health care personnel?
5. How can we make the best use of the new paraprofessionals? Where exactly do they fit into the present medical care team?
6. Discuss the five major types of health insurance. Which one do you feel would best suit you and your family?

7. Compare and contrast the health care system of the United States with those of other western nations. Which one do you feel is superior, and why?

8. Of the recent proposals for national health insurance, which one would you like to have seen initiated in the United States? Which one(s) has the best chance of being adopted?

9. Who are the forces opposed to national health insurance? What are their reasons for opposition?

10. Differentiate between the Medicaid and Medicare programs. Are they living up to their original expectations?

11. How does the concept of preventive medicine fit into your life-style?

12. What are HMOs? How do they promote preventive medicine?

Readings

Books and pamphlets

Crichton, Anne. *The Community Health Centre in Canada: Health Care Organization of the Future.* Montreal: Canadian Printco, 1973.

Elling, Ray H., ed. *National Health Care.* New York: Atherton Press, 1971.

Health Insurance Institute. *Modern Health Insurance.* New York: The Institute, 1969.

————. *Source Book of Health Insurance Data.* New York: The Institute, 1970.

McTaggart, Aubrey C. *The Health Care Dilemma.* Boston: Holbrook Press, 1971.

Articles

Andreopoulos, Spyros, ed. "Medical Cure and Medical Care," *The Milbank Memorial Fund Quarterly* 50 (1972).

Clarkson, J. Graham. "Community Integration of Health and Welfare Services," *Canadian Journal of Public Health* 63 (1972): 203–06.

Coburn, A. Stephen. "Health Care Myths: Another View." *Hospital Progress,* December 1973, pp. 50–53.

Davis, Karen. "Hospital Costs and the Medicare Program." *Social Security Bulletin,* August 1973, pp. 1–19.

Falk, I. S. "Medical Care in the U.S.A.—1932–1972. Problems, Proposals and Programs from the Committee on the Costs of Medical Care to the Committee for National Health Insurance," *Health and Society, The Milbank Memorial Fund Quarterly,* 51 (1973): 1–32.

Flash, William S. "National Health Insurance Responses to Health Care Issues." *Public Administration Review* 31 (1971): 507–18.

Greenhill, Stanley. "Alberta Health Care Utilization Study (1968 and 1970)." *Canadian Journal of Public Health* 62 (1971): 17–22.

Hacon, William S. "Health Manpower Development in Canada." *Canadian Journal of Public Health* 64 (1973): 5–12.

Hodgson, Godfrey. "The Politics of American Health Care." *The Atlantic,* 1973, 45–61.

Hogness, John R. "Toward a National Health Manpower Policy." *Journal of Medical Education* 48 (1973): 19–26.

Lewis, Irving J. "Government Investment in Health Care." *Scientific American,* April 1971, pp. 17–25.

Madison, Donald L. "Recruiting Physicians for Rural Practice." *Health Service Reports* 88 (1973): 758–62.

———. "The Structure of American Health Care Services." *Public Administration Review* 31 (1971): 518–27.

McDonald, Alison D., *et al.* "Physician Service in Montreal before Universal Health Insurance." *Medical Care* 11 (1973): 269–86.

Mott, Basil J. F. "The Changing Health Care Scene." *Public Administration Review,* 31 (1971): 501–06.

Mueller, Marjorie Smith. "Private Health Insurance in 1973: A Review of Coverage, Enrollment, and Financial Experience." *Social Security Bulletin,* February 1975, pp. 21–40.

Navarro, Vicente. "National Health Insurance and The Strategy for Change." *Health and Society, The Milbank Memorial Fund Quarterly* 51 (1973): 223–51.

Reinhardt, Uwe E. "Proposed Changes in the Organization of Health-Care Delivery: An Overview and Critique." *Health and Society, The Milbank Memorial Fund Quarterly* 51 (1973): 169–222.

Rogatz, Peter. "Some Reflections on the Costs of Health Care." *Bulletin of the New York Academy of Medicine* 49 (1973): 430–42.

Wilson, Vernon E., and Myers, Beverlee A. "Health Care Policy Issues in the 1970's." *Health Service Reports* 87 (1972): 879–85.

Wolfe, Samuel. "Consumerism and Health Care." *Public Administration Review* 31 (1971): 528–36.

Notes

1. Jack C. Ebeler, "Health Care Expenditures and Prices," Library of Congress, Congressional Research Service (Washington, D.C., 1977), p. 2.

2. Thomas N. Chirikos, *Allied Health Manpower in Ohio* (Columbus: Ohio Advisory Council for Vocational Education, 1972), p. 21.

3. Edward Klebe, "National Health Insurance," Library of Congress, Issue Brief #IB7305, Congressional Research Service (Washington, D.C., 1977), p. 2.

4. Daniel M. Wilner, Rosabelle Price Walkley, and Lenore S. Goerke, *Introduction to Public Health* (New York: Macmillan Co., 1973), p. 94.

5. Chirikos, *Allied Health Manpower,* p. 41.

6. Marjorie Smith Mueller, "Private Health Insurance in 1973: A Review of Coverage, Enrollment, and Financial Experience," *Social Security Bulletin,* February 1975, pp. 21–22.

7. Committee for Economic Development, *Building a National Health-Care System* (New York: The Committee, 1973), p. 59.

8. Marc Lalonde, *A New Perspective on the Health of Canadians* (Ottawa, Canada: Department of Health and Welfare, 1974), p. 11.

9. Elliot Richardson, Testimony before House of Representatives Committee on Appropriations, Feb. 17, 1971.

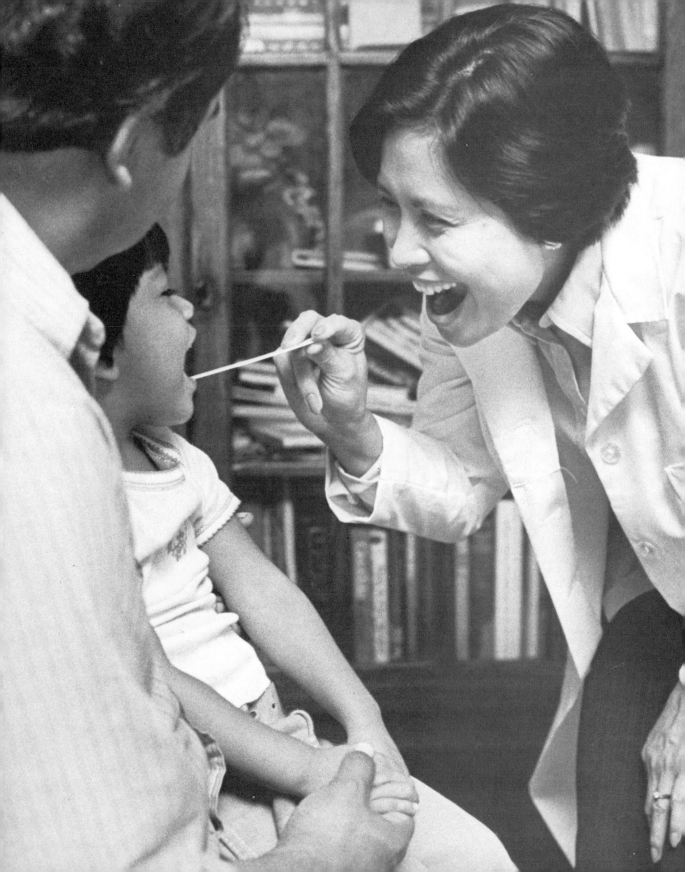

Community Health: Organization and Activities

21

Up to this point the focus of discussion in this book has been upon the personal health problems of the college student. Those problems that are particularly unique and of concern to you, the reader, have been dealt with. Hopefully, as various issues and concerns have been examined, new insights and adaptive procedures have been conveyed to you.

However, none of us lives in a vacuum; very few of our activities each day are conducted in isolation. Our health status and well-being have an effect upon others in our society and our surroundings. Obviously, the reverse of this is true; the well-being of others affects our health.

Many health problems are created because of the interaction of each of us with various groups. The improvement of group or community health is beyond the ability of just one individual. Therefore, historically wherever people have come together in a culture or a society, some efforts at community action have resulted. These actions have been directed to make life more healthful, sanitary, and free of disease. The study of man's efforts along these lines, from earliest times until the present, is a study in community efforts at adaptations to health concerns, differing from culture to culture and from one period of time to another.

Each of us interacts within several groups every day. At this moment you may be part of a community known as a class. Between now and tomorrow at this time you will have been part of several, perhaps even a great number of, societal groups. Within any society there are varying "communities." All too often we use this term to signify a political subdivision, such as a city, county, township, state, or province. However, in the broader context of community, there are many such social interacting groups in the world.

In discussing the scope for resolution of health problems, the National Commission on Community Health Services emphasized the concept of a "community of solution."[1] It was the position of this commission that a "community of solution" was established "by the boundaries within which a problem can be defined, dealt with, and solved." A health concern may be limited to a rather small geographic entity, possibly a classroom with several children having a mildly contagious illness. Few people might be affected, and a relatively narrow scope of involvement might result. On the other hand, a health concern may be much broader in scope. It may involve an entire city, a region, or maybe a nation.

Two examples might be given to illustrate how "communities of solution" may differ, depending on the specific problem. The first health-related problem

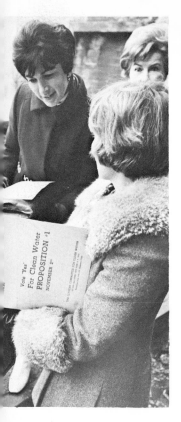

Fig. 21.1. These women are involved in a health campaign to get out the vote on a Clean Water Proposition by providing educational materials on clean water to the public.

that might be suggested is control of rodents in a low socioeconomic area of the inner core of a large city. Our concern is with the poor sanitary conditions that attract rodents, lack of understanding by many citizens of rodents and their effects, and the failure of civic authorities to bring together forces to help resolve this problem. When the problem has been identified, efforts must be taken to ascertain what measures could best be brought together to resolve or at least improve the situation. Educational measures, sanitary activities, and community involvement might be incorporated within a given "community of solution" to improve these conditions. Usually such a problem is a specific concern to a rather limited section of the community. Many people, particularly those living in suburban areas, fail to realize the problem exists, let alone to be concerned about it.

Concern over problems of air pollution in the same metropolitan area presents us with a different "community of solution." Air pollution cannot be isolated to a given city, town, or village. Involvement must be broader to include an entire region. Possibly several counties and cities are a part of this problem area. Location of the major sources of air pollution, the prevailing winds, traffic patterns, and types of industrial development are all considerations that must be given in identifying the particular "community of solution." As can be seen for each specific problem, the region, population, facilities, and citizens can be different.

Each health problem must be examined and understood in relationship to the specific population group involved. Regardless of the magnitude of a given health problem, the resolution is important, as it contributes to the goal of providing a healthful society in which better personal health can be experienced by the individual.

Historically, activities designed to improve the health of the public were programs centered upon *communicable disease control* and efforts to provide a *sanitary environment*. These activities have been a concern not only in America, but throughout the world. Today in most of the developing nations of the world, disease control and sanitation are of paramount importance. It should be quite obvious that these two components of community health are interrelated and complementary. As better sanitary conditions develop in a community, the possibilities for reducing communicable diseases are increased.

Expanding community problems have resulted in a broadening of the scope of community health activities beyond communicable disease control and sanitary activities. Today we must be concerned with problems related to chronic diseases, to safety prevention and control, and to the provision of maternal and child health services. Alcoholism, drug abuse, and mental illness necessitate corporate community activity to meet the needs of many individuals. The availability of needed services for dental care, nutrition, and nursing becomes more important as the scope of community health programs expands.

The importance of community health activities is not limited to a specific age group. Maternal and child health programs are designed with the health concerns of the individual before birth, when still a fetus, in mind. School health programs and occupational and industrial health are concerned with the important years of a person's life when he or she is in school and then earning a livelihood. Greater

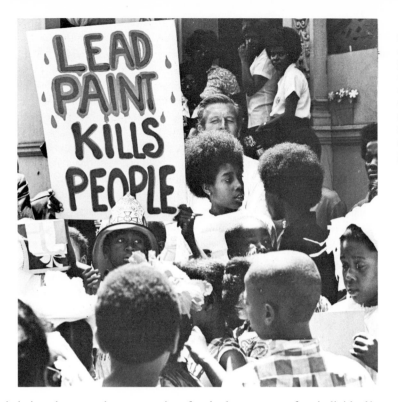

concern is being shown at the present time for the latter years of an individual's life, that period of time when one is retired, a senior citizen.

Two very important activities of many health departments, which play an important role in community health programming, are vital statistics collection and the operation of a public health laboratory. Vital statistics provide us with a determination of the number of deaths, births, and other important morbidity data in a given locality. It is required by law that records of deaths and births be kept in each state. Vital statistics become increasingly important in program planning in a community because specific needs can be identified from the study of vital statistical data. A health laboratory is very important for the many biomedical activities necessary to help protect the health and well-being of the community. The microbiologic laboratory is important in communicable disease control programs. Testing of culture samples of water, milk, and other foodstuffs are a part of the sanitation program of the health department.

The organizations for community health activities have traditionally been classified as *official* health organizations, *voluntary* health agencies, and *professional* associations.

Official health organizations are those offices of government at the local, state, and national level with special responsibility for health programs. The health activities of these agencies are supported by official (tax) funds. The programs

Official Health Organizations

and services provided are outgrowths of the constitutional and legislative requirements established for meeting the health needs and the well-being of the population.

Within the framework of the United States federal government the Department of Health, Education and Welfare (HEW) has specific responsibilities for problems related to health. Although the constitutional responsibility for health rests with each state, the federal government has become more and more involved in concerns related to health. Many health activities are a part of the programs of many different agencies within the federal government. These activities fall within the various departments of government and are specific to the responsibilities of their particular department. For example, the operation of hospitals for military personnel is a part of the program of the Department of Defense. School lunch programs are supported to some degree by the Department of Agriculture. The Department of Labor is involved in programs relating to the occupational safety and well-being of the working individual.

As people have demanded more health services to meet the many health needs of our society, it has been the role of the federal government to undertake many of these programs. The major responsibility for fulfilling the health missions of the federal government rests with the Public Health Service (PHS). The Public Health Service is under the direction of the Office of Assistant Secretary for Health.

Two basic health missions have been assigned to HEW: (1) to maintain and protect the health of the American people, and (2) to develop resources for improving the level of health of all Americans.

At present the Public Health Service consists of six agencies. An examination of the scope of these agencies will give some indication of the types of the federal government's involvement in health programming. There has been frequent change in the organizational structure of the various bureaus, departments, and divisions of government. Therefore, the structure of the Public Health Service as presented may actually be different at the time this chapter is read; nonetheless, the activities themselves will still remain somewhat constant.

The six agencies of the Public Health Service are:

1. Food and Drug Administration (FDA)
2. Health Services Administration (HSA)
3. Health Resources Administration (HRA)
4. National Institutes of Health (NIH)
5. Center for Disease Control (CDC)
6. Alcohol, Drug Abuse, and Mental Health Administration (ADAMHA)

Food and Drug Administration It is the responsibility of the Food and Drug Administration to protect the public from harmful and falsely labeled foods, drugs, and cosmetics. This is done by inspections, by laboratory testing, and by action taken to remove from the marketplace those foods, drugs, and cosmetics not meeting regulations. Any new drug that is manufactured to be sold in interstate commerce must be approved by the FDA.

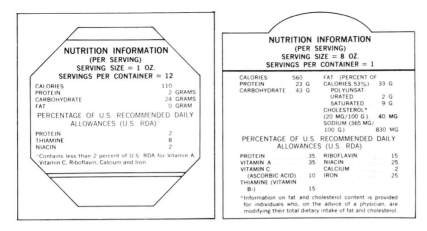

NUTRITION INFORMATION		
(PER SERVING)		
SERVING SIZE = 1 OZ.		
SERVINGS PER CONTAINER = 12		
CALORIES		110
PROTEIN		2 GRAMS
CARBOHYDRATE		24 GRAMS
FAT		0 GRAM
PERCENTAGE OF U.S. RECOMMENDED DAILY ALLOWANCES (U.S. RDA)		
PROTEIN		2
THIAMINE		8
NIACIN		2

Contains less than 2 percent of U.S. RDA for Vitamin A, Vitamin C, Riboflavin, Calcium and Iron.

NUTRITION INFORMATION			
(PER SERVING)			
SERVING SIZE = 8 OZ.			
SERVINGS PER CONTAINER = 1			
CALORIES	560	FAT (PERCENT OF	
PROTEIN	23 G	CALORIES 53%)	33 G
CARBOHYDRATE	43 G	POLYUNSAT-	
		URATED	2 G
		SATURATED	9 G
		CHOLESTEROL*	
		(20 MG/100 G)	40 MG
		SODIUM (365 MG/	
		100 G)	830 MG
PERCENTAGE OF U.S. RECOMMENDED DAILY ALLOWANCES (U.S. RDA)			
PROTEIN	35	RIBOFLAVIN	15
VITAMIN A	35	NIACIN	25
VITAMIN C		CALCIUM	2
(ASCORBIC ACID)	10	IRON	25
THIAMINE (VITAMIN B₁)	15		

*Information on fat and cholesterol content is provided for individuals who, on the advice of a physician, are modifying their total dietary intake of fat and cholesterol.

Fig. 21.3.   The Food and Drug Administration sets regulations
for labeling foods, drugs, and cosmetics.
The minimum information (left) that must appear on a nutrition label.
Optional listings (right) for cholesterol, fats, and
sodium may also appear at the manufacturer's discretion.

Fig. 21.4.   The Indian
Health Service provides
at-home health services
for people living on
United States Indian
reservations.

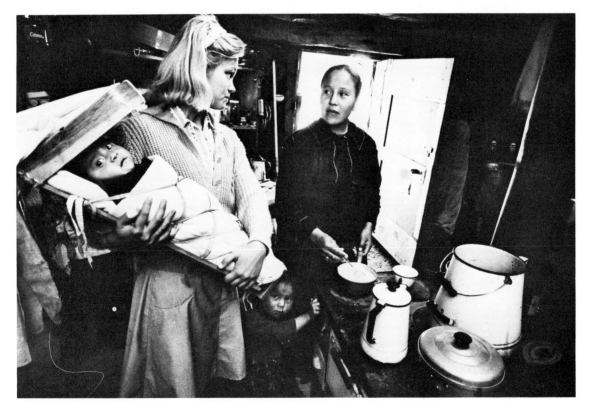

Health Services Administration   Programs designed to provide various health services are administered by this division. Two programs have been established in recent years to help make health care available to all Americans: Health Maintenance Organizations (HMO) and Emergency Medical Services (EMS). Health Maintenance Organizations provide comprehensive health services on a prepaid basis. This topic was examined in the previous chapter. Emergency Medical Services programs help local communities develop effective emergency services that are available in times of accident, sickness, and injury. The Indian Health Service, which is responsible for health services on Indian reservations, operates hospitals, health centers, and other health facilities. Also, federal efforts to provide family planning services for the entire American population are an important part of the HSA program. Other services provided by the HSA are: (1) community health service, (2) maternal-child health service, and (3) federal health programs service.

Health Resources Administration   Programs of research, training, and planning take place in the Health Resources Administration. Through the various sections in this administrative unit comprehensive health planning is funded. Emergency medical services, health manpower programs, and the national center for health statistics are other activities of importance.

National Institutes of Health   Research designed to improve the health of mankind takes place within the ten different National Institutes of Health. The different institutes and their general areas of research are indicated in table 21.1.

Center for Disease Control   Efforts designed to conduct epidemiologic study of disease have been centered in this division of the Public Health Service. In addition to efforts directed toward the reduction of disease, all federal programs that are an outgrowth of the Occupational Safety and Health Act of 1970 (OSHA) are now administered by this federal agency. This act created a national institute, known as the National Institute of Safety and Health (NIOSH).

Alcohol, Drug Abuse, and Mental Health Administration   The basic objective of this agency is to prevent and treat mental illness and the misuse of alcohol and drugs. This is accomplished by the support of alcohol treatment programs throughout the country. Also, local programs of treatment of drug addicts and abusers are supported by ADAMHA. Efforts to identify new and more effective means of treating the mentally ill are funded by this agency of government.

Since 1953, when HEW was organized, all health programs at the federal level have been centered in this department. There is continuing desire on the part of many public health personnel and some members of the United States Congress to form a cabinet-level department devoted entirely to health. Those who support such a proposal feel that all health responsibilities of HEW should become a part of a separate department of health. It is felt that greater control and emphasis could result from such an administrative change.

Table 21.1 The National Institutes of Health
and Specific Areas of Research

Institute	Area of Research
National Institute of Arthritis, Metabolism, and Digestive Diseases	Rheumatoid diseases and digestive conditions
National Cancer Institute	Cancer and related conditions
National Institute of Child Health and Human Development	All aspects of child health from prenatal concerns to infant health problems
National Institute of Dental Research	Conditions relating to the teeth and oral hygiene
National Institute of Environmental Health Sciences	Problems caused by environmental conditions that are detrimental to health
National Eye Institute	Conditions affecting the ability to see and resulting in blindness
National Institute of General Medical Sciences	Numerous medical problems; genetic diseases and acupuncture research are examples
National Heart and Lung Institute	All cardiovascular and lung diseases
National Institute of Neurological Diseases and Stroke	Conditions relating to the neurological system and to stroke

State and Local Health Departments

Each of the states in the United States has a health department. These state health departments are headed by health commissioners, with policy-making decisions and overall program planning the responsibility of a board of health.

Various health services are provided by each of these individual health departments. Activities such as communicable disease control and environmental sanitation control are found in most departments. Health nursing services, maternal-child health services, and laboratory services are almost always available in state health departments. The normal functions of a public health laboratory involve work in pathology, bacteriological work, and virology.

The public health nurse is probably the most visible employee of a health department as she goes about the community providing needed basic nursing services. The work of the public health nurse involves home visits, school health service activities, educational and service activities as part of the maternal-child health program, and many other responsibilities.

Required vital statistics—births, deaths, morbidity—are kept by the health department. Programs designed to educate the public in health matters that influence health behavioral patterns in a positive manner are a part of the health education sections' responsibilities.

Even though the constitutional responsibility for maintaining the health status of the people lies with the state governments, historically these bodies of government have delegated the actual day-to-day working operations to city, county, or township entities. Most state health programs are supportive of the activities and programs of the local health department. The organization and structure of most local health departments are very similar to the state health department. There is a health commissioner, who is legally responsible for all health matters under his jurisdiction, a board of health, and the various working departments and services.

Fig. 21.5. Local health departments play a major role in maintaining community health. These photos show some of the many facets of the work of the Chicago Board of Health. (1) As part of a city-wide immunization program, a nurse administers a dose of oral polio vaccine. (2) The Board maintains a comprehensive pediatric program which includes audiology among a large spectrum of tests. (3) A lab technician prepares blood samples for identification of blood-lead levels in child patients. The Board screens more than 60,000 children annually for lead poisoning.

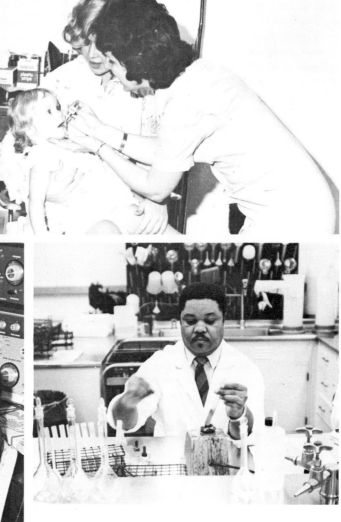

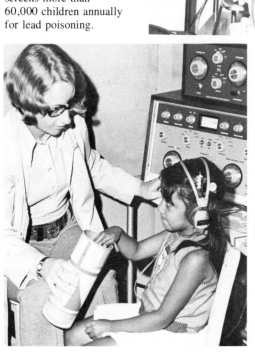

Local health departments provide the various services already listed for state departments. Sanitary services and health education activities are particularly important in local departments.

For many, particularly the poor, the dental and health clinics operated by some local departments of health are the primary source of health care. Such services are provided through taxation and are available to anyone living in the area. Other health services that usually are found in a local health department clinic are family planning services and immunizations and vaccinations for children.

Often the activities of a health department are determined by local need and the availability of state and federal funds to support a given program. In recent years in the United States, funds have been available to develop programs designed to identify and reduce incidence of lead poisoning in children. This condition is particularly a problem for those who live in older homes with chipping and peeling paint on the walls and the floors.

Venereal disease has reached epidemic proportions in much of North America. Programs designed to identify the contacts and to treat patients with VD have expanded to many local health departments in the past few years.

Programs often are established for meeting the health needs of a particular population group. One example of this type of local health department activity involves programs for migrant families. The health of the migrant is often rather poor. This is partially due to mobility, partially due to cultural differences, and almost always due to poverty. In addition to the normal health problems that all people experience, the migrant often is forced to live in poor sanitary surroundings, which results in dysentery and diarrhea. Many very basic personal health needs must be met by the health department activities for the migrant.

Numerous other special programs could be identified. Nutritional programs established for the expectant or new mother, health services for the elderly, and screening programs for schoolchildren are but a few of the programs often found. Wherever a need is strong enough for community action and where support is present, the local health department will be the agent to perform the task.

Many college students have little understanding of the role that the local health department plays within the community. Often this agency of government is seen as providing services to only a selected population group. As we better understand the roles played by local and state health departments, the role of these agencies in contributing to better personal health for everyone becomes clearer.

International Health Concerns

Just as an accumulation of individual personal health problems leads to concern for the health of a community, so we must become aware of the health of the nations. No nation can exist in total isolation in the latter part of the twentieth century. The health problems and concerns of one nation can very easily affect the well-being of individuals in a neighboring country.

All nations of the world have some activities designed to improve the health of its citizens. However, in many of the Third World nations, where health problems are the greatest, the resources are very inadequate. Health manpower, financial resources, and basic knowledge are very often lacking in these countries. As a result, nations often are forced to rely upon others for support and help in combating disease, controlling population growth, improving health care delivery systems, and solving the thousands of other health problems unique to each nation.

Throughout history man has not been particularly known for his ability to organize and coordinate efforts designed to solve international health problems. Since 1948, the major efforts at worldwide cooperation to improve the health and well-being of the more than 4 billion people on earth has been centered in the World Health Organization (WHO), an agency of the United Nations. Its central headquarters is in Geneva, Switzerland, with six regional offices located throughout the world (table 21.2). In 1977 there were 152 members and associate members of the World Health Assembly, which is the governing body of WHO. Each member nation of WHO has representation on this governing body.

The basic objective of WHO is to help nations to help themselves when dealing with health concerns. This concept is followed as attempts to make available needed medical supplies and attempts to train health personnel take place.

Disease control activities have been an important aspect of WHO activity through the years. Malaria has been one of the most widespread diseases in the world. Efforts to eradicate this condition have included programs of spraying in areas, such as Afghanistan, Mexico, the British Solomon Islands Protectorate, and throughout Africa, Asia, and Latin America.

Smallpox is an example of another disease that WHO efforts have been very successful in reducing. In 1967 smallpox was endemic in thirty nations of the world. By means of surveillance, screening, vaccination, and education, smallpox has been virtually eliminated in all of the nations of the world. An outbreak of smallpox in Somalia is all that kept WHO from being able to declare in 1977 that smallpox had been eradicated.

The World Health Organization makes available funds and training personnel to help prepare those health professionals who can meet the health needs of the various nations. For example, nurses have been trained in over 100 countries with assistance from WHO. Dental training has also been supported by WHO.

The organization has also been active in programs designed to improve the quality of the environment. Over the past several years an international network designed to monitor air pollution has been established. It is the objective of these

Table 21.2 Regional Offices of the World Health Organization

Region of World	Office Location
Africa	Brazzaville, Zaire
Americas	Washington, D.C., U.S.A.
Asia (Southeast)	New Delhi, India
Europe	Copenhagen, Denmark
Middle East	Alexandria, United Arab Republic
Pacific (Western)	Manila, Philippines

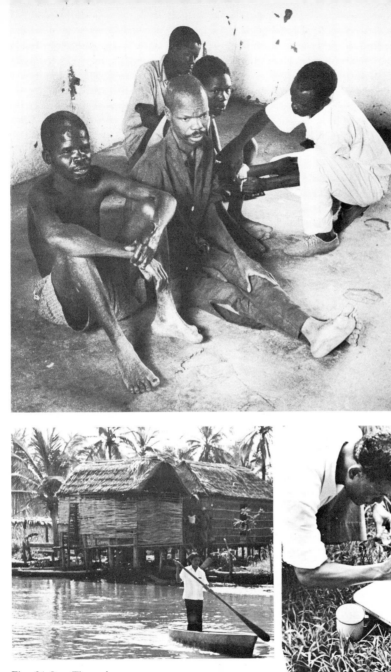

Fig. 21.6. The World Health Organization, in a study of the epidemiology of sleeping sickness in Africa, treats patients at Li Rangu hospital near Yambio, Sudan.

Fig. 21.7. Malaria is one of the most widespread diseases. One of the first steps to eradicate it in a specific area involves investigating the density of mosquito larvae in watery areas.

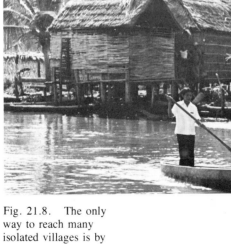

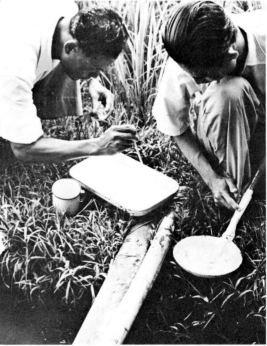

Fig. 21.8. The only way to reach many isolated villages is by water. This medical auxiliary is traveling to a village on Lake Maracaibo in Venezuela.

monitoring stations to include the promotion of comparable methods of measurement, the introduction of reliable and effective procedures for the calibration of routine sampling and analytical methods, and the development of acceptable procedures for handling and statistically analyzing data.

The World Health Organization has working arrangements with other international agencies such as the United Nations Children's Fund (UNICEF) and the Food and Agricultural Organization (FAO). The first-named agency conducts programs for children in developing nations, programs designed to meet the nutritional needs of the children and to control communicable diseases; FAO is concerned with programs to relieve hunger and malnutrition.

Voluntary Health Organizations	The voluntary health organization plays an important role in the overall community health programs. These agencies are supported by private contributions and donations; tax monies are not used. Usually fund-raising campaigns provide the operating money for the voluntary health agency.

Voluntary health organizations usually have a specific focus of concern and program. The focus might be a specific disease, such as cancer (the American Cancer Society) or arthritis (the Arthritis Foundation). The agency might concern itself with a particular structure of the body, such as the heart (American Heart Association) or the eyes (National Society for the Prevention of Blindness). Another classification consists of a broader-based interest for a special group of individuals, such as mental health (National Association of Mental Health) or safety (National Safety Council).

The activities of the various voluntary health agencies are numerous and diversified. Many of them provide direct health services to the citizens of the community. The Arthritis Foundation makes available needed services to the arthritic patient. The American Red Cross provides such services as home nursing, sickroom supply services, and a national blood transfusion service (see also picture opposite chapter opener). Research activity and support is a major part of the programs of many voluntary health agencies. Usually the research is not conducted by the agency, but funds are provided to those researchers who are involved in specific activity of interest to that health organization.

Probably the most observable activities in the eyes of the general public are the public educational activities of many agencies. Efforts to inform the public better about a particular health problem have been a major concern of these agencies for years. In addition to educational programs and activities conducted for the general public, many voluntary health agencies now include extensive programs of a continuing educational nature for the health professionals.

Some of the voluntary health agencies have been active in the political arena by lobbying for specific legislation. An example of these attempts can be seen in many of the activities of the National Lung Association, which has been rather effective in lobbying for legislation relating to the establishment of air pollution control standards and antismoking regulations.

Most voluntary health organizations operate at the local, state, and national level. Usually there is a board of directors that is responsible for setting policy

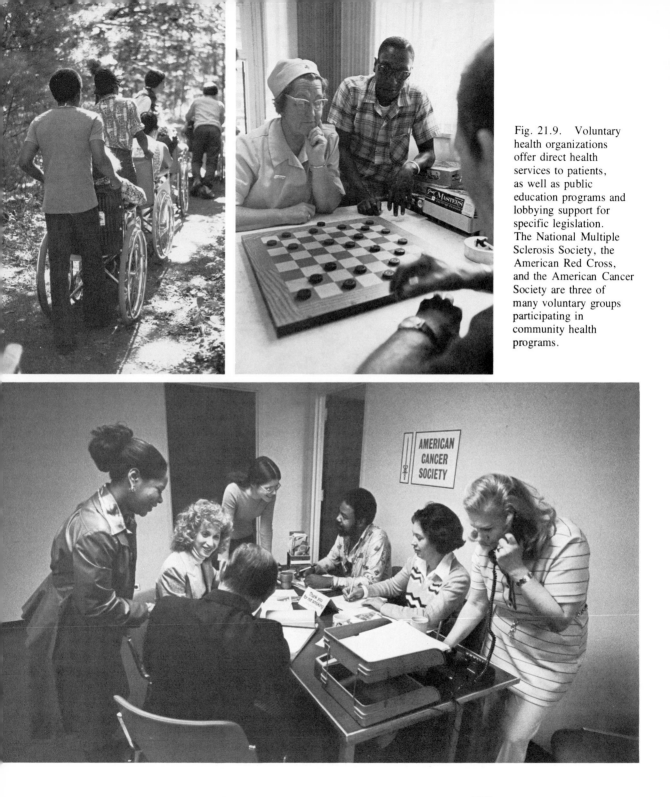

Fig. 21.9. Voluntary health organizations offer direct health services to patients, as well as public education programs and lobbying support for specific legislation. The National Multiple Sclerosis Society, the American Red Cross, and the American Cancer Society are three of many voluntary groups participating in community health programs.

and direction for the organization. The voluntary health agency, while supported financially by contributions and gifts and using a great amount of voluntary staff help, still employs a professional staff. It is this staff that performs the daily functions of the agency. Such personnel usually include administrative directors, health educators, nurses, and other pertinent individuals.

Voluntary health agencies are not supported financially by tax funds. Funds are obtained through private contributions and donations. In some instances the agency provides certain services for which a minimal fee is charged. For the most part, monies are obtained through fund-raising campaigns.

Fund raising usually takes place in one of two ways. A joint effort with many agencies participating is held in most communities. These joint community efforts are known by such names as the United Way, United Appeal, or Community Chest. Their joint campaigns are usually efficient administratively, and such an effort eliminates numerous calls upon citizens during the year by each individual agency.

Some agencies prefer not to be involved in the community fund-raising drive. They feel that their specific identity is lost in the joint community approach. They would suggest that one of the objectives of the fund-raising campaign, in addition to obtaining funds, is to educate the public about the services rendered by the particular agency. Part of this educational process includes informing the public about the particular problem with which they are concerned.

The voluntary health organization is a vital part of the community health program. Probably everyone at some time has had contact with some aspect of this phase of the community health program. As an individual, you can benefit from the educational activities of these agencies; you may receive direct services from them; also you can help the health activities of voluntary health organizations by providing financial contributions or working time to support these agencies.

Professional Associations

Most health-related professions are represented by some professional health association. These professional health organizations are usually national in scope, with state and local affiliates.

Such associations play several roles in contributing to the overall health of the community. Most serve an educational role for the members as well as for the general public. For example, the American Medical Association publishes monthly a general-interest magazine, *Today's Health,* which includes information about a wide number of health topics. All of the professional organizations publish a more technical or professional journal of interest to the members. Newsletters supply updated information in many instances.

Many of the professional organizations have established standards of training for those entering the profession. Such is true of the American Dental Association, the American Nurses Association, and the American Medical Associations.

All of these professional organizations have at least an annual meeting, plus numerous other local, regional, and state gatherings. It is at these professional meetings that recent research of interest, programming, and activity of the members of the specific association are presented. These meetings serve as a valuable in-service educational experience for the professional, as well as providing a time when official action can be taken in the form of policy statements and professional resolutions. In 1974 the American Public Health Association acted on some twenty resolutions at its annual meeting.[2] These resolutions covered such topics as abortion, emergency health services, need for home health services, comprehensive health planning, nursing home registration, and standardizations of certificates for recording births and deaths.

Often the actions and support of the professional health organizations have been instrumental in bringing about change in the community. For example, for years the American Dental Association has played a leading role in the support of community programs for fluoridation of the public drinking water.

The scope and interest within a professional health organization may be very broad, as in the case of the American Public Health Association. These organizations are composed of a cross-section of many public health fields. On the other hand, the American Academy of Pediatrics has basically one objective, that is, to improve the health of children by stimulating interest in pediatrics.

Fig. 21.10. The American Dental Association, like many professional health associations, sponsors educational programs on health issues, such as the use of fluoride on the teeth and in public drinking water.

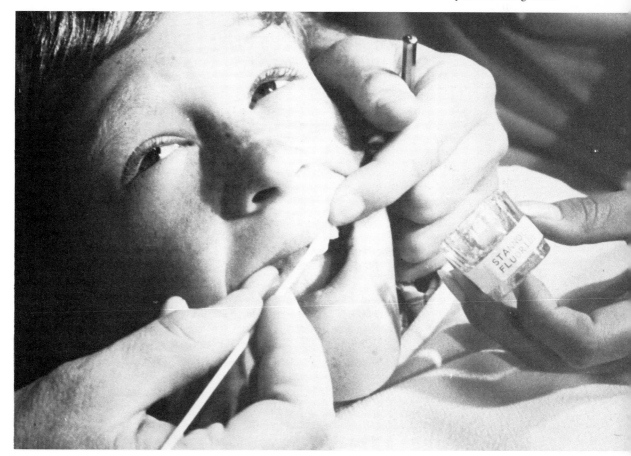

Table 21.3   Some Professional Health Organizations

American Association of Pediatrics
American Dental Association
American Hospital Association
American Medical Association
American Nurses Association
American Public Health Association
American School Health Association

This objective, though narrow in scope, is met by a number of activities identified as follows:[3]

1. Stimulation of interest in pediatrics among premedical and medical students
2. Improvement of pediatric health services
3. Increase in the number of child health facilities
4. Reduction of the infant mortality rate
5. Promotion of immunization programs for children
6. Improvement of school health services

The professional health associations have played a major role at times in influencing national health care policies and programming. The American Medical Association traditionally has stood in opposition to major efforts to bring about national health care programs. On the other hand, in Canada, the Canadian Medical Association and the Canadian Hospital Association have played an important role in gaining acceptance of the national hospital and medical insurance programs among the various health professionals.

To identify all professional health organizations would be beyond the scope and space of this section. However, table 21.3 lists several of the better-known associations in the United States.

Summary

Within North American society there are various organizations, programs, and projects designed to help meet health needs. These community health activities usually fall within the scope of a number of different program directions. They may be funded by tax monies (official health organizations), by voluntary contributions (voluntary health organizations), or they may be professional in nature.

Unless you personally cannot cope with your own health problems for individual or financial reasons, it is altogether possible that you never have had direct contact with the programs of community health organizations. Yet, as we live in the community, we cannot escape the activities and programs of community health. This certainly will be more true in future years as we see a broadening of governmental involvement in the health fields.

Sanitation and disease control have always been a focus of community health activities; this focus will increase as we attempt to cope with the health care and environmental concerns of our present time.

1. List as many community health and health-related agencies and programs as you can think of. What benefits have you received as a result of their work?
2. Differentiate between official, voluntary, and professional health agencies and associations. List a few specific names of agencies or associations in each category.
3. What are the functions of HEW in the United States?
4. How are voluntary health organizations funded?
5. What is WHO? How has it attempted to help nations solve their health concerns?
6. What contributions do professional health associations make to the overall health of a community?
7. What priorities should medical research be given in the United States? Are we doing enough in the medical research field today?

Readings

Hanlon, John J. *Principles of Public Health Administration*. St. Louis: C. V. Mosby Co., 1974.
National Institutes of Health. *1972 Annual Report*. Bethesda, Md.: The Institutes, 1972.
Wilner, Daniel M.; Walkley, Price Rosabelle; and Goerke, Lenore S. *Introduction to Public Health*. New York: Macmillan Co., 1973.

Notes

1. National Commission on Community Health Services, *Health Is A Community Affair* (Cambridge, Mass.: Harvard University Press, 1967), p. 4.
2. *The Nation's Health*, October 1974, pp. 3–10.
3. American Academy of Pediatrics, *An Introduction to the American Academy of Pediatrics* (Evanston, Ill.: The Academy, 1967).

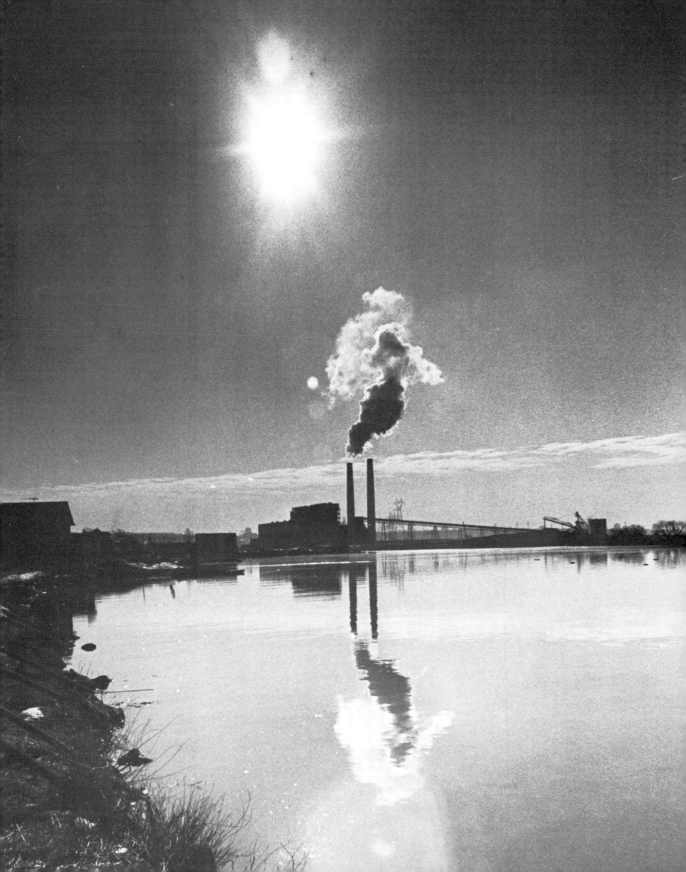

Environmental Health: Air and Water

22

Before the 1960s a college student studying health would have expressed little interest in environmental conditions as they pertained to his or her personal health. By the middle and latter part of that decade, extensive interest had developed in the problems of a deteriorating environment. Concern was expressed by thousands of college students about the damage done to man as the result of polluting the environment. This booming concern reached its zenith in 1970 with what became known as Earth Day. On a day in April, programs, speeches, marches, and numerous other activities took place throughout North America as an indication of the concern over deteriorating environmental conditions in our world.

For some, this increased public awareness of the problems of environmental quality in our world was a passing fad. It provided many with an opportunity to express opposition to the Establishment. For others it created a greater awareness of the problems we are faced with as we attempt to adapt to the increasing amount of pollution in so much of the environment about us.

There are many definitions of pollution. We would like to suggest a definition not very profound or professional, but yet quite accurate. In talking about pollution at dinner one evening, the author's four-year-old son was asked what pollution was, because he had been using the word during the conversation. The child's response was, "That is when you litter things up." In a very succinct way that is what the environmental crisis is all about. Through the centuries there has been an ever-growing amount of litter put into the natural state of our environment. Whether in the air, in the water, or on the land, the litter all too often has a detrimental effect on the health and well-being of the inhabitants of our globe.

Just as there appeared to be some initial positive actions taken for better environmental conditions, a new concern developed in the latter part of 1973. Throughout the industrialized, Western nations of the world a shortage of oil for energy purposes became apparent. The catalyst for this crisis was the action taken by the Arab nations of the Middle East in stopping the flow of oil to Western nations. This action was principally in response to these nations' political support of Israel.

Because of the shortage of oil, it became necessary to begin to search for other means of energy production. In a matter of several months in 1973 and 1974, many actions were taken by government and industry counter to measures that would protect our environment. Industries were encouraged to transfer from oil or high-grade coal to lower-grade coal as a source of energy. This meant an increase in air pollution resulting from the burning of lower-grade fossil fuels. The building of a pipeline from the northern slopes of Alaska, held up for some time because of the concern over its potential damaging effects to the environment, was approved in a matter of days by the United States Congress in response to the energy crisis. The first oil began to flow through the completed pipeline during the summer of 1977. To improve gas mileage on automobiles, many felt that pollution control devices required by law should be removed. As new demands for energy increase, the role of nuclear power, with all of its accompanying problems related to the environment, will become more important.

As you read this chapter, no doubt your daily newspaper carries the current dialogue between the concern for the environment on one hand and the problems of energy conservation on the other. We can only surmise as to what effects the problems related to the shortage of energy will have on environmental conditions. For this reason, it would seem all the more important, as we examine the various environmental problems and their relationship to our personal health, to consider what adaptations mankind must perform in the years ahead.

Another stumbling block to the control of worldwide environmental problems is opposition by some of the Third World developing nations. These nations, who are just now beginning to enter the industrial age, see the environmental movement with its emphasis on control of pollution as economically antidevelopmental for them. They suggest that it is an attempt by the industrialized nations, principally white European and North American, to prohibit and inhibit growth by other newer nations, normally nonwhite Asian and African nations. Whereas the present industrial nations had no opposition to their growth, and in fact such development was encouraged, now the newly developing or Third World nations feel that the "haves" are using the issue of environmental control to prevent their economic development.

Not only are environmental concerns political and social in nature throughout the worldwide community, but the environment in which we live is at all times affecting the total well-being of the individual. We must understand how it does so. Dangers to the health of mankind must be examined.

As early as 1962 Rachel Carson directed the attention of some to the danger of pesticides in our environment.[1] Many have considered her work to be a classic; others felt she was simply an alarmist. Nevertheless, she did create an atmosphere of concern that since the writing of the book has been shown to be accurate. Other well-known writers who have focused attention on environmental factors include Paul Ehrlich,[2] Barry Commoner,[3] and René Dubos.[4]

Our examination of the environmental crisis will not be from a technological or philosophical perspective, but from an individual outlook. We need to know how various pollutants affect our health and then to consider what action we can take to help resolve the environmental problems of our day. As a person studies the problems of the environment and their effects upon the health of people, one should be moved to some kind of action, either individual or corporate. This action must be positive in nature. Let us not get mired in the politics of assessing blame for our present state of being, but let us examine positive and creative avenues of corrective behavior.

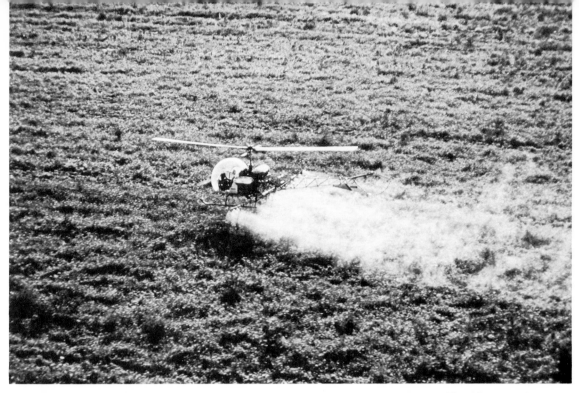

Some have suggested that with continued exposure to various pollutants man will in time adapt and become resistant to the detrimental conditions associated with such exposure. However, Dubos feels that there is no basis for such hope.[5] He points out that what really occurs "is not true adaptation but a form of tolerance achieved at the cost of functional impairment."

In discussing the need for action to help improve the environmental situation of our day, Dubos directs our attention to the latter part of the past century. During that period of time, environmental reforms were necessary to help stem the tide of cholera outbreaks throughout Europe and America. Seriously needed reforms of that day took three approaches:

1. Enlightened and dedicated laymen organized campaigns for cleaning up the urban mess and for providing the multitude with pure air, pure water, and pure food.
2. Public health officers organized boards of health and enforced a number of sanitary regulations, often against public resistance.
3. Scientists organized new research institutes to study the problems of microbial pollution that were characteristic of the period.

Dubos feels that such approaches can serve as a pattern for action with relation to the environmental problems of our day. We may well need a dedicated and enlightened lay citizenship to bring about the needed changes. It is in this spirit that we examine some of the environmental concerns in the world as we enter the 1980s.

Fig. 22.1. Aerial crop-dusting is one potential source of air pollution. Scientists still do not know what long-term effects many chemicals will have on the environment.

Air Pollution   Without oxygen no life can exist in the universe. This fact emphasizes the importance of having available a clean, healthful supply of air.

Normal air about us consists of nitrogen, oxygen, carbon dioxide, and several other lesser-known gases. Approximately 21 percent of the air we breathe is oxygen that is necessary for the maintenance of life. But our air supply is limited. It must be reused, and nature provides ways to replenish the air by the process of exhalation.

Wind and rainfall play an important role in cleaning the air. Man with his industries, automobiles, and many other methods for overloading the air with polluted gases and solid matter has made it almost impossible in many localities to find healthy air to breathe. This creates problems related to health, because we must breathe whatever air is available. It is impossible to reject the air about us for another source.

From the beginning of recorded history, man has dumped pollutants into the atmosphere. However, it has only been in the past twenty years or so that serious concern has been expressed regarding the deteriorating quality of the air we breathe and its effect upon the well-being of people. It is the continuing, everyday exposure to increasing levels of pollutants with which we must be concerned. While the human organism can adapt to subtle and ongoing changes in the quality of the air that is breathed, it cannot function optimally with continual exposure to polluted air.

The catastrophic episodes involving air pollution have been well documented. At various times in history serious occurrences have taken place that brought illness, discomfort, and even death to citizens living in the geographic regions involved. Most serious has been the blanketing of areas with heavy air pollution, most often the result of unusual meteorologic conditions. Such an episode took place in December 1973 in the Meuse River Valley in Belgium. Some sixty deaths were recorded, and over 6,000 people became seriously ill. Those who died or became ill were older individuals, most of whom already had lung or heart disorders.

A classic situation involving serious air pollution took place in 1948 in Donora, Pennsylvania. In October of that year almost half of the people of the region had some type of eye, nose, or throat irritation. Headache, nausea, cough, and breathing difficulties were very common during the period of extreme air contamination. Twenty people died as the direct result of the situation.

London had such an episode in 1952, when nearly 4,000 people died. In 1956 London experienced a similar problem resulting in the deaths of some 1,000 individuals.

A number of conclusions have been reached from analyzing the physical effects of these major catastrophic occurrences of air pollution. The National Tuberculosis and Respiratory Disease Association (now known as the American Lung Association) has suggested that the following generalizations can be made:

1. The effects of the incidents were anatomically localized and limited to the respiratory tract.

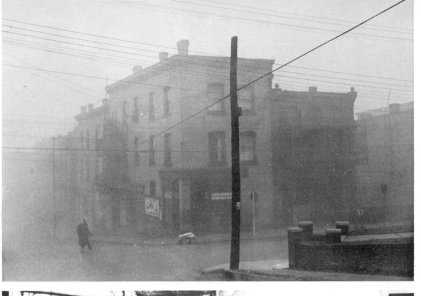

Fig. 22.2. Even the streetlights of the main business street in Donora were obliterated by the daylight ''death smog.''

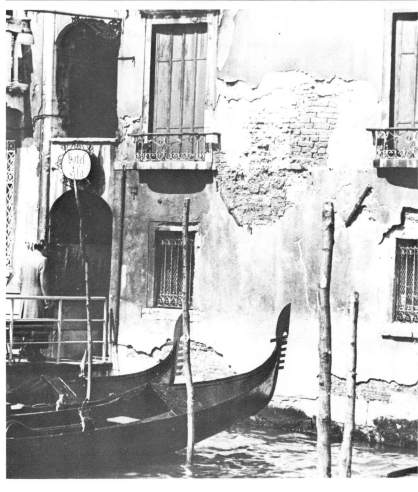

Fig. 22.3. Air pollution is a world-wide problem. This crumbling wall in Venice, Italy, (left) is being gradually eaten away by acid fumes. A bicyclist (below) in downtown Washington, D.C., wears a mask for protection against smog.

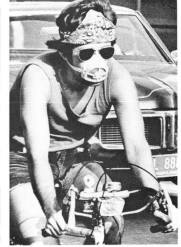

2. The people most vulnerable were the elderly and those with preexisting disease of the cardiorespiratory system.
3. Meteorological conditions were an important factor.
4. Not one but two or more interacting pollutants were responsible.[6]

Temperature
Inversion

The meteorological conditions that were present in all of these cases and have been repeated in similar, less well-documented instances should be understood. Each of the catastrophic situations took place during the winter season, when power generating plants and home heating units were usually working at their maximum. Winds were nonexistent; hence any dispersion of pollutants was negligible. A high-pressure system created an inversion layer over the entire region. As a result, cooler air became trapped under the warmer layer of air. This layer became heavily polluted with particulate matter and other pollutants. Such occurrences are known as "temperature inversions."

Under normal conditions the temperature of air becomes cooler as it rises. For every 1,000 feet in altitude the temperature of air averages 3.5° F or 2° C cooler. When warm air from near the surface of the earth is pushed upward or a warm layer of air moves over a specific area, we find inversion. A layer of warm air above traps the cooler air beneath. Since the meteorological conditions causing the temperature inversion cannot be altered, it becomes obvious why control of air pollution in these situations is so important.

Fig. 22.4. During a *temperature inversion*, particulate matter is trapped by a layer of warm air above cooler air. Polluted air cannot escape and serious pollution often results. (Below) Denver is shown under such an inversion.

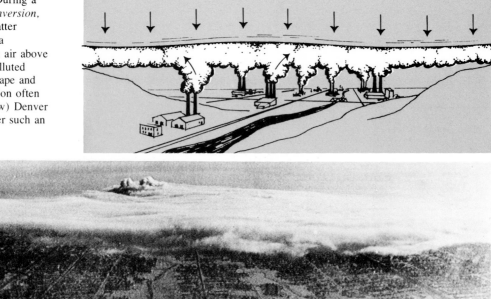

The inversion condition will remain until the warm layer of air moves out of the area. Air movement is a necessity to return conditions to normal.

Temperature inversion is particularly prevalent and likely to occur in mountainous regions. Where an industrial city is located in a valley with surrounding mountains, the terrain helps to trap the polluted air beneath the warmer layer of air, as shown in figure 22.4. Until the warmer layer moves beyond the valley, serious problems may result.

Numerous pollutants are in the air at all times. They have varying degrees of effect on people. Some have little or no effect; others are more detrimental to plants, leaves, flowers, and vegetation than to man and animals. Material and metals are sometimes damaged, marred, and even destroyed by certain pollutants.

Principal Air Pollutants

The principal air pollutants in the world today are: (1) carbon monoxide, (2) sulfur oxides, (3) nitrogen oxides, (4) hydrocarbons, (5) photochemical oxidants, particularly ozone, and (6) particulate matter. For each of these pollutants the United States Environmental Protection Agency (EPA) has established air quality standards in an effort to improve the quality of the air throughout the North American hemisphere.

The major source of air pollution results from combustion of fossil fuels. Natural gas, coal, and the various petroleum products are the fossil fuels that produce most of the air quality problems.

Carbon Monoxide   Carbon monoxide (CO) is an odorless, colorless, tasteless, and poisonous gas that is the result of incomplete combustion of organic materials. Approximately half of all air pollutant emissions are carbon monoxide, with the internal combustion engine of the automobile the principal source. Figure 22.5 shows the various sources of carbon monoxide and indicates what percent of the carbon monoxide in the air is emitted by each.

Carbon monoxide is absorbed in the lungs and enters the red blood cells. Because of hemoglobin affinity for carbon monoxide, the normal oxygen supply is replaced by the gas. Extremely large amounts of carbon monoxide will result in a lack of oxygen supply to the various body cells, particularly the brain. With failure to receive the vitally needed oxygen, suffocation and death result.

Exposure to smaller amounts of carbon monoxide over extended periods of time has often not been of particular concern to many people. However, there is definite indication that long-term exposure may reduce one's physical and mental effectiveness.

Specific concern is expressed for those with respiratory and circulatory problems. For example, continued exposure to carbon monoxide may be a serious problem for the individual with a heart condition. Because the body cells need oxygen and carbon monoxide infiltrates the blood's hemoglobin, it is necessary for the heart to work harder to supply the oxygen. As a result, further potential damage is done to an already weakened heart.

There is little doubt that a person driving in busy traffic is exposed to many times more carbon monoxide than would be considered normal. The effect that

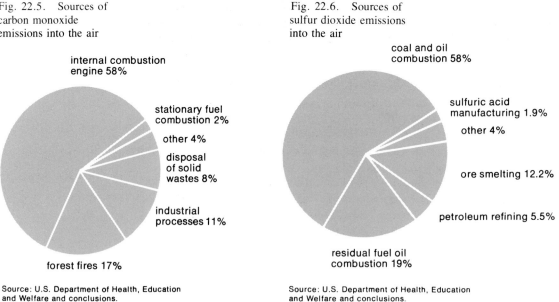

Fig. 22.5. Sources of carbon monoxide emissions into the air

internal combustion engine 58%

stationary fuel combustion 2%

other 4%

disposal of solid wastes 8%

industrial processes 11%

forest fires 17%

Source: U.S. Department of Health, Education and Welfare and conclusions.

Fig. 22.6. Sources of sulfur dioxide emissions into the air

coal and oil combustion 58%

sulfuric acid manufacturing 1.9%

other 4%

ore smelting 12.2%

petroleum refining 5.5%

residual fuel oil combustion 19%

Source: U.S. Department of Health, Education and Welfare and conclusions.

such exposure has on one's mental performance is of some concern. Laboratory studies show that people may get headaches or may become dizzy or show other signs of illness upon exposure to 100 ppm (parts per million) of carbon monoxide.[7] In heavy traffic in many urban areas, this concentration of carbon monoxide is often observed. Impairment of vision and judgment have been observed when people are exposed to low levels of the gas. In Montreal levels that could cause eye, ear, and brain damage in certain individuals were found to exist at times.[8]

Harmful effects of carbon monoxide may be multiplied in areas of higher altitude. In Denver it was noted that the "levels [of carbon monoxide] in nonsmokers exceeded the maximum allowable levels set by the Environmental Protection Agency. Smokers had levels almost four times the permitted maximum." This research suggested that "we should be concerned about the possible harmful interactions between carbon monoxide and low oxygen levels."[9]

Sulfur Oxides   Sulfur oxides are another common pollutant in the air. They are the result, for the most part, of the combustion of fuels containing sulfur. For example, coal when burned releases sulfur. This sulfur when combined with oxygen in the air forms sulfur dioxide. In addition to coal, the burning of residual oil, paper, rubber tires, and other solid wastes adds sulfur dioxide to the atmosphere. Sulfur dioxide is a heavy, colorless gas that is partly converted to sulfur trioxide in the atmosphere. In the presence of water vapor or moisture, sulfur trioxide is converted to sulfuric acid, which has been shown to destroy vegetation and to corrode stone and metal.

Most sulfur dioxide emission is caused by the combustion of coal, particularly in electric power generation and in home and industrial heating processes. Figure 22.6 shows the sources of sulfur dioxide contributions to air pollution.

The major effect of the various sulfur oxides upon the health of people is irritation of the respiratory system. Some airway constriction is caused by exposure to these gases. Both laboratory and epidemiological studies have suggested there are detrimental effects of sulfur dioxide on humans when accompanied by particulate matter.

As coal becomes increasingly important again as a source of energy, it is vital that measures be taken to reduce as much as possible the amount of sulfur oxides released into the air during combustion. The technology to burn coal in a clean manner is available. There must be a willingness to insist that this technology be used.

Nitrogen Oxides Approximately 78 percent of the air we breathe contains a gas known as nitrogen. This is a colorless, odorless, and tasteless gas. Two oxides of nitrogen are considered to be pollutants. These are nitric oxide and nitrogen dioxide. The oxides of nitrogen are the product of high-temperature combustion of several sources of energy: coal, oil, and gasoline.

The automobile is the major source of nitric oxide. Nitric oxide in the atmosphere is converted to nitrogen dioxide. This gas is yellow-brown in color. For this reason it has a detrimental effect on visibility.

Nitrogen dioxide in combination with water vapor in the air produces nitric acid, which can corrode metal surfaces and damage vegetation.

The initial problems associated with exposure to nitrogen oxides for humans are irritation of the eyes and the respiratory passages. Longer exposure results in damage to the respiratory tract and accompanying lung disease. For the individual who smokes, there is an additional consideration in light of the fact that the smoke from cigarettes contains several hundred ppm of nitrogen dioxide. When this is combined with oxides of nitrogen in the atmosphere, the problems for health are magnified.

Hydrocarbons Hydrocarbons are compounds containing carbon and hydrogen. The most commonly found hydrocarbons in air pollution monitoring are methane, benzene, toluene, propane, and ethylene. The sources of hydrocarbon emissions can be seen in figure 22.7.

No direct effects on the health of human beings from exposure to hydrocarbons have been identified. However, they are a major factor, along with the nitrogen oxides, in the formation of smog found in areas such as Los Angeles.

Photochemical Oxidants Photochemical oxidants are the result of a series of chemical reactions in the atmosphere that are initiated by the natural rays of the sun. Two chemical compounds are specifically of concern as they relate to air pollution. These are ozone and peroxyacyl nitrates (PAN).

These compounds are the result of the interaction between hydrocarbons, nitrogen oxides, and the ultraviolet from sunlight. Hydrocarbons and nitrogen oxide compounds are broken up, and oxygen atoms are released. These oxygen atoms join other oxygen atoms already in the atmosphere to form ozone, a very unstable gas. It is formed in the atmosphere naturally by electrical discharge

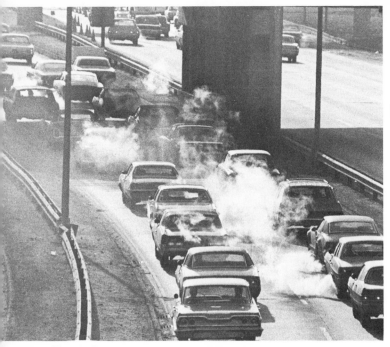

transportation 52%

solid waste disposal 5%

fuel combustion 2%

industrial
processes 14%

organic solvent
evaporation 27%

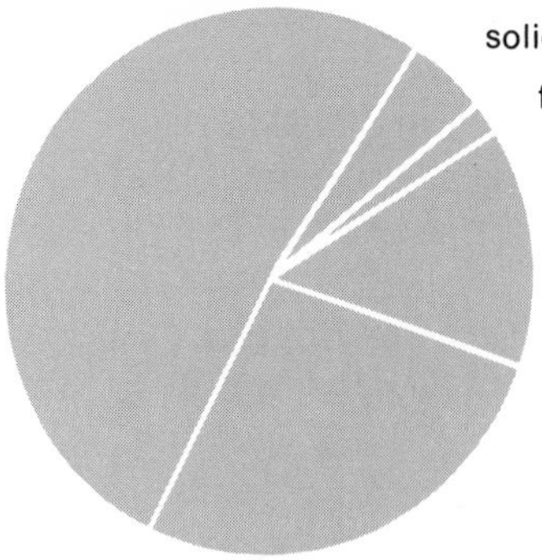

Source: U.S. Department of Health, Education
and Welfare and conclusions.

Fig. 22.8. Sources of
hydrocarbon emissions
into the air

Fig. 22.7. It is easy to
see why automobiles are
the major source of air
pollutants.

(lightning), and in the stratosphere it is formed by solar radiation. Ozone is an
irritant to the lungs, eyes, and throat. Headache, cough, shortness of breath, and
airway resistance are symptoms that often accompany its presence in the air.

It has been observed that ozone does damage to plants. In animals it has been
known to cause a thickening of the bronchiolar walls. Another concern regarding
ozone is that it causes rubber to crack and to decompose.

Peroxyacyl nitrates may well be the main cause of eye irritation caused by
photochemical smog. Eyes have a tendency to burn and tear in the presence of
PAN. It also has been shown that this gas produces damage to plants and to
vegetation.

Particulate Matter Not all air pollutants are necessarily gases. Many airborne
particles are a part of the pollution of the air. Any matter in the air, either solid or
liquid, is referred to as particulate matter. Soot, dirt particles, dust, and fly ash
are found abundantly in the air. Any person who has lived in a large industrial
city knows what it is like to leave the window open at night and awaken in the
morning with the windowsill covered with the results of particulate matter in the
air. Though suspended particles in the air may not be toxic in nature, they certainly are detrimental to a clean air environment.

Other particulate substances present in the air have toxic effects upon people
when certain elevated levels are reached. Fluorides, lead, asbestos, and beryl-
lium are examples of such toxic particulate substances.

The real danger in particulate matter is the damage done to the surfaces of the
respiratory system. Very great concern should be expressed as to how extensive

chronic respiratory conditions are affected by prolonged exposure to increased levels of particulate matter. Exposure to particulate matter results in respiratory damage, especially to the cilia. The cilia are important in protecting the respiratory system from pathogenic microorganisms and dirt. When damaged or destroyed, they no longer function properly, and the underlying cells of the respiratory system structures are vulnerable to damage.

In 1963 the United States Congress passed a Clean Air Act. Since the passage of this Act, other federal legislation has been passed that is designed to strengthen the programs of air quality control. On December 31, 1970, the Clean Air Act was amended. This legislation broadened earlier control programs. Under the law the state and local governments had primary responsibility to control air pollution. However, the responsibilities for approving and enforcing standards at the federal level of government were strengthened. Through the Environmental Protection Agency (EPA) several regulations for enforcement were developed.

Legal Efforts
to Control
Air Pollution

It was the responsibility of the EPA to establish national air quality standards. Each state was to develop and adopt implementation plans for its particular regions. The state standards were not developed until public hearings had been held. After holding public meetings, each state submitted a plan for approval to the EPA that was to show how the national standards would be achieved by the mid-1970s.

The national standards consisted of two parts: *primary standards* and *secondary standards*. The primary standards were designed to set limits that were considered to be safe for the health and well-being of people. The secondary standards established limits that would be considered safe for vegetation, material, and crops.

The Clean Air Act of 1970 created the mechanism for enforcing clean air standards. If for some reason, particularly one related to adverse weather control, a pollution emergency occurs in a given locality, the EPA may take whatever action is necessary to shut down the sources of pollution in the area. Such action is to take place when it is felt that air conditions are in fact harmful to the health of people in the region. The first such emergency occurred in November 1971 in Birmingham, Alabama.

Other mechanisms are available in the Act for forcing compliance with state implementation plans, for hazardous emission standard violations, and for violations of new-source performance standards. New-source performance standards were established in an effort to control pollution from new buildings, factories, and production plants.

The Clean Air Act of 1970 contained several requirements directed at reducing the amount of pollutants from motor vehicles. Over half of the pollutant matter that enters the air comes from motor vehicles; this is basically the result of the internal-combustion engine. The standards established in this Act required a 90 percent reduction in carbon monoxide, hydrocarbon, and nitrogen oxide emissions by the mid-1970s from levels recorded in 1970.

However, there has been an increasing effort to reduce or postpone implementation of these standards. The automotive industry claims it is impossible to meet the car production standards until well into the 1980s. Deadlines have come and gone with new dates set when the standards must be met.

In 1977 the automotive industry threatened to discontinue production of its 1978 models until the required standards were revised. They said that it would be necessary to shut down their manufacturing assembly lines and put many people out of work. The industry claimed it was not possible to meet the clean air standards for 1978 automobiles.

As a result the United States Congress agreed to postpone the implementation of these standards until 1980. If past performance is any indication, the same scenario will no doubt be replayed in 1980. The increasing need to produce fuel-efficient automobiles and inflationary costs in recent years have both worked in a negative way to bring about national clean air compliance.

Temperature Change

There are scientists in the world who feel that serious problems will arise as a subtle, but continuing rise in global temperatures occurs. This is the result of an increased concentration of carbon dioxide in the atmosphere, retarding normal heat loss from the earth. This has been referred to as the "greenhouse effect."

Under normal conditions the light rays from the sun strike the surface of the earth as ultraviolet radiation. These shortwave radiations are reflected back as longer wavelength infrared radiation (or heat) energy. But in the presence of carbon dioxide, the heat energy radiation is absorbed and not reflected off into the stratosphere. With an increase in carbon dioxide in the air, it is felt that there will be greater absorption of long-wave radiation (or heat). As a result, the average temperature of earth may well rise several degrees. This could create serious problems, in that polar ice caps will melt with a rise of only a few degrees in earth's temperature. Extensive, widespread flooding in many regions of the world would be catastrophic.

Fig. 22.9. Which do you feel is more likely to occur? (Left) A cooling trend in the world ("Ice Age" development) or (right) a warming trend in the world ("greenhouse effect")?

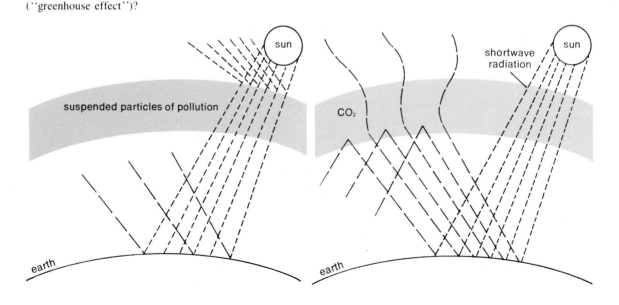

The opposite effect has been hypothesized by many concerned about the effects of an increase in particulate matter and other pollutants in the atmosphere. Those holding to this opposite view suggest a cooling effect on earth's temperature. The rays from the sun strike the various suspended particles in the atmosphere and are partially reflected back into space without ever arriving on the earth's surface and changing into heat energy. The effect might well be a significant drop in temperature. Certainly, with increasing disposal of debris into the air, earth temperature could be lowered, creating the potential for a new Ice Age.

Both possible situations are shown in figure 22.9. The potential for damage to the well-being of mankind is awesome in either case. The human body might well adapt to many subtle changes relating to air pollution, but when potential for catastrophic changes in the earth's structures is present, the problems for people become quite obvious.

Where would you go to find a clear, sparkling, cool, nonpolluted stream? It is altogether possible that for some the location of such a body of water may be beyond the bounds of one's immediate geographic locality. Each passing year, with a few exceptions, pollution of our waters increases. For many the enjoyment of being able to drink from a cool stream or river or the opportunity to swim in a clear body of water is no longer a possibility.

Water Pollution

Water is an indispensable resource for mankind. Not only is it the habitat of aquatic life, but it is an essential resource in the maintenance of all life. The human body consists of approximately 60 percent water, and substantial loss of this water results in dehydration. Dehydration may result in serious physical effects and may even produce death. The importance of water is further understood when it is realized that phytoplankton (minute aquatic life) is responsible for the generation of 70 percent of our world's oxygen supply.[10]

For far too long the supply of good water has been taken for granted. The daily use of water per person averages 125 gallons. Some estimate that by the year 2000 this per capita daily use will be between 300 and 350 gallons.[11] The average water intake of the American adult is one and one half to five quarts a day. We use water, giving little consideration to its quality unless it looks dirty, is odorous, or does not have a satisfactory taste.

Five main factors are responsible for the problems of increased water pollution: (1) population growth, (2) urbanization and suburbanization, (3) industrial expansion, (4) higher individual incomes and expectations, and (5) new and increased use of technology.[12]

Water pollution involves the adding of undesirable foreign matter, either living or nonliving, to the water. These foreign substances cause a deterioration of the quality of the water so that in time it may not be suitable for drinking or for other uses.

A flowing body of water, such as a stream or a river, has a natural ability to purify itself. The process of water movement plays some role in this purification process. In addition, microscopic plants, bacteria, algae, and other plants and animals contribute to the breakdown and consumption of foreign matter. However, streams and rivers become overloaded as man dumps his wastes into them. Natural plant and animal sources are destroyed, further contributing to the deterioration of the water quality.

A nonflowing body of water, such as a lake, does not purify itself as does a stream or a river. In lakes there is a natural, continual aging process. This aging process may take thousands of years; it is nature's way for lakes to purify themselves. When this process is accelerated, it is called *eutrophication*. As the result of man-made pollutants being dumped into the water, the life and vitality of the body of water is diminished, and what results is a dying lake or tributary. One of the five Great Lakes bordering the United States and Canada is Lake Erie, where serious changes have occurred in recent years. In the last fifty years as much eutrophication has occurred in Lake Erie as would have taken place naturally in an estimated 15,000 years.[13]

Eutrophication is a process that leads to a lack of oxygen in the water. As a result, forms of life useful to man, such as game fish, cannot survive. Less desirable aquatic life, such as catfish and other scavenger fish, thrive and replace those fish normally found in the body of water.

Algae are aquatic plants that derive energy from photosynthesis. They consume carbon dioxide and release oxygen. Inorganic nutrients, such as nitrogen, sulfur, iron, potassium, and phosphorus, are needed by the algae. As inorganic nutrients become more abundant, the algae grow faster. What results is a surface covering of algae that we know as slime. When the algae die, they serve as food for bacteria in the water. In turn, bacterial decomposition consumes oxygen. This results in a deficit of oxygen and of aquatic life that is able to survive.

Two specific factors set in motion this rapid acceleration of the eutrophication process. One of these factors is an increase of nutrients in the water. The other is the introduction of minerals, particularly nitrogen and phosphorus.

Increase of pollution in the water often results from the addition of plant nutrients. Agricultural fertilizers are examples of such plant nutrients. When they run off as silt into a river or stream, these fertilizers serve as nutrients. Organic matter is decomposed in the water by bacteria, protozoa, and other organisms, a process that utilizes oxygen. As a result, the oxygen is depleted more rapidly than it can be replaced from the atmosphere. Therefore, the quality of the water deteriorates.

Modern detergents have contributed to the process of eutrophication. Detergents are synthetic and contain plant nutrients. Phosphates, added to detergents to soften wash water and clean clothes more satisfactorily, are replenished in the body of water and increase the nourishment of algae, accelerating growth not only of algae but also of other aquatic plants. There have been many attempts to reduce the use of phosphates. A fairly simple process for removing phosphorus at wastewater treatment plants has been developed. This process involves adding chemicals that cause the phosphates to settle out of the wastewater.

Organic wastes are a common cause of water pollution. Most organic wastes result from untreated human and animal wastes.

More than half of the water pollution is the result of industrial wastes. A great variety of waste products are discharged into rivers and streams by industry. Pulp

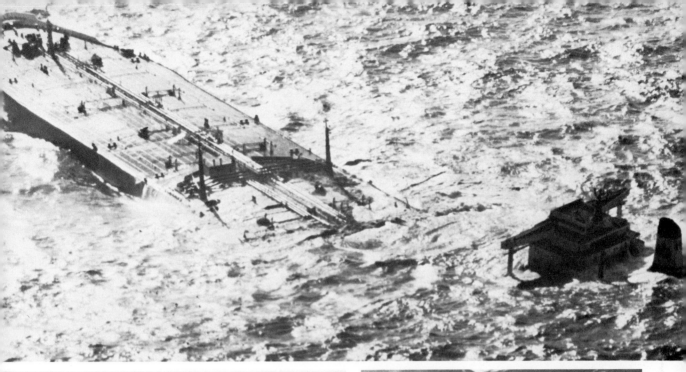

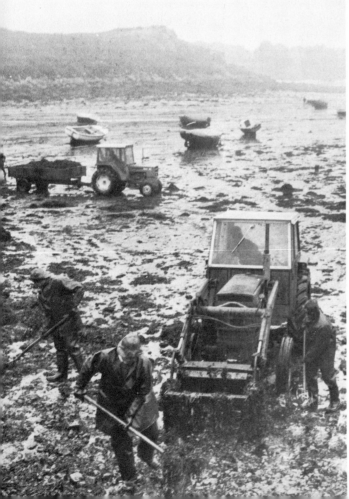

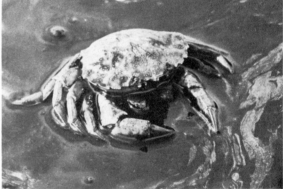

Fig. 22.10. On March 23, 1978, the steering mechanism failed on the Amoco Cadiz, a tanker loaded with 80,000 tons of crude oil. The ship broke in two on the shoals of Portsall, France. French farmers (left) helped soldiers clean up seaweed in the port of Portsall, and sea animals, such as the crab above, died in the polluted waters. As of that day, it was the worst oil spill in history.

and paper mills that break down wood into fibers to make paper are among the major industrial polluters of our rivers. The wastes from this pulping process are usually dumped into local streams and rivers.

Some industrial wastes are toxic. The harmful effects of others are less obvious, but still disturb the quality of the water. Lead and mercury are examples of metals that are poured into the water as the result of industrial processing, which causes health problems for humans.

Mercury   Mercury is a metal that has very serious effects on humans when large amounts accumulate in the body. This metal is found throughout our environment. It is found only in trace concentrations in natural water supplies. The human body has been able to adapt to the mercury found in nature. However, it is the buildup of large concentrations of the metal in the body that is of concern to us.

Unlike other metals, mercury has an extremely low melting point. For this reason it is seen at ordinary temperatures as a liquid. It has been given the name quicksilver because of this characteristic.

Historically, mercury has presented occupational hazards to people coming in contact with its fumes. The best-known of these were the nineteenth-century hat makers in the felt hat industry. Fur pelts were dipped into vats with mercuric nitrate solution, a process that made the animal skins more pliable for shaping. The individuals working with these skins absorbed the mercury compounds through their skin or inhaled the vapor. As the result of such exposure, fatigue, headache, and irritability, accompanied by tremors, difficulty in walking, and mental disability, were commonplace.

Today there are thousands of uses for mercury. In agriculture mercury compounds are used on seeds to protect them against fungus growths during storage. Grain spoilage is reduced by using mercury as a fungicide.

In industry there are numerous uses for mercury. Pulp and paper mills use it very extensively. Mercury is used in these industries to help control microorganisms that tend to damage machinery. Mercury inhibits the growth of bacteria and mildew, and for this reason it is widely used in paint manufacturing. Paints used on boats or on surfaces that will receive a great amount of moisture use mercury. Mercury is also used with certain kinds of floor waxes and furniture polishes and in the production of plastics. Fluorescent la. .ps are activated by mercury vapor. The National Institute of Occupational Safety and Health estimates that at least 150,000 persons in the United States are routinely exposed to mercury in their daily places of employment.

Mercury is used as a component in tooth fillings. Millions of people have fillings that contain a 50 percent mercury amalgam.

Serious concern over the effects of mercury on humans was not expressed until the early part of the 1950s. One of the earlier incidents showing the dangers of mercury occurred in an area in Japan known as Minimata Bay, where numerous fishermen and their families became ill. First, fish were weakened and began to float to the surface. Next, all the cats in the town died. People became easily fatigued and had headaches accompanied by a numbness in the extremities and the mouth. Vision became blurred and constricted. Hearing was affected, and

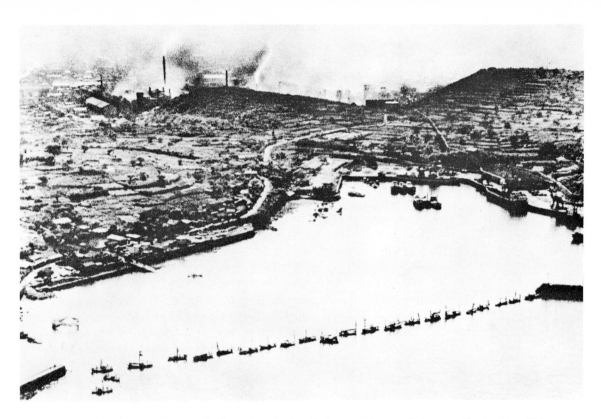

muscular coordination was impaired. Seven hundred and ninety-eight people became ill, and 2,800 more were suspected of having the disease. One hundred and seven people died.

Initially the cause of this illness was not known. Research into the problem indicated damage to the nervous system, particularly to the neurons, the cells of the cerebrum and the cerebellum. In addition to the fatalities that occurred, an abnormally high number of infants were born with congenital defects during this time. Many survivors are mentally and physically as helpless as infants and must be bathed, dressed, and fed.

Further investigation uncovered the cause to be methyl mercury in the fish eaten by the people of this region. Research showed that "metallic mercury and inorganic mercury compounds can be methylated (converted to methyl mercury) by anaerobic bacteria in the mud of lake bottoms."[14] They then enter the food chain and eventually become toxic for humans. For example, the shellfish in the mud became affected; then the fish that lived on shellfish received increased levels of mercury. The effect on the people came about through eating contaminated fish. Autopsies of those who died in the Minimata disaster revealed mercury levels of 13 to 144 ppm in kidney tissues. The mercury content of mud in the bay ranged from 12 to 2,010 ppm.[15]

It was discovered that the mercury had been dumped into the water by a petrochemical company. In 1973 the company was ordered by the court to pay to

Fig. 22.11.   Fishermen tied their boats together in a long line to block the mouth of Umedo Port as they demanded compensation for illness and death caused by mercury pollution of water.

each victim between $60,000 and $68,000, in addition to a monthly allowance of $150. By now the company has paid more than $80 million to victims of the disease.[16]

Other tragedies from mercury poisoning similar to the one at Minimata Bay have been recorded throughout the world. In the mid-1960s a second incident occurred in another area of Japan. In Sweden, Iraq, and Pakistan other problems relating to mercury have been noticed. Recently, high concentrations of mercury were found in the English-Wabigoon River in Ontario.

Possibly the most tragic documented incident in North America of acute mercury poisoning occurred in 1970 in New Mexico. In this situation a man had fed waste grain to his hogs. This grain had been treated with a pesticide that contained methyl mercury. The hogs did not show any signs of illness; however, later research indicated that mercury had concentrated in their bodies. After one hog had been slaughtered and eaten, several children in the family suffered severe nerve damage. One child lost his sight, speech, and muscle control. The mother was pregnant, and the child she was carrying at the time was born blind and retarded.[17]

The Canadian and American fishing industry has been affected by the problems related to mercury. In 1970 a graduate student at the University of Western Ontario showed that fish taken from Lake St. Clair, between Michigan and Ontario, and from Lake Erie contained extremely high levels of mercury. Fish were found to have levels of mercury higher than 0.5 ppm. As a result, restrictions were placed on fishing in Lakes Huron, Erie, and St. Clair. The same has been done in many other parts of the world.

Physiologically, what happens after exposure to high levels of mercury? Inorganic mercury settles in the liver, kidneys, and small intestines. Damage to these organs results in problems of reabsorption and secretion and of diarrhea. General muscular incoordination due to brain damage has occurred.

Organic methyl mercury affects mainly the brain. Those parts of the brain controlling vision, hearing, and balance are particularly affected. Loss of hair, teeth, and fingernails has also been observed.

There are a number of questions about the effect on the human body of exposure to mercury. What is a safe level of exposure? There is a great difference of opinion. The United States government says that 0.5 ppm in seafood is dangerous. On the other hand, many scientists consider 0.2 ppm in human blood to be dangerous. The World Health Organization has warned that more than 0.05 ppm is harmful. It becomes obvious that extensive research into this problem must be performed to learn what level of exposure can be considered to be safe for humans.

Other questions are of concern: How long does mercury remain in the environment? How fast does it dissipate? Does it become more toxic over a period of time? What is the effect of mercury in the bottom of rivers and lakes? Little is known about the life span of mercury in these environmental settings.

Can some effective antidote be found? There is hope that one can be developed in the near future. Treatment at the present time consists basically of withdrawal of the mercury from the body.

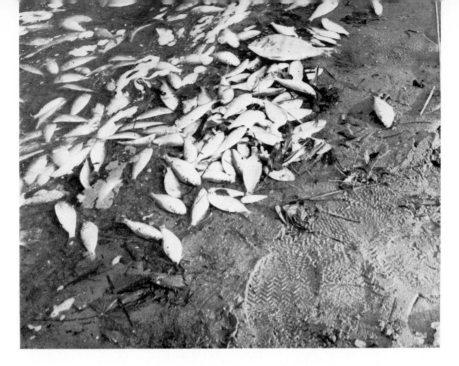

Fig. 22.12. Fish cannot adjust to changes in normal water temperature. Many fish die and eutrophication is hastened when water that is used to cool industrial machinery is returned to its source hotter than it was originally.

Thermal Pollution

Water is used as a coolant of machinery in many industrial settings. Over 80 percent of water used by industry is used for cooling.[18] The water is usually taken from the stream, river, or lake and used to cool heated equipment. When the water is returned to its source, it is warmer than normal, raising the temperature of the principal water supply. Warmer water absorbs less oxygen, which results in a slowing down of the decomposition of organic matter.

The problem of thermal pollution of water is particularly important in power-generating plants. With the development of more nuclear power plants, the problems associated with thermal pollution will no doubt be increased.

Fish cannot adjust to changes in normal water temperature. The life cycle of many fish is closely related to change in water temperature. Some fish, for example, spawn when water temperature drops in the fall; others spawn when temperatures rise in the spring. Imagine the problems for fish that are created by upsets in normal water temperature.

Agriculture

Agriculture makes an extensive contribution to water pollution. The use of inorganic fertilizers in agriculture presents serious problems, as has already been said. Up to one fourth of the fertilizers used are lost in surface runoff before the plants can utilize them. They simply enter the stream or river and may become part of the next town's water supply. Associated with this problem is the matter of siltation from erosion. As the soil is plowed for agricultural purposes, it is exposed to erosion. Erosion, as well as damaging the terrain and removing badly needed soil, removes the nutrients from the eroded areas. We have already discussed the relationship of nutrients to the development and acceleration of the eutrophication process.

Animal wastes present another problem of water pollution. The use of animal feedlots where cattle are brought for the purpose of fattening has created a particularly vexing problem. A feedlot with 10,000 head of cattle produces as much waste as a community of 160,000 people. Runoff from these feedlots produces increasingly serious problems of water pollution.

Municipal
Water Systems

There are 30,000–40,000 municipal water supply systems in the United States. In an effort to understand the quality of water available in community water supplies, the Department of Health, Education, and Welfare conducted a study in 1969–70. This study included an inspection and evaluation of 969 community water supply systems. Several of the findings of this study are rather interesting and somewhat disconcerting as one goes to the drinking fountain for another drink of "nice, clean, healthy water."

1. Eight million people receive impure drinking water from community water systems. A majority of these individuals live in smaller communities.
2. Another estimated 30 million people obtain water from wells and springs.
3. Thirty-six percent of the individual tap-water samples examined in the study contained one or more bacteriologic or chemical constituents that exceeded the limits of the 1962 Federal Drinking Water Standards.
4. Fifty-six percent of the systems had some deficiency of equipment design, construction, or condition of the plant.
5. Seventy-seven percent of the plant operators were not adequately trained in water microbiology.
6. Seventy-nine percent of the systems had not been inspected by local authorities in the calendar year preceding the study.
7. Smaller systems were found to have more deficiencies than the larger ones.
8. Of the twenty-two communities with population greater than 100,000, only 36 percent satisfied surveillance criteria.[19]

What actions can be taken by the individual in a community to insure that the quality of water available to him is not unsafe? The United States Environmental Protection Agency has suggested the following:

1. Know what constitutes good treatment of drinking water and then find out how your water is treated.
2. Know how your water is tested.
3. Insist that the pipes that bring water to your tap be examined and are free from contamination.
4. Check well and spring water on a routine basis.
5. Be familiar with local and state laws governing safe drinking water.
6. Make your concern for safe drinking water known by local, state, and federal authorities.[20]

Water Purification
Systems

With an increasing population in the urban centers of the United States, a major concern of water pollution control involves efforts to reduce pollution from municipal sewage. The Environmental Protection Agency estimates that there are approximately 13,000 municipal sewer systems in the United States. Munic-

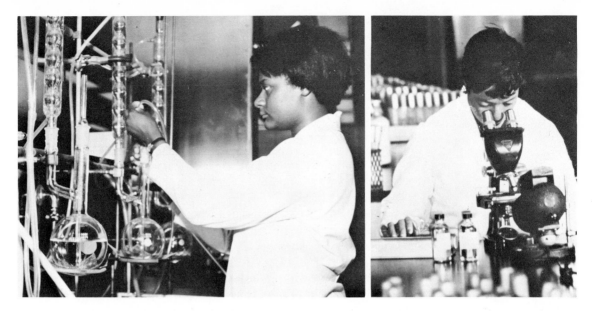

Fig. 22.13. Chicago's water system is world renowned for the research and development work carried on in its laboratories. Water is tested chemically, bacteriologically and microscopically through all phases, from the raw lake water to the consumer's tap. Over 450,000 tests and analyses are performed yearly.

ipal water purification systems should contain both the primary and secondary treatment processes.

Primary sewage treatment is a process of screening and sedimentation. Water is placed in a tank where the large impurities, such as sand, trash, and other suspended solids, will settle. There is also a filtration process that removes large objects as the water passes through a series of screens. About one third of the communities in the United States are served by systems providing only primary treatment of water prior to returning it to the original source. After this the water does not look bad, but it still contains microorganisms and organic nutrients.

The secondary sewage treatment process is important because it is here that microorganisms and organic nutrients are removed. For particles too small to filter, a coagulation process is used. These small particles are made larger through coagulation so that they will settle or can be filtrated.

During this secondary process the water is sprayed over a bed of stones. While it is trickling around the stones, the nutrients are reduced by bacterial action. During this process the water is biologically purified. Aerobic bacteria, air, and sunlight help oxidize and purify the water.

The final step in the secondary process involves disinfection of microorganisms by means of chlorination. This process reduces the bacterial content.

During the latter part of 1974, concern was expressed regarding the possible presence of carcinogenic chemicals in public drinking water. An EPA study of the drinking water in New Orleans revealed small quantities of several dangerous organic chemicals. The cause was felt to be chlorine gas. Chlorine is widely used to disinfect water by killing bacteria. When it is combined with chemicals in the water, a hazardous situation seems to arise. In the New Orleans study, sixty-six organic chemicals were found in the water. The two chemicals that had caused the greatest concern were chloroform and carbon tetrachloride. Both are considered to be possible cancer-causing agents. Further study of the water supply of other large cities is being undertaken to learn more about the relationship of chlorinated water to cancer.

Legislation

The United States Congress passed significant legislation in 1972 to help control water pollution. At that time the Federal Water Pollution Control Act became law. The purpose of this law was to establish a national system of permits aimed at controlling discharges of pollutants by industries, municipalities, and other sources. The implementing of various standards that were designed as a result of this act has been very slow. A half-decade later only six toxic effluent limitations have been established.

The purpose of this federal legislation was to make waterways fishable and swimmable by the year 1983. The intent of this legislation has been to require communities to develop plans that will guarantee clean, unpolluted water in the years ahead. In support of these efforts to improve the nation's water quality, President Carter promised in 1977 to take steps to make water pollution "unprofitable as well as illegal." This is to be accomplished by imposing penalties on industries that fail to meet standards on schedule.

Health Effects

From an esthetic point of view, contamination of a body of water is very degrading. However, it would seem important to understand the effects of water pollution on the health of people. Historically there have been outbreaks of waterborne illnesses, such as typhoid, cholera, dysentery, gastroenteritis, and infectious hepatitis, which result from the action of microorganisms in the water. Treatment of drinking water and improved sewage systems have helped to eliminate many of these diseases. However, they still occur from time to time when proper sanitary procedures are not taken. Because of the fact that we are not accustomed to having these diseases, when they do occur, serious consequences often follow. In 1973 a cholera outbreak occurred in Italy. Near panic struck several regions, and immunization protection against the disease was unavailable to many who requested and wanted it.

Some individuals are able to adapt to the presence of microorganisms in their normal source of water supply. Any North American who has traveled to Mexico knows of the importance of protecting against dysentery. Drinking improperly boiled water can result in a very serious case of diarrhea for the visitor. On the other hand, the citizens of Mexico have adapted to the water condition and do not experience the dysentery. This is the situation for travelers in many of the nations of the world.

There also have been cardiovascular conditions related to the drinking of contaminated waters. Increased sodium intake from polluted waters has been shown to put a strain on the heart. A statistical association between cardiovascular mortality and corrosiveness of water has been noted. The corrosiveness of the water may cause more metals to be ingested.[21]

Sewage and wastes from domestic animals, from land fertilized with agricultural chemicals, and from garbage are common sources of nitrates. Aquatic

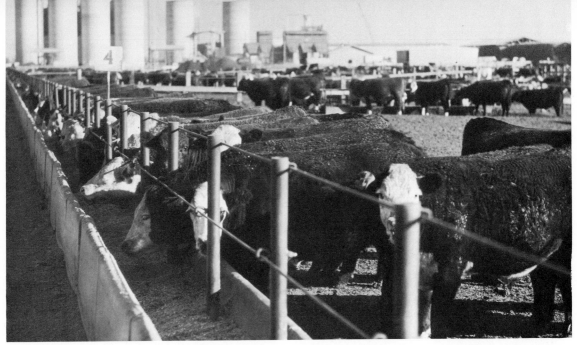

plants take in nitrates almost as soon as they are in the water. There continues to be an increase in nitrates in both surface and ground waters located below the surface of the ground. Wells and springs are common sources of supply of ground waters. When underground sources of water become contaminated, it is a serious problem because purification of such water is almost impossible. The EPA has pointed out the particular danger to newborn babies up to three months of age who receive drinking water contaminated by nitrates. Infants of this age ''suffer the principal risk of damage as a result of drinking water high in nitrates, damage that includes a blood disease that if not treated can result in death.''[22]

In 1977 President Carter instructed the Environmental Protection Agency to develop standards that would control the amount of chlorinated hydrocarbons found in drinking water. The reason for this concern about chlorinated hydrocarbons is due to increasing evidence that they may be carcinogenic.

Much must be done to improve the water quality in our land. The United States federal government has identified several activities that will be important if we are to have better water supplies.

1. Techniques for monitoring viruses in drinking water are needed. This is particularly important in light of the fact that there is a relationship between viruses and the incidence of hepatitis.
2. A clarification of the role of chlorination and other types of disinfection of drinking water to help eliminate viruses is needed.
3. Ways must be developed to protect water supplies from radioactive wastes.
4. Epidemiologic studies of relationships between disease and water quality are needed.
5. Methods for improving water treatment processes must be developed.[23]

Fig. 22.14. Wastes from domestic animals, particularly large numbers of animals confined in small areas such as feedlots, are common sources of nitrates. These nutrients contaminate both surface and ground waters.

Can the quality of our waters be improved? It is very easy to become depressed and begin to wonder if pure water is another depleted resource, never to be regained. This is particularly true when one remembers what happened during the summer of 1969 on the Cuyahoga River near Cleveland, Ohio. The Cuyahoga became so contaminated that fire resulted. The river caught on fire!

Because of the need for water, uncontaminated water, in the life cycle of human beings, it seems absolutely necessary that man make major adaptations in his behavioral patterns toward eliminating wastes that go into our water systems. Major polluted water systems *can* be restored. By the early 1960s the Willamette River in Oregon had become a seriously polluted body of water. It was so contaminated that even scavenger fish could not exist. By implementing legislation and striving for cleanup programs of the river, the people of Oregon have returned this body of water to a very productive state. For example, the waste discharged into the river has been reduced by 90 percent. Water quality now meets state and federal standards; salmon, trout, and other fish have returned; and the water can again be used for water sport activities.[24]

What was done in Oregon and is now being done in many other localities must become the norm as man strives to eliminate the filth and contamination that has despoiled so many of the bodies of water throughout the world.

Summary

Without clean air and an adequate supply of good water, the quality of life of man is seriously jeopardized. Throughout history societies have been concerned about the quality of air and water. Disease and death have been closely allied with despoilment of these resources.

Increase in population, urbanization, industrialization, and other factors have brought an accelerated rate of pollution to our air and water in the mid-1970s. This pollution is not only esthetically disturbing, but also is a danger to our health and well-being.

Legislation of changes in life-style has been attempted to improve air and water quality. These legislative regulations have created problems. To meet them, industry finds that its costs must increase. This in turn contributes to the inflationary costs to consumers. As a result many today are asking whether it is feasible to continue to enforce environmental standards.

You will need to face these issues in the years ahead. Not only is this true of air and water concerns, but also in regard to other environmental issues that have become apparent in the 1970s. These we shall examine in the next chapter.

Review Questions

1. How has the current energy crisis hindered efforts to clean up the environment?
2. What factors are responsible for the condition known as a "temperature inversion"? Where are they most likely to occur?

3. Since we know that the internal combustion engine is the major source of carbon monoxide pollution, what action would you take to reduce this?

4. How would you convince a community of the importance of implementing public or mass transportation?

5. How is photochemical smog formed? What is its major contributor?

6. Give examples of particulate matter. How do some of these pose hazards to the body?

7. How has the government taken steps to protect our air? Have they been effective?

8. What is the "greenhouse effect"? How can particulate matter possibly cause an opposite effect?

9. Describe the process of eutrophication.

10. Why is there a major concern about detergent soaps polluting our waters?

11. What steps can be taken to deal with the problem of water pollution caused by industrial wastes?

12. How does mercury physiologically affect the body? How does it outwardly manifest itself?

13. From where do you receive your water supply? Have you ever been concerned about its purity?

14. Discuss diseases that are associated with unclean drinking water. How many are still a threat to us today?

15. What steps can individual consumers take not only to stop water pollution but also to conserve our water supply?

Readings

Environmental Health (General)

Books and Pamphlets

Boughey, Arthur S. *Man and the Environment*. New York: Macmillan Co., 1971.

DeBell, Garrett. *The Environmental Handbook*. New York: Ballantine Books, 1970.

Environmental Protection Agency. *Action for Environmental Quality*. Washington, D.C.: The Agency, 1973.

———. *Toward a New Environmental Ethic*. Washington, D.C.: The Agency, 1971.

Phillips, John. *Environmental Health*. Dubuque, Iowa: William C. Brown Co., 1971.

The Progressive. The Crisis of Survival. Glenview, Ill.: Scott, Foresman and Co., 1970.

Schaeffer, Francis A. *Pollution and the Death of Man: The Christian View of Ecology*. Wheaton, Ill.: Tyndale House Publishers, 1970.

Waldbott, George L. *Health Effects of Environmental Pollutants*. St. Louis: C. V. Mosby Co., 1973.

Articles

Dubos, René. "Health and Environment." *American Lung Association Bulletin* 59 (1973): 10–12.
Hanlon, John Jr. "Environmental Health—Concerns and Issues." *Archives of Environmental Health* 20 (1970): 72–76.

Air Pollution

Books and Pamphlets

Environmental Health Service. *Air Quality Criteria for Carbon Monoxide.* Washington, D.C.: HEW, 1970.
———. *Air Quality Criteria for Hydrocarbons.* Washington, D.C.: HEW, 1970.
———. *Air Quality Criteria for Particulate Matter.* Washington, D.C.: HEW, 1970.
———. *Air Quality Criteria for Photochemical Oxidants.* Washington, D.C.: HEW, 1970.
———. *Air Quality Criteria for Sulfur Oxides.* Washington, D.C.: HEW, 1970.
Environmental Protection Agency. *Clean Air. It's Up to You, Too.* Washington, D.C.: The Agency, 1973.

Articles

Ahmed, A. Karim, "Unshielding the Sun—Human Effects," *Environment* 17 (April-May 1975): 6–14.
Kerrebijn, K. F., and others, "Study on the Relationship of Air Pollution to Respiratory Disease in Schoolchildren," *Environmental Research* 10 (1975): 14–28.
Hardy, George E.; Pate, Paul; Robison, Charles B.; and Willis, W. T. "First Use of the Federal Clean Air Act's Emergency Authority." *American Journal of Public Health* 64 (1974): 72–76.
League of Women Voters. "Air Pollution." September, 1970, pp. 1–3.
Lillie, Victoria, "Clean Air Act of 1970: Where Do We Stand in 1975?" *Environment Midwest,* June 1975, pp. 3–5.
O'Sullivan, Dermot A. "Air Pollution." *Chemical and Engineering News,* 8 June 1970, pp. 38–46.
Thompson, Donovan J. "Air Pollution, Weather, and the Common Cold." *American Journal of Public Health* 60 (1970): 731–39.
Zapp, John A. "Man, Air, and Environment." *Archives of Environmental Health* 20 (1970): 96–99.

Water Pollution

Books and Pamphlets

Department of Health, Education, and Welfare. *Community Water Supply Study: Analysis of National Survey Findings.* Washington, D.C.: Public Health Service, 1970.

League of Women Voters of the United States, Lake Erie Basin Committee.
Lake Erie: Requiem or Reprieve? Cleveland, Ohio: The League, 1966.

Marx, Wesley. *The Frail Ocean.* New York: Coward-McCann, 1967.

World Health Organization. *Aspects of Water Pollution Control.* Geneva: The
Organization, 1967.

Articles

Chemical and Engineering News. "Mercury Stirs More Pollution Concern."
Chemical and Engineering News, June 1970.

Clark, John R. "Thermal Pollution and Aquatic Life." *Scientific American,*
March 1969, pp. 19–27.

Oesnoyers, Patricia A., and Chang, Louis W., "Ultrastructural Changes in
the Liver After Chronic Exposure to Mercury," *Environmental Research*
10 (1975): 59–75.

Notes

1. Rachel L. Carson, *Silent Spring* (Boston: Houghton Mifflin Co., 1962).
2. Paul R. Ehrlich, *The Population Bomb* (New York: Ballantine Books, 1968).
3. Barry Commoner, *The Closing Circle* (New York: Alfred A. Knopf, 1972).
4. René Dubos, *So Human an Animal* (New York: Charles Scribner's Sons, 1968).
5. René Dubos, "Health and Environment," *American Lung Association Bulletin* 59 (1973): 11.
6. *Air Pollution Primer* (New York: National Tuberculosis and Respiratory Disease Association, 1969), p. 61.
7. Ibid., p. 38.
8. J. W. MacNeill, *Environmental Management,* Constitutional Study Prepared for the Government of Canada (Ottawa, Canada: Information Canada, 1971), p. 145.
9. Cropp, G. J. A. "Effects of Air Pollution on Health," *Journal of Environmental Health* 35 (1973): 556.
10. MacNeill, *Environmental Management,* p. 12.
11. Ibid., p. 100.
12. Jacob I. Bregman, "Man, Water, and Environment," *Archives of Environmental Health* 20 (1970): 100–101.
13. National Geographic Society, *As We Live and Breathe: The Challenge of Our Environment* (Washington, D.C.: The Society, 1971), p. 18.
14. Amos Turk, Jonathan Turk, and Janet T. Wittes, *Ecology, Pollution, Environment* (Philadelphia: W. B. Saunders Co., 1972), pp. 125–26.
15. Richard H. Wagner, *Environment and Man* (New York: W. W. Norton & Co., 1971), p. 248.
16. W. Eugene Smith and Aileen M. Smith, *Minimata: Words and Photographs* (New York: Holt, Rinehart & Winston, 1975).
17. John J. Putman, "Mercury: Man's Deadly Servant," *National Geographic Magazine,* October 1972, p. 518.
18. Wagner, *Environment and Man* (1971), p. 133.
19. Environmental Protection Agency, *A Drop to Drink: A Report on the Quality of Our Drinking Water* (Washington, D.C.: The Agency, 1973), pp. 2–8.
20. Ibid., p. 13.
21. Environmental Protection Agency, *Health Effects of Environmental Pollution* (Washington, D.C.: The Agency, 1973), p. 9.
22. Ibid.
23. Environmental Protection Agency, *A Drop to Drink,* pp. 7–10.
24. Ethel A. Starbird, "A River Restored: Oregon's Willamette," *National Geographic Magazine,* June 1972, pp. 818–34.

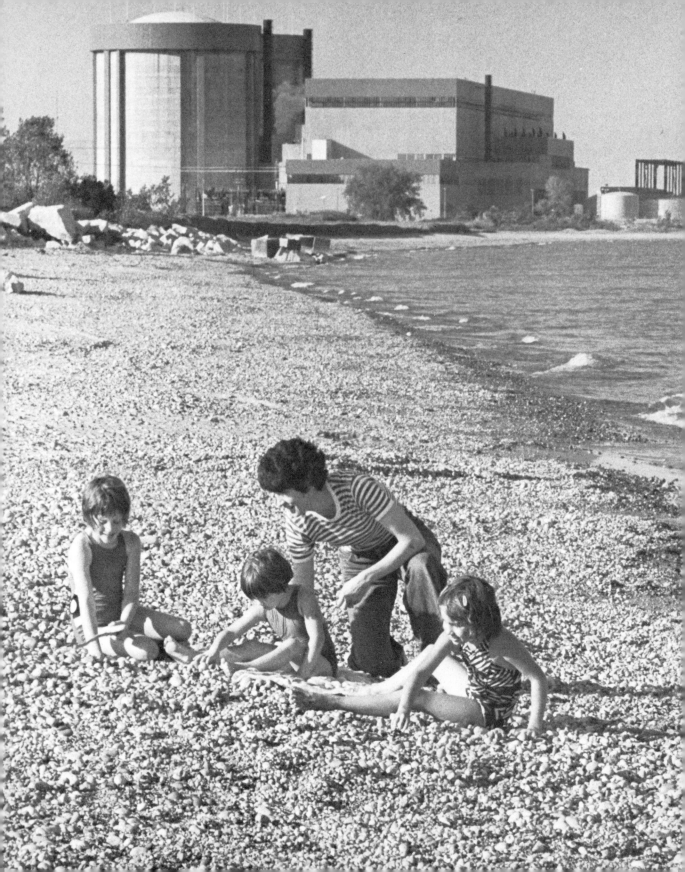

Environment: Continuing Concerns

23

There has always been some pollution of the air and the water. From earliest recorded time mankind has become ill and died as the result of drinking impure water. The industrial revolution brought about conditions that have led to pollution of the air about us.

Today, however, other pollutants pose serious problems in the ecosystem of mankind. Pesticides, fluorocarbon aerosol propellants, and radiation have presented society with new and different problems in the past thirty years, and the continuing increase of solid waste materials makes their disposal a problem. Greater urbanization and industrialization makes the continuing increase of noise of greater concern than ever before.

Each pollution problem discussed in this chapter is no less serious than air or water pollution. All of them require society in the latter 1970s to be prepared to act if conditions are to improve. These problems have created the need for us in North America to examine what we value and feel to be important in our society. Each of us must consider what adaptations need to be made if some order is to come out of continuing increase in environmental pollution.

The average person in our society today has a "throw-away" mentality. That for which we have no need we discard. With the development of disposable, non-returnable containers and the rapid increase in population, solid waste disposal is a mounting environmental problem that may very well affect the health and well-being of all people.

Tremendous amounts of solid wastes are produced each year in North America. As we travel anywhere in this land, we see evidence of this in dumps, junkyards, and trash on the highway. The Environmental Protection Agency (EPA) says that over 4 billion tons of solid wastes are produced annually in the United States. Table 23.1 shows a general breakdown of the total amount of waste material.

Of this total amount of solid waste, 190 million tons are hauled away for disposal. On a per capita basis, 5 to 6 pounds of solid wastes are generated each day in the United States. By 1985 this amount may rise to 8 pounds per person per day.

Problems of solid waste removal have been amplified in recent years by the manufacture and extensive use of disposable containers made of plastics and other materials that do not burn or decay.

Solid Wastes

549

Table 23.1   Solid Wastes Produced in the United States

Source	Tons
Agricultural wastes	2,300,000,000
Mineral wastes	1,700,000,000
Household, municipal, and industrial wastes	360,000,000
Total	4,300,000,000

Source: Environmental Protection Agency data.

Waste Disposal
Procedures

Agricultural wastes, including animal manures and orchard prunings, account for more than half the amount of solid wastes produced each year. One head of cattle, for example, produces as much waste as sixteen people.[1] When one realizes that cattle feedlots may contain 5,000 to 10,000 head of cattle, it becomes clear that a single feedlot may produce as much waste as a city of 160,000 people.

Dumps   Probably the oldest and most traditional method of solid waste disposal is dumping. Waste material is brought to a given location and thrown away. No effort is made to cover the waste, but it is usually burned to reduce the bulk of the waste material. Wind scatters the paper and other light objects, rodents and other scavengers search for food, and mosquitoes and flies reproduce in the open dump. Open dumping has in no way vanished from the American scene. Approximately 82 percent of all collected solid waste is disposed of in unsanitary open dumps.[2]

Dumps are an eyesore in a community. They also may add to other environmental problems such as air pollution because of burning; rodent-related problems, particularly disease; and water contamination. The overall bulk of waste deposit at an open dump is reduced in several ways, however. Burning, either purposeful or spontaneous, almost always occurs in dumps. Organic matter that is not consumed by insects, rodents, and other animals is reduced by decomposition. Many human scavengers visit dumps to pick up useful waste materials left there by others. A friend of this writer is extremely proud, and possibly rightly so, of the fact that most of the furniture, including rugs, in his lake cottage was found in visits to various dumps.

Sanitary Landfill   A much better procedure for the removal of solid wastes is the development of an adequate, well-designed, and well-engineered sanitary landfill. At a properly operated sanitary landfill the waste material is compacted when dumped, after which dirt is placed over it. Usually one part dirt is used to four parts refuse. After the landfill area is covered with dirt each day, the site is compressed and smoothed by large bulldozers.

A major advantage of a sanitary landfill is that the waste is buried each day. Burning and blowing of the material is at a minimum and rodents are few. Land that is of little use otherwise may be reclaimed by being filled and then developed into a park, recreation site, golf course, or housing area.

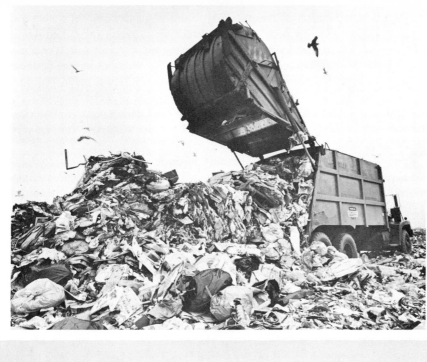

Fig. 23.1. Open dumps are invitations to unwanted birds, rodents, insects, and other animals, yet communities continue to use this form of solid waste disposal.

Fig. 23.2. A properly engineered and operated sanitary landfill is possibly the best means of solid waste removal. Large bulldozers are used to compact the waste and cover it over with dirt each day.

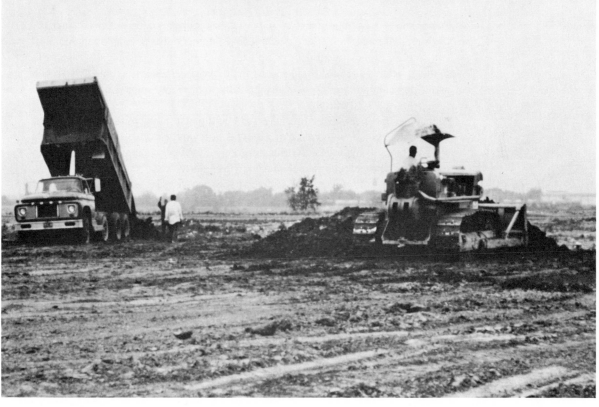

There are numerous problems that may arise if a sanitary landfill is not properly engineered and operated, however. Anaerobic decay of the buried wastes may lead to continual settling of the land for many years. As a result, it becomes rather difficult to use the reclaimed area until the possibility of settling has been minimized. It is also extremely important that the landfill area be well planned and operated to protect against possible contamination of water supplies. The Environmental Protection Agency has said that less than 6 percent of sanitary landfill sites in the United States meet minimum federal standards of engineering, operation, and area management.

Many problems are presented in finding adequate and available land for landfill purposes. Numerous geological considerations are important in site selection. Water-table levels are crucial, since areas with high water-table levels are not satisfactory as landfill locations. Esthetic and political considerations often come into play in finding a suitable location for a landfill. Most people, when informed that a site in their neighborhood has been selected for use as a sanitary landfill, will object vehemently to such development. Who wants to live near a sanitary landfill? If these residents realized that a sanitary landfill is not a dump and in the long-range view may in fact be an asset to their locality, there might not be as much opposition. Nevertheless, landfill site selection often creates heated city council debates and produces many "letters to the editor" before the problem is resolved.

Incineration　The burning of solid wastes has probably been practiced since the beginning of mankind. Today one still finds incinerators operated by municipalities, private homes, apartment complexes, and industries. Incineration is useful in that it destroys solid substances and in the process reduces volume by as much as 80 percent.[3] However, as a result of burning, soot, smoke, and particulate matter are released into the air.

Increasing concern is being expressed about plastics that go through the incineration process.[4] A component of plastic is polyvinyl chloride (PVC), and when PVC is burned, hydrogen chloride is produced. After combining in the air with moisture, hydrogen chloride produces hydrochloric acid.

The process of incineration is somewhat expensive. To serve a community of 100,000 persons it could cost as much as 6 million dollars just to build an adequate incinerator. Operation costs of community incinerators have been found to run as high as $12.12 per ton.[5] This is over twice the cost of using a sanitary landfill. The use of incinerators is not economical in cities with fewer than 55,000 people.[6]

Incineration could be used to generate heat and energy if properly developed. As of now, this process has had rather limited application in the United States. However, numerous European cities use heat and energy generated by incineration. With increased shortages of energy supplies, such as have been experienced during the 1970s, some efforts must be directed toward using incineration of solid wastes to generate steam, which in turn can be used to produce electrical energy.

If incineration is to be an effective means of solid waste removal, municipalities with such plants will have to improve their operations. The EPA

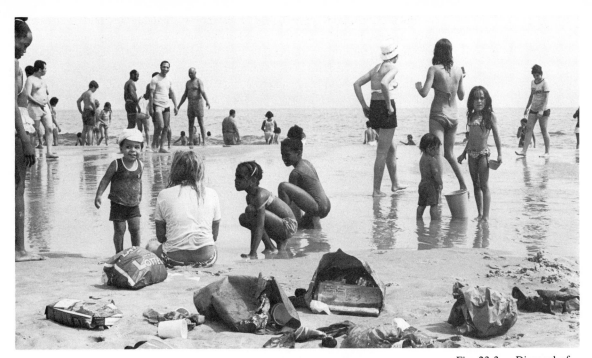

Fig. 23.3. Disposal of trash is everyone's concern in a country where citizens produce nearly 12 million tons of solid wastes a year.

has pointed out that in terms of today's needs and technology most municipal incinerators are obsolete and ineffective.

Composting   Composting as a means of recycling waste material has been used extensively in some European countries. Organic garbage and refuse are aerobically decayed by bacterial decomposition and then used as conditioners of the soil. No unpleasant odors result from this composting process.

Composting has not been particularly popular in the United States because the organic garbage must be separated from paper, glass, cans, and other such trash. Such separation is best done by the individual prior to having the waste material collected, and it is not a part of most people's pattern of living to take the time to separate out organic wastes as is necessary for the composting process to occur.

Recycling   Greater efforts must be made at recycling for refuse of much of our present waste. Thousands of us will have to stop thinking in terms of throwing away our waste products and start thinking of ways to reuse it. In the past it has not been economical to recycle, and the availability of resources for production processes have made recycling unnecessary.

Many products can be recycled today. Paper is one solid waste product that can and must be recycled. We must not permit the natural resource from which paper comes, trees, to become depleted. Millions of tons of paper products are recycled at the present time. However, only about 20 percent of waste paper is reused today, as compared with some 35 percent during the years of World War II.

Metals, including copper, lead, and zinc, are another resource that can be recycled. Metal recycling would help solve another continuing and expanding problem—what to do with old and abandoned automobiles? Since an owner no longer can receive a reasonable amount of money for an old car, thousands of automobiles are simply abandoned. The EPA estimates that 7 million old cars and trucks are junked each year; a large portion of these are abandoned. In large urban areas this is an ever-increasing problem. In New York more than 50,000 abandoned vehicles were removed in a recent year.[7]

Glass is another product that can be recycled quite effectively. It is possible to recycle glass completely. By means of grinding, glass can be reduced to particles that can then be used in numerous processes. Reground glass can be used as a soil conditioner in compost and as a road-surfacing material. The Owens-Illinois Company, a glass manufacturing industry, has developed what is known as "glasphalt." Their experimental road surface includes the use of glass not just in the surface layer but also in each layer beneath.

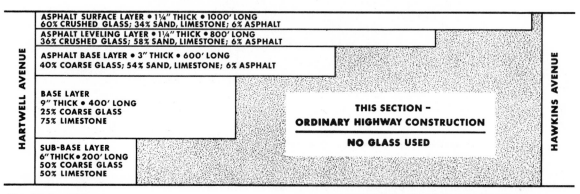

Fig. 23.4. This cross section of glasphalt indicates the composition of the various layers.

*ALL PERCENTAGE FIGURES ARE APPROXIMATE.

Recreational Use An interesting approach to using waste material for new and creative purposes is exemplified by the development of a recreational site in DuPage County, Illinois. Here a 150-foot mountain with a basal area of forty acres was built from waste material that was dumped into a sanitary landfill in an old gravel pit between November 1965 and October 1973. Refuse was dumped straight from the compaction trucks. No items were removed. Today this location is a beautiful park with three lakes used for swimming, boating, and fishing. Overlooking the entire recreational site is the artificial mountain.

Noise

Through the mechanism of sound the human being maintains contact with a major part of the surroundings within which he lives and moves. We communicate on a person-to-person basis by sound; warnings of impending danger are drawn to our attention by sound; we relax to the sound of enjoyable music; and much of our education is acquired by way of sound. Without sound and the ability to hear sound, we become isolated from a significant portion of the world around us.

At some point, however, sound becomes a nuisance or a distraction, and we are faced with the problem of noise. Noise has been identified as "meaningless, unwanted, and irregular" sound. There are differences of opinion as to what noise is. An acoustical engineer may suggest that if a sound is one we like, it is not noise; if it is disliked, it would probably be labeled noise. An electric guitar might not be noise to you, but to your neighbor trying to sleep or to read, it certainly is a nuisance. Whether we perceive a sound as noise or not, our real concern centers upon the loudness of the sound.

Except for the disturbing nature of noise, many people give little thought to the problems it creates. Nevertheless, noise is increasing in our society today. We usually think of it as an urban concern. Modes of transportation, such as trucks, planes, trains, and cars are major contributors to the noise level. In urban areas the sounds of heavy traffic combine with the sounds of construction—air hammers, compressors, bulldozers, and the like—to produce a cacophony that is exceedingly disturbing.

Noise is becoming a problem in suburban localities and in rural areas, too. The increasing popularity of motorcycles, snowmobiles, and other noise-producing machines raises the sound level in many nonurban areas.

Exposure to noise produced by various types of farming equipment also has been shown to have a detrimental effect on hearing. In a study conducted in Alberta, Canada, it was found that farmers exposed to farm machinery noise had a greater hearing loss than would be expected from normal aging.

Sound has two characteristics: pitch and loudness. Pitch is the height or depth of the sound. It is measured in units known as cycles per second (cps). The human ear can detect sound as low as 16 cps and as high as 16,000 cps.[8] Loudness or intensity is recorded in units called decibels (dbs). Zero decibel is the weakest sound level that can be detected by the human ear.

Characteristics of Sound

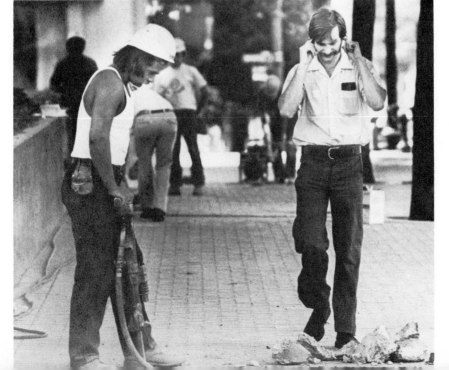

Fig. 23.5. Noise can be a nuisance and a distraction, but worst of all, it can lead to premature hearing loss.

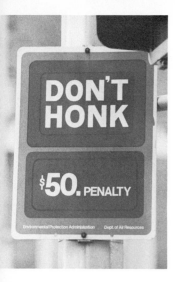

Decibels are logarithmic, not linear, units of measurement. For this reason there is a sharp increase in loudness of sound with each single decibel increase. For example, ten decibels of sound is ten times more intense than one decibel. However, twenty decibels is one hundred times more intense than one decibel. Thirty decibels is one thousand times as intense as one decibel, and so forth. If one continues this progression, one hundred decibels is ten billion times as intense as one decibel of sound.

Most sound that the human being encounters ranges between 50 and 90 dbs. The level at which most people begin to feel pain is about 120 dbs. The sound level of a two-person conversation may be around 60 dbs, and traffic noise in a city has been found to range from 70 to over 90 dbs. If you have ever been on the ground near a jet airplane when it is taxiing for takeoff, you will recall the ear-shattering noise. The sound level being generated by that plane is near 140 dbs.

Concern must be expressed for individuals who are exposed to high levels of sound in their places of daily employment. There is little doubt that many people are exposed to both continuous and intermittent sound levels that are injurious to their hearing over an extended period of time. According to federal regulations, the highest level of sound that a worker can be exposed to over an eight-hour working day is 90 dbs.

Physiology of Noise

Sound waves enter the ear and pass through the ear canal to the eardrum. Behind the eardrum are three tiny bones, known as the ossicles. The sound waves cause the eardrum to vibrate, which sets the ossicles into motion. This action is the mechanism by which the sound is transmitted to the inner ear.

The ossicles perform another interesting function. By means of "the acoustic reflex," tiny muscles disengage the ossicles from contact with the eardrum in the presence of extremely loud sounds, thereby protecting the inner ear from damage. When exposed to continual loud sounds, these small muscles cease to function properly. Like any set of muscles, if they are used continuously without time for rest, fatigue and inability to function normally will occur. Then excessive sound pressure is transmitted to the inner ear, setting up vibrations in the cochlea. This structure is filled with fluid and has microscopic hair cells. Normally these small cells move back and forth in the fluid. The energy created by this movement goes to the brain, where the sound is interpreted.

Exposure to 85 dbs of sound may cause these tiny hair cells to become fatigued. If they are given time to recover, no permanent hearing loss will result. However, when exposed to continual loud sound, these hairs may become permanently damaged. Once this happens, they can never repair themselves.

These tiny hair cells respond differently to various frequencies of sound. Those sensors for high-frequency sounds are the most susceptible to damage. For this reason, after continual exposure to excessively high levels of sounds, one may begin to experience hearing loss in the upper octaves.

Effects of Noise

Numerous physiological effects occur as the result of continued exposure to high levels of sound. The EPA, in summarizing some of the physical effects of exposure to sound, identified the following:

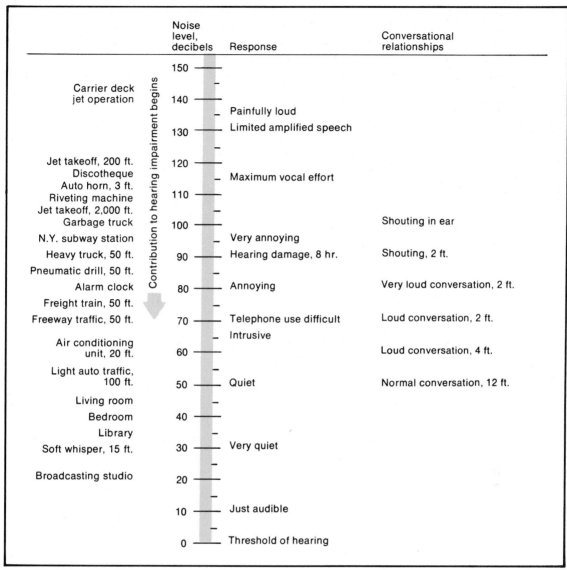

	Noise level, decibels	Response	Conversational relationships
	150		
Carrier deck jet operation	140	Painfully loud	
	130	Limited amplified speech	
Jet takeoff, 200 ft.	120		
Discotheque		Maximum vocal effort	
Auto horn, 3 ft.			
Riveting machine	110		
Jet takeoff, 2,000 ft.			
Garbage truck	100		Shouting in ear
N.Y. subway station		Very annoying	
Heavy truck, 50 ft.	90	Hearing damage, 8 hr.	Shouting, 2 ft.
Pneumatic drill, 50 ft.			
Alarm clock	80	Annoying	Very loud conversation, 2 ft.
Freight train, 50 ft.			
Freeway traffic, 50 ft.	70	Telephone use difficult	Loud conversation, 2 ft.
		Intrusive	
Air conditioning unit, 20 ft.	60		Loud conversation, 4 ft.
Light auto traffic, 100 ft.	50	Quiet	Normal conversation, 12 ft.
Living room			
Bedroom	40		
Library			
Soft whisper, 15 ft.	30	Very quiet	
Broadcasting studio	20		
	10	Just audible	
	0	Threshold of hearing	

Contribution to hearing impairment begins

Source: Chart adapted from Environmental Protection Agency data.

Fig. 23.6. Sound levels and human response

1. Blood vessels in the brain dilate.
2. Blood pressure rises.
3. Blood vessels in other parts of the body constrict.
4. Pupils of the eyes dilate.
5. Blood cholesterol level rises.
6. Various endocrine glands pour additional hormones into the bloodstream.

With continued exposure to excessively loud sound, some permanent loss of hearing will result. If we take as an example frequent exposure to 90 dbs of sound at a frequency of 2,000 cycles, we can say that hearing ability may be depressed over a period of ten years by as much as 15 dbs.[9] The seriousness of this exposure can be seen when it is realized that 95 dbs of sound is about as much as a power lawn mower puts forth.

Noise must be considered a stress agent upon the human body. Headaches, tension, disruption of sleep, and other psychological effects are often the result of noise exposure. It becomes increasingly evident that efforts must be made to reduce the levels of sound in our environment before serious physical and psychological problems arise. Such efforts will involve better use of acoustical engineering procedures. Sound that is necessary must be muffled. Pipes in our homes and buildings must be made of a material that keeps sound to a minimum. In industrial settings, workers must learn to wear ear mufflers. Industrial safety experts tell us that one of the biggest problems is educating and convincing employees of the need to protect their hearing while on the job.

As with so many other environmental concerns, it will cost money to protect people from noise pollution. To help muffle noise from airplanes using National Airport in Washington, D.C., it was necessary to install 5 million dollars' worth of extra soundproofing in the John F. Kennedy Center for the Performing Arts.[10] On the other hand, it is conceivable that for as little as $25 per car a quieter muffler could be developed that would reduce noise on our roads and highways.

Lead Poisoning

An increasing concern in older, usually blighted, neighborhoods today is the problem of lead poisoning. Lead poisoning is specifically a problem among preschool children living in very old, deteriorating homes where lead-base paint has peeled from walls, floors, doorways, and other building parts.

Lead is a toxic element that causes several health problems. The body does not totally and adequately rid itself of lead. As a result, continual exposure over an extended period of time results in a high concentration of lead in the body. Under normal circumstances the level of lead in the blood will range between 0.05 and 0.4 parts per million (ppm). Above 0.8 ppm, serious lead poisoning will result. The average level in the United States is about 0.25 ppm.[11] The matter of real concern to medical specialists is whether this "average" amount is safe or if there is already too high a level of lead in the bloodstreams of many people. At exactly what level does harm result, below which there is no problem? At what rate does lead accumulate in the human body? How rapidly is it lost through normal physiological processes? These are just a few of the questions concerning the effects on the health and well-being of people exposed to lead.

Lead is ingested and absorbed in soluble form into the bloodstream. It is eliminated from the body through the feces and urine and by means of perspiration. However, some lead accumulates in the bones and tends to replace badly needed calcium.

Lead poisoning in the early stages produces signs of anemia. The person experiences headaches, weakness, fatigue, and pain. The kidneys can be affected, and nephritis often occurs. The nervous system may become affected. If the person is left untreated, blindness, paralysis, coma, and death can result.

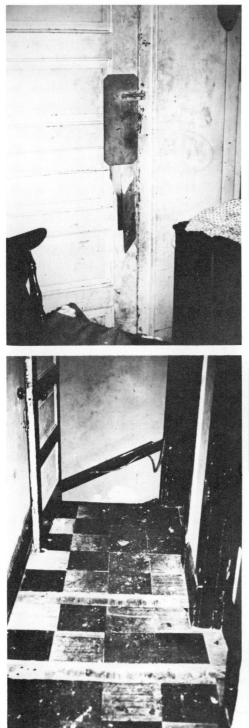

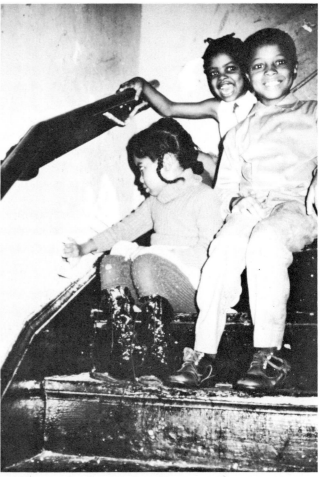

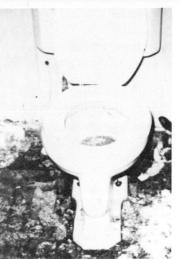

Fig. 23.7. Lead poisoning has become an increasing problem for young children who live in older, blighted neighborhoods. Eating paint chips containing toxic lead can lead to death if the child does not receive treatment.

Lead poisoning is a particular problem among children who suffer from pica. Pica is the habit of ingesting materials that normally are considered inedible. There are two theories about the cause of pica. One maintains that the child has some specific nutritional deficiency and is searching for compensation by ingesting inedible substances. The other theory asserts that pica is primarily the result of psychological factors, that the child has an unmet oral need probably connected with the inadequacy of his affective relationship with his mother.[12]

The extent of the problem of lead poisoning is not known. It is felt that many children who are mentally retarded or suffer some form of brain damage may be so because of toxic lead ingestion in their preschool years.

During the early 1970s much concern developed over lead poisoning in children. Stimulated in part by the surgeon general's guidelines for a campaign against lead poisoning, many local health agencies requested and received funding for programs to help resolve this problem. These programs usually involved: (1) diagnosis and screening of children in the suspected population to identify as many cases as possible of lead poisoning, (2) treatment of those having blood lead levels above that considered to be dangerous, and (3) education of the entire public about lead poisoning, its effects, cause, treatment, and prevention.

In a further action directed to help resolve the problem, the Food and Drug Administration in 1972 banned the use of lead in all household paints. The objective of this action was to prohibit the use of any household paint containing more than 0.06 percent lead.

Pesticides

It has always been the desire of mankind to control those pests that destroy food crops, cause disease, or are a detriment in some way to one's life-style. Many insects and other organisms do cause great problems. However, a great number of insects are not detrimental in nature, but are helpful and even necessary in the ecological cycle of life.

Since the latter part of the 1930s chemicals that do not occur in nature have been synthesized in the laboratory for use in pesticides. These pesticides include insecticides, miticides, rodenticides, fungicides, and herbicides. Over 900 basic chemical compounds are used in commercial pesticides. The public usually identifies them by their trade names, such as Aldrin, Dieldrin, Endrin, Malathion, Parathion, and others. Probably the best known is dichlorodiphenyltrichloroethane, or DDT.

It must be emphasized that pesticides also have been very helpful to mankind. In agriculture they have been beneficial in killing insects that would otherwise destroy food crops. This has been particularly important in those parts of the world where food shortages exist. In many of the Third World nations insects destroy up to one third of the potential food crops if various insecticides are not used.

Pesticides have been extremely valuable in the eradication and control of numerous diseases. Malaria has been one of the most widespread diseases in the world. The use of DDT is the basic control measure for malaria, as well as for yellow fever, the plague, and other diseases that are transmitted to man by insects.

Little thought was given to the widespread use of pesticides until the early 1960s. In 1962 Rachel Carson wrote a book entitled *Silent Spring*, which has become a classic in its effort to alert the general public to the toxic dangers of continued use of pesticides in the environment. As a result, greater understanding and concern have developed regarding pesticides and their effects.

There are three basic reasons for concern regarding the continued use of pesticides: (1) they are universal poisons; (2) they degrade slowly; and (3) they are fat-soluble.[13] As universal poisons, pesticides kill not only the pest insects but also fish, birds, animals, and beneficial insects in the area sprayed. Many beneficial insects are needed to maintain a given ecosystem. Most insecticides are nonselective in nature, destroying beneficial and valuable organisms along with the destructive pests.

Some insects build up a resistance to pesticides after continued exposure over a period of time. What often happens is that greater quantities of a given pesticide are needed to kill the detrimental pests that have built up resistance and immunity to the pesticide. A chemical that previously posed no threat for other organisms in the environment may become lethal for them in greater quantities.

The two kinds of pesticides that are most harmful in the environment are organophosphates and organochlorines. Acute exposure to the organophosphates interferes with the transmission of nerve impulses in human beings. Under normal physiological conditions, only one impulse at a time crosses the gap between adjoining nerve fibers. In the presence of organophosphates, impulses continue to pass uninterrupted along the nervous system. This results in such conditions as cramps, spastic incoordination, muscle twitching, paralysis, convulsions, and occasionally death as the outcome of paralysis of the respiratory system. Nausea and sweating may signify an accidental exposure to or ingestion of an organophosphate. Most organophosphates are much more toxic than the organochlorides. The most common organophosphate is probably Parathion.

The organochlorines are the better known of these two pesticides. They include, for example, Aldrin, Dieldrin, and DDT. They are known as chlorinated hydrocarbons because they contain carbon, hydrogen, and chlorine.

Chlorinated hydrocarbons decompose very slowly. Most chemical compounds that occur in nature are biodegradable, that is, broken down by normal processes in nature. However, compounds synthesized by science often have a half-life (the time required for half of the original quantity to decompose) of ten to fifteen years. In normal agricultural practice, fields are sprayed at least annually. As a result, concentrations of pesticides build up in the soil.

Chlorinated hydrocarbons are fat-soluble, that is, they mix with fatty tissue. Therefore, they build up and are stored in the body. As early as 1948, it became clear that these compounds could accumulate in fatty tissue.[14] This creates a question: What is the long-term effect of a buildup of such substances in the human body? The average American has a concentration of 12 ppm of DDT in his system. At present there is no direct evidence that this level of concentration is harmful to humans.[15]

Another problem created by chlorinated hydrocarbons is the body's inability to metabolize calcium properly. Several species of birds are in danger of extinction because of the production of eggs with thin shells that break or crack before a new chick can be born. The brown pelican on Anacapa Island, off the coast of California, is an example of such a bird probably doomed to extinction.[16] Since calcium is so important in human bone growth, there is concern as to what bone damage may be done in man by long-term exposure to chlorinated hydrocarbons.

As of 1973 the United States Environmental Protection Agency placed extensive controls on the use of DDT. DDT is only to be used for public health quarantine purposes. In agriculture it may still be used to protect three crops—green peppers, onions, and sweet potatoes since there are no effective alternative insecticides available for these crops. For any other agricultural use, DDT is now banned.

It is the concern of long-term exposure to all pesticides in the environment that is important. Today's middle-aged population is the first generation that has lived entire lives with pesticides in the environment. Previous generations were born prior to the development of these substances. It is doubtful whether any death has ever been recorded from normal usage of pesticides. However, what physiological adaptations the human body is having to make and what future adaptations will be necessary can only be conjectured at this time.

The need for increased food output in the world today, the desire to continue reducing or eliminating hundreds of disease causing organisms, accompanied by the realization of the dangers associated with continued unobstructed use of many pesticides leaves one uncertain about how adaptation will take place. Certainly biological control must play a greater role. The introduction of natural predators of unwanted pests into ecosystems must be accomplished. Attempts at sterilization of unwanted male pests have been somewhat successful at eliminating certain harmful insects. The development of varieties of crops that naturally are resistant to pests may be somewhat effective. Regardless of whether these measures or others are developed, we cannot continue to rely upon pesticides that in turn create a serious environmental problem for all mankind.

Toxic Substances

The Environmental Protection Agency reports that every year some 30,000 new chemicals are introduced into our environment. What will be the effect of these chemicals individually or in combination, today and in the years ahead? Many people have called for increased actions to protect against the introduction of chemicals that are a risk to health and the environment. In January 1977 a federal law, the Toxic Substance Control Act, was enacted to protect against the release of dangerous chemicals into the environment. This act provides various measures that should help eliminate the use of those chemicals that constitute an unreasonable health risk.

One chemical compound was specifically noted in this act. The chemical was polychlorinated biphenyl (PCB). PCBs are to be eliminated from all commerce by mid-1979.

In the early 1970s PCBs were detected in fish, the air, water, eggs, cheese, animal feeds, and a variety of other dairy products. They also have been observed in human tissues and in the milk of nursing mothers. Concern and attention regarding PCBs was aroused when these chemical compounds began to have physically observable effects on humans. This often has been the case with compounds that persist in the environment.

One of the most tragic instances of food contamination occurred during the mid-1970s in the state of Michigan. A chemical known as polybrominated biphenyl (PBB) was first produced in 1971 and marketed as a fire retardant. In 1973 PBB was mistakenly mixed with bags of magnesium oxide, a livestock feed additive. The two products were similar in appearance.

As the result, the PBB was accidentally sold to a number of farmers throughout the state of Michigan. The cattle, pigs, and poultry began to exhibit several physical signs of contamination about two months after the food was introduced. Milk production was reduced, the hoofs of cattle developed abnormal growths, skin changes occurred, and overall food consumption decreased.

The PBB was stored in the fat of the contaminated animals. As a result, it entered the human food chain when the meat of the contaminated animals was eaten. Thousands of head of livestock had to be destroyed. Examination of people suspected of PBB poisoning continues.

Whether the Toxic Substance Control Act implemented in 1977 can reduce the possibility of a PBB tragedy in the future is an open question. Certainly toxic substances that are detrimental to the health of people should not be on the commercial market, if this act fulfills its purpose.

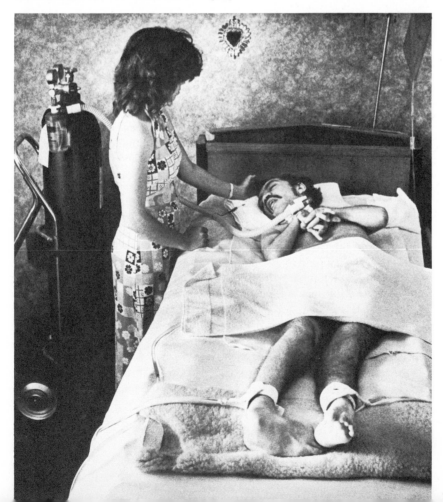

Fig. 23.8. Toxic substances pose a health threat to people who work with them. Scot Fox, overcome by hydrogen sulphide gas at an oil refinery in January 1974, has lain unconscious ever since in a Joliet, Illinois, nursing home. Hydrogen sulphide, when inhaled, goes directly into the bloodstream and paralyzes nerve centers in the brain that control breathing. Fox's brain, robbed of oxygen for a time, is now irreparably damaged.

Fluorocarbons   In 1974 it was suggested for the first time that the fluorocarbons used as propellants in aerosol cans might be endangering the life of all organisms on our planet. A study by the Australian Commonwealth Scientific and Industrial Research Organisation (ACSIRO) released in mid-1974 revealed a steady decline from 1965 to 1973 in the ozone concentrations about 10 to 20 miles above the earth's surface. Although these concentrations were known to have varied before, their fluctuations were accounted for by changes in the solar cycles.

The ozone that envelops the earth absorbs ultraviolet rays from the sun and protects all living matter from the effects of radiation. Ultraviolet rays cause sunburn and possibly skin cancer in humans.

Soon after the announcement of the ACSIRO data, F. S. Rowland of the University of California proposed the following theory to explain the depletion of the ozone layer. Man-made, relatively inert fluorocarbons (specifically chlorofluoromethanes) drift into the upper atmosphere where ultraviolet rays break them down into their various atoms. One product of this reaction is chlorine, which in turn combines with and transforms the free ozone in the atmosphere.

Fluorocarbons are used extensively as propellants in aerosol containers. As early as 1963, aerosols surpassed in popularity all other ways of packaging cosmetics. Now aerosols are used throughout the home for spraying such diverse products as paints, plastics, waxes, cleansers, room deodorizers, foods, and medicines.

Within months of the publication of Rowland's theory, manufacturers began substituting other propellants for the fluorocarbons in aerosols or packaging fluids for spraying in old-style atomizers. Meanwhile, scientists continue to measure fluctuations in atmospheric ozone and to devise tests of the Rowland theory.

In 1976 three governmental agencies (the Food and Drug Administration, the Consumer Product Safety Commission, and the Environmental Protection Agency) announced plans to phase out the use of fluorocarbons as propellants in aerosol products. By April 1979 all products containing fluorocarbon propellants must be removed from interstate commerce. It is estimated that this action will reduce by 60 percent the fluorocarbon emissions in the United States.

Radiation   Most environmental hazards stimulate the senses in some manner. They can be seen, touched, heard, or smelled. However, a very serious pollutant of increasing concern in the world today, nuclear radiation, cannot be identified by the senses.

Certainly the effects of radiation may be seen. However, radiation itself is little understood by many college students as well as the general population. Many misunderstandings are presently based upon the effects of the atomic bombings in Japan during World War II and subsequent development of nuclear power sources. Many people have great fear of radiation and what it can do to the human being.

Radiation is the result of the splitting of atoms. This activity is known as *fission*, which occurs when the core of an atom (the nucleus) is struck by a

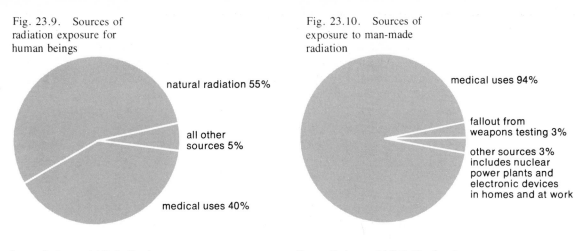

Fig. 23.9. Sources of radiation exposure for human beings

natural radiation 55%

all other sources 5%

medical uses 40%

Source: Environmental Protection Agency, *Toward a New Environmental Ethic*, 1971.

Fig. 23.10. Sources of exposure to man-made radiation

medical uses 94%

fallout from weapons testing 3%

other sources 3% includes nuclear power plants and electronic devices in homes and at work

Source: Environmental Protection Agency, *Toward a New Environmental Ethic*, 1971.

neutron. This splitting of the atom results in two new atoms being formed, each with more neutrons that strike other atoms. When atoms split, they release great amounts of energy and radiation. The release of radiation is known as radioactivity. Radioactivity is the basis of our concern as it relates to the health of mankind.

Exposure to radiation may cause leukemia and other types of cancer. Also, numerous genetic defects seem to be related to it. The extent of harm to the individual depends upon the particular part of the body exposed to radiation, the potency of the dose received, and the rate at which it is received.

There are three kinds of radiation that concern us: (1) alpha particles, (2) beta particles, and (3) gamma rays. Though alpha particles are more harmful than either beta particles or gamma rays, they cannot penetrate solid matter. A sheet of paper normally can stop these rays. Hence, they do not affect internal organs of the body because they cannot penetrate the skin. They would be very dangerous if they entered the body, either through inhalation or through a cut in the skin.

Some beta particles can penetrate the skin, but usually this penetration is not deep enough to damage internal organs. It is the gamma rays that present the real problems because of their penetrating ability. Gamma rays are similar to X rays. X rays are electromagnetic waves, whereas gamma rays, as has been explained, are streams of physical particles.

Radiation in the air at a given point is measured by a unit called a roentgen (r). This unit of measurement is named for Wilhelm Konrad Roentgen, who discovered X rays in 1895. Roentgen's first use of X rays was in relationship to his studies of bone structure.

The human being has always been exposed to some small amounts of radiation in nature. Some radioactive gases are released by soil and by rock formations such as uranium. Also, cosmic rays that are measurable on earth are given off by the stars in outer space. There are many radioactive agents in the atmosphere that result from sun flares, which give off solar particle beams. It is estimated that the average amount of natural radiation to which an individual is subjected is about 175 millirems a year.[17]

Since the splitting of the atom by man and the entrance of our civilization into the nuclear age, a number of new sources of radiation have been introduced. The one that comes to mind first is the fallout from nuclear weapons use and testing. Certainly, as a source of radiation, weapons are the most awesome and hold the greatest potential for the destruction of mankind. However, nuclear weapons are not important at the present time as a source of radiation.

Radioactive fallout resulting from nuclear detonation is not always localized where the detonation has occurred. The entire world must be concerned. In 1966 the Chinese government produced a nuclear explosion. A week to ten days later increased deposits of fresh fission products were identified in the United States. The heaviest concentrations of fallout were noticed in Arkansas. It is believed that this was the case because of a heavy rainfall during the period of time when the radioactive cloud was passing over the United States.[18] As additional nations develop nuclear armament capabilities, fallout might well become a matter of greater concern in the future. Somehow mankind must learn to live without reliance on nuclear weaponry to resolve differences between nations, or civilization could well be faced with problems of adaptation about which we today cannot even speculate.

Fig. 23.11. The map shows the locations of presently operating nuclear power reactors and sites of proposed nuclear plants in the United States.

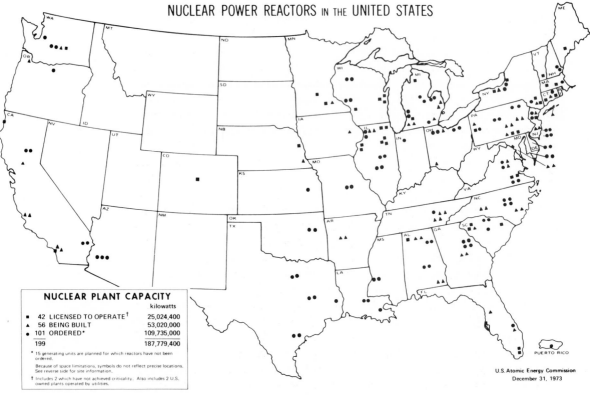

NUCLEAR POWER REACTORS IN THE UNITED STATES

NUCLEAR PLANT CAPACITY	
	kilowatts
■ 42 LICENSED TO OPERATE[†]	25,024,400
▲ 56 BEING BUILT	53,020,000
● 101 ORDERED*	109,735,000
199	187,779,400

* 15 generating units are planned for which reactors have not been ordered.

Because of space limitations, symbols do not reflect precise locations. See reverse side for site information.

† Includes 2 which have not achieved criticality. Also includes 2 U.S. owned plants operated by utilities.

U.S. Atomic Energy Commission
December 31, 1973

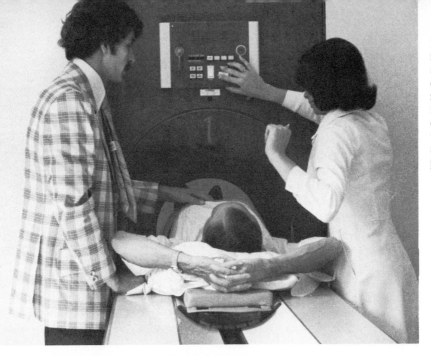

Fig. 23.12. While medical uses account for about 94 percent of all exposure to man-made radiation, careful, infrequent use of X ray can provide the physician with valuable information at little risk to the patient.

Exposure to radioactive material occurs in the home. Numerous household appliances are radioactive to a small extent. For example, television tubes, luminous wristwatches of certain kinds, and the shoe-fitting fluoroscopes that were so popular a few years ago are radioactive.

By far the greatest source of man-made radiation is X rays used in medicine. The EPA has pointed out that medical uses account for about 94 percent of all exposure to man-made radiation. Many of these X rays are being administered out of carelessness and ignorance. All too often no one asks if the patient has been exposed to X rays within the past few months. This is of particular concern to the pregnant woman, who should not be X rayed during pregnancy, particularly during the first trimester.

Exposure to large doses of radiation injures human tissue. These injuries are known as *somatic effects*. Somatic effects may occur as the result of the radiation striking a molecule in the tissue and damaging it. Exposure to between twenty-five and fifty roentgens (r) may affect white blood cells. Radiation sickness, a condition resulting in nausea, fatigue, anemia, sore throat, diarrhea, and even loss of hair, occurs as the result of exposure to 100–200 r. When one is exposed to 350–500 r, death may result. Exposure to 600–700 r is almost always fatal.

More subtle, but every bit as much of a concern, is exposure to low levels of radiation over a long period of time, often the result of occupational exposure in a number of different industries. Simply living in an environment with increasing amounts of radiation may affect us. We do not know as much as we would like about long-term effects of continuous or intermittent exposure to low levels of radiation. There is evidence that leukemia, lung cancer, skin cancer, bone cancer, and skeletal abnormalities can be caused by such exposure. Of particular concern is the damage to bone marrow that results from radiation. Eye problems have also been identified with exposure to radiation, especially the development of cataracts.

There is increasing concern about the damage that may be done to reproductive cells over a long period of time. Such exposure may result in damage or alteration of human genes, leading to the possibility of mutations. Damage can be done to the chromosomes as well. The real problem here lies in the fact that such damage will not be revealed until future generations are born.

Nuclear power can be used for beneficial purposes. In a time when sources of energy are at a critical stage in many parts of the world, attention must be turned to the use of nuclear power in the production of energy. However, any use of nuclear power raises the specter of environmental pollution, particularly disposal of radioactive substances and wastes. In the development of new power plants to help resolve the shortage of energy or in the use of nuclear energy for propelling nuclear ships, submarines, or rockets, the environmental concerns remain basically the same.

Nuclear power stations are presently being built in some twenty-five or more countries of the world. Nuclear energy is used to generate electrical power. When nuclear fission takes place, heat is generated; this heat turns water into steam, which spins an electrical turbine, which spins a generator to produce electricity.

At the present time approximately 100 nuclear power plants are either in operation or under construction in the United States. The EPA predicts that there will be about 450 such plants in operation by 1990.

It must be admitted that there is rather strong opposition to the construction of nuclear power plants in many localities. Small amounts of radiation are released from the reactors. The amount is very minute; however, any increase in radiation may present greater long-term risks for people.

Another consideration is that there is always a potential for accidents when large amounts of radioactivity are released into the environment. The Atomic Energy Commission has stressed that safety has been built into the construction of all nuclear power plants. Yet the possibility of a catastrophic accident is always present.

With the increased use of nuclear power, there will be more need for disposal of radioactive wastes. Such wastes are buried in isolated locations in concrete vaults. Continuous monitoring of waste disposal areas must be maintained to make sure that leakage does not occur.

In addition to the problem of disposal of radiation wastes and the danger of radiation escaping from the power site, attention must be given to the effects of thermal pollution of the water. Great amounts of water are needed to cool the reactors. Many nuclear power plants use a million or more gallons of water per minute in the cooling process. Unless this water is placed in a cooling pond before being returned to the river or the lake from which it was taken, serious problems can occur. The problem of thermal pollution of water was discussed in the previous chapter.

We have discussed the process of splitting atoms (fission). *Fusion* reaction also needs to be understood. Fusion of atoms produces energy, a reaction that requires a temperature of hundreds of millions of degrees. Yet fusion produces much less radioactivity than fission. Research suggests that fusion may be the solution to the world's energy shortage. However, because of many technological problems, fusion power may not be a reality until the turn of this century.[19]

Nuclear power presents our civilization with a number of very difficult alternatives. On the one hand, there are many benefits to be derived from nuclear energy. Yet, for each benefit there are potential dangers. Whether man's demands for energy will result in nuclear development that in turn lowers the quality of life for everyone remains to be seen. Certainly, as we understand the alternatives, it is hoped that we will be able to make sound decisions that will make adaptation easier.

Summary

With increased numbers of people and increased industrial development there has been accelerated growth in the amount of solid wastes produced in America. Also, greater noise, the use of potentially harmful pesticides and fluorocarbons, and the continuing use and development of nuclear energy with its accompanying problems of radiation have raised ecological concerns not faced in past decades.

Each of these environmental concerns has varying effects on the health and well-being of people. Many, such as exposure to noise or to radiation over a long time, are somewhat subtle. It is difficult to ascertain just exactly what level of exposure is harmful to one's well-being. Others, such as an ugly dump or a buildup of solid wastes, are not so subtle.

Changes in life-style and coordinated efforts to reduce these environmental problems will come about only as we realize that the little each of us can do will have a positive, wide-ranging effect. As we learn to adapt and adjust, we will be able to cope with other health-related issues as we progress through life.

Review Questions

1. How were solid wastes disposed of in the past? What problems did this create?
2. Describe new techniques of waste disposal that are becoming commonplace.
3. What is recycling? How would you promote a recycling program in your community?
4. With the arrival of new supersonic transport planes, what steps must be taken to preserve the environment from noise pollution?
5. If pesticides have been vital in the production of crops, why is there such concern about them today?
6. What would be the effect on food production if pesticides were banned? Is this a logical answer to this environmental problem?

7. What problems or dangers are associated with the use of nuclear power plants? Do you believe the laws are protective enough?
8. What limitations would you place on nuclear testing?

Review Questions

Noise

Books and Pamphlets

Burns, William. *Noise and Man*. London: John Murray, 1968.
Environmental Protection Agency. *Noise Pollution*. Washington, D.C., 1972.
Kimber, Diana Clifford, et al. *Anatomy and Physiology*. 15th ed. New York: Macmillan Co., 1966.
Report of the Panel on Noise Abatement. *The Noise Around Us*. Washington, D.C.: Department of Commerce, 1970.

Articles

Baron, Robert Alex. "Noise and Urban Man." *American Journal of Public Health* 58 (1968): 2060–66.
Beranek, L. L. "Noise." *Scientific American,* December 1966, pp. 66–76.
Falk, Stephen A., and Farmer, Joseph C. "Incubator Noise and Possible Deafness." *Archives of Otolaryngology* 97 (1973): 385–87.
Goldsmith, John R., and Jonsson, Erland. "Health Effects of Community Noise." *American Journal of Public Health* 63 (February 1973): 782–93.
Johnson, Eric K. "Noise, Health and the Community." *Ohio's Health* 25 (December 1973): 23–26.
Konopa, Valerie O., and Zimering, Stanley. "Noise—The Challenge of the Future." *Journal of School Health* 62 (1972): 172–77.
Kryter, K. D. "Psychological Reaction to Aircraft Noise." *Science* 151 (1966): 1346–55.
Smith, L. K. "Noise in the News." *Canadian Journal of Public Health* 60 (1969): 299–306.
Wayshak, Gary. "Construction Equipment Noise Is Above Ear Damaging Level." *Journal of Environmental Health* 36 (1973): 147–51.
Weinstein, Neil D. "Effect of Noise on Intellectual Performance." *Journal of Applied Psychology* 59 (1974): 548–54.

Solid Wastes, Radiation, Lead, and Pesticides

Books and Pamphlets

Blatz, Hanson. *Introduction to Radiological Health*. New York: McGraw-Hill Book Co., 1964.
Carson, Rachel. *Silent Spring*. Boston: Houghton Mifflin Co., 1962.
Lindell, Bo, and Dobson, R. Lowry. *Ionizing Radiation and Health*. Geneva: World Health Organization, 1961.

Mayneord, William Valentine. *Radiation and Health*. London: Nuffield
Provincial Hospitals Trust, 1964.

Articles

Barber, Donald E. "Changing Patterns in Radiological Health." *American
Journal of Public Health* 59 (1969): 2251–56.
Duel, Ward. "Solid Waste: Health Concerns." *Journal of Environmental
Health* 38 (July-August 1975): 31–35.
Irving, George W. "Agricultural Pest Control and the Environment."
Science 168 (June 1970): 1419–24.
Niering, William A. "The Effects of Pesticides." *Bioscience* 18 (1968):
869–75.
Novick, Robert E. "Man, His Environment and Lead." *Journal of
Environmental Health* 35 (1973): 363–67.
Taylor, David A.; Amos, Rosemary R.; Stevens, James T.; and Thomas,
John A. "Pesticides and the Environment." *Journal of School Health*
62 (1972): 82–85.
Van Dam, André. "The Limits to Waste." *Futurist* 9 (February 1975):
18–21.

Notes

1. League of Women Voters of the United States, *Solid Waste—It Won't Go Away*, Publication No. 675 (Washington, D.C.: The League, 1971), p. 5.
2. National Geographic Society, *As We Live and Breathe: The Challenge of Our Environment* (Washington, D.C.: The Society, 1971), p. 182.
3. Amos Turk, Jonathan Turk, and Janet T. Wittes, *Ecology, Pollution, Environment* (Philadelphia: W. B. Saunders Co., 1972), p. 142.
4. Richard H. Wagner, *Environment and Man* (New York: W. W. Norton & Co., 1971), p. 420.
5. League of Women Voters, *Solid Waste*, p. 11.
6. MacNeill, *Environmental Management*, p. 98.
7. League of Women Voters, *Solid Waste*, p. 4.
8. Eva Hammond, "Hearing Defects of School Age Children," *Journal of School Health* 60 (1970): 405.
9. Turk, Turk, and Wittes, *Ecology, Pollution, Environment*, p. 198.
10. National Geographic Society, *As We Live and Breathe*, p. 139.
11. Wagner, *Environment and Man*, p. 254.
12. Robert H. Woody, "Controlling Pica Via an Environmental-Psychobehavioral Strategy: With Special Reference to Lead Poisoning," *Journal of School Health*, December 1971, p. 548.
13. Turk, Turk, and Wittes, *Ecology, Pollution, Environment*, p. 43.
14. Environmental Protection Agency, *Toward a New Environmental Ethic* (Washington, D.C.: The Agency, 1971), p. 22.
15. Ibid., pp. 22–23.
16. National Geographic Society, *As We Live and Breathe*, p. 54.
17. Robert Plant, "The Dangerous Atom," *World Health*, January 1969, p. 17.
18. Ann B. Strong, Charles B. Porter, Melvin W. Carter, and Edward F. Wilson, "Localization of Fallout in United States from May, 1966 Chinese Nuclear Test," *Public Health Reports* 82 (1967): 487.
19. National Geographic Society, *As We Live and Breathe*, p. 101.

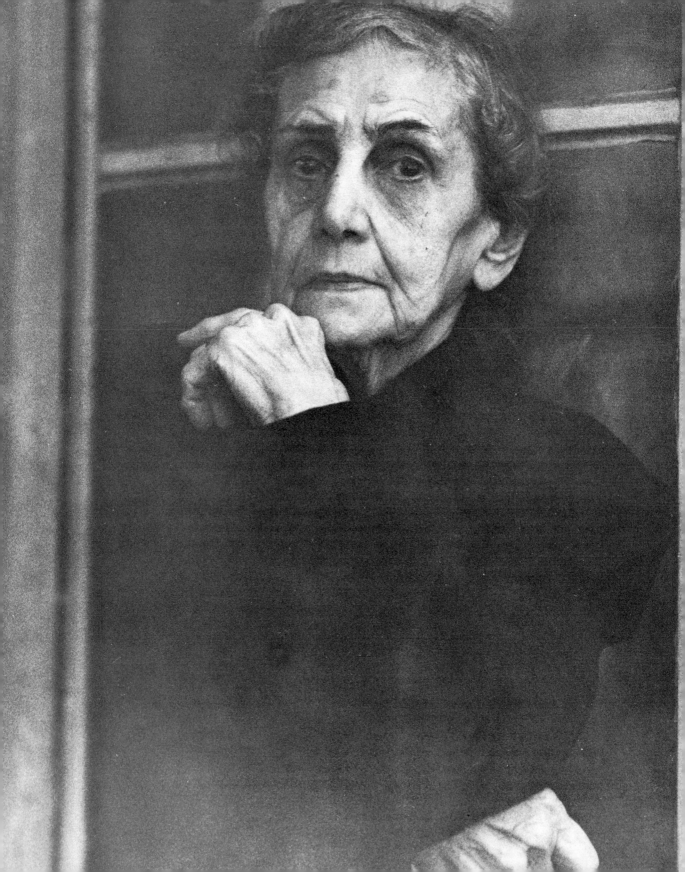

Aging: The Challenge Lies in Adapting

24

The individual is a biological, psychological, and social constellation moving forward in time. The dynamics of the transformation of the individual from childhood through adulthood are such that mixtures of stability and change, persistence and adaptation, and emergence of new features are seen in the wide range of human characteristics.[1]

Increased longevity, early retirement, diminished morbidity, and the determination of an aging population to be recognized, respected, and received have all combined to create renewed interest in aging and the aged. This chapter seeks to investigate problems relating to aging: to determine the nature of the current dilemma and to answer the charges of discrimination currently posed by older people in America.

The definitions of the terms *young* and *old* are largely determined by custom and life-style. In the United States the aged are generally considered those who have reached sixty-five years of age. Certainly nothing magical occurs on one's sixty-fifth birthday that initiates the aging process or signifies that one is physically old. This figure was arbitrarily selected as the retirement age when the federal social security program was established in 1935. Thus, this figure represents a social index of age that allows us to determine retirement periods as well as dates of eligibility for supportive services to the elderly.

Over the past several years the retirement age has changed somewhat. In 1956 the Social Security Administration allowed women to opt for reduced benefits at age sixty-two, and in 1961 they extended the same option to men. In 1973 the optional retirement age dropped to sixty years with the passage of the Older Americans Comprehensive Services Amendment to the Social Security Act. Nevertheless, age sixty-five represents the most common age for retirement in the United States, and persons over this age are those most often represented in government statistics concerning the elderly.

The number of persons sixty-five and over in the United States is approximately 22,935,000, or roughly 10.5 percent of our population. The Bureau of the Census tells us that the number of older people in the United States will continue to increase, at least through the year 2020. It is estimated that there will be 24 million elderly people by 1980, 28.8 million by 2000, and 40.2 million by

Who Are the Aged?

Aging is a social problem in the United States, which is a particularly youth-oriented society. The aged are often deprived of both social status and purpose of life.

2020. It is further projected that this latter figure will represent 15 percent of the United States population.

The number of elderly persons in the United States has increased considerably since the beginning of this century when the elderly population numbered little more than 3 million persons, or 4 percent of the population. The increase in the American aged that has occurred from 1900 to the present represents a much larger gain than that for the total population, which increased from 76 million to 220 million over the same period of time. What factors are related to such increases? And why should we be concerned with the growing numbers of older Americans? Let us examine the answers to these questions.

According to the Population Reference Bureau, the immigration of large numbers of young adults prior to World War I contributed to the large number of older adults seen in recent years. Also, the large number of births that occurred in the late nineteenth and early twentieth centuries affected the size of the aged population we see today. A third contributing factor is the reduced death rate that has come about as a result of advances in medicine and improvements in sanitation. Reduced infant and childhood death rates were especially important.[2]

Since 1900, declining infant and childhood death rates have contributed significantly to an increase in life expectancy in the United States. Life expectancy refers to the average number of years that a person can look forward to living. It generally applies to the number of years that a newborn is expected to live. For example, an individual born in 1900 could expect to live approximately forty-eight to fifty years, while a person born today can expect to live over seventy years. In reference to the sixty-fifth year of life, only 39 percent of the infants born in 1900 could expect to survive to this age that now marks the difference between middle and old age. Seventy-two percent of the infants born today are expected to celebrate their sixty-fifth birthdays.[3]

Expectation of life can be computed for any age. When it is calculated for today's middle-aged or elderly person and compared with such a calculation for persons born in 1900, the life span has not been significantly extended. For instance, a sixty-five-year-old in 1900 could anticipate living another 11.9 years compared with a sixty-five-year-old in 1973 who could expect to live another 15.3 years.

We do note variations in life expectancy in the United States based on sex and race. Women live longer than men, and whites live longer than nonwhites. Life expectancy has continued to be highest for white females and lowest for non-white males.

Our concern with life expectancy and the number of elderly individuals has illustrated that a sizable proportion of Americans is considered aged and that the proportion is expected to grow over the next several years. We must study the numbers and needs of this group if we are to provide for them.

| Redefining the Generation Gap | Over the life span of any individual, not only are the organism, the personality, and the age-appropriate roles changing, but also the structure of society and the roles it affords, which change as norms, mores, attitudes, and knowledge |

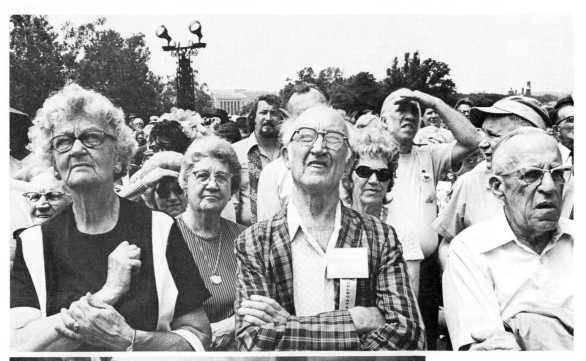

Fig. 24.1. Increasing numbers of senior citizens in the 1970s refuse to allow their complaints to be ignored. These people are attending a senior citizens rally in front of the Capitol in Washington, D.C.

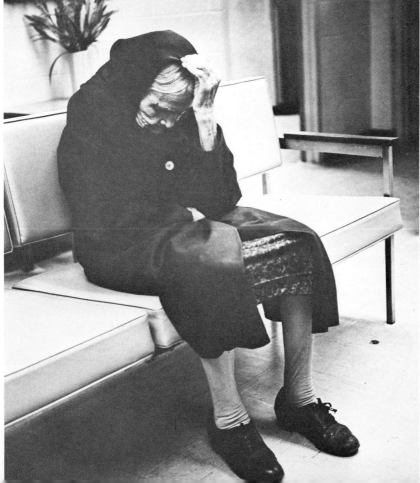

Fig. 24.2. If we wish to increase our life span, we must find ways to reverse or arrest the biological aging process. People die from diseases, but they also die because a part or parts of their bodies have literally "run down."

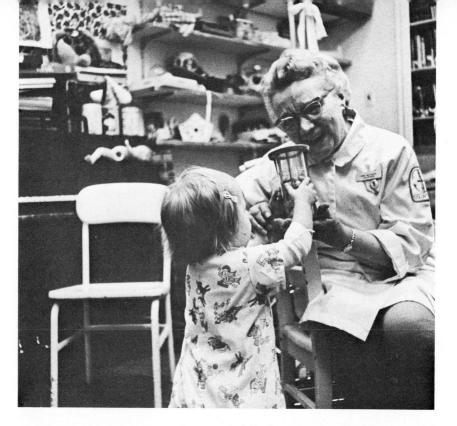

Fig. 24.3. One way to fight the aging process and the boredom that frequently comes after retirement is to keep active and interested in life. Many senior citizens find volunteer work is rewarding.

change, or as wars and depressions occur.[4] Each generation has its own set of problems, and just as the nature of individuals varies, so does the nature of social interaction. Similarly, just as the generation gap divides adults and youth, so it separates the middle-aged from the aging, and the later division is every bit as subtle as the earlier one.

Probably the greatest single event marking the later generation gap is retirement, for it signifies the end of public occupation and transfers the individual from the role of "giving" to that of "receiving." Retirement frequently means pension, travel, hobbies, and rest—in short, the good life, albeit at varying levels. The key point is that the productivity level is probably low, and although youth recognize and even support the reward system, they find it difficult to support the aged on the one hand and accept direction from them on the other.

Social interaction between generations only compounds the problems, although an interesting inverse relationship seems to exist: the greater the gap between generations, the better they seem to get along. The aged get along far better with children than even the children's parents do. Undoubtedly this effect is due to the degree of threat one generation represents for the other. Grandparents are little threat to their grandchildren, and vice versa; cast the grandparents into the parental role, however, following the death of the real parents, and the generation gap may suddenly grow quite troublesome.

To some degree, the threat theory may help explain the resentment many middle-aged people feel toward their own parents. The parents expect deferential treatment and make demands on their offspring, a complete role reversal from earlier days.

The generation gap is further intensified by educational factors. Whereas the myth of any direct correlation between aging and declining intelligence has almost been put to rest,[5] the fact remains that virtually every new generation in this century has achieved a higher level of formal education than its predecessor, and obviously more recent education. Although adult training centers and gerontological education ventures are increasing, the educational advantage will probably always reside with youth. The key concept here is that education does not necessarily indicate intelligence.

> "...this is one thought that has impressed me, Govinda. Wisdom is not communicable. The wisdom which a wise man tries to communicate always sounds foolish."
>
> "Are you jesting?" asked Govinda.
>
> "No, I am telling you what I have discovered. Knowledge can be communicated, but not wisdom. One can find it, live it, be fortified by it, do wonders through it, but one cannot communicate and teach it. I suspected this when I was still a youth and it was this that drove me away from teachers."[6]

Recency of education will probably always be a factor, as younger people tend to be more active in the total learning process. To some extent, this may explain

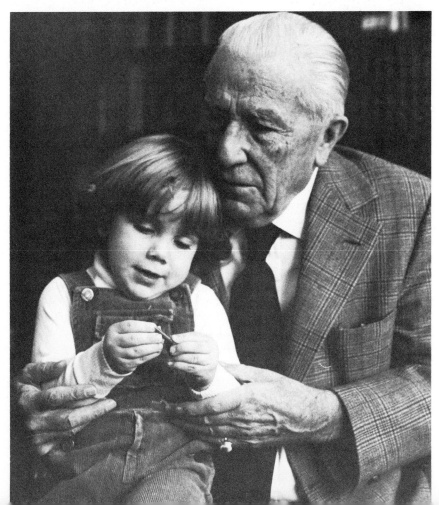

Fig. 24.4. Grandparents and grandchildren often enjoy a special relationship. Since they are on opposite ends of the generation gap, they represent no threat to one another.

conservative tendencies among the elderly to stick with their "tried and proven" ways. Their stubbornness may represent a simple reaction formation developed to help them cope with change: they ignore it.

Economics is increasing in its importance as a generation-gap factor. Fewer and fewer people are working beyond the age of sixty-five. The median incomes for people in their late fifties and early sixties are below those of their thirty-five to forty-five-year-old counterparts. Further, Social Security, life insurance, retirement benefits, and pensions make up an increasingly greater portion of the total income as age progresses. To a large extent, then, advertising for consumer spending is largely focused on the young, and even the "old folk" claim they prefer it that way. But at what cost to their self-concept? Already deprived of active commercial pursuit, they are further overlooked as potential spenders, except by the shrewd. And the shrewd are often more devious than considerate.

Age itself may soon provide an interesting shift in the societal structure. Whereas the tremendous baby boom of the forties created a youth movement, almost overnight the current decline in new births will soon create a relative vacuum in the younger groups and important consequences within the age structure of society. Where social interaction is essential, particularly between generations, problems intensify—and the more urgent the interaction, the more intensified will become the generational differences.

The following chart schematically demonstrates the problem. Given any specific task that affects all three groups, for example the Canada Pension Plan, diverse opinions begin to interact. The youngest generation is usually not enthusiastic; it is they who must pay for the plan over the longest period of time, and for whom the benefits are most remote. Those in the middle group, on the other hand, support the idea, but wish to keep the payments low. Those in the oldest group, who expect the most immediate gain, support the plan most strongly and seek even higher benefits. They believe they have paid their dues to society and should now reap the rewards. Youth, on the other hand, value a one-to-one ratio between achievement and reward, and are not likely to accept either deferred payment or compensatory remuneration for the masses.

Fig. 24.5. The aging process, showing selected generations over time.

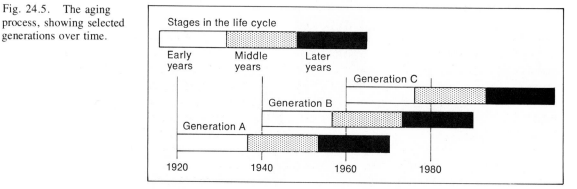

Adapted from a schematic used by Riley and Associates, 1968: 2.

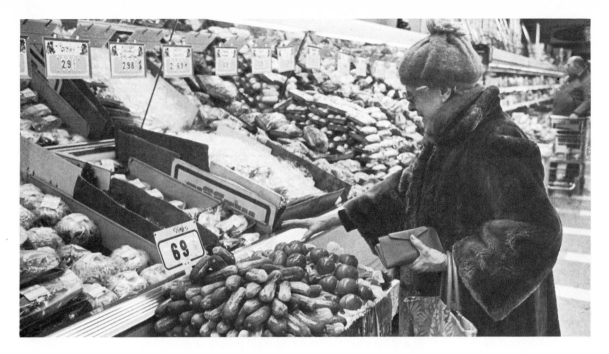

Fig. 24.6. Economics is an issue of concern to the elderly. Rising costs of basic goods often strain their small incomes to the limit.

Every society has an age structure; contemporary America has a broadened one. Whereas the proportion of the population over sixty-five was around 3 percent in 1850, it is over 9 percent today. And the proportion between forty-five and sixty-four has increased from 10 to 20 percent.[7] There are close to a million persons in North America today who are over eighty-five! This rapid increase in the proportion of aged people has created unprecedented problems for planners. The economic, social, recreational, political, educational, and even religious institutions are faced with significant tasks in adapting to a proportionately aging population. Nor is the shift temporary. The slow, steady decline in birth rates across the continent will soon provide the population over forty-five with majority status and create marked shifts in emphasis. Generation gaps will always exist, but the shift in societal prestige may soon move beyond youth, and into middle age. In time, even Americans may learn to venerate the aged.

Those persons who study aging are known as gerontologists, and their field of study is called gerontology. The scope of this study is very broad, and for that reason it represents a subspecialty in many different fields. Thus gerontologists with a biological background may be concerned with age-associated changes that take place at the cellular level or with immune reactions that are characteristic of old age. Housing, transportation, and changes in status and role are among the concerns of the social gerontologist. The anthropologist who calls himself a gerontologist may focus on the differential effects of aging on ethnic and racial groups or the comparative position of the aged in Western and non-Western societies.

The Study of Aging

Scholars in various other disciplines also study aging. Psychologists may be concerned with perceptual changes that occur over time, differences in memory between the young and old, or the psychological impact of retirement. The economist might focus on the operation of the social security program and the support of future generations of older Americans. Indeed, the study of aging involves many fields, and one should identify each gerontologist's approach if one is to view that scholar's work in proper perspective.

It is necessary to differentiate between *gerontology* and *geriatrics*. As already indicated gerontology is the study of aging, while geriatrics refers to treatment of the elderly. Traditionally geriatrics has been used to refer specifically to the medical treatment of health problems peculiar to old age. However, in recent years the term has been used more flexibly. For example, a person who delivers services that alleviate the social problems of old age might be called a geriatric social worker. Those in the field of recreation who devote themselves to developing and directing leisure-time activities for older persons may be said to be involved in geriatric recreation. Today the term is frequently used as a modifier, indicating an applied field that is aimed at age-related problems.

Where does health education fit in the study of aging? We believe it has a unique and important role to play in integrating and disseminating health information from these many avenues of study. Health education helps us understand changes that accompany aging and the significance of those changes. With such an understanding we may be able to deliver services that are more appropriate to the needs of older persons. Likewise, health education in aging can prepare us for our own old age. Aging does not consist of changes that commence at age sixty-five. It is a lifelong process that begins at conception and ends with death, and it is one in which we and all other living things participate.

Avoid Stereotypes— Dispel Myths

In concentrating on the aged as a population group we must guard against establishing stereotypes. The aged are not all alike any more than are all thirty-five-year-olds alike. The aged are a heterogeneous group of people.

In general, our society has come to view old age negatively and to equate each dread adult birthday with another step in the downhill descent to death. This over-the-hill concept stems from our youth orientation. We often equate youth with attractiveness, activity, productivity, health, and sex appeal and maturity with the opposite qualities. Certainly youth does not have a monopoly on positive traits. As Butler and Lewis have expressed it, youth depends on the piece-by-piece accumulation of personality and experience, while old age can enjoy the finished product—a completed human being.[8]

In an introduction that preceded her speech, an older woman was referred to by the host as being seventy-five years young. Much to the dismay of her audience and host, she emphatically stated that she did not want to be thought of as seventy-five years young. "I am seventy-five years *old,* and I am not ashamed of it," she said. The host probably felt that he was paying her a compliment by his remarks, but such remarks reflect a negative view of old age. We must learn to recognize the accomplishments of people regardless of their age. To refer to

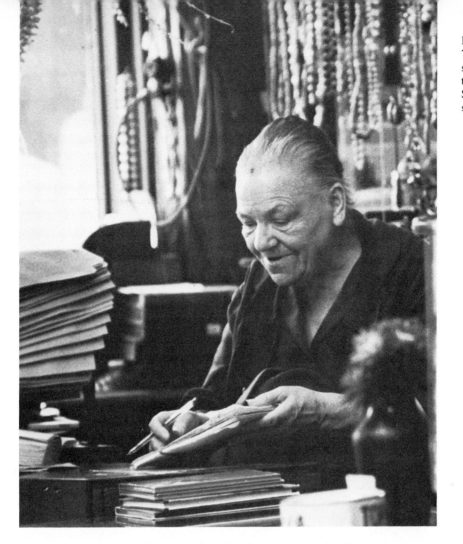

active, attractive, intelligent, or productive persons of advanced years as "young" because they do not fit our stereotype of old age is an insult to the dignity of us all.

Perhaps our negative view of aging stems partially from the knowledge that many of our nation's elderly are alone, poor, sick, or disabled. But we do not improve their lot or the destinies of today's young but aging citizens by equating these conditions with their being old. Most older people are not isolated, poor, sick, or disabled. However, we do need to improve the lot of those who are and to reduce their number in the future.

A common myth associated with aging is that most elderly people either live alone or in an institution. Neither of these assumptions is correct. Approximately 70 percent of our nation's elderly live in families. By living in a family is meant that they either live with their spouses or with close relatives. More elderly men than women live in families; one-third of our older women live alone. These differential residence patterns reflect the fact that, in general, women live longer than men. Therefore, there are more widows than widowers and hence more women living without their spouses.

Ninety-five percent of the American elderly reside outside of institutions. That means that at any given time 5 percent of our elderly live in nursing homes or long-term care facilities. On the average one in four of us will spend some time in our lives in such an institution. We need to improve the quality of care for those who live in nursing homes, but we also need to develop more programs for home care of the elderly.

In general, the income situation for older Americans is dismal. On retirement, income drops considerably for many of them. Forced retirement and longer life mean that fewer elderly persons are part of the labor force. Retirement benefits are a predominant and important source of income, with approximately 95 percent of the elderly being eligible for social security benefits. Although these benefits have increased through the years, so has the cost of living. For many of these people, benefits are barely enough to keep them going. Approximately 16 percent of older Americans are living below the official poverty level.

Their income, coupled with their greater need for medical services, makes medical expenses a special financial burden for the elderly. Dollars for health must compete with dollars for food, clothing, and shelter. Even special health insurance programs such as Medicare and Medicaid leave many elderly persons with health expenses. These programs do not fund all health needs, nor do they always pay the total cost of covered services.

Although certain diseases become more prevalent with age, it should not be assumed that the older years are characterized by sickness and disability. Such assumptions are dangerous for individuals and health professionals alike, because assumptions can become expectations.

The person who expects pain, discomfort, or disability to occur as part of aging may wait too long before seeking medical care. The health worker who expects his older patient to suffer pain and dysfunction may respond minimally when the patient displays such symptoms. If a person is not expected to be any healthier or any more comfortable than he is, little effort may be expended to improve his health or to alleviate his discomfort.

Although 86 percent of older persons have long-term health problems, 67 percent do not have problems that presently interfere with their mobility.[9] Hence, any notion that most elderly persons are confined to their homes due to immobility is false. Of the 95 percent of the aged who reside outside of institutions, 5 percent are homebound due to long-term afflictions.

Finally, we must be aware that the group we call aged includes people of varying ages. Conditions for a sixty-five-year-old may be quite different than those for a ninety-five-year-old. Therefore, we must guard against lumping these persons under one blanket term. The American aged have recently been referred to as "young old," those between sixty-five and seventy-four, and "advanced old," those over seventy-five. Our older population is aging, and we see that the proportion of the aged in the seventy-five and above category is increasing.

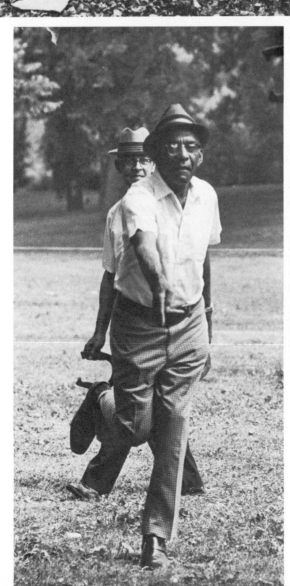

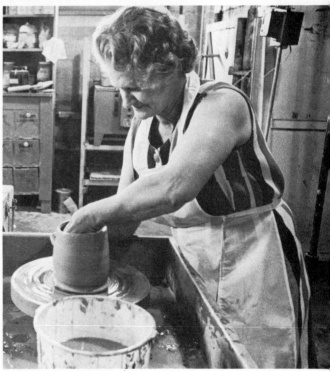

Fig. 24.8. Reaching the age of 65 needn't mean giving up enjoyable activities. Many retirees even take up new sports and hobbies, such as chess, horseshoes, and pottery making.

If we escape the hazards of youth and continue to grow older, we must accept some functional decline. Aging always ends in death, and as we age, we become more vulnerable to accidents and disease. Recognizing age-associated changes in the body and patterns of illness can lead us to a more relevant approach to the care of the elderly. At this point let us concentrate on the manifestations of illness in the aged and possible implications for the delivery of health care to them.

Chronic conditions represent the key health problems affecting middle-aged and older adults. Such conditions are long term and generally lead to irreversible changes. Heart disease, cancer, and cerebrovascular disease resulting in stroke are chronic conditions that also happen to be the three leading causes of death among the elderly.

Definite causes for chronic diseases are generally unknown, and cures are often unavailable. This factor has important implications for the delivery of health care services to the aged. Modern medicine focuses on disease cures, and physicians are highly trained in curative medicine. Disease is to be combated and conquered. Such efforts are noble and appropriate, but today's elderly ill cannot wait for cures. They need supportive care that helps them live more comfortably. This area of health care needs greater development.

Long-term chronic illness leads not only to treatment and management problems but also to financial problems. Long-term monitoring of a condition or continued drug therapy to maintain one's health state are expensive. Average annual medical expenses for the older population are three times those of our younger Americans. As mentioned earlier, Medicare and Medicaid do not offer complete coverage of health bills. Routine physical examinations and prescription drugs are among the services excluded from these programs.

Diagnostic efforts are usually geared toward the identification of a single problem. However, among elderly patients a single problem is not the rule. Degenerative changes, as well as the incidence of certain diseases, increase with age. Thus, an older patient may be suffering from multiple physical problems rather than a single dysfunction.

The presence of symptoms that may accompany various disorders may lead to confusion in accurate diagnosis and may also be important warning signs that go unheeded. For example, one individual may have heart disease, gastrointestinal disorders, and esophageal problems all at the same time. Chest pain may be associated with all of these conditions. Thus, when a chest pain occurs, one disorder may be uncovered and the others may go undiagnosed.

Let us cite another example involving a change in bowel habits. Such change is a well-known danger sign of cancer. Yet, it may be ignored by the family or physician of an older person who has been preoccupied with bowel problems and constipation. Even rectal bleeding, which may signal cancer, may be unheeded because it is confused with previously existing hemorrhoids.

In addition, diagnosis may be made difficult by age-related alterations in the traditional clinical picture associated with a given disease. For example, pain ordinarily motivates us to seek help. In the case of the cardiovascular disease angina pectoris, a suffocative pain in the chest may be an important warning sign of an impending heart attack. Such pain symbolizes to us and to our physician

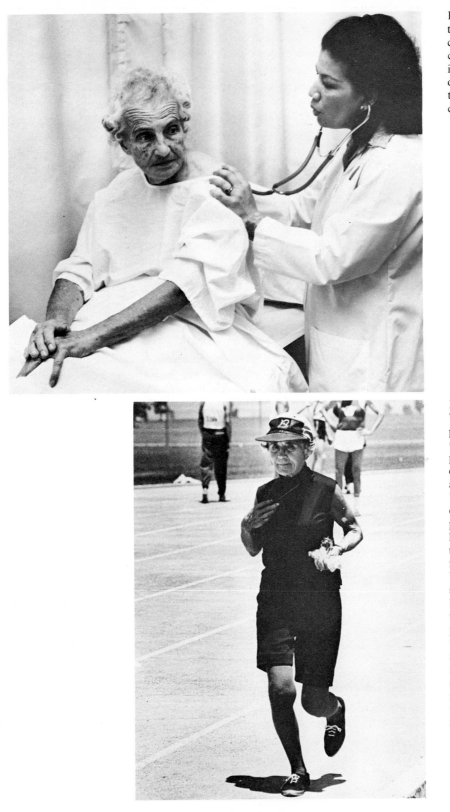

Fig. 24.9. Older people tend to suffer from chronic physical conditions. This woman is being examined by the doctor before admission to a nursing home for care and treatment.

Fig. 24.10. Mrs. Eula Weaver, 89, and a participant in the California LFC Study, is proof that the chronic conditions caused by aging can be alleviated. The LFC program is an exercise program that promotes cardiovascular health and a special diet that restricts the intake of fats and cholesterol. When she entered the study at 81, Mrs. Weaver had severe angina, various cardiovascular problems, arthritis, and was on eight types of medication. Forty-eight months later she was off all drugs and jogging, riding a bike, and working out in a gym regularly.

that something is wrong. In the elderly the pain of angina pectoris may be absent. Approximately one-fifth of older persons feel no pain when a heart attack occurs.

When pain does accompany a disorder, it may be less severe. In some people who are mentally confused, the pain may be easily forgotten. Furthermore, some persons may dismiss pain as a necessary burden of old age. Pain is not a normal accompaniment of aging, and it should not be ignored.

Elderly persons are more likely to develop mental manifestations of their physical problems. For instance, hardened and narrowed arteries that serve the brain poorly may produce disorientation, deficits in memory, shifts in mood, and impaired intellectual function. Likewise, the side effects of some drugs associated with long-term therapy for chronic disorders include transient dizziness, giddiness, or confusion. Mental depression may also accompany irreversible and chronic ill health. The trauma and drugs that accompany surgery, electrolyte imbalances, and nutritional disorders can also impair nutritional and oxygen supplies to brain tissues. Unfortunately, mental confusion and senility are too often considered normal accompaniments of aging, and a search for their cause may not be made.

Certainly there are elderly persons in whom inadequate blood flow to the brain due to cerebral arteriosclerosis results in irreversible, senile brain disease. This condition is significant and is probably associated with about half of the cases of mental disorders in old age. However, mental confusion should not be summarily dismissed as an irreversible manifestation of the aging process.

We have viewed some factors that are important in the care of elderly patients. But, once again it must be emphasized that not all elderly persons are patients. The later years are not typically filled with pain and ill health. Certainly aging eventually results in death, and in the absence of sudden accident, death must be preceded by some dysfunction and underlying disorder.

Summary

The growing proportion of the population in the age group over sixty-five has demanded increasing attention from government at all levels. Aging has been discussed in both a demographic context and a functional one. Retirement for some brings a welcome change in life, a new era, a fresh beginning. For others it is the end of an era, the completion of productivity, the first day of the last phase in the life cycle. For some it is exciting; for others depressing. The fault for such ambivalence lies both in man and in culture. Now we will turn to the last phase of the life cycle—death: coping with it and preparing for it.

Review Questions

1. For what reasons have social scientists begun to examine the status of older people?
2. What is meant by the statement, "The process of aging is entire, rather than particular"?

3. Do you believe that aging begins after an organism has attained maturity or that it begins with the commencement of life?

4. What is gerontology?

5. What are some stereotypes that many people have about the aged?

6. Discuss the concept that the aged are usually sick and ill.

7. What are some chronic diseases that tend to affect the elderly?

8. What is senility?

9. Should younger generations be held responsible for the care and welfare of the elderly? If so, what are their responsibilities?

10. Compare and contrast the attitudes toward aging in Eastern and Western cultures.

11. What effects do retirement bonuses have on the aging?

12. As life expectancy increases, how can society restructure itself to accommodate the elderly?

Readings

Butler, R., and Lewis, M. *Aging and Mental Health*. St. Louis: The C. V. Mosby Co., 1977.

Kart, C.; Metress, E.; and Metress, J. *Aging and Health: A Biological and Social Perspective*. San Francisco: Addison-Wesley, 1978.

Mendelson, M. *Tender Loving Greed*. New York: Vintage Books, 1974.

Woodruff, D., and Birren, J. *Aging: Scientific Perspectives and Social Issues*. New York: D. Van Nostrand Co., 1975.

Zarit, S., ed. *Readings in Aging and Death*. New York: Harper and Row, 1977.

Notes

1. J. Birren, *The Psychology of Aging* (Englewood Cliffs, N.J.: Prentice-Hall, 1964), p. 1.

2. Population Reference Bureau, "The Elderly in America," *Population Bulletin* 30 (1975): 3.

3. Ibid.

4. M. Riley et al., *Aging and Society*, vol. 1 (New York: Russell Sage Foundation, 1968), p. 1.

5. Carole Offir, "At 65, Work Becomes a Four-Letter Word," *Psychology Today*, March 1974, p. 40.

6. Hermann Hesse, *Siddhartha*, translated by Hilda Rosner. Copyright 1951 by New Directions Publishing Corporation. Reprinted by permission of New Directions Publishing Corporation, New York.

7. Riley et al., *Aging and Society*, vol. 3, p. 3.

8. R. Butler and M. Lewis, *Aging and Mental Health* (St. Louis: The C. V. Mosby Co., 1977).

9. J. Kelly et al, "What the family physician should know about treating elderly patients, Part 1," *Geriatrics* 32, no. 9 (1977): 97–102, 105, 109–10.

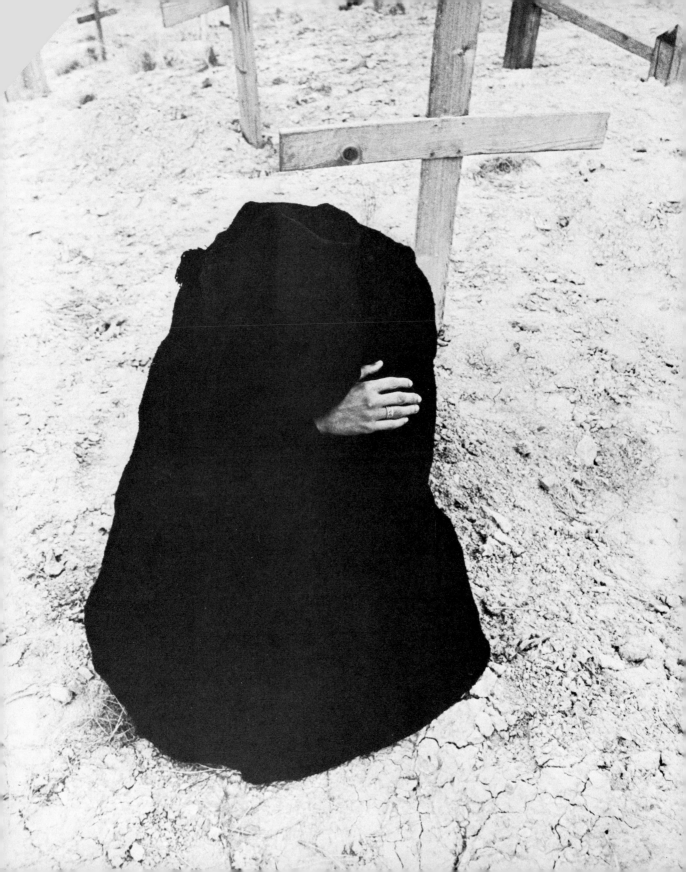

Death and Dying: Completion of the Life Cycle

25

Perhaps the ultimate human adaptation is the acceptance of death, the termination of life. Although the process of dying and the event of death for many people are taboo topics of investigation and consideration, they are nevertheless integral parts of the human life cycle. There can be no birth without death. Likewise, there can be no death without life.

Ideally, awareness and anticipation of death help prepare the individual to focus on life, to set priorities in living, and to appreciate the here-and-now of each precious moment. Preparation for death may thus be a growth and maturation experience for the living. In a most sublime way, a realization of our own mortality intensifies the human capacity for love.[1] We are more likely to focus on those relationships that build rather than destroy, to strive against petty resentment and argument, and to see that meaningful human relationships can transcend death.

Our anxieties and natural fears of death have been increased by the rather impersonal ways in which we die today.[2] Dying in hospitals and nursing homes—where a majority of deaths occur—has become lonely, psychologically isolated, mechanical, and even dehumanized to some degree, despite the advances of modern medical care. The terminally ill patient, divorced from the culture and community that defined life, is too often seen only in terms of heart rate, pulse, pulmonary function, and urinary output. Rarely are the feelings, concerns, opinions, or desires of the dying considered. And because medical specialization usually offers sequential and discontinuous care, many will die without a true medical advocate.

It is probably true that most of us acknowledge the reality of death—for the other person. We infrequently accept the possibility of our own deaths, except as the result of accident. The thought of just wearing out and dying of natural causes in old age is barely tolerated. And yet, as science and technology successfully extend human life, just such a death is the probable fate of nearly two thirds of our aging population.

Our perceptions of death vary and reflect diverse values and philosophies. Death may be seen as punishment for our sins, an act of atonement, or a judgment of a just God. For some, death means loneliness and a destruction of personality with a total loss of identity. Of course, death may be viewed as a cruel interruption of

Death in Modern Society

Differing Perceptions of Death

the human quest for happiness in which death itself is the common denominator for all men and women. Others think of death as redemption, a relief from pain and from the trials and tribulations of earth. Some embrace death and welcome it as a friend, the gentle night, the necessary end of the human experience. Still others perceive death in terms of fulfillment, completion, or accomplishment. Rather than the fearful termination of life, death is that grand conclusion to a beautiful story. To some extent, then, how we depart from this earthly abode is influenced by how we have lived. According to Leonardo da Vinci, "As a well-spent day brings happy sleep, so a well-spent life brings happy death."[3]

Denial and Avoidance of Death

Although attitudes toward death may vary, a general and current reaction to the necessity of dying is one of *denial* and *avoidance*. Such denial takes various forms:[4, 5]

- The tendency of the funeral directing industry to gloss over death and to fashion greater lifelike qualities in the dead.
- The adoption of euphemistic language for death, such as "exiting," "passing on," "never say die," and "good for life," which implies forever.
- The reduction of death from a necessity and essentiality to a mere mishap, the ultimate misfortune in the scientific quest for permanence.

Fig. 25.1. Attitudes toward death vary among people, but death is an event we all must eventually accept.

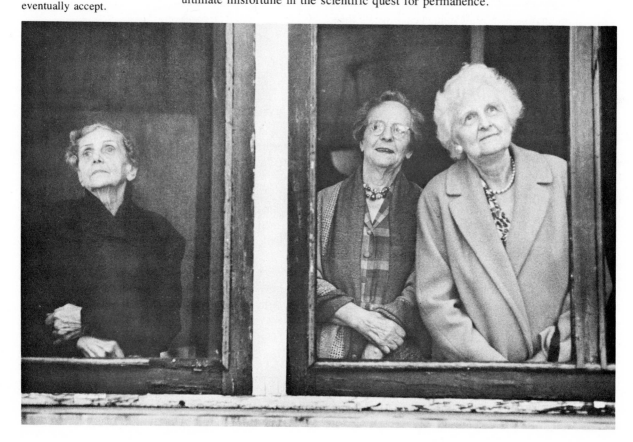

Chapter Twenty-Five

- The persistent search for the "fountain of youth" as expressed in clothing styles, effects of cosmetics, and the visible effects of dieting.
- The rejection and isolation of the aged and aging who remind us of death.
- The adoption of the concept of a pleasant and rewarding "afterlife," thus giving rise to immortality.
- The fixation on and preoccupation with sexual expression and proving one's potency. As long as we can do it, we are still vital, and not dead yet.[6]
- The emphasis of the medical profession on the prolongation of biological life rather than on diminishing human suffering.
- The frequent shielding of children from the "horrors" of death.
- The attempt to conquer death through expressions of violence, strength, cruelty, and aggression, all of which exert some control over the lives of others—and their deaths too.

In many ways, then, we are death-avoiders and death-deniers. However, the denial of death is responsible in part for the countless empty and purposeless lives lived today. As Kübler-Ross notes,

> When you live as if you'll live forever, it becomes too easy to postpone the things you know that you must do. You live your life in preparation for tomorrow or in remembrance of yesterday, and meanwhile each today is lost. In contrast, when you fully understand that each day you awaken could be the last you have, you take time that day to grow, to become more of who you really are, to reach out to other human beings.[7]

Thus, to grow, we must learn to die to our confining chains of restraint and be open to the possibilities of experiencing life and loving others.

Many persons prefer not to think about their own deaths because they feel powerless about the inevitable. They fail to see that the reality of death provides each individual with numerous opportunities for adaptation—choices to be made and options or alternatives to be exercised. In a real sense, we can prepare for death if we perceive it as a stage of growth rather than as the enemy.

Worden and Proctor[8] and Draznin[9] identify several facets of our mortality and approaching death, all of which can be influenced by personal actions and decisions. For instance, we can choose how we view our own deaths and the deaths of loved ones. We can have some input into how we want to be remembered by friends and family. We can indeed choose to fear death less, order our lives on the basis of a limited life span, and begin to intensify and improve our present relationships.

We can indicate where we would prefer to die (at home, in a hospital, or in a nursing home), what to do with our bodies once we are finished with them, and we can decide whether or not to carry life insurance or prepare a will.

Presently, as an individual, you may choose among several alternatives for funeral arrangements and body disposition. You can even develop resources for confronting death in your own family and among your friends, and prepare your spouse for widowhood in the future—a reality which three out of four wives will

Preparing for Death: Choices and Decisions

eventually experience. You can achieve the psychological upper hand over your own terminal illness if you have the need and the desire to do so!

While thousands of persons exercise the option of self-destruction or suicide each year, many others simply prefer to let nature take its course. In the event of serious debilitation in a terminal illness, they desire not to have their lives extended by artificial life support systems when there is no likelihood of recovery. Such individuals seek a dignified and natural death, and a legal means of implementing their right to die.

The state of California has taken the lead in permitting terminally ill patients to have some legal influence over their own dying. The California Natural Death Act authorizes persons to give their prior consent to have artificial life-support systems, such as respirators and kidney dialysis machines, withdrawn under certain specified conditions. Several legal safeguards are provided, however, for the patient's own protection. The consent document is a legal document, considered to be a form of "living will," which will be discussed later in this chapter.

Hoping to have part of themselves live on in someone else, millions of Americans have voluntarily donated their body organs for transplants. Others have made plans to give their entire bodies upon death to institutions for medical education and research. Kidneys, corneas of the eyes, pituitary glands, ear bones, and other body tissues and organs can be designated as gifts under the provisions of the Uniform Anatomical Gift Act or similar state laws. Organ donors typically carry a special Uniform Donor Card or have such information on their drivers' licenses. The common options include the donation of (1) any needed organs or parts, (2) only designated organs or parts, or (3) the whole body, for anatomical study, if necessary.

If your own state does not make provision for such donations on its driver's license, you can obtain a free Uniform Donor Card from the National Kidney Foundation, the Eye-Bank Association of America, and the American Medical Association. Of course, special forms for body donation can be procured from medical schools and state anatomical boards. Your own family physician will probably be able to assist you in getting the necessary forms.

Just because you have designated yourself a donor does not mean that an appropriate recipient will be located for your organs and tissues. In addition, you should not consider body donation as the perfect cure for the high cost of funerals and burial. If your body is not suitable, that is, too large, too diseased, or too traumatized by accident, or not needed by the medical school at the time of your death, your survivors will have to finance the disposition of your remains.

| Dimensions of Death and Dying | The final human experience is marked by a cessation of vital bodily functions. |

Functional Death   Evidence of this *functional,* or *somatic, death* includes the absence of heartbeat and spontaneous breathing. However, due to modern medical technology that has made possible the resuscitation of both cardiac and pulmonary functioning, many medical authorities now include the death of the brain among the criteria for determining the termination of life.[10]

Brain Death   This type of death is established by the absence of electrical impulse activity in the brain as shown on an *electroencephalogram* (EEG). Other indicators of brain death are unresponsiveness to pain, unreceptiveness to stimulation, and the absence of reflexes.

Several states have recently defined death legally in terms of the absence of brain waves.

Cellular Death   Although vital body organs cease to function, many cells in the body continue to live for some time after somatic death. Muscles continue to respond, and certain groups of cells removed from a dead body may be kept alive indefinitely in tissue cultures.[11] Thus, cellular death, as manifest in rigor mortis (the death-stiffening of the body's muscles), can be distinguished from functional death.

Spiritual Death   Some professionals who care for the dying now recognize a fourth type of death, that is, spiritual death, or death of the being.[12] This concept is based on the association of meaningful life or being, including responsiveness to others, with the activity of the brain and consciousness. While physical processes can be maintained, sometimes through extraordinary medical procedures and life-support systems, meaningful personhood beyond the vegetative state is impossible.

While the biological aspects of death are often emphasized and confirmed by an *autopsy* or postmortem examination of the human remains, the process of dying is also a psychological experience. The crisis of death is marked by a genuine fear of the unknown, coupled with the fear of loneliness. What is perceived as strange and undesirable, but which cannot be fully anticipated, fosters a deep fear in the individual. This "basic death anxiety" is often reinforced by the isolation of the hospital room and the removal of the patient from decision-making processes and the familiar surroundings of home and community.

Fear of death also includes the fear of abandonment, and the loss of family and friends. If body image is distorted by disease or injury, patients may think of themselves as unlovable and rejected—even by physicians and nurses—thus contributing to their emotional isolation. The death fear also encompasses the fear of loss of control, fear of loss of personal identity, and fear of regression, the instinct to death (the Freudian construct of Thanatos) that pushes the individual ". . . to retreat from the outer world of reality to a primal world of fantasy and bliss."[13]

Psychological reactions or adaptations to the reality of impending death have been researched by Elisabeth Kübler-Ross in interviews with hundreds of terminally ill patients. She has divided the behavior of dying patients into five stages described as follows.[14] It should be emphasized that these stages do not always follow one another in the precise order listed and that the several stages often overlap one another. Patients sometimes go back and forth from one stage to another.[15]

Psychological Experience

Psychological Reactions or Adaptations

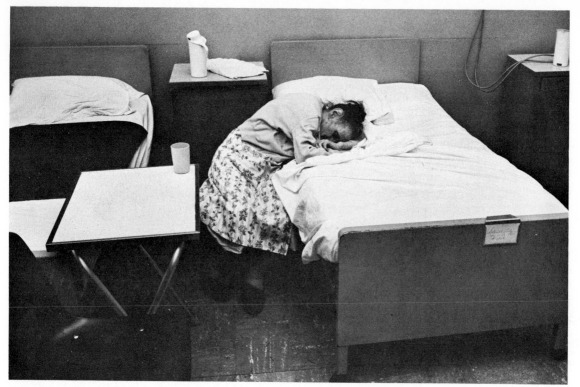

Fig. 25.2. Some people welcome death as an end to suffering or as the beginning of a new "life," while others fight death to the very moment it occurs. Depression is a normal stage in the process of accepting death.

First Stage: Denial and Isolation   Commonly, the initial reaction to awareness of a terminal illness is one of shock and denial. Often, the patient responds with such statements as, "No, it can't be me. It is not true. It's not possible." Denial, though, is usually a temporary defense and is soon partially replaced with acceptance when patients are confronted with financial matters or unfinished business and begin to worry about their surviving children.

Second Stage: Anger   When denial can no longer be maintained, it gives way to feelings of anger, resentment, rage, and envy. Now the patient's question is: "Why me?" The patient becomes increasingly difficult to care for as the anger is displaced and projected on to physicians, nurses, hospital staff, family members, and even God. The realization of loss is great, and those persons and things that symbolize life, energy, and functioning are particular targets of resentment and jealousy.

Third Stage: Bargaining   Sometimes originating in unexpressed guilt, the dying patient enters into a brief period of negotiating—often with God— in an attempt to postpone death or relieve pain and physical discomfort. Psychologically, the patient is saying, "Yes, me, but . . . ." In exchange for a few more days, weeks, or months of life, the patient promises to lead a reformed life dedicated to God or in service to others as part of the bargain.

Fourth Stage: Depression With the realization of the certainty of death, patients often enter a period of "preparatory grief," during which they become very silent, refuse visitors, and spend much of their time in crying or grieving. Such normal behavior is actually an effort to disconnect the self from all love objects. Attempts to cheer up patients at this stage should be discouraged because they have a real need to contemplate their impending death.

Fifth Stage: Acceptance If a patient has progressed through the stages described above, a final period is usually experienced. It is marked by peace, a unique acceptance of one's fate, and a desire to be left alone. While this stage is not precisely a happy one—it is often devoid of feelings—physical pain and discomfort tend to be absent. It has been characterized as the end of the struggle, the final resting stage before undertaking a long journey. According to one observer, this acceptance is like the very beginning of life,

> when a person has physical needs and needs only one person to give him some tender, loving care and compassion—who can be with him but doesn't have to talk all the time.[16]

Although many observers cite a decline in the belief in an afterlife as increasing the fear of death, the belief or hope in some form of life after death has been nearly universal until the present age. Some contend that such a belief is foolish and superstitious; others base their firm belief on faith and find that the promise of life beyond the grave is reassuring and comforting.

The Afterlife and Near-Death Experiences

Concepts of the afterlife vary, with some placing greater emphasis on the survival of the spirit or mind while others focus on some form of renewed physical existence. Some more common interpretations of life after physical death include the survival of the soul of the person; the immortality of one's genes through reproduction; an ever-evolving purification and growth of the spirit; reunion with the Godhead; the general resurrection of the body; everlasting rewards of heaven and the punishments of hell; rebirth of the soul in another person or object (reincarnation); and a cosmic consciousness or eventual unification of all minds, as proposed by Koestler.[17]

While theologians and philosophers debate the possibilities and nature of life after death, an increasing amount of evidence has been reported suggesting that the end of the body is not necessarily the end of life experiences. One researcher, Raymond Moody, studied the condition of near death in three categories of subjects: (1) persons who had been resuscitated after being pronounced clinically dead; (2) those who had come very close to physical death through severe injury or illness; and (3) individuals who told of their experiences as they died.[18]

Moody's findings, substantiated in part by other researchers, revealed a common pattern of near-death phenomena. Those persons who were studied reported having experiences of

- Hearing oneself being pronounced dead by a doctor or some other person.
- Feelings of peace and quiet after the physical distress of dying.

- Hearing noises, such as loud buzzing sounds or ringing sounds, sometimes reported as musical.
- Feelings of rapid movement through a dark space or tunnel.
- Being out-of-body, that is, viewing one's own body from a distance.
- Meeting other spiritual beings who were prepared to ease the transition into death for the newly deceased.
- Encountering very bright lights, often interpreted as beings of light.
- Undergoing a panoramic review of one's life events in conjunction with an evaluation.
- Approaching a form of border or limit between earthly life and the life beyond life.
- Coming back to oneself, or the reunion of self with one's physical body.

Although some persons have used Moody's findings as evidence of life after death, he maintains that testimony about near death is not proof that we survive death. In an evaluation of Moody's research, one critic concludes that:

> Even if such cases can be documented, a skeptic could still argue that a person had these experiences before death, as the brain was losing its oxygen supply, not during the period of the flat EEG. As yet there is simply no sure way to know. This is one scientific debate of which each of us, in the end, is the final judge.[19]

Prolongation of Life
Advances in medical science and innovations in medical technology have made possible the maintenance of heart action and breathing in the dying patient for considerable periods of time. Diseased and malfunctioning body organs can be replaced in some instances by synthetic and mechanical parts and, in limited circumstances, by organ transplantation from human donors. Indeed, it appears as if some measure of immortality is being achieved through the prolongation of life now made possible by medical technology.

Such miracles of medicine now pose new dilemmas for physicians, theologians, lawyers, and society in general, to say nothing of the terminally ill patient. Should hopelessly ill persons in agonizing pain be kept alive? What about the person whose brain has been irreparably damaged by a lack of oxygen or the trauma of a bullet or grenade? How long should resuscitation procedures be continued? The ultimate question regarding the value of life might be posed as follows:

> Is the extra life span and the degree of rehabilitation worth the discomfort, the psychological hazards, the long hospital stay, the enormous cost, and the tying up of a large part of a hospital staff when other patients need care?[20]

A "Living Will"
Traditionally, the medical profession has dictated that every possible skill be used to ease pain and extend life. Such has been the expectation of the lay public. However, there is a growing tendency to view the right to die with dignity as equally valid as the right to live. Evidence of this belief is seen in the requests of thousands of persons for free copies of the so-called "living will" from the Euthanasia Educational Council.

TO MY FAMILY, MY PHYSICIAN, MY LAWYER, MY CLERGYMAN
TO ANY MEDICAL FACILITY IN WHOSE CARE I HAPPEN TO BE
TO ANY INDIVIDUAL WHO MAY BECOME RESPONSIBLE FOR MY HEALTH, WELFARE OR AFFAIRS

Death is as much a reality as birth, growth, maturity and old age—it is the one certainty of life. If the time comes when I, _____, can no longer take part in decisions for my own future, let this statement stand as an expression of my wishes, while I am still of sound mind.

If the situation should arise in which there is no reasonable expectation of my recovery from physical or mental disability, I request that I be allowed to die and not be kept alive by artificial means or "heroic measures." I do not fear death itself as much as the indignities of deterioration, dependence and hopeless pain. I, therefore, ask that medication be mercifully administered to me to alleviate suffering even though this may hasten the moment of death.

This request is made after careful consideration. I hope you who care for me will feel morally bound to follow its mandate. I recognize that this appears to place a heavy responsibility upon you, but it is with the intention of relieving you of such responsibility and of placing it upon myself in accordance with my strong convictions, that this statement is made.

Signed _____

Date _____

Witness _____

Witness _____

Copies of this request have been given to _____

_____

_____

_____

Fig. 25.3. "A Living Will," The Euthanasia Educational Council, 250 West 57th Street, New York, N.Y. 10019.

Such a living will appears in figure 25.3. Although this and similar documents such as the Christian Affirmation of Life are considered legal, they have no legal force at present. The living will represents an assertion of the individual's right to self-determination over his or her own body. The recently passed California statute pertains only to the withdrawal of life-sustaining treatment, and says nothing about the administration of pain relievers that could hasten death.

Euthanasia   The term *euthanasia* has been used synonymously with mercy killing, and during the Nazi reign in Germany, it assumed the dimensions of genocide or legalized mass murder. However, euthanasia actually means a "good death," an easy, painless, and happy death.[21]

Two general types or categories of euthanasia are now recognized:

- Direct or active euthanasia in which a physician administers a large dose of medicine which, while easing pain, depresses the central nervous system to such an extent that the brain centers controlling heart action and breathing no longer function. At present, this form of deliberately terminating a suffering person's life is not legal in any civilized nation.
- Indirect or passive euthanasia in which specific medical procedures or techniques, such as oxygen administration, intravenous feeding, and heart surgery—all of which could prolong life—are either omitted or withheld from a terminally ill patient. Surveys indicate that this form of euthanasia is practiced by more than a few physicians.[22]

Convincing arguments for and against euthanasia exist. Proponents hold that extreme suffering is degrading and demoralizing. To maintain an individual in a vegetative state when there is no hope of recovery is not only immoral but places a severe burden on the family of the patient and on society in general. Opponents cite the biblical commandment prohibiting killing and thus perceive euthanasia as murder. Furthermore, there is great concern over who would exercise control over life and death and the abuses of power that could result. Would there ever be a temptation to eliminate the aged, the inefficient, and those whose beliefs and practices represented a threat or burden to the ruling class?[23]

Grief and Mourning   The death of a loved one often precipitates a psychological crisis in the survivors. Such mental suffering or *grief* is characterized by a profound sense of loneliness, fear, and despair. These reactions are normal and are commonly experienced by the bereaved—those who have lost a close relative or friend.

Several factors influence the nature, duration, and reactions of grief, including the specific relationship between the survivor and the deceased, the meaning of the dead person, the functions of the dead person in the life of the survivor, and the nature of the changes in the survivor's life that result from the death.[24] Sometimes a narcissistic response surfaces in an individual whose son or daughter has just been killed in an automobile accident. The parent might ask, "Why did this tragedy happen to me?" Perhaps less narcissism would be revealed in the response, "Why did this terrible thing happen to my child?" Guilt reactions can be common too, especially if the relationship between the survivor and the deceased was marked by resentment as well as affection or if the survivor secretly wished for the death of a terminally ill patient.

Three Stages of Grief   The main tasks of the mourner are freeing oneself emotionally from the deceased, readjusting to a life in which the dead person is missing, and the forming of new relationships with other persons. This grief work is facilitated by the progression of the survivor through a predictable course of ordinary behavior defined in three somewhat distinct stages.[25]

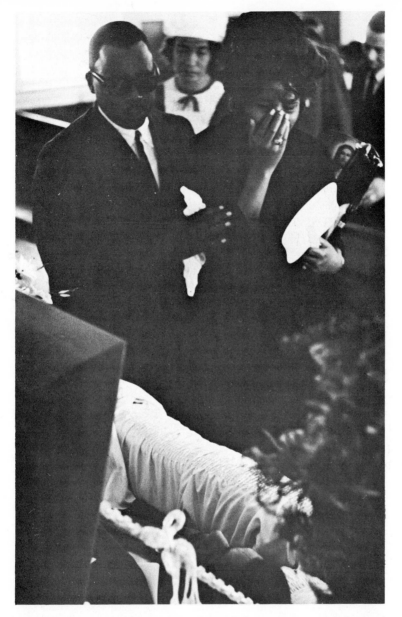

Fig. 25.4. The outward
expression of grief helps
the mourner adjust
to the loss of a friend
or relative.

Stage 1 This stage is manifest by shock, disbelief, numbness, weeping and wailing, and agitation. It often begins immediately after death and usually lasts from one to three days. This stage of grief is similar to the denial and anger stages in the Kübler-Ross classification of the stages of dying.

Stage 2 This stage is characterized by painful longing for the dead, memories and visual images of the deceased, sadness, insomnia, irritability, and restlessness. Beginning shortly after death, this stage of grief peaks between the second and fourth weeks, subsides after three months, but may persist for up to one year. Elements of bargaining for the return of the deceased person as well as depression may be detected, again corresponding to the stages of dying.

Stage 3 Usually this stage occurs within a year after death. Analogous to the acceptance or last stage of dying, this grief-resolution phase is marked by the resumption of ordinary life activities, the ability to recall the past and the deceased with interest and pleasure, and the establishment of new relationships with others.

Some persons never recover completely, as the grief may linger, especially when a child is lost. On occasion, survivors even develop neurotic depression, false euphoria, psychosomatic illnesses, self-destructive impulses, and the physical symptoms experienced by the deceased. Medical assistance and psychological counseling can be helpful in resolving such manifestations of grief.

Funeral Ritual   In most cultures, people have found that the grieving process is facilitated through the funeral ritual. Although the funeral is most often a communal act that recognizes the unique value of a particular dead person, it nevertheless serves many needs of the survivors.

Indeed, the funeral "... is a time for the living to face the fact of their mortality, that they for a time live a life measured by space and time."[26] Additionally, funerals help separate the physical and emotional bonds between the deceased and the survivors, accomplish the transition to life without the deceased, and serve to bind the bereaved to the group of the living. Group participation in the funeral ritual can be a rich source of emotional support and strength for the mourner.[27]

When someone dies, the survivors often experience an unconscious threat to their own "body image." Seeing the remains of the other person helps reduce such fear and reaffirms the viability of the survivors. Funerals also help assure the bereaved that when they die, their bodies will be disposed of properly and in a dignified manner. The rituals associated with a funeral also remind the survivors that despite the mental chaos of grief there remains a certain structure and order in the social system and that life continues.

It is unfortunate that in a society that largely denies death, the vital and wholesome work of grief is actually discouraged. While for a few days after a death there are still some rituals to be followed, such as the sending of flowers and of food to the bereaved, donating money to specific charities, and home visitations,

the general attitude, either implied or actually spoken, is, "Think about something else. That's the best way," a poor approach were it possible to follow it. For it is harmful psychologically to interrupt the helpful work of mourning.[28]

Thus, by adapting to death through denial, we tend to interfere with the normal grieving process and to prolong it unnecessarily or suppress it as if it were a personal weakness.

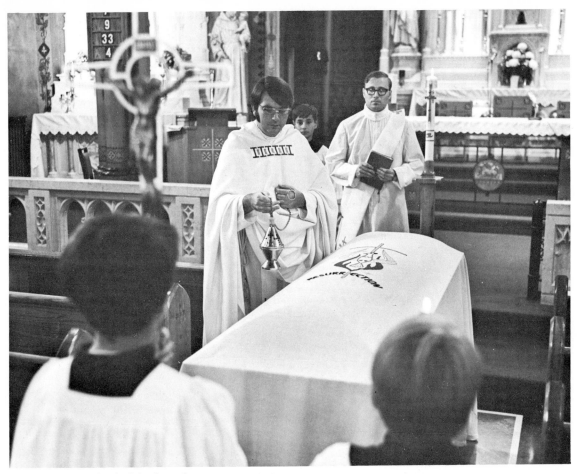

Fig. 25.5.   The ritual of the funeral
itself allows for the expression of grief in
a communal setting.

Increasing numbers of individuals are concerned about the relatively high cost of
funerals and body disposition. Many people make funeral and burial arrangements in advance of actual need, either with a reputable funeral director or
through a memorial society. (The memorial society is a cooperative organization
that assists members in selecting needed funeral services by advance planning.)
Others plan with family members so that the survivors can follow the general or
specific wishes of the deceased in providing a dignified, simple, yet economical
funeral.

Most Americans, however, will face the expenses of the funeral and body
disposition only when a family member has died. This is usually a time marked
by many pressures, emotional distress, diluted bargaining power, and lack of
experience in making informed and rational decisions. Unfortunately, the deep
sense of guilt on the part of some survivors, their reluctance to ask about various

options, and their desire to put a loved one away in style often increase the likelihood of their purchasing unnecessary services and merchandise.

Various choices are available in funerals, cemetery burials, and grave markers. As the Federal Trade Commission's Seattle Regional Office reports, prices for such services and merchandise sold by the death-related industries vary substantially, and inexpensive arrangements can be made. However,

> . . . because of the shroud of secrecy these businesses have historically thrown over their industries and prices, consumers must aggressively seek out information, especially price information, in order to make an informed funeral, cemetery, and grave marker purchase.[29]

Those who are planning a funeral or arranging for body disposition should be aware of the several categories of conventional expenses.[30]

- Basic services of the funeral home staff; embalming; use of facilities and equipment; restoration of the body and casketing; transportation of the body; arrangements for clergy and ground burial; acquisition of death certificates; assistance in obtaining certain governmental benefits from the Veteran's Administration or from social security
- Casket or body container
- Vault or liner, an encasement for the casket often required by local cemeteries to prevent settling of the ground around the casket
- Cemetery plot, mausoleum crypt, urn garden or columbarium niche
- Charges for opening and closing the grave at the time of burial
- Grave marker, or urn for cremated remains

It is not uncommon for the average funeral and body disposition expense to exceed $2,000. Of course, some pay less, while many pay much more.

Alternatives to traditional funeral and body disposition methods are available. Besides donation of the body to medical science, there is cremation of the body, or reducing the body to ashes by means of heat. Cremation may occur immediately after death and be followed later by a memorial service. Sometimes, though, cremation follows the usual funeral ritual. Regardless of when cremation takes place, it costs considerably less than ground burial.

Although the number of cremations is increasing somewhat, many persons will prefer ground burial for personal, religious, or philosophical reasons. Without regard to which options are chosen, the obvious advantage of preplanning is that it permits a reasonable consideration of choices and alternatives, and even comparison shopping, if one so desires. Thus, survivors will not be forced to make so many and such costly decisions at the last minute.

Behavioral Adaptations with the Dying and the Survivors

When you interrelate with dying family members or friends who are terminally ill, remember that they are still living, for dying is part of living. Those persons still have value as human beings and still have many human needs, physical and mental. They will likely be going through one or more of the psychological stages described by Kübler-Ross, but do not attempt to move them from one psychological stage to another. Accept them as they are.

Price alone does not tell consumers everything they might want or need to know about death arrangements...Consumers may, for example, prefer a given funeral home or cemetery on the basis of reputation, prior service, location, religious or ethnic identification, physical facilities or any of several other considerations. While these nonprice factors can be important, consumers must decide for themselves just how important they are in terms of dollars and cents.

Source: Seattle Regional Office, Federal Trade Commission

The purpose of embalming is to make the corpse presentable for viewing during a funeral. If viewing is not desired or if a corpse is to be viewed only during the period immediately after death, embalming may not be necessary. Embalming fluid preserves the body for only a few days. It is a mistake to think that the fluid retards deterioration for any significant amount of time.

Embalming requirements vary from state to state. Many states require embalming only if the person has died of a communicable disease or if the body is to be transported over state lines. If the body is held for more than 24 hours (not buried or cremated immediately), embalming is often required. Some states do not require embalming if the funeral home holding the deceased has adequate refrigeration facilities.

Since embalming may be performed by a funeral home, even when it is not required by law, check out the laws or rules for embalming in your area. If embalming is not required, you may be able to decline an unnecessary expense.

The purchase of a casket for cremation is usually not required by law. However, some container may be required by the funeral home, cemetery or crematory. A fiberboard or plain wooden box may be adequate.

Cremation-after-viewing does not always require the purchase of a casket. Sometimes the deceased may be placed on a day bed or couch, or a casket may be loaned for viewing purposes. While some states do not allow the re-use of a casket, some do. Check this in your state!

After cremation, the deceased's remains may be scattered or placed in an urn or other container for burial or housing in a columbarium—a special building or wall for above-ground storage of cremated remains. Urn prices vary substantially, just as the costs of caskets do.

Most cemeteries require the purchase of a grave liner, a concrete container into which a casket is placed, to prevent the earth from caving in. Vaults are more elaborately designed and more expensive than grave liners but are used basically for the same purpose. However, vaults are alleged to be airtight and watertight and are sold to people with the belief that the sealing of a casket within a vault will preserve the deceased and the casket from deterioration and disintegration. While the casket may disintegrate more slowly within a vault, human remains deteriorate regardless of attempts to preserve them. Vaults are not required by state law, and any cemetery regulation can usually be satisfied by either a vault or a liner. Vaults can be an unnecessary expense and will greatly increase the total funeral and cemetery bill.

Often cemeteries have grave marker requirements as to material, size, style, etc., which may severely limit a consumer's choices. Consumers may find that some cemeteries will not permit installation of a monument purchased from an independent monument dealer. Alternatively, buyers may find some cemeteries charge a higher installation fee if a monument is purchased from an independent monument dealer. Therefore, it would be wise to check the cemetery's rules regarding markers before purchasing a lot or a marker. If the cemetery's rules are restrictive, its prices may be higher than others. Shop around!

Fig. 25.6. Learning the facts about funeral and body disposition expenses before a family member dies can protect the consumer from purchasing unnecessary services and merchandise later.

Dying and death are scary topics to be sure. Admit that you too are afraid, and drop the pretense that death will not occur. However, as many thanatologists and grief therapists suggest, always maintain hope for the dying. Attending physicians can assure patients that everything medically possible is being done to give them a fighting chance. You can assure the dying that you will be there as long as you are needed. This assurance can be proven by your presence, by holding and touching the dying, by mourning and weeping with them, and by recognizing how hard it is for them to die.

Ask if there is anything you can do to make dying persons more comfortable. Give them every opportunity to make even the smallest decision affecting their own care and comfort. Let them decide for themselves how much light there should be in the room, what position in bed is most comfortable for them, in what sequence to eat foods, if you are feeding them. You may also offer to help get final things in order—messages written and directions given. If you are willing and able, offer to help survivors cope with their problems after their loved ones have died. You may even be able to help the terminally ill resolve old conflicts with others. Certainly, you can listen while they reminisce about happy times and about people they remember with fondness.

If dying persons express rage, do not make them ashamed of such anger. If they are severely depressed, do not try to cheer them up. Accept their behavior, rude or strange as it may seem, without taking offense or threatening to leave them as a punishment for their being bad. Above all else, do not make others feel guilty about dying. After all, it is normal and natural to die. Do not induce guilt feelings in dying persons by implying that you consider their deaths acts of desertion. Recognize that crying and asking questions about death are normal expressions of feeling in the dying. Be willing to share their emotions and fears with them openly and honestly.

There is no one way to respond to the bereaved individuals who have lost their loved ones through death. There are, however, some ways you can help the grieving survivors recover from the shock of death.[31]

1. Permit and help bereaved persons put into words or otherwise express their feelings of pain, sorrow, and loss. Review with them their relationship with the deceased.
2. Help bereaved persons understand the changes they may be undergoing in their emotional reactions.
3. Help grieving individuals find the words to describe their future relationship with their memory of the deceased.
4. Act as a "primer or programmer" of activities for bereaved persons, and organize among your friends flexible, modest schemes for including the bereaved in your activities.
5. Assist the bereaved in dealing with such situations as doing household chores, notifying class instructors, procuring temporary financial or transportation resources.
6. Offer grieving persons your assistance in making future plans for the weeks immediately following the funeral.

7. Avoid interpreting the defensive behaviors of the bereaved as being abnormal. Also avoid excessive caring for and overprotection of survivors.

Not all of these actions will be available to you in consoling, soothing, and giving solace to your friends and relatives. If you can do nothing but listen responsively and display your sincere concern, you will have helped the bereaved adjust to the present situation. Do not encourage grieving friends to suppress their normal reactions of fear, anger, guilt, hostility, and loneliness. Instead, the National Funeral Directors Association recommends:

> Encourage the mourner to tell you what he feels, rather than trying to prescribe how he should feel.
> It is no help to say, "Don't talk about it." The survivor . . . may need to speak and act out his feelings—denial, turning slowly to bewilderment, and finally to the weeping, despairing confrontation with the truth of his loss.
> It is not necessary to say a great deal to the bereaved. The most significant approach may be non-verbal. A firm shake of the hands, a look into their eyes—will show that you care.[32]

Unfortunately, as Kastenbaum observes, "We are reluctant to pause for death. Thinking about the dead is a waste of time."[33] Our society has too often withdrawn support from the bereaved. In an abnormal manner, the world continues to move on as if nothing has happened, with little tolerance for or recognition of grieving. Perhaps we can contribute to the health of the bereaved by saying we care, we share your loss, and we are sorry. Maybe we too can learn, like the bereaved, that the pain and hurt of grief is the price we must pay for love and commitment. This too may be our final adaptation as we approach death, the final stage of life and growth.

Summary

Death has been portrayed as the ultimate human adaptation—a natural event in the life cycle. There can be no life without death. Yet our culture tends to be death avoiding and death denying.

Various dimensions of death were identified as: functional, brain death, cellular, and spiritual. Since the end of life is also a psychological experience, the five stages of death as defined by Kübler-Ross were also discussed. Problems of prolonging life and the controversy of euthanasia were explored, as well as the processes of grief and mourning.

The functions and the costs of funerals and body disposition were examined in terms of benefits to the survivors or to those who want to preplan for such events. The concluding section dealt with approaches to helping the terminally ill person and bereaved friends and family members.

Review Questions

1. As opposed to the past, why is death such an impersonal act today?
2. Give examples of how denial is used as a reaction against death.
3. Distinguish between cellular death and functional death.
4. Discuss Kübler-Ross's five stages of death.
5. Should terminally ill patients be allowed to die rather than be kept alive by machines?
6. Differentiate between active and passive euthanasia. Which could you support?
7. Why are funerals psychologically helpful for the bereaved?
8. List several categories of expense usually associated with funerals and body disposition.
9. Explain how you might help terminally ill persons live until they die. Be specific.
10. Which of the guidelines for dealing with bereaved survivors do you think would be the most difficult to put into practice? Why? Can you identify any other ways of helping bereaved persons?

Readings

Goleman, Daniel. "Back from The Brink," *Psychology Today,* April 1977, pp. 56, 58–59.

Grollman, Earl A. *Concerning Death: A Practical Guide for the Living.* Boston: Beacon Press, 1974.

Kübler-Ross, Elisabeth. *Death: The Final Stage of Growth.* Englewood Cliffs, N.J.: Prentice-Hall, Inc., 1975.

——————. *Questions and Answers on Death and Dying.* New York: Collier Books, 1974.

Mannes, Marya. *Last Rights.* New York: New American Library, Inc., 1973.

Mitford, Jessica. *The American Way of Death.* Greenwich, Conn.: Fawcett Publications, Inc., 1963.

Moody, Raymond A., Jr. *Life After Life.* New York: Bantam Books, Inc., 1975.

Morgan, Ernest, ed. *A Manual of Death Education and Simple Burial.* Burnsville, N.C.: Celo Press, 1975.

Notes

1. John P. Brantner, "Death and the Self," *Death Education: Preparation for Living,* ed. Betty R. Green and Donald P. Irish (Cambridge: Schenkman Publishing Co., 1971), pp. 24–26.
2. Elisabeth Kübler-Ross, *On Death and Dying* (New York: Macmillan Publishing Co., Inc., 1969), pp. 8–10.
3. John Langone, *Death Is a Noun* (Boston: Little, Brown and Co., 1972), p. 54.

4. Herman Feifel, "The Meaning of Death in American Society," *Death Education: Preparation for Living*, pp. 4–9.
5. Kübler-Ross, *On Death and Dying*, pp. 11–16.
6. Rollo May, *Love and Will* (New York: W. W. Norton & Co., Inc., 1969), pp. 105–7.
7. Elisabeth Kübler-Ross, *Death: The Final Stage of Growth* (Englewood Cliffs, N.J.: Prentice-Hall, Inc., 1975), p. 164.
8. J. William Worden and William Proctor, *PDA* Personal Death Awareness* (Englewood Cliffs, New Jersey: Prentice-Hall, Inc., 1976), p. 17.
9. Yaffa Draznin, *How To Prepare For Death: A Practical Guide* (New York: Hawthorn Books, Inc., 1976), pp. 3–7.
10. "O Death, Where Is Thy Definition?" *Medical World News*, 25 January 1974, pp. 35–36.
11. Arnold Toynbee et al., *Man's Concern with Death* (New York: McGraw-Hill Book Co., 1969), p. 19.
12. Langone, *Death Is a Noun*, p. 21.
13. E. Mansell Pattison, "The Experience of Dying," *American Journal of Psychotherapy*, January 1967, p. 40.
14. Kübler-Ross, *On Death and Dying*, pp. 38–137.
15. Elisabeth Kübler-Ross, "What Is It Like to Be Dying," *American Journal of Nursing*, January 1971, p. 56.
16. Ibid., p. 59.
17. Arthur Koestler, "Cosmic Consciousness," *Psychology Today*, April 1977, pp. 53–54, 104.
18. Raymond A. Moody, Jr., *Life After Life* (New York: Bantam Books, Inc., 1975), p. 16.
19. Daniel Goleman, "Back from the Brink," *Psychology Today*, April 1977, pp. 56, 58–59.
20. American Friends Service Committee, *Who Shall Live? Man's Control over Birth and Death* (New York: Hill and Wang, 1970), p. 45.
21. Florence Clothier, *Euthanasia—The Physician's Dilemma* (New York: The Euthanasia Educational Council, 1972), p. 1.
22. Daniel C. Maguire, "Death by Chance, Death by Choice," *Atlantic Monthly*, January 1974, p. 64.
23. Langone, *Death Is a Noun*, p. 62.
24. Eli Marcovitz, "What Is the Meaning of Death to the Dying Person and His Survivors?" *Omega* 4 (1973):19.
25. Robert B. White and Leroy T. Gathman, "The Syndrome of Ordinary Grief," *American Family Physician*, August 1973, p. 97.
26. Edgar N. Jackson, *The Christian Funeral* (New York: Channel Press, 1966), p. 33.
27. Paul E. Irion, *The Funeral: Vestige or Value?* (New York: Abingdon Press, 1966), p. 99.
28. Sarah Morris, *Grief and How to Live with It* (New York: Grosset and Dunlap Publishers, 1972), p. 60.
29. Federal Trade Commission, Seattle Regional Office, *The Price of Death: A Survey Method and Consumer Guide for Funerals, Cemeteries and Grave Markers* (Seattle: The Commission, 1975), p. 2.
30. Maryland Center for Public Broadcasting, *Consumer Survival Kit—The Last Rights: A Look At Funerals* (Owings Mills, Md.: The Center, 1975), p. 1.
31. Irwin Gerber et al., "Brief Therapy to the Aged Bereaved," in *Bereavement: Its Psychosocial Aspects*, eds. Bernard Schoenberg et al. (New York: Columbia University Press, 1975), pp. 313–14.
32. National Funeral Directors Association, *The Condolence or Sympathy Visit* (Milwaukee: The Association, n.d.), pp. 2–3.
33. Robert J. Kastenbaum, *Death, Society, & Human Experience* (St. Louis: The C. V. Mosby Company, 1977), p. 262.

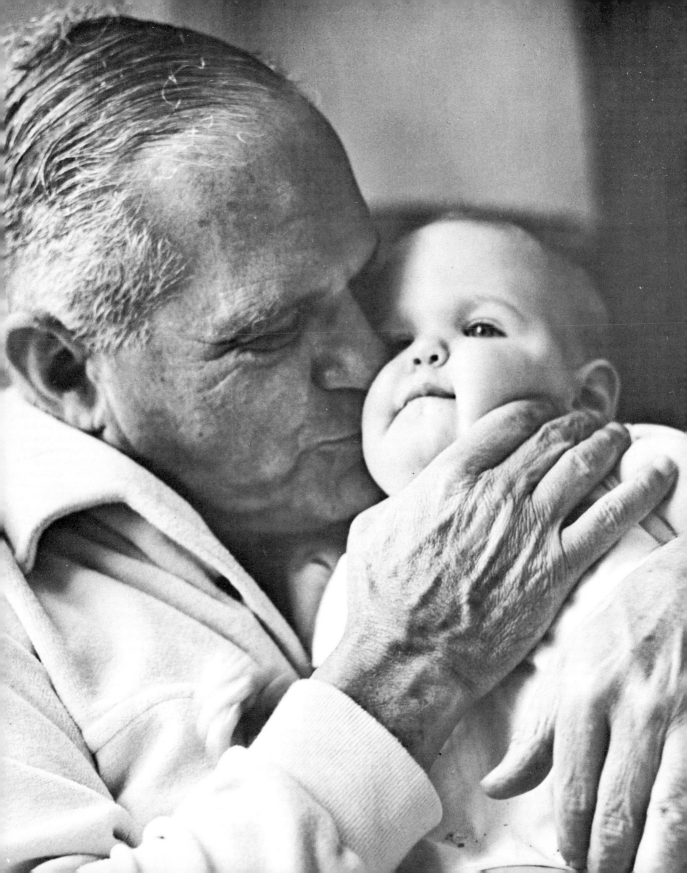

Quality Life:
The Ultimate Goal

26

If you were assigned the task of writing a paper explaining what adaptations will be necessary for you personally to make as you face the next month, the next year, or the next decade, what specific entities would you present? Change is ever present in the world. Each of us is uncertain as we contemplate the future. Yet meeting challenges is what makes living exciting and interesting.

Not one of us knows what will happen in the future. As we think of those changes in health and medicine that have occurred in the past generation, we can only surmise as to what will take place in the next. With ever-increasing attempts to develop new and better medicines and medical procedures and to improve the health care delivery system, we are assured that changes are inevitable. The effect of these changes will certainly have positive and possibly negative effects on the personal health and well-being of everyone.

Throughout the various parts of this textbook, it has been our desire to suggest ways in which mankind will need to adapt and consequences that might result if adaptation does not occur. Hopefully, future adaptations will contribute to a better quality of life for everyone. Only as individual health and quality of life are enhanced will the character of society improve.

A positive force that is receiving considerable attention today is the concept of preventive health care. This concept should have been paramount in our thinking and actions through the past years. However, most Americans have been crisis-oriented with regard to their health. Traditionally, medical care has been sought only when the person was ill or the possibility of sickness was imminent. It is being realized more each year that costs and long-range health problems might be reduced or eliminated if ongoing preventive measures are taken to protect one's personal health and well-being.

The concept of life-style was presented in an earlier chapter. Most people have given little thought to the role that personal life-styles play in their well-being. Hopefully, as more emphasis is directed to preventive health care, the individual will evaluate his or her life patterns and make those adjustments that will contribute to a better quality of life. Such adjustments may well mean eating less or differently than at present, giving up a habit that is hard to break yet certainly harmful to health (i.e., smoking), becoming more active in a physical sense (walking or riding a bicycle to work, jogging, etc.), or having a yearly physical examination. Many more personal adjustments could be identified.

Preventive
Health Care

The individual in future years must be motivated to *want* to adapt his or her life-style in ways that will result in a more positive level of health and well-being. This becomes quite difficult as we find ourselves attempting to cope with varying value systems. Such motivation will only come about as people become more knowledgeable concerning health. All the health services in the world might be available, but without the desire or personal motivation to use them, they will be of no value. For example, one of the best procedures to identify early signs of uterine cancer in the female is the Pap smear. This is well known by many women. However, why aren't more women motivated to have an annual Pap test? It is this kind of motivation that must be better understood in the years ahead and can then be used to modify behavior for more positive health.

What do you see as a change in life-style that you should make that will necessitate some adaptive process and yet is necessary for better personal health? Are you, your family, and your friends prepared to make those needed adjustments in life-style? Have there been any changes in your health behavior since the beginning of this school term and your reading of the first chapter of this book?

Right to Environment Free from Dangers to Health

An increasing emphasis upon preventive health care and the *right* to live in a healthful environment will lead to some interesting individual as well as community adaptations. Smoking has long been considered a right that an individual has if he or she so desires. However, little thought or consideration has been given to what right the nonsmoker has to live and work in areas free from air polluted by smoke. It would seem as though the nonsmoker has a right to travel in an airplane, bus, or train; to listen to a lecture or attend a concert in an auditorium; to work; or to eat at a restaurant, without being exposed to air filled with the smoke from cigarette, pipe, or cigars. This will call for major changes as separate areas for the smoker and the nonsmoker will be demanded.

The right to a pollution-free environment will be one that you should come to expect in your adult years. The past generation has basically focused upon industrial development; little thought was given to the condition of the environment in which we live. To bring about a pollution-free environment, a number of life-styles in America will need to be changed. Some of these changes were discussed in previous chapters on the environment. If we fail to make needed changes, both as individuals and collectively as a society, one can only suggest, as René Dubos pointed out in 1973, that "we shall experience some disastrous problems of disease or, at least, a progressive degradation of public health if we continue to accept . . . that pollution is one of the facts of life."[1]

The Baby Boom and the Future

In the years immediately following World War II, the latter part of the 1940s, the 1950s, and into the early 1960s, a great number of individuals were born. This became known as "the baby boom." At every stage of life since birth, this large influx of persons has created serious problems and upheavals for various societal institutions involved. When they entered elementary and then secondary school, there was a tremendous shortage of classrooms, teachers, and resources to meet

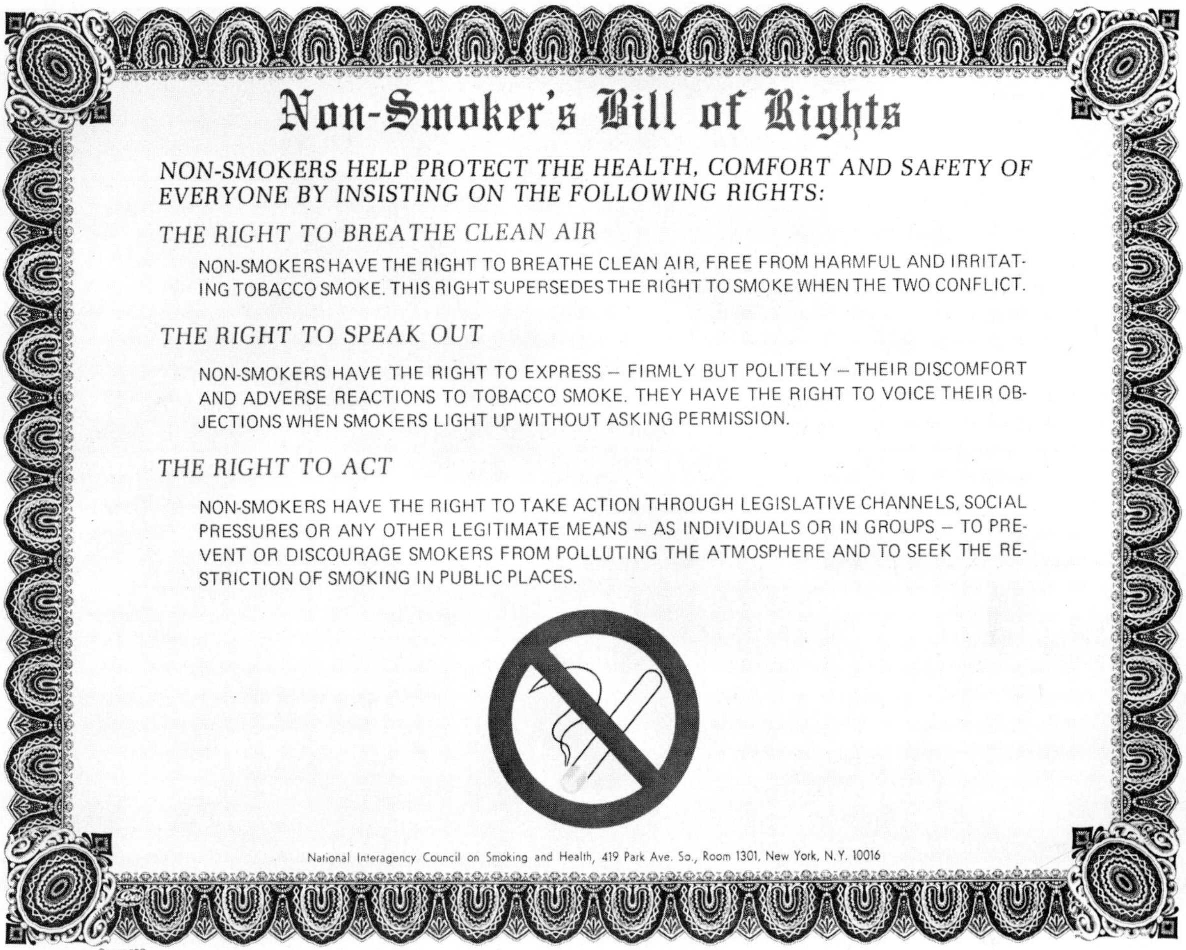

Non-Smoker's Bill of Rights

NON-SMOKERS HELP PROTECT THE HEALTH, COMFORT AND SAFETY OF EVERYONE BY INSISTING ON THE FOLLOWING RIGHTS:

THE RIGHT TO BREATHE CLEAN AIR

NON-SMOKERS HAVE THE RIGHT TO BREATHE CLEAN AIR, FREE FROM HARMFUL AND IRRITATING TOBACCO SMOKE. THIS RIGHT SUPERSEDES THE RIGHT TO SMOKE WHEN THE TWO CONFLICT.

THE RIGHT TO SPEAK OUT

NON-SMOKERS HAVE THE RIGHT TO EXPRESS — FIRMLY BUT POLITELY — THEIR DISCOMFORT AND ADVERSE REACTIONS TO TOBACCO SMOKE. THEY HAVE THE RIGHT TO VOICE THEIR OBJECTIONS WHEN SMOKERS LIGHT UP WITHOUT ASKING PERMISSION.

THE RIGHT TO ACT

NON-SMOKERS HAVE THE RIGHT TO TAKE ACTION THROUGH LEGISLATIVE CHANNELS, SOCIAL PRESSURES OR ANY OTHER LEGITIMATE MEANS — AS INDIVIDUALS OR IN GROUPS — TO PREVENT OR DISCOURAGE SMOKERS FROM POLLUTING THE ATMOSPHERE AND TO SEEK THE RESTRICTION OF SMOKING IN PUBLIC PLACES.

National Interagency Council on Smoking and Health, 419 Park Ave. So., Room 1301, New York, N.Y. 10016

Fig. 26.1. The right to a pollution-free environment is a right you should come to expect in your adult years.

the educational needs of these young people. New schools were built, and educational facilities multiplied. As this crowd of humanity started to come of college age in the mid-1960s, colleges and universities grew rapidly, with many institutions of higher education doubling or tripling their enrollments in a very few years. Associated with this rapid growth of colleges and universities were times of revolt and upheaval, particularly on the campus in the latter part of the 1960s and the early 1970s. Today we find this "baby-boom" group entering the job market. Problems have been created: many jobs, such as teaching, are hard to find; unemployment has risen; and other related concerns are present. Up to this point in the life cycle of this group, adaptation by societal institutions to resolve the problems created by numbers has been necessary.

As we look ahead, we can start to see what will occur as this population group enters middle age and retirement. With the onset of middle age will come the inevitable health problems related to that stage of life. As we found shortages of schools and jobs in the past, we must wonder if there will exist the needed health

Fig. 26.2. Any positive and creative steps you take now to improve the health and well-being of the human race will increase the world's chances of meeting the challenges of overpopulation, starvation, and disease.

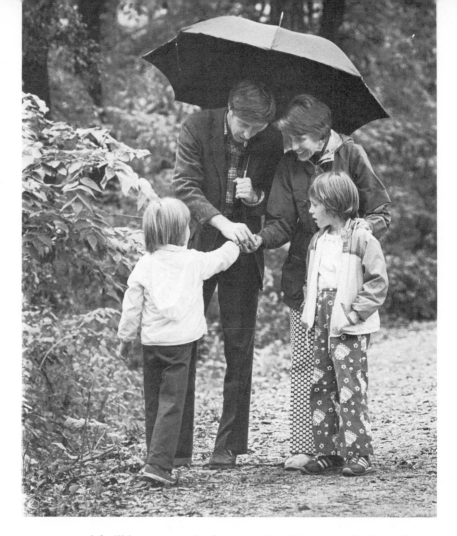

manpower and facilities to meet the future needs of these people. Early in the next century this group of people will be retiring, and many will be in need of facilities for the aged such as nursing homes. Will we have adequate and properly administered nursing-home facilities for all, or will shortages and overcrowding exist at that stage of life as they have at earlier stages? With the increased numbers and the increased expectations of quality of life, challenges will be presented to those health institutions that serve the elderly. Hopefully, we will be better prepared at that point than we were at earlier stages in the life cycle of those born during the baby boom.

That the human being will adapt to changes in his environment and his lifestyle is of little doubt. The quality of the life we will live in the years between now and the turn of the century cannot necessarily be assumed to be better. Simply because the quality of life has seemed to improve in the last century and the centuries prior to that for people living in America does not mean that the same will hold true in the years ahead.

It seems to us as we think of the years ahead that, regardless of medical research development and scientific advances, our personal value systems will play a significant role in the application and use of what we have examined. A value system that focuses upon quality human life will present conflict at times. How are we to cope with change from the perspective of the values each of us feels to be important?

Much would seem to indicate that the quality of life will improve. On the other hand, as one thinks of overpopulation, starvation, malnutrition, and other problems, the outlook can become very pessimistic.

It is doubtful if even a prophet could foretell exactly the quality of life we will experience in the years ahead. Our hope is that having an awareness of what directions life might take in the future will help each person reading this book to be better informed and better able to make those judgments and decisions that will contribute to an improved quality of human life. This is what we all want, but it cannot be purchased, nor will it ''fall into our laps.'' Hopefully, you will become motivated to do your part in your personal life so that your life-style will in fact lead to a more positive quality of life and then work for an improved society for yourself and your generation throughout the world. Any positive and creative steps we take to improve the health and well-being of the human race in the years ahead should of necessity begin now with you and your generation. Such a focus will take ''new and concerted human effort.''[2] That is the challenge we hope you will accept.

Review Questions

1. What role does the health educator play in preventive health care?
2. Do you believe there is a need for preventive health care?
3. Do you believe the human organism can adapt to a rapidly changing environment?
4. What is meant by the concept, health is a right of all persons?

Notes

1. René Dubos, ''Health and Environment,'' *American Lung Association Bulletin*, September 1973.
2. Glenn T. Seaborg, ''The Recycle Society of Tomorrow,'' *Futurist*, 8, no. 3 (June 1974).

Glossary

abdomen portion of the body located between the chest and the pelvis.

abortion spontaneous or induced termination of a pregnancy before the fetus can survive by itself outside the womb.

abscess inflammation of tissue accompanied by collection of pus.

absorption passage of substances through the walls of the digestive tract into the bloodstream.

acidosis poisonous systemic condition caused by a decrease of insulin in the body.

acoustic reflex mechanism disengaging bones of the middle ear from contact with the eardrum in the presence of extremely loud sound.

acupuncture treatment of certain diseases and alleviation of pain by inserting fine needles into the body at specific points called loci.

acute having rapid onset, severe symptoms, and short course.

adenosine diphosphate (ADP) product resulting from the breakdown of ATP.

adenosine triphosphate (ATP) enzyme found in all cells that when broken down releases energy necessary for muscular contraction and other energy-requiring reactions.

adenovirus virus that causes the common cold and other upper respiratory infections.

adrenal glands pair of endocrine glands positioned on top of the kidneys that produces epinephrine, norepinephrine, and cortisone.

aerobic exercises physical activities that require immediate and constant use of oxygen over an extended period of time.

alcoholism chronic abuse of alcohol to the extent that it interferes with the drinker's health or functioning.

alcometer instrument used to check the amount of alcohol in a person's blood.

aldosterone hormone that promotes retention of salt and water by the kidneys.

alleles paired genes located in corresponding chromosomes that determine inherited characteristics.

allergen substance capable of producing an allergy.

allopathy treatment of disease by using medicines that produce effects different from those of the disease treated.

alveoli tiny air sacs in the lungs in which the exchange of gases between the blood and lungs takes place.

amino acids nitrogenous compounds that are the building blocks of proteins and the end products of protein digestion.

amnesia loss of memory.

amniocentesis removal of some amniotic fluid from the amniotic sac for tests and analysis.

amnion membrane surrounding the developing fetus and containing life-protecting fluid.

amniotic fluid clear fluid that surrounds and helps protect the growing fetus.

amphetamines drugs that stimulate the central nervous system.

anaerobic exercises physical activities that do not require the use of great quantities of oxygen over long periods of time.

anal stage the Freudian stage of psychosexual development during which a young child's primary pleasure is associated with the anal activities of holding and expelling fecal matter.

analgesic medicine that relieves pain.

anaplasia condition in which cells lose their normal appearance, a characteristic of cancer cells.

androgen hormone that stimulates growth of male secondary sex characteristics.

androgyny a situation free of sex-role differentiation in which both males and females share desirable personal qualities formerly associated with either maleness or femaleness.

anemia reduction in red blood cells or in hemoglobin.

anesthesiology administration of anesthetic drugs during surgical or diagnostic procedures.

anesthetic agent that produces insensibility to pain or touch.

aneurysm saclike bulging of a weakened arterial wall.

angina pectoris   chest or arm pains caused by a decreased supply of blood to the heart muscle.

antabuse   drug that interferes with alcohol oxidation and is used in the treatment of alcoholism.

antibiotic   substance that inhibits growth of or destroys microorganisms and is used to treat infectious diseases.

antibody   substance produced in blood that provides immunity to certain types of viruses and other microorganisms.

anticholinergic   reducing muscle tone and contractility and constricting the blood vessels; sedative, tranquilizing.

antigen   substance that stimulates production of antibodies.

antihistamine   chemical substance that inhibits production of histamine by the body.

antimetabolite   drug used to interrupt the growth of cancer cells.

anxiety   abnormal state of fear and dread marked by extreme tension and nervousness.

aorta   main artery that carries oxygenated blood from the left ventricle of the heart to the body.

aphrodisiac   substance that stimulates one's sexual appetite.

appendectomy   surgical removal of the appendix.

arteriosclerosis   thickening and hardening of the artery walls that causes them to lose their elasticity; hardening of the arteries.

artery   thick-walled blood vessel that carries oxygenated blood away from the heart to various parts of the body.

arthritis   inflammation of the joints.

artificial insemination   injection of sperm into a female by means other than coitus for the purpose of conception.

asceticism   a coping skill of defense that involves the denial of instinctual drives, such as enjoyment, sleep, and eating.

asphyxiation   loss of consciousness in humans due to lack of oxygen.

asthma   bronchial spasms caused by allergic reaction, infection, or particle irritation.

astigmatism   inability to keep entire visual field in focus.

atherosclerosis   circulatory disease caused by deposits of cholesterol and fats inside large and medium-sized arteries that decrease the inside diameter of the vessels.

athlete's foot   fungus infection of the foot that causes itching and scaling of skin.

atrioventricular node   small bundle of specialized heart muscle fibers situated underneath the right atrium that sends impulses from the pacemaker to the ventricles.

atrium   one of pair of upper chambers of the heart that receives blood from the veins.

autopsy   postmortem examination of a body to determine cause of death.

autosomes   paired chromosomes that are not sex chromosomes.

autosuggestion   acceptance of thought arising from within oneself that brings about some mental or physical action or change.

barbiturates   drugs that depress the central nervous system to produce sleep or a quieting effect.

Barr body   dark area (chromatin mass) found in the nuclei of cells in normal females.

Bartholin glands   two tiny glands on either side of the vagina that secrete a precoital fluid during sexual excitement.

basal body temperature (BBT)   temperature of a body at complete rest.

basal metabolism (or BMR—basal metabolic rate) minimum amount of energy a person uses during a resting, postabsorptive state.

behavior therapy   (also behavior modification) a treatment for mental disturbances based on the learning of less bizarre, more effective coping behaviors.

benign tumor   localized, nonspreading, and usually nonlife-threatening growth.

benzopyrene   recognized carcinogen found in coal smoke and cigarette smoke.

bile   secretion of the liver that helps in the digestion of fats in the small intestine.

biodegradable   able to be broken down into smaller parts, the result of normal processes of nature.

biopsy   removal of a small piece of tissue from the body for the purpose of microscopic examination.

blackout   temporary loss of consciousness.

bladder   sac that stores urine.

blastocyst   hollow, fluid-filled sphere formed by the cells of a fertilized egg in early pregnancy.

blood   red liquid that flows through the circulatory system carrying nourishment and oxygen to the body cells and carbon dioxide and wastes from the cells.

blood plasma   liquid part of the blood.

blood pressure   pressure of the blood on the walls of the blood vessels, especially the arteries.

blood type   characteristic of red blood cells determined by one or more of its antigenic properties.

blue baby   infant suffering from congenital heart defect that allows blood to circulate without being oxygenated in the lungs.

BMR   see **basal metabolism.**

bowel   intestine.

brain death   absence of electrical impulse activity in the brain.

bronchiole   small subdivision of a bronchus.

bronchogenic carcinoma   cancer of the lung that originates in the lining of the bronchial tubes.

bronchus   one of the two large branches of the trachea that transports air to the alveoli; bronchial tube.

bursitis   inflammation of a bursa, or sac, between a tendon and bone.

calorie   unit used to express the energy content of food; the amount of heat required to raise the temperature of a kilogram of water (2.2 pounds) one degree centigrade.

cancer   uncontrolled, malignant cellular tumor.

cannabis sativa   Indian hemp plant from which marijuana is made.

capillary   small blood vessel located between an arteriole and venule where oxygen is exchanged for carbon dioxide.

carbohydrates   group of foods, such as sugars and starches, that contain only carbon, hydrogen, and oxygen. Carbohydrates are the major source of calories in an average diet.

carbon monoxide (CO)   a colorless, odorless gas that may cause death by asphyxiation.

carcinogen   substance that causes cancer.

carcinogenesis   production of cancer.

carcinoma   cancer of the epithelial cells that can spread to other parts of the body through the blood and lymph.

cardiopulmonary resuscitation (CPR)   basic emergency life support technique involving mouth-to-mouth breathing, or other ventilation technique, and chest compression.

cardiovascular   pertaining to the heart and blood vessels.

cardiovascular diseases   noncommunicable diseases that affect the heart and blood vessels, such as atherosclerosis, hypertension, rheumatic heart disease, and congenital heart defects.

cardiovascular endurance   ability of the heart, lungs, and blood vessels to function efficiently.

caries   deterioration of bones or teeth; tooth decay.

cartilage   dense, fibrous connective tissue that constitutes a part of the skeleton.

cataract   cloudiness or opacity of the lens of the eye that interferes with vision.

cell   small body of protoplasm containing a nucleus; the basic structure of all plants and animals.

cellular death   death of body's muscles as evidenced by rigor mortis.

central nervous system   system of the body that controls all voluntary acts; the brain and spinal cord.

cerebrovascular accident (CVA)   reduced supply of blood to the brain; stroke; apoplexy.

cerebrovascular disease   sickness affecting the blood vessels of the brain (cerebrum).

cervix   narrow end of the uterus that opens into the vagina.

cesarean section   method of childbirth in which surgical incision is made in the abdominal and uterine walls to allow delivery of the fetus.

chancre   painless ulcer or sore that appears at the site of a syphilitic infection.

chancroid (soft chancre)   an acute bacterial infection transmitted sexually and characterized by painful genital ulcers and swelling of the lymph nodes.

chemotherapy   use of drugs to treat disease.

chickenpox   infectious viral disease usually affecting children.

chiropractor   one who manipulates the spine.

chlorpromazine   tranquilizing drug used to treat major and minor psychotic conditions; trade name is thorazine.

cholera   acute bacterial infection that affects the small intestine.

cholesterol   substance found in the fatty parts of animal tissue and in egg yolks that contributes to atherosclerosis and gallstones.

choriocarcinoma   a rare form of uterine cancer.

chromatin   part of the cell nucleus that carries the genes.

chromosomes   threadlike structures within the nucleus of the cell that carry DNA and protein and are responsible for transmitting all hereditary characteristics of the cell.

chronic   long lasting and often permanent.

chronic bronchitis   respiratory disease with recurring inflammation of the bronchial tubes and excessive mucus production.

chronic obstructive pulmonary disease (COPD)   a debilitating condition combining emphysema and chronic bronchitis; commonly found in long-time cigarette smokers.

cilia   tiny hairlike projections lining the bronchial tube that sweep mucus and other debris out of the lungs; similar projections lining the fallopian tube that sweep mature ovum from ovary to uterus.

circumcision   surgical removal of the prepuce or foreskin of the penis.

cirrhosis   degenerative disease of the liver characterized by the destruction of liver cells and the formation of fibrous connective tissue.

clitoris   small sensory structure at the junction of the labia minora that is the most sensitive part of the female's sexual organs.

cloning   asexual reproduction of a new human being from the multiplication of a single body cell.

cocaine   stimulant drug derived from the coca bush that causes psychological dependence.

cochlea   spiral-shaped, fluid-filled structure of the inner ear.

codeine   narcotic drug derived from opium.

coitus   sexual intercourse or copulation.

coitus interruptus   sexual intercourse that ends with the withdrawal of the penis from the vagina prior to ejaculation.

coitus reservatus   sexual intercourse without ejaculation.

colitis   inflammation of the lining of the colon.

collagen   protein found in bones and connective tissues.

collateral circulation   blood flow through smaller vessels, bypassing an infarct in a larger vessel.

colon   large intestine from the end of the ileum to the anus.

colostrum   secretion from the breast a few days before or after childbirth.

columbarium   a structure for aboveground accommodation of cremated remains.

communicable disease   infection transmitted from human to human or animal to human.

compensation   a coping skill of defense in which an individual develops a desirable personal trait to overcome an undesirable trait.

composting   planned bacterial decomposition of wastes for the purpose of disposal and land conditioning.

compromise   a coping skill involving the acceptance of an available or attainable substitute goal when the original goal cannot be achieved.

compulsion   the persistence of certain actions that a person cannot resist performing.

conception   fertilization of an ovum by a spermatazoon thereby forming an embryo.

condom   thin sheath worn over the penis during sexual intercourse as a contraceptive to prevent sperm from entering the vagina and as a prophylactic to prevent the spread of venereal disease.

congeners   substances, such as dextrins, maltose, certain soluble minerals and vitamins, organic acids, and salts, found in beer and wine.

congenital   characteristic present at birth but not necessarily inherited.

congestion   excessive amount of blood or fluid in an organ or a tissue.

conjunctivitis   inflammation of the membranes under the eyelids and over the eyeball.

contagious   easily spread from person to person.

contraception   prevention of fertilization or conception.

conversion reaction   a type of hysterical neurosis in which an individual's voluntary nerve system and/or spinal senses are affected, causing paralysis, convulsions, or loss of speech or sight—all without any physical basis.

coping skills   the methods or techniques used to adjust or adapt to the demands of stress.

cornea   clear, transparent portion in the front of the eye.

coronary artery   one of two arteries arising from the aorta and feeding blood to the heart itself.

coronary heart disease (CHD)   atherosclerosis of the coronary arteries that supply the heart muscle.

coronary occlusion   total or diminished flow of blood through an artery to the heart that is caused by a spasm or a blood clot.

coronary thrombosis   formation of a clot in a coronary artery that obstructs the flow of blood to the heart causing a heart attack.

corpus cavernosum   spongy body in the penis that fills with blood upon sexual stimulation causing an erection.

corpus luteum   yellow body in the ovary formed by an ovarian follicle that has released an ovum; it secretes the hormone progesterone.

cortisone   hormone secreted by the adrenal glands that is sometimes used to treat asthma and arthritis.

couvade   male "pregnancy."

cowper's glands   pair of pea-shaped glands beneath the male urethra that secrete a preejaculatory fluid.

cremation   process by which the human remains are reduced to ashes by means of heat.

cross-tolerance (cross-dependence)   ability of one narcotic to eliminate withdrawal sickness caused by lack of a second narcotic.

crude birth rate   number of registered live births per 1,000 population.

crude death rate   number of recorded deaths per 1,000 population.

crypt   a concrete chamber in a mausoleum into which a casket is placed.

culdoscopy   female surgical sterilization procedure.

curettage   surgical cleaning of tissue by scraping with a curette.

cutaneous lesion   eruption or break in the skin.

CVA   see **cerebrovascular accident.**

cyanosis   blueness of skin caused by low oxygen content of the blood.

cystic fibrosis   inherited disease causing thickening of secretions from the mucous glands of the body, particularly the pancreas, lungs, and liver,

cystitis   inflammation of the bladder.

decibel (db)   unit of measurement used to record the intensity or loudness of sound.

defense mechanisms   coping skills that tend to protect the self from insult, devaluation, and disorganization.

delirium tremens   involuntary shaking of the body, restlessness, mental confusion, and possible hallucinations caused by alcohol dependency.

Demerol   synthetic narcotic drug.

denial   a coping skill of defense that involves the clear refusal to believe that an anxiety-producing event is true.

deoxyribonucleic acid (DNA)   double-strand coil of chemicals responsible for the production of body proteins and containing all the biological directions for man's hereditary characteristics.

depressant   agent or substance that depresses the central nervous system.

depression   abnormal state of sadness or feeling of dejection.

dermatology   diagnosis and treatment of diseases of the skin and scalp.

DES   see **diethylstilbestrol.**

detoxification   process of removing the poisonous quality of a substance from the body.

detumescence   loss of vasocongestion or swelling, particularly in the genitals.

diabetes mellitus   inherited disease in which the pancreas fails to produce sufficient insulin, causing an increase in blood-sugar level.

diagnosis   use of scientific and skillful methods to identify the cause and nature of a sick person's disease.

diaphragm   contraceptive device resembling a dome-shaped cap that covers the opening to the cervix.

diastolic pressure   arterial pressure while the heart relaxes and refills with blood.

diethylstilbestrol (DES)   synthetic hormone used in animal feed to promote growth, found as residue in meat, and thought to cause vaginal cancer in humans.

differentiation   in the embryo, the development of specialized forms or functions in cells.

diffusion   passage of substance through a membrane.

dilation and curettage (D and C)   procedure in which the cervical opening is dilated and the uterine wall is gently scraped; most often used for diagnosing cervical problems; may be used for early abortion.

diphtheria   acute infectious disease that affects the upper respiratory system.

disacharide   complex sugar molecule capable of being split into two monosacharides; sucrose is the most common one found in the normal diet.

displacement   a coping skill of defense in which an individual transfers socially unacceptable feelings from the actual stressor to some unrelated object or person.

disposition   final placement or disposal of a dead person.

dissociative reaction   a type of hysterical neurosis in which disturbing memories, thoughts, and feelings are separated from one's consciousness, resulting in amnesia, sleepwalking, or the development of a multiple personality.

diuretic   increasing the production of urine: any substance that has a diuretic effect.

DNA   see **deoxyribonucleic acid.**

Down's syndrome   congenital, chromosomal abnormality that causes mental retardation, slanted eyes, flattened forehead, and poor muscle tone; mongolism.

drug   chemical substance that, when taken into the body, may modify one or more of the functions of the body.

dysentary   term used to describe a number of intestinal disorders that are usually caused by bacterial or viral infection and are marked by abdominal cramps and diarrhea.

ecology   study of the relationship between living organisms and their environment.

ecosystem   group of organisms interacting with each other and their environment to maintain a constant balance of life.

ectomorphy   a type of body build described by Sheldon as fragile and slender with slight development of muscles, bones, and organs of the viscera.

edema   swelling of body tissues caused by accumulation of excess fluids.

ego   that subpart of the personality that satisfies the demands of the id within the realities of the external world, according to Freud.

ejaculation   expulsion of semen from the penis.

electrocardiogram (ECG)   graphic recording of the electrical activity produced by contractions of the heart.

electroencephalogram   graphic recording of the electrical impulses in the brain.

embalming   temporary preservation of the human body by means of chemicals.

embolus   circulating clot that is carried in the bloodstream until it plugs a small blood vessel.

embryo   developing child in the uterus during the first eight weeks after conception.

emphysema   respiratory disease causing loss of elasticity and rupturing of the alveoli.

encephalitis   inflammation of the brain.

endemic   constant presence of a communicable disease in a particular region or among a specific group of people.

endocarditis   inflammation of the membrane within and around the heart.

endocrine glands   glands that secrete hormones directly into the bloodstream; ductless glands.

endoderm   the innermost layer of cells in the blastocyst.

endodontics   treatment of interior tooth tissues.

endometrium   mucous membrane that lines the inside of the uterus.

endomorphy   a type of body build described by Sheldon as round and short, tending toward fatness and softness.

epidemic   sudden increase in a communicable disease in a given locality.

epidemiology   study of the occurrence and distribution of diseases in human populations.

epididymis   elongated structure located on top of each testis in which sperm cells mature and are stored.

epilepsy   chronic condition of the nervous system that may cause convulsions, loss of consciousness, and psychic or sensory malfunction.

epinephrine   hormone secreted by the adrenal glands that acts as a vasoconstrictor, cardiac stimulant, and bronchial tube relaxer; adrenaline.

episiotomy   surgical incision in the vagina to prevent tearing of the vaginal walls during childbirth.

epithelium   layer of cells forming the epidermis of the skin and the surface layer of mucus membranes.

Epstein-Barr virus (EBV)   a member of the herpes virus group thought to cause mononucleosis.

erythroblastosis fetalis   anemia of a fetus or newborn infant caused by transfer through the placenta of maternal antibodies that are formed as a result of incompatibility between blood groups of mother and child; hemolytic disease.

erythrocyte   see **red blood cell.**

esophagus   muscular canal extending from the pharynx to the stomach through which food passes.

estrogen   female hormone that promotes sexual development.

ethyl alcohol   alcoholic beverage produced by fermentation.

etiology   study of the causes of disease.

euphoria   feeling of well being.

eustress   pleasant or healthy stress.

euthanasia   putting to death a person who is hopelessly ill or injured; mercy killing; true meaning is an easy, painless, and happy death.

eutrophication   accelerated aging process in water due to an excess in nutrients.

exoderm   the outermost layer of cells in the blastocyst.

fallopian tube   tube extending from an ovary to the uterus through which an ovum travels.

fantasy   a coping skill of defense involving the satisfaction of personal frustration and the achievement of specific goals through imaginary accomplishments.

fats   substances that are found in most foods, are high in caloric content, and are a source of energy.

feces   body waste consisting of food residues, bacteria, and intestinal excretions that is discharged from the intestines by way of the anus.

fecundity   capable of producing offspring frequently and in large numbers.

fermentation   natural chemical process whereby yeast cells convert sugar to carbon dioxide and alcohol.

fertility   ability to produce offspring.

fertilization   union of a spermatozoon with an ovum, producing a zygote; conception.

fetus   developing child in the uterus from the third month after conception until birth.

fibrillation   see **ventricular fibrillation.**

fimbria   fringelike end of fallopian tube nearest the ovary.

fission   splitting of the core of an atom when it is struck by a neutron.

flashbacks   recurrence of certain features of a drug experience, usually without apparent cause, days or months after the last dose.

follicle-stimulating hormone (FSH)   hormone produced by the anterior lobe of the pituitary gland that stimulates the Graafian follicles of the ovaries.

foreskin   see **prepuce.**

fraternal twins   siblings born at the same time from two separate ova.

functional death   see **somatic death.**

fungus   parasitic, cellular organism that lacks chlorophyll.

fusion   combining atoms to produce huge amounts of energy.

gamete   a mature germ cell.

gamma globulin   blood proteins that contain antibodies and resist infection.

gastric   pertaining to the stomach.

gastrointestinal   pertaining to the stomach and intestine.

general adaptation syndrome (GAS)   a series of physical and chemical reactions identified by Selye that protect the threatened body and help it regain homeostasis.

generic name   nonproprietary name of a drug or pharmaceutical preparation.

genes tiny protein structures found in chromosomes that transmit all hereditary characteristics and genetic information.

genetics science dealing with the study of genes and heredity.

genital herpes a type of infectious disease caused by a herpes simplex virus and characterized by painful blisters and lesions in the genital areas of both men and women.

genital stage the Freudian stage of psychosexual development marked by an evolving interest in adult heterosexuality and in the needs of others rather than in one's own needs.

genitalia reproductive organs.

genotype combination of genes specific to every individual.

germ cell sex-determining cell; ovum and sperm; gamete.

German measles see **rubella.**

gerontology study of the aging process.

gestation period from fertilization to birth; pregnancy.

gland specialized group of cells that produces a secretion for use elsewhere in the body.

glasphalt a road-surfacing material made of recycled glass.

glaucoma increased pressure of fluid within the eye that is a leading cause of blindness.

glucose simple sugar formed by the breakdown of carbohydrates, carried in the blood, and used as a source of energy.

glycogen form in which the body stores glucose.

goiter enlargement of the thyroid gland due to lack of iodine in the diet.

gonad sex gland; testis in the male and ovary in the female.

gonococcemia presence of gonococci (bacteria causing gonorrhea) in the blood.

gonorrhea venereal disease that affects the genitourinary tract and is spread primarily through sexual intercourse.

Graafian follicles small sac in the ovary in which the ovum matures and from which the ovum is released during ovulation.

granuloma inguinale a chronic and progressive ulcerative disease of the skin and lymphatics of the genital and anal regions thought to be caused by bacterialike microorganisms known as Donovan bodies.

greenhouse effect continual rise in global temperatures caused by an increased concentration of carbon dioxide in the atmosphere that retards normal heat loss from the earth.

gynecology diagnosis and treatment of diseases of the female reproductive system.

half-life length of time it takes for 50 percent of the atoms of a radioactive sample to decay.

hallucinogens drugs that produce distortions of the senses or hallucinations; examples are LSD, mescaline, and DMT.

hashish dark brown resin collected from the flowering tops of the cannabis plant.

HCG (human chorionic gonadotrophic hormone) a secretion in the placenta that stimulates production of ovarian hormones essential to fetal development.

health insurance insurance that covers health-care expenses.

health maintenance organization (HMO) prepaid group program for comprehensive health care, including preventive medicine.

heart attack damage to the heart due to blockage of a coronary artery by a thrombus or embolus.

hemoglobin substance in red blood cells that carries oxygen from the lungs to the tissues and gives blood its red color.

hemolytic affecting the red blood cells.

hemophilia hereditary disease in which blood fails to clot normally, causing excessive bleeding.

hemorrhage abnormal bleeding from a ruptured artery or vein.

hepatitis inflammation of the liver caused by infection.

hernia protrusion of an organ or part of an organ through the wall of the cavity that normally contains it; rupture.

heroin narcotic synthesized from morphine.

herpes simplex infectious viral disease characterized by small blisters on the skin and mucous membranes; cold sore.

heterosexual behavior sexual attraction to or sexual activity with individuals of the opposite sex.

heterozygous possessing different alleles for a certain characteristic.

histamine chemical release by body tissues in allergic reactions.

Hodgkin's disease cancer of the lymph nodes.

homeopath one who treats disease by drugs, given in small doses, which produce in a healthy person symptoms similar to those of the disease.

homeostasis the inner state of constancy in which there is an equilibrium of body functioning, thought processes, emotions, and feelings.

homeostatic mechanism process that maintains the body's internal environment in a state of constancy.

homogamy marriages between persons of similar social, economic, racial, or religious backgrounds.

homosexual behavior   sexual attraction to or sexual activity with individuals of the same sex.

homozygous   possessing identical alleles for a certain characteristic.

hormone   chemical substance secreted by an endocrine gland that acts elsewhere in the body.

Huntington's disease (HD)   hereditary disease in adults characterized by jerking, twitching, difficulty in speaking, and mental deterioration.

hydrocarbon   compound composed only of hydrogen and carbon.

hydrogen chloride   highly corrosive chemical produced when polyvinyl chloride is burned.

hydrops   abnormal accumulation of fluid in the body.

hypergamy   marriage to one of equal or higher status.

hyperkinetic   abnormally active.

hyperopia   difficulty in focusing on near objects; farsightedness.

hyperplasia   increase in the number of layers of basal cells.

hypertension   high blood pressure.

hypnotherapy   treatment of disease by hypnotism.

hypochondriasis   a form of anxiety reaction characterized by preoccupation with one's body and fear of presumed disease.

hypothalamus   tiny section of the brain lying just above the pituitary gland that regulates such basic body functions as water balance, temperature, appetite, and sleep.

hysterectomy   surgical removal of the uterus.

id   that subpart of the personality that is the source of psychic energy expressed as basic, primitive instincts, according to Freud.

identical twins   siblings born at the same time from the same ovum.

identification   a coping skill of defense in which a person behaves and acts as if he or she were some other person, who is often perceived as a model.

idiopathic   relating to disease with no known cause.

immunity   resistance to disease and infection.

immunosuppressive drug   substance administered to transplant patient to reduce the body's tendency to reject a new organ or tissue.

immunotherapy   treatment that promotes production of immunity by tricking the body's natural defenses into fighting disease, as in cancer.

implantation   attachment of the blastocyst to the wall of the uterus.

impotence   inability of the male to have satisfactory sexual intercourse, usually due to an inability to attain or maintain an erection.

incineration   burning of solid wastes as a means of disposal.

incubation period   period of time between initial infection and appearance of symptoms of a communicable disease.

infarct   damaged or dead tissue caused by decreased blood circulation or complete blockage of an artery.

infection   invasion of the body by a pathogen.

influenza   severe viral respiratory disease.

inpatient   person who receives prolonged medical observation or care in a hospital.

insulin   hormone produced by the islets of Langerhans in the pancreas that regulates sugar metabolism.

intellectualism   a coping skill of defense in which the person directs his or her attention to intellectual or philosophical issues to avoid some basic anxiety.

interferon   protein produced chemical substance that functions as an antiviral defense.

internship   one-year hospital training period that a newly graduated physician must fulfill to qualify for state licensure.

intoxication   temporary state of apparent malfunctioning or mental chaos caused by the presence of alcohol in the central nervous system.

intrauterine   within the uterus.

intrauterine device (IUD)   small plastic or metal device inserted into the uterus to prevent pregnancy.

intravenous   within or into a vein.

introjection   a coping skill of defense in which identification with another results in the adoption of that person's values and aims.

jaundice   yellowing of the skin and the whites of the eyes caused by an excess of bile.

joint   place where two bone ends meet.

karyotype   a typical arrangement of chromosomes in a single cell.

Klinefelter's syndrome   male chromosomal abnormality associated with an XXY chromosome combination.

kwashiorkor   nutritional disease caused by a diet high in carbohydrates and low in proteins.

labia   lips of the female external genitalia.

lactation   production of milk.

lactic acid   end product of glucose metabolism produced during anaerobic work.

laparoscopy   female surgical sterilization procedure.

laryngitis inflammation of the larynx causing hoarseness and sometimes temporary loss of voice.

latency stage the Freudian stage of psychosexual development during which no significant personality changes occur.

Legionnaires' disease a sometimes fatal ailment resembling pneumonia that attracted worldwide notice during a 1976 American Legion convention in Philadelphia.

lesion site of any diseased or injured tissue of the body.

lethal causing death; fatal.

leukemia cancer of the blood-forming organs.

loci specific points on the exterior of the body where tiny needles are inserted during acupuncture.

longevity length of life.

luteinizing hormone (LH) hormone secreted by the pituitary that in the female causes the Graafian follicle to rupture and release a mature egg, and in the male is involved in production of testosterone.

lymph node small, round body that is located along the lymphatic vessels and produces lymphocytes.

lymphocyte type of white blood cell manufactured largely in the bone marrow whose function is to protect the body from foreign substances that invade it.

lymphogranuloma venereum a systemic infection of the lymph nodes and lymph channels caused by sexually transmitted bacteria and characterized by small ulcers on the penis, vagina, or rectum.

lymphoma tumor of the lymph nodes; Hodgkin's disease.

lysergic acid diethylamide (LSD) a partially synthetic; potent hallucinogen; "acid."

lysozyme chemical substance that dissolves the cell walls of certain bacteria.

malaria infectious disease caused by protozoan parasites within the red blood cells and transmitted by the bite of a mosquito.

malignant tumor cancerous tumor.

mammography X-ray examination of the breast.

marijuana hallucinogen derived from the dried leaves and flowering tops of the Indian hemp plant, cannabis sativa.

mastectomy surgical removal of the breast.

masturbation self-stimulation of one's genitals, usually to the point of orgasm.

mausoleum a structure for above-ground accommodation of a casket.

measles see **rubeola.**

meiosis cell division occurring only in sex cells whereby the number of chromosomes is reduced by half.

meiotic nondisjunction occasionally during meiosis the chromosomes of a particular pair fail to separate, leaving one cell deficient while the other cell receives both chromosomes.

melanoma cancerous skin tumor filled with dark pigment, often black in color.

membrane thin, soft, layer of tissue that lines a cavity of the body or covers and separates one organ from another.

menarche beginning of menstruation indicating that puberty has been reached.

meningitis inflammation of any of the three membranes enveloping the brain and spinal cord.

menstruation discharge of blood from the uterus through the vagina that is caused by the breakdown of the endometrium when fertilization does not take place.

mentation mental activity or rational thinking.

mescaline hallucinogenic oil extracted from the peyote cactus that alters consciousness.

mesoderm the middle layer of cells in the blastocyst.

mesomorphy a type of body build described by Sheldon as athletic and characterized by heavy shoulders, firm muscles and bones, and upright physique.

metabolism process of making energy available to the body through chemical and physical changes.

metastasis transfer of cancerous cells through the bloodstream and lymphatic system to form a growth in another part of the body not directly connected to the original cancerous site.

metazoa animal organisms that can infect humans.

methadone synthetic narcotic drug used as a substitute for heroin to prevent withdrawal symptoms.

methyl mercury organic compound of mercury widely used as a fungicide and extremely toxic to humans.

microorganism tiny living plant or animal that is not visible to the eye; microbe.

minerals inorganic substances found in nature.

miscarriage see **spontaneous abortion.**

mitosis cell division in which a somatic cell is duplicated and receives the exact number of chromosomes and characteristics of the parent cell.

modeling a form of learning whereby one imitates another person's behavior; one of many influencing factors in personality development.

mongolism see **Down's syndrome.**

monogamy marriage between one man and one woman.

mononucleosis acute infectious disease thought to be caused by a virus of the herpes group.

monosaccharide simple sugar that cannot be decomposed by hydrolysis and is absorbed directly from the intestine.

morbidity condition of being diseased.

morphine narcotic derived from opium.

mucus protective fluid secreted by the mucous membranes and glands that contains white blood cells, inorganic salts, and other materials.

multiple sclerosis disease of unknown causation characterized by loss of the insulating myelin sheath that normally covers nerve fibers.

mumps contagious viral disease with inflammation and swelling of the parotid and other salivary glands, fever, and pain.

muscular dystrophy progressive weakening and wasting of the muscles.

mutation a basic change in an organism that makes it unlike its parents.

myocardial infarction heart attack.

myocarditis inflammation of the walls of the heart.

myocardium heart muscle.

myopia failure to see distant objects; nearsightedness.

naprapath one who treats diseases as if they are caused by connective tissue and ligament disorders.

narcissistic erotic feeling aroused by one's own body and personality.

narcosis stuporous anesthetic condition.

narcotic drug that relieves pain and induces sleep.

naturopath one who treats diseases with sunlight, manipulation, exercise, water, air, organic foods, and naturally occurring drugs.

nausea uncomfortable sensation in the stomach with an inclination to vomit.

neonatal mortality number of infants who die during the first four weeks after birth.

neoplasm see **tumor.**

nephritis inflammation of the kidney.

nephron basic filtering unit of the kidney that produces urine.

neurology diagnosis and treatment of diseases of the nervous system.

neurosis a minor personality disorder or less severe mental problem in which the individual usually stays in touch with reality.

neuron basic structural unit of the nervous system that consists of a cell body, an axon, and one or more dendrites.

nicotine poisonous alkaloid that is the dependency-producing component in tobacco smoke.

nitrogen colorless, odorless gas making up most of the atmosphere and found in all living things.

nitroglycerine drug used to alleviate pains of angina pectoris.

nocturnal emission involuntary discharge of semen during sleep; "wet dream."

nonspecific urethritus any inflammation of the male or female urethra (the passage for urine) not caused by gonorrhea organisms.

norepinephrine hormone secreted by the adrenal glands that acts as a stimulant to the sympathetic nervous system.

nucleus spherical body found in most plant and animal cells that contains a number of organelles, including the chromosomes, and is necessary for growth and reproduction.

nutrient substance found in foods that supplies nourishment and energy to the body.

obesity weighing more than 20 percent over normal skeletal and physical requirements.

obsession an unwilling repetition of unwanted thoughts.

obstetrics care of women during pregnancy and immediately following childbirth.

operant conditioning a form of learning whereby correct responses are rewarded and thus become more likely to be repeated.

ophthalmia neonatorum eye infection in newborns caused by gonorrhea.

ophthalmology diagnosis and treatment, including surgery, of diseases and defects of the eye.

opiates drugs derived from opium.

opium narcotic derived from the dried juice of the unripe oriental poppy pod.

optometrist one who examines eyes, prescribes corrective lenses, and conducts visual training.

oral contraceptive pill containing synthetic female hormones to prevent pregnancy; birth control pill.

oral stage the Freudian stage of psychosexual development in which an infant derives pleasure by means of the mouth.

organelles ministructures found within the cells that are responsible for specific functions. Such structures include the nucleus, ribosomes, mitochondria, endoplasmic reticulum, and golgi bodies.

organochlorine pesticide containing chlorinated hydrocarbon.

organophosphate pesticide containing phosphorus.

orgasm climax of sexual excitement.

orthodontics dental development and proper alignment of teeth.

orthopedics diagnosis and medical or surgical treatment of the bones and joints of the body.

ossicles three bones of the middle ear that vibrate and thereby produce sound.

osteoarthritis progressive deterioration of the joints.

otitis media bacterial infection that damages the eardrum and bones of the middle ear.

otolaryngology diagnosis and treatment of diseases of the ear, nose, and throat.

otosclerosis abnormal growth of spongy tissue in the middle ear that leads to hearing loss.

outpatient person who receives medical or dental care but who does not occupy a hospital bed.

ovarectomy surgical removal of the ovaries.

ovary one of two reproductive glands in the female that produce ova and sex hormones.

overweight weighing more than 10 to 20 percent over the normal desirable weight.

ovulation release of a mature egg from the Graafian follicle of the ovary.

ovum mature female reproductive cell capable of being fertilized by a sperm cell.

oxidation combining with oxygen to form water and carbon dioxide and produce heat and energy.

ozone photochemical oxidant formed when atomic oxygen combines with oxygen already in the atmosphere that irritates the lungs, eyes, and throat, damages plants, and causes rubber to crack and decompose.

pacemaker see **sino-atrial node.**

pancreas gland that secretes digestive enzymes and the hormone insulin.

pandemic sudden increase in a communicable disease in many countries at the same time.

panophthalmitis inflammation of the whole eye.

Pap test microscopic examination of vaginal fluid to test for cancer of the cervix and uterus.

paranoia a major psychotic disorder marked by delusions of persecution and grandiosity.

parasite plant or animal that lives on or in a host organism and receives its nourishment at the expense of the host.

parathyroid two pairs of glands near the thyroid whose secretion affects the metabolism of calcium and phosphorus.

parturition process of childbirth.

pathogen disease-producing microorganism.

pathogenticity capable of causing disease.

pathology identification of diseases through analysis of changes of body organs, tissues, and cells, and alterations of body chemistry.

patriarchal family social pattern in which the family group is dominated by the father.

pediatrics prevention, diagnosis, and treatment of children's diseases.

pediculosis ("crabs") an infestation of the pubic area by crawling, blood-sucking lice that look like crabs when magnified.

pedodontics treatment of children's dental problems.

penicillin widely used antibiotic drug produced by several species of molds.

penis male organ of sexual intercourse and urination.

pericarditis inflammation of the fibrous sac surrounding the heart.

perihepatitis inflammation of the tissues around the liver.

periodontics treatment of gums and bones supporting the teeth.

periostitis inflammation of tissue covering the bone, marked by tenderness and swelling.

peripheral nervous system division of the nervous system that includes the cranial and spinal nerves and the autonomic nervous system.

peroxyacyl nitrates (PAN) photochemical oxidant formed by a series of chemical reactions in the atmosphere that causes the eyes to burn and tear and damages plants and vegetation.

personality the consistent ways in which a person reacts in adjusting to problems and fulfilling various needs.

pertussis whooping cough.

pesticide chemical sprayed on crops to kill insects.

peyote hallucinogenic stimulant derived from the mescal cactus.

phagocytes white blood cells that surround and destroy pathogens.

phallic stage the Freudian stage of psychosexual development in which the manipulation of one's sexual organs is the child's source of pleasure.

pharmacogenetics study of the effects of drugs on heredity and the unborn child.

pharmacology study of the interaction of chemical agents with living organisms.

pharyngitis inflammation of the pharynx; sore throat.

phenotype visible expression of a person's genes.

phenylalanine hydroxylase enzyme produced in the liver that is needed to convert phenylalanine into tyrosine.

phenylketonuria (PKU) metabolic disorder caused by absence of the enzyme phenylalanine hydroxylase.

phlegm thick mucus found especially in the respiratory passages.

phobia an overpowering fear of some specific object or situation that a person willingly acknowledges as harmless in the light of reality.

photochemical exidants chemical compounds created in the atmosphere by the sun.

photosynthesis process whereby in the presence of light plants convert carbon dioxide to oxygen and produce sugar.

phytoplankton minute aquatic life responsible for generating most of our oxygen supply.

pica ingesting materials that normally are considered inedible.

pinocytosis process of liquid absorption by cells.

pituitary gland small gland located at the base of the brain that secretes hormones for body growth, development, and regulation; sometimes called the "master gland."

placebo inactive substance given to a patient to satisfy the demand for medicine; also used in controlled drug studies.

placenta spongy structure in the uterus that connects the fetus to the mother by means of the umbilical cord through which the fetus receives nourishment.

plaque whitish film on the teeth containing bacteria and conducive to tooth decay; calculus or tartar.

plaques soft fatty deposits that line the interior walls of arteries in atherosclerosis.

plastic surgery surgical correction or repair of deformed or mutilated body parts or surgical improvement of facial or body features.

platelet colorless disk found in blood that is involved in blood coagulation and clot formation.

pneumonia inflammation of the lungs caused by bacteria, viruses, chemical irritants, and allergens.

podiatrist one who diagnoses, prevents, and treats foot disorders; chiropodist.

poliomyelitis (polio) acute, systemic, infectious disease that occurs in varying degrees of severity.

polychlorinated biphenyls (PCB) chemical compounds found in industrial products and wastes that may accumulate in animal tissue and do cause birth defects and liver damage in animals.

polygamy form of marriage in which a man has more than one wife or a woman has more than one husband at the same time.

polyvinyl chloride component of plastic that produces the corrosive hydrogen chloride when it is burned.

postnatal occurring shortly after birth.

pregnancy period from conception until birth when the child is developing in the uterus.

prepuce fold of skin that extends over and covers the glans in the male and is usually removed in circumcision; foreskin. In the female, a hood of skin over the clitoris.

preventive medicine study, prevention, and control of epidemic, environmental, and occupational hazards and diseases.

proctitis inflammation of the rectum.

proctosigmoidoscope slim, lighted tube through which a physician can look directly inside the rectum and bowel.

progesterone hormone produced by the corpus luteum that prepares the uterus for the implantation of the fertilized egg.

projection a coping skill of defense in which the blame for personal problems is shifted to another person or group of individuals whose imagined faults are responsible for your own difficulty.

promiscuity engaging in indiscriminate or casual sexual intercourse with many people.

prophylactic disease-preventing; a condom used for disease prevention.

prostate gland gland in the male that surrounds the urethra and bladder and secretes a preejaculatory fluid.

protein class of complex organic compounds containing amino acids which are found in plants and animals, and are essential for the growth and development of all living cells.

pseudocyesis imaginary pregnancy

psilocybin hallucinogen extracted from the psilocybe mushroom that produces effects similar to LSD and mescaline.

psychedelic drug, usually a hallucinogen, that produces altered states of consciousness.

psychiatry diagnosis and treatment of emotional disturbances and mental disorders.

psychoactive drug drug that chemically alters mood, thought, feeling, or behavior.

psychoanalysis classical Freudian psychotherapy featuring techniques of free word association, interpretation of dreams, and the recall of early childhood conflicts.

psychoanalytic psychotherapy a type of psychotherapy widely used today that emphasizes a helpful and supportive verbal exchange about specific internal conflicts of a patient.

psychodrama extemporaneous acting out by one or more persons of events in one's life for the purpose of relieving tension or relearning social reactions.

psychologist one who studies the nonmedical science of human behavior.

psychosis a major personality disorder or more severe mental problem in which an individual appears to have lost contact with reality.

psychopath an individual with a personality disorder that manifests itself in an apparent lack of conscience and in antisocial behavior.

psychosomatic disorder a physical disorder that is psychological in origin and the result of unexpressed, protective physiological reactions.

psychotherapy   a particular treatment for mental disturbances that features verbal interchange between a patient and trained therapist.

psychotropic   affecting the mind or mental activity; psychoactive.

puberty   stage of life when secondary sex characteristics develop, reproductive organs become functional, and sexual maturity is reached.

pulmonary embolism   obstruction of a blood vessel in the lungs.

pus   liquid product of an infection composed of albuminous substances and dead leukocytes.

pyelonephritis   inflammation of the kidney.

pyorrhea   periodontal disease that can cause loosening of the teeth.

quack   one who falsely represents ability and experience in diagnosis and/or treatment of disease.

quickening   first detectable movements of the fetus in the uterus.

quinine   drug used primarily to treat malaria.

radiation   emission of energy caused by the splitting of an atom.

radioactivity   release of radiation.

radiology   diagnosis and treatment of disease by using radiant energy, such as X rays.

rationalization   a coping skill of defense that involves the formulation of a socially acceptable reason for holding an attitude or performing a behavior when the real reason would be unacceptable to one's conscience.

reaction formation   a coping skill of defense in which your behavior and self-expression are exactly the opposite of your true feelings.

recycling   processing of solid wastes for reuse.

red blood cell   small cell that lacks a nucleus and contains hemoglobin which carries oxygen to and carbon dioxide from the tissues; erythrocyte.

reference group   those persons, real or imaginary, with whom one identifies and whose expectations, real or imaginary, one tries to meet.

reflex   an involuntary movement or action made in response to a stimulus.

regression   a coping skill of defense that involves the readoption of a behavior that was characteristic of an earlier phase in one's life.

remission of symptoms   temporary, periodic absence of symptoms.

renal   pertaining to the kidney.

repression   a coping skill of defense that involves keeping anxiety producing events at a subconscious level.

reserpine   drug that reduces tension.

reservoir   human, animal, plant, or inanimate matter in which an infectious agent normally lives and multiplies.

Rh disease   disease of the blood cells in infants arising from the presence of Rh blood factor in the child and its absence in the mother; hemolytic disease.

rheumatic fever   inflammatory condition often attacking joints, lungs, brain, or heart following streptococcal infection.

rheumatic heart disease   disease of the heart caused by rheumatic fever.

rheumatoid arthritis   inflammatory joint disease affecting the whole body.

rickets   nutritional disease caused by lack of vitamin D in the diet.

rickettsiae   microorganisms that must rely on other organisms to complete their life cycles; some cause illness in humans.

rigor mortis   stiffening of skeletal muscles after death.

ringworm   fungus skin infection marked by a red-ringed patch that causes itching, pain, and scaling.

roentgen   basic unit of radiation; rad.

role expectations   approved personality traits and behaviors traditionally associated with various social roles, such as parent and child, student and teacher, male and female.

rubella   infectious disease causing eruption of small red spots on the skin; German measles.

rubeola   infectious disease causing eruption of small red spots on the skin.

saddleblock   an anesthetic affecting the part of the lower torso that would normally contact the saddle in horseback riding.

sanitary landfill   site where solid wastes are buried in layers under dirt as a means of waste disposal and land reclamation.

sarcoma   cancer of the connective tissues, such as bones, muscle, cartilage, and fat cells.

scabies   an infectious skin disease caused by a small mite and characterized by intense itching and by the appearance of pimples and blisters.

schizophrenia   one of the most serious and least treatable of the psychoses, characterized by serious disturbances of thinking and behavior.

sciatica   leg condition characterized by a sharp, shooting pain running down the back of the thigh.

scrotum   external sac that contains the gonads or testicles and related structures.

sedative   depressant drug that acts to slow down the central nervous system function and is used medically to induce sleep and to reduce nervousness, anxiety, and convulsions.

sedativism drug dependency resulting from multiple sedative abuse.

seizure an epileptic attack characterized by loss of consciousness, as in petit mal (mild seizure); sometimes accompanied by involuntary convulsions, as in grand mal (severe seizure).

self-actualization Maslow's term for personality growth behavior concerned with developing proficiencies and increasing capabilities.

semen thick fluid discharged from the urethra of the male that is composed of secretions from various glands plus sperm stored in the seminal vesicles.

seminal vesicles two pouches in the male located between the bladder and the rectum that produce a secretion which serves as a liquid vehicle for the sperm.

seminiferous tubules tiny tubules located in the testes in which sperm develop and mature.

senescence process of growing old.

septicemia presence of toxins in the blood; blood poisoning.

sex role the outward expression of one's sexual identity as revealed in speech, mannerisms, sexual arousal and response, and interrelationships.

sex-role stereotype behavior traditionally associated with either the male or female.

sexual identity the private inner sense or awareness of self as male or female.

sexual intercourse sexual union of a male and a female in which the penis is inserted into the vagina; copulation; coitus.

Siamese twins identical twins with bodies joined at some point.

siblings children born of the same parents; brothers or sisters.

sickle-cell anemia hereditary disorder found mostly among blacks that affects the hemoglobin of red blood cells.

silicosis lung-damaging disease suffered by miners.

silver nitrate antibacterial solution that is placed in the eyes of newborn infants to protect them from gonorrhea-induced blindness.

sino-atrial node small mass of specialized cells in the right, upper chamber of the heart that gives rise to electrical impulses that initiate contractions of the heart; pacemaker.

smallpox acute, contagious viral disease characterized by fever, headache, abdominal pain, and lesions of the skin.

somatic cells cells other than germ cells that form all tissues and organs; body cells.

somatic death absence of heartbeat and spontaneous breathing.

somatic theraphy the use of physical agents in the treatment of mental disorders, particularly psychoses.

somatotype a classification of body build as described by Sheldon, such as endomorphy, mesomorphy, and ectomorphy.

specific dynamic action (SDA) used of food in reference to the energy expended by the body in processing it.

speed methamphetamine (meth); drug abused for its stimulating effects.

spermatazoon male sex or germ cell capable of fertilizing an ovum; sperm.

spermatogenesis production and development of sperm.

spermicide chemical that destroys sperm and is used as a contraceptive.

sphygmomanometer instrument for measuring arterial blood pressure.

spina bifida congenital defect allowing the spinal column to protrude through the skin.

spinal an anesthetic administered through the spine to anesthetize the lower portion of the torso.

spinal subluxation improper alignment or derangement of the vertebral column which, according to the chiropractic theory, causes a disturbance to the nervous system.

spirochete slender, spiral-shaped microorganism capable of burrowing into the skin.

spleen organ located directly underneath the diaphragm on the left side of the body whose functions are blood formation, storage, and filtration.

spontaneous abortion nonintentional expulsion of the fetus prior to the third month of life; miscarriage.

sporadic occasional occurrence of a communicable disease.

stereotype simplified idea or attitude held by a group of people about the way other people or events are or should be.

sterility incapable of fertilization and reproduction.

sterilization rendering a person incapable of fertilization, usually by surgically severing the tubes that carry reproductive cells.

stillbirth birth of a dead fetus.

stimulant drug or agent that increases the activity of the central nervous system.

strabismus imbalance of the muscles controlling eye movements.

strep throat sore throat produced by streptococcal bacteria; sometimes followed by rheumatic fever.

stress a condition of disturbed inner equilibrium or stability that demands some adjustment or adaptation.

stressor a stress-producing agent.

stroke impeded blood supply to the brain.

subluxation improper alignment or derangement of vertebrae.

superego that subpart of the personality that functions as the conscience, according to Freud.

superfecundity successive fertilization of two or more ova formed during the same menstrual cycle and leading to a multiple birth.

surgery treatment of disease, injury, or deformity by manual or operative procedures.

syndrome group of signs and symptoms identifying a particular disease.

synergists drugs that taken together have an exaggerated effect out of proportion to that of each drug taken separately.

synesthesia phenomenon, usually drug related, in which one sensation may be translated into another, e.g., sounds may be seen, smells may be felt.

synovial fluid clear lubricating fluid secreted by the membranes of a joint.

synovium smooth lining membrane of a joint.

syphilis venereal disease that may involve any organ or tissue and is spread by sexual contact.

systolic pressure pressure exerted against the arteries during the heart's pumping stroke.

Tay-Sachs disease enzyme deficiency in infants caused by a recessive gene and characterized by severe physical retardation and blindness.

temperament a particular set or group of personality characteristics.

temperature inversion meteorological condition whereby cooler air becomes trapped under a warmer layer of air and the cooler layer becomes heavily polluted.

tendon fibrous connective tissue that attaches muscles to bones.

tenosynovitis inflammation of the sheath around a tendon.

teratogen agent that causes an abnormality or malformation of the fetus.

testes male gonads which produce spermatazoa and testosterone.

tetanus acute infectious disease caused by the toxin *Clostridium tetani;* lockjaw.

tetrahydrocannabinol (THC) basic active ingredient in marijuana and hashish thought to be responsible for their psychoactive properties.

thalidomide tranquilizing drug taken by many pregnant women during the late 1950s that caused severe birth defects.

thermography heat-sensitive photographs of the breast to detect cancer.

thoracic pertaining to the chest.

thromboembolism blockage of a blood vessel by a clot (thrombus) formed elsewhere.

thrombophlebitis inflammatory condition caused by a blood clot that obstructs a vein.

thrombus clot that forms at the site of an obstruction in an artery.

thyroid gland at the base of the neck that produces hormones affecting growth and metabolism.

TMR see **total metabolic rate.**

tonsillectomy surgical removal of the tonsils.

total metabolic rate (TMR) a measure of the total energy expenditure of one's body, including BMR, SDA, and activity.

toxic pertaining to or caused by a poison.

toxins poisonous chemicals.

toxoids preparations of altered bacterial poisons that stimulate production of antibodies.

trachea large cartilaginous tube extending from the larynx to the bronchial tubes; windpipe.

trademark name name of a drug used on the competitive market by a manufacturer.

tranquilizer central nervous system depressant that helps relieve anxiety or extreme emotional states.

translocation occurs when a piece of one chromosome slides into another, noncorresponding chromosome.

trauma injury or wound.

trichomoniasis infection of the vagina caused by the microorganism *Trichomonas.*

trigonitis inflammation of the mucous membrane at the base of the bladder.

triticale high-protein grain that is cross between wheat and rye.

tubal ligation severing the fallopian tubes as a method of sterilization.

tubercle healed lesion that forms a firm lump resembling knots on tuberous plants.

tuberculosis communicable disease primarily affecting the lungs and caused by a bacillis which forms tubercles in the affected areas.

tumescence process of becoming swollen.

tumor abnormal, nonfunctional cell mass that grows independent of surrounding structures.

Turner's syndrome chromosomal disorder in which the female has only one X chromosome.

typhoid fever acute contagious disease characterized by headache, fever, constipation, and rose-colored spots on the skin.

typhus fever acute infectious disease usually prevalent in unsanitary locations.

ulcer   open sore or lesion of the skin or mucous membrane.

umbilical cord   tubelike structure that connects the fetus to the placenta and through which the fetus receives nourishment from the mother.

urethra   tube that transports urine out of the body from the bladder and carries semen in the male.

urn   a container for cremated remains.

urogenital   having to do with the organs or functions of excretion and reproduction.

urology   diagnosis and treatment of diseases and disorders of the kidneys, bladder, ureters, and urethra, and the male reproductive system.

U.S.P.   United States Pharmacopeia, a reference book containing official standards for identity, strength, and purity of various drugs.

uterus   hollow pear-shaped organ in the female within which the fetus is nourished and grows.

vaccine   preparations of weakened or killed pathogens that stimulate antibody formation without causing observable signs of disease.

vacuum aspiration   abortion procedure whereby a thin, flexible tube is inserted into the uterus to suck out the fertilized egg along with the menstrual lining.

vagina   canal in the female that extends from the vulva to the cervix.

vaginitis   inflammation of the vagina.

varicose veins   condition in which veins become dilated, causing pain, especially in the legs.

vas deferens   tube that carries sperm from the testes to the seminal vesicles.

vasectomy   male surgical sterilization procedure.

vasocongestion   congestion of the blood vessels, especially the veins in the genital area.

vasoconstriction   constriction of the blood vessels.

vasodilation   dilation of the blood vessels.

vector   an organism that transmits a disease-producing microorganism.

vegetarian   person who eats no animal meat or by-products but lives on vegetables alone.

vein   thin-walled blood vessel that carries blood from various parts of the body back to the heart.

venereal disease (VD)   communicable disease transmitted primarily through sexual intercourse.

venereal warts   virus-caused warts that appear on the external genitalia of males and females, usually within one to three months after intercourse with an infected partner.

ventricle   one of the pair of lower chambers of the heart that receives blood from the atrium and pumps it out of the heart.

ventricular fibrillation   complete incoordination of heart contractions, often leading to sudden death by heart attack.

vertebrae   small, movable bones of the spinal column.

viral hepatitis   see **hepatitis.**

virility   male sexual potency.

virus   microscopic infectious organism that is parasitic and depends on nutrients inside cells for its metabolic and reproductive survival.

vitamin   general term for any of a group of organic substances which are essential for normal metabolism, growth, and development.

volatile substances   easily vaporized chemicals that produce a state of intoxication when inhaled, usually solvents found in airplane glue, lighter and cleaning fluids, and gasoline.

vulva   external female sex organs.

"wet dream"   see **Nocturnal emission.**

white blood cell   small, colorless cell found in blood, lymph, and tissues whose major function is to destroy microorganisms that may cause infection; leukocyte.

withdrawal   a coping skill involving escape from or avoidance of a stressor; cessation of drug use, sometimes accompanied by debilitating physical and psychological symptoms.

X chromosome   sex-determining chromosome found in all the female gametes and in one half of the male gametes.

Y chromosome   sex-determining chromosome found in one half of the male gametes and in none of the female gametes.

yellow fever   acute viral disease that affects the liver and is transmitted only by certain mosquitoes.

zygote   fertilized egg cell.

Index

Day care for children, 299
DDT, 560–562
Death, 589–607
  acceptance of, 590, 595
  afterlife, 595–596
  brain, 593
  from cancer, 372–373
  causes of, 10–13
  cellular, 593
  denial and avoidance of, 590–591
  differing perceptions of, 589–590
  euthanasia, 598
  functional, 592
  of loved one, reactions to,
    598–600
  patient's influence over, 592
  preparing for, 591–592
  psychological adaptations to,
    593–595
  spiritual, 593
  Sudden Infant Death Syndrome,
    389
  suicide, 168–171
  survivors, interacting with,
    604–605
Death rates
  for cardiovascular disease, 358
  decline in, 574
  and population growth, 332
  and smoking, 188, 189, 192
  for United States, 14
Decibels, 555–556
Decision-making
  behavioral, and reference groups,
    141–142
  respect and responsibility in, 137,
    138
Defense mechanisms
  of body, 70–71
  psychological, 154, 158–162
Deficiency diseases, 10
Delirium tremens, 225
Delivery, 31–36
Delusions, 253
Demerol, 258, 467
Denial
  of death, 590–591, 594, 600, 601
  as defense mechanism, 159
Dental caries, 392
Dentist, 458–459
Depressants, prescriptions for, 467
Depression, 165
  in dying patient, 595
Dermatologist, 449
Detergents and eutrophication, 534
Detumescence, 296
Developing countries
  and environmental movement,
    522
  health programs for, 511–514
  population growth in, 329
  view of family planning, 338

Dexedrine, 252
Diabetes mellitus, 58
  causes, 390, 391
  fake treatments, 475
  and heart disease, 355
  and obesity, 391
  treatment, 391
Diaphragm, 314–315
Diarrheal disease, epidemic, 65
Diastolic pressure, 348
Diet
  adequate, 408–414
  balanced, 359
  and cancer, 374
  fad, 410, 412–414
  and heart disease, 355–356
  high-fiber, 413
  low-carbohydrate, 412–413
  quackery, 479–480
  Recommended Dietary
    Allowances, 410, 412
  vegetarian, 413–414
  for weight control, 412–413,
    435, 436
  Zen-macrobiotic, 414
Digestive system disorders, 14, 433
Dietary drinking, 209
Diethylstilbestrol, 27, 374
Dilation and curettage, 323
Diphtheria, 65, 73, 76
Directory of Medical Specialists,
  451
Disability insurance, 491, 492
Disease(s), 1–2, 8–11
  in aged, 584, 586
  cardiovascular, 345–367, 584,
    586
  causes of, 8–10
  and cigarette smoking, 184,
    185–194, 195
  communicable, *see*
    Communicable diseases
  control activities, 510–511,
    512–514, 561
  definitions, 8
  general resistance to, 70
  genetic, 50–60
  and life-style, 345, 356–360
  noncommunicable, 369–397
  and obesity, 430, 433
  pulmonary, 184, 190–191
  and water pollution, 542
Displacement, 160–161
Dissociative reaction, 164
Distilled spirits
  alcohol content, 213
  and blood-alcohol level, 214
  making, 211
Divorce rate, 293
DMT (dimethyltryptamine), 254
DNA (deoxyribonucleic acid), 46,
  50

Dominant traits, 48, 60
Dose-response relationship, 189
Double standard of sexual behavior,
  282–283, 284, 286
Double-funnel theory of courtship,
  280–281
Douches, 42
"Downers," 250
Down's syndrome, 29, 31, 56, 58
Drinking, *see* Alcohol; Alcoholism
Drug abuse, 233, 234–273
  abstinence syndrome, 239–240
  and adaptive behavior, 246–247
  adulterated drugs, 238
  alcohol, *see* Alcoholism
  alternatives to, 268–269
  causes of, 241–247
  deaths and injuries due to, 249
  definition, 234
  dependence, 238–240
  in the future, 267–268
  legal aspect, 236–237, 266–267
  medical aspect, 235
  patterns and trends in, 247–250
  polydrug abuse, 258
  psychoactive drugs, 250–262
  risks, 237–240
  and search for identity, 128
  social aspect, 235–236
  solutions, 248, 250
  symptoms, 264–265
  terms, 264
  treatment and rehabilitation,
    262–263, 266
Drugs, therapeutic, 465, 469, 470
  abuse, *see* Drug abuse
  advertising, 465, 466, 470–472
  allergy to, 78
  against common cold, 79
  definition, 233
  effects on fetus, 27–28
  for epilepsy, 395
  fertility, 18
  generic vs. brand names, 445,
    467–468
  labeling, 466–467
  misuse, 233–234, 235, 237
  multiple, interaction of, 237
  for obesity, 252
  over-the-counter, 465–466
  prescription, 466–467
  prices, 445
  psychoactive, 173, 234
  restrictions on, 467
  self-medication, 468–470
  side effects, 78, 467, 586
  in treatment of disease, 9, 78,
    84–85, 89, 173, 233, 364,
    383, 386–387, 393
  use with alcohol, 216, 251, 467
  use in pregnancy, 237
Dumps, 550, 551

inadequate, 455–456
primary-care, shortage of, 487–488
selecting, 448–454
specialties, 449–450
staff, of hospitals, 452
using wisely, 453–454
Physician's assistant, 489
Pica, 560
Pill, the, 316
side effects, 317–318
Pitch of sound, 555
Pituitary hormones, 97, 98, 101, 102, 104, 316–317
Placenta, 32
Plateau phase, sexual, 296
Podiatrist, 459
Poliomyelitis, 66, 73, 76
Pollution
air, 191, 378, 512, 514, 524–533
definition, 521
doing away with, 610
fluorocarbons, 564
noise, 554–558
nuclear wastes, 568
pesticides, 560–562
water, 533–544
Polychlorinated biphenyls (PCBs), 27, 562–563
Polydactyly, 58
Polygenic traits, 48
Polyposis, intestinal, 376
Polyunsaturated fats, 356, 359
Polyvalent vaccines, 81
Polyvinyl chloride, incineration, 552
Population
baby boom, effects of, 610–612
doubling time, 327–328
growth, causes and results, 329, 332, 333–335
growth, possible solutions, 336–342
in urban areas, 329–331
Portal of entry, 68
Portal of exit, 66, 68
Postal Service, United States, 481–482
Pragmatism, 138
Preejaculate, 105, 107
Pregnancy
alcohol use during, 216
diagnosis, 19–20
drug use in, 27–28, 216, 237
expected rate per year, 311
imaginary, 20–21
nutrition in, 24, 412
sexual intercourse during, 38
stages of, 21–23
X ray use during, 567
Premarital sex
attitudes toward, 140–141

history of, 281–285
in 1970s, 285–286
North American vs. European, 285
Prematurity, 58
Premenstrual tension, 103
Prepuce, 106
of clitoris, 296
Prescription drugs, 466–467
Preventive health care, 78–79, 444, 496–498, 609–610
Principle of least interest, 278–280
Problem drinking, 217, 219–220
Proctologist, 450
Prodromal stage of disease, 69
Professional health associations, 516–518
Progesterone, 102–103, 312, 316–318
Projection, 158
Propinquity and mate selection, 287, 290
Prostate gland, 103, 104, 105
Protein-calorie malnutrition, 400–401
Proteins, 405–406
antibodies, 46
body's production of, 46
calories in, 408
deficiency, 10, 400–401
functions and sources, 409
Recommended Daily Dietary Allowance, 412
Protozoa, 66, 67
Pseudocyesis, 20–21
Psilocybin, 254
Psychiatrist, 450
Psychic space, 161–162
Psychoactive drugs, 234–240
abuse, see Drug abuse
Psychoactive effect, 177
Psychoanalysis, 172
theories of alcoholism, 222, 224
theory of repression, 159
Psychological tensions, see Stress
Psychologist, 459
Psychomotor seizure, 393–394
Psychoses, 165
symptoms, 166
types of, 166–167
Psychosexual development, 118–119
Psychosomatic disorders, 167–168
Psychosurgery, 173
Psychotherapy, 171, 172
for alcoholism, 226
for drug abuse, 262
Puberty, 97–108
Public health
government programs, 505–509
laboratories, 505, 509
sanitary measures, 78

Public health nurse, 509
Public Health Service agencies, 506–508
Puffery, 470–471
Pulmonary embolism, 362

Q fever, 66
Quackery, health, 472
arthritis, 476–477
cancer, 477–479
consumer protection from, 480–482
consumer's contribution to, 474–475
devices, 473, 475, 476, 478
food faddism, 479–480
recognizing a quack, 473–474
Quality of life, future, 609–613
Quickening, 22
Quinacrine, 322
Quinine, 78

Race
and blood type, 50
differences in cancer, 373–374
and hypertension, 354–355
and life expectancy, 574
and mate selection, 287, 288, 289
and sickle-cell anemia, 8, 51–53
and venereal disease, 87
Radiation
and cancer, 374–376, 378
in cancer treatment, 382
effect on chromosomes, 568
effects on fetus, 26–27
genetic damage from, 568
natural, 565–566
nuclear, as environmental hazard, 564–569
sickness, 567
Radical mastectomy, 382
Radioactive wastes in water, 543
Radioactivity, 565–569
Radioisotopes, 382
Radiologist, 450
Rationalization, 158
Reaction formation, 159
Recessive traits, 48, 60
Recommended Dietary Allowances, 410, 412
Recycling of wastes, 553–554
Red Cross work for aged, 579
Reference groups and premarital sexual behavior, 141–142
Refractive errors of eye, 394
Regression, 159–160
Religion
and birth control, 338
and food patterns, 402
and mate selection, 287, 288
REM sleep, 251
Remarriage, 293

Credits

Jean-Claude Lejeune: 116, 119, 121, 127, 129, 147, 154, 163, 167, 579, 583 bottom left

Magnum Photos, Inc.: Bob Adelmann, 295 top right; Leonard Freed, 240, 243; Michael Hanulak, 236, 239; Dave Healey, 205; Hirogi Kubota, 295 bottom left; Constantine Manos, 137; Chris Maynard, 295 top left

March of Dimes: 29, 30, 40, 51, 53 bottom, 235

Medical Illustration Service, Syracuse VA Hospital: 361 bottom, 391 left, 447 top left, top right

Monkmeyer: Irene Bayer, 585 top; Eric L. Brown, 599; Paul Conklin, 575 top; Mimi Forsyth, 105, 110, 286, 289 bottom right, 295 bottom right, 488; Fujihira, 263; Michal Heron, 575 bottom; Mahon, 289 bottom left; Hugh Rogers, 437, 466, 505, 551 top; Leonard Lee Rue, 403 top; Sybil Shackman, 134; Sybil Shelton, 304

National Institute of Health, University of Oregon: 34 top

National Library of Medicine: 166

Chicago Chapter National Multiple Sclerosis Society: 515 top left

National Retired Teachers Association-American Association of Retired Persons: 438 left

The National Tuberculosis and Respiratory Disease Association: 391 right

Northwestern Memorial Hospital: 356, 457, 484, 567

Ortho Pharmaceutical Corporation: 314 left, bottom center, bottom right, 316 left

Parke, Davis & Company: 316 top right

Pfizer, Inc.: 62

David Reed: 559

Rush-Presbyterian-St. Lukes Medical Center, Chicago: 9, 53 top, 349 top, 363 left, 497, 576

Jos. Schlitz Brewing Co.: 211 left

Landrum B. Shettles, M.C.: 41 bottom

Arthur Siegel: 326

Howard Simmons: 452

Rick Smolan: 588

State Historical Society of Wisconsin: 288

Taurus Photos: Eric Kroll, 553; Shirley Zieberg, 577

Turtox/Cambosco: 47

United Nations: 335, 339; J. Frank, 334; ILO, 337; M. Tzovaras, 341

United Press International: 131 right, 220, 525 bottom left, bottom right, 526, 530, 537

U.S. Department of Health, Education and Welfare: 34 bottom; Center for Disease Control, 65, 67 top left, top center, top right, middle center, bottom center, bottom right; Center for Disease Control, Venereal Disease Branch, 88, 90; Food and Drug Administration, 473, 476 left, 478

U.S. Department of Justice: Drug Enforcement Administration: 234, 237, 238, 246, 252, 254, 255, 256, 257, 259, 260, 262

U.S. Signal Corps, National Archives: 181

WHO: 513 bottom right; P. Almasy, 513 bottom left; D. Henrioud, 513 top

Wide World Photos: 403 bottom, 525 top, 535 bottom left, 539, 555; AP Newsfeatures Photo, 245

wcb

ISBN 0-697-07382-3